Textbook of

Anatomy
and
Physiology
for Health Professionals

Textbook of
Anatomy
and
Physiology
for Health Professionals

Dr Indu Khurana MD
Professor, Department of Physiology
Pt. B.D. Sharma Postgraduate Institute of Medical Sciences
Rohtak, Haryana (India)

Arushi Khurana MD
School of Medicine
University of Connecticut
USA

CBS

CBS Publishers & Distributors Pvt Ltd

New Delhi • Bengaluru • Chennai • Kochi • Kolkata • Mumbai
Bhopal • Bhubaneswar • Hyderabad • Jharkhand • Nagpur • Patna • Pune • Uttarakhand • Dhaka (Bangladesh)

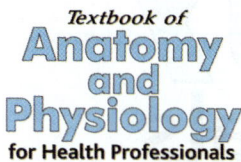

Textbook of
Anatomy and Physiology
for Health Professionals

ISBN: 978-81-239-1656-9

Copyright © Authors

First Edition: 2009
Reprint: 2010, 2014, 2015, 2017, 2019

Published by Satish Kumar Jain and produced by Varun Jain for
CBS Publishers & Distributors Pvt Ltd
4819/XI Prahlad Street, 24 Ansari Road, Daryaganj, New Delhi 110 002, India.
Ph: 23289259, 23266861, 23266867   Fax: 011-23243014   Website: www.cbspd.com
e-mail: delhi@cbspd.com; cbspubs@airtelmail.in.
Corporate Office: 204 FIE, Industrial Area, Patparganj, Delhi 110 092
Ph: 4934 4934   Fax: 4934 4935   e-mail: publishing@cbspd.com;   publicity@cbspd.com

Branches

- **Bengaluru:** Seema House 2975, 17th Cross, K.R. Road,
  Banasankari 2nd Stage, Bengaluru 560 070, Karnataka
  Ph: +91-80-26771678/79   Fax: +91-80-26771680   e-mail: bangalore@cbspd.com
- **Chennai:** 7, Subbaraya Street, Shenoy Nagar, Chennai 600 030, Tamil Nadu
  Ph: +91-44-26680620, 26681266   Fax: +91-44-42032115   e-mail: chennai@cbspd.com
- **Kochi:** 42/1325, 1326, Power House Road, Opp. KSEB Power House
  Ernakulam 682 018, Kochi, Kerala
  Ph: +91-484-4059061-65   Fax: +91-484-4059065   e-mail: kochi@cbspd.com
- **Kolkata:** 6/B, Ground Floor, Rameswar Shaw Road, Kolkata-700 014, West Bengal
  Ph: +91-33-22891126, 22891127, 22891128   e-mail: kolkata@cbspd.com
- **Mumbai:** 83-C, Dr E Moses Road, Worli, Mumbai-400018, Maharashtra
  Ph: +91-22-24902340/41   Fax: +91-22-24902342   e-mail: mumbai@cbspd.com

Representatives

• **Bhopal** 0-8319310552	• **Bhubaneswar** 0-9911037372	• **Hyderabad** 0-9885175004	• **Jharkhand** 0-9811541605
• **Nagpur** 0-9021734563	• **Patna** 0-9334159340	• **Pune** 0-9623451994	• **Uttarakhand** 0-9716462459
• **Dhaka (Bangladesh)** 01912-003485			

Printed at Magic International Pvt. Ltd., Greater Noida, UP, India

Preface

A sound knowledge of anatomy and physiology of the human body is most essential for all the health science graduate students. An effort has been made in this Textbook of Anatomy and Physiology to provide the essential matter in a thorough yet concise manner. The book has been written primarily for the students of nursing and other allied health sciences to help them understand the fundamental basics of the subject. Material provided is aimed at providing an insight into how the body is structured and how it functions and how the alterations in normal structure and functioning results in disease. To achieve this aim the text matter on pure and applied aspects of human anatomy and physiology has been skillfully intermingled and presented in an adorned form. Care has been taken to include the material as per syllabi prescribed by Council for Nursing and Council for other allied health sciences. It is hoped, the book will be useful in laying a strong foundation for health science graduate students.

The book has been organized into twelve sections and each section has been subdivided into various chapters. Section 1 is devoted to general anatomy and physiology and the rest eleven sections describe the human body system by system.

Salient Features

- The text has been organized in such a way that the students can easily understand, retain and reproduce it. Various levels of headings, subheadings, bold face and italics given in the text will be helpful in quick revision of the text.
- A brief list of contents given in the beginning of each chapter provides a clear layout of the text.
- The exposition of the text is such that an average student will not find any difficulty in conceptulizing it.
- The text has been well illustrated with a high quality clear line diagrams which provide vivid and lucid details.
- To further enhance the lucidity of the book the text and figures are presented in an attractive colour format.
- To emphasize the clinical significance of anatomy and physiology, the relevant applied aspects have been covered adequately in each chapter.
- The important information has been highlighted with the help of plenty of tables and flowcharts.

An arduous task like this is never possible without the unending blessings of teachers and parents, to whom we shall ever remain indebted. We wish to express gratitude to our esteemed teachers Prof. Inderbir Singh and Prof. P.I. Singh for their valuable guidance.

We acknowledge, with profound gratitude, the contribution of Prof. A.K. Khurana who has not only guided and helped during each and every step during preparation of this book, but has also authored a chapter on Anatomy and Physiology of Eye and Vision. We also wish to express our gratitude to Dr. (Mrs.) Sushma Sood, Prof. & Head,

Department of Physiology and Prof. S.S. Sangwan, Director, PGIMS, Rohtak for providing an excellent academic and working atmosphere.

It is our special pleasure to acknowledge with gratitude the most assured cooperation and skill of M/s CBS Publishers & Distributors in general and Mr. S.K. Jain, Managing Director, and Mr. Vinod Jain, Production Director, in particular. Dr. Aashima and Dr. Saurav deserve a special slot in the preface for their artistic touch which we feel has provided a considerable beauty to this book.

Mr. Y.N. Arjuna and Mr. Dharmvir from CBS Publishers need a special appreciation for their generous help. Ventures like this are never entirely free from human errors, some inaccuracies, ambiguities and typographical mistakes. We would, therefore, welcome feedback and suggestions from teachers and students for further improvement of the book.

Indu Khurana
Arushi Khurana

PREFACE

Contents

General Principles of Anatomy and Physiology

General Principles of
Anatomy and
Physiology

Introduction to Human Anatomy and Physiology

1.1

ANATOMY AND PHYSIOLOGY

ANATOMY

Anatomy is the branch of biology which deals with the study of structure of the body. It has following subdivisions :

Gross anatomy is the macroscopic structure of body parts that can be seen with the unaided eyes.

Comparative anatomy is the study of similarities and differences in the structure of body parts of the various species of animals.

Surface anatomy or topographic anatomy is the study of deeper parts of the body in relation to the skin surface. It is helpful in clinical practice and surgical operations.

Developmental anatomy or embryology refers to the study of development of animal body from the one cell stage to the period of growth and development before birth.

Histology is the study of minute structure of body parts that can only be seen with the aid of a microscope, and therefore is often called *microscopic anatomy or microanatomy.*

Radiographic anatomy is the study of deeper organs by plain and contrast radiography and by other imaging techniques like CT scan, and MRI.

PHYSIOLOGY

Physiology, in simple terms, refers to the study of normal functioning of the living structures. The human physiology is concerned with the way the various systems of the human body function and the way each contributes to the functions of the body as a whole. In other words, the human physiology is concerned with specific characteristics and mechanisms of the human body that make it a living being and the mechanisms which help in adaptation and homeostasis which are the two fundamental features of life. The term physiology includes following subdivisions :

1. General physiology. This term envisages the general concepts and principles that are basic to the functions of all the systems.

2. Systemic physiology deals with the functioning of different systems of the body, e.g. respiratory physiology includes different physiological aspects of respiration. *Cell physiology* is the study of the individual cells themselves, as they live out on a small scale all the activities that characterise the larger organisms.

Before studying the general biophysiological processes and the cell physiology, it will be worthwhile to have a brief knowledge about the regional and functional organization of the human body.

REGIONAL ORGANIZATION OF HUMAN BODY

ANATOMICAL REGIONS AND CAVITIES OF THE BODY

Anatomical regions. For convenience of anatomical description the human body can be divided into following regions (Fig.1.1-1) :
- Head and neck region,
- Thorax,
- Abdomen, and
- Upper and lower extremities

Cavities of human body. The organs that make up the different systems of the body are contained in four cavities:
- Cranial cavity,
- Thoracic cavity,
- Abdominal cavity, and
- Pelvic cavity

Head and neck region and cranial cavity

Head is the uppermost part of the body.
Face is the part of the head which includes the regions of forehead, eyes, nose, cheeks and chin.
Cranial cavity refers to that part of the head which is bounded by the bones of skull and contains the brain.
Neck is that part of the body which connects the head with the trunk. Trunk refers to combined thorax and abdomen.

Thorax or thoracic cavity

Thorax refers to the chest which is a cage formed by a bony framework and supporting muscles. This bony cage is also called thoracic cavity. It contains:

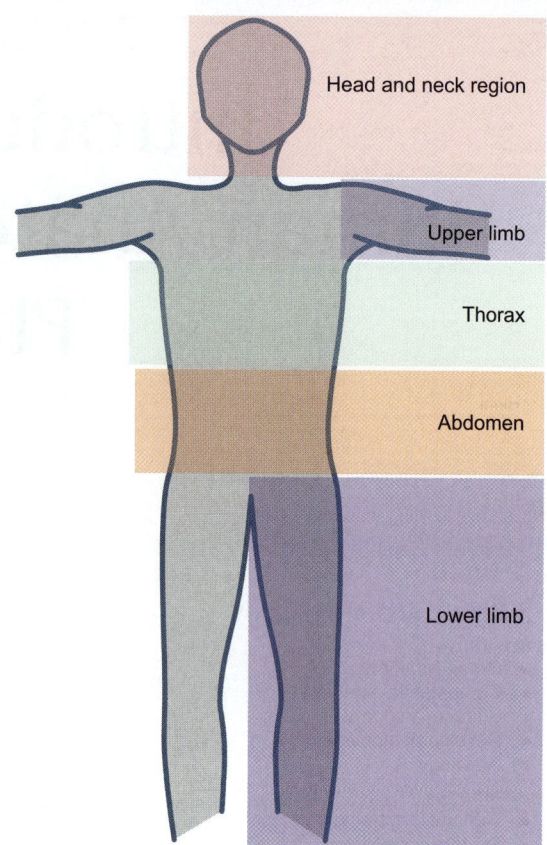

Fig. 1.1-1. Regions of the body

- Lungs, trachea and bronchi;
- Heart and major blood vessels,
- Oesophagus,
- Lymph vessels and lymph nodes, and
- Nerves

The thoracic cavity is divided into right and left cavities, each containing one lung.
Mediastinum is the name given to the space between the lungs and the structures found there such as heart, oesophagus and blood vessels.

Abdomen

Abdomen is the anatomical term used for the region of the trunk which lies below the thorax. The region of abdomen can be divided into two cavities—abdominal cavity and pelvic cavity.
Abdominal cavity. It is separated from thoracic cavity by a muscular structure called diaphragm.
Contents. The abdominal cavity contains several organs of vital importance to body, such as :
- Stomach, small and large intestines
- Liver, gall bladder pancreas and spleen
- Kidneys and adrenals
- Vessels, nerves, lymphatics and lymph nodes.

Regions. The abdominal cavity can be divided into following nine regions (Fig.1.1-2) which facilitate the description of the positions of the organs and structures it contains :

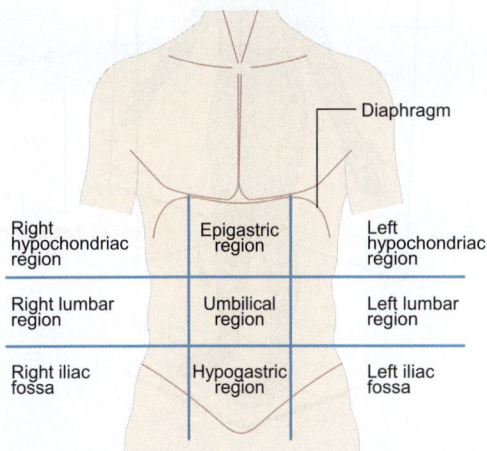

Fig. 1.1-2. *Regions of abdominal cavity*

- Right hypochondriac region (1),
- Epigastric region (2),
- Left hypochondriac region (3),
- Right lumbar region (4),
- Umbilical region (5),
- Left lumbar region (6),
- Right iliac fossa (7),
- Hypogastric region (8), and
- Left iliac fossa (9)

Pelvic cavity refers to a funnel shaped cavity which extends from the lower end of the abdominal cavity. It is bounded by pelvic bones.

Contents of pelvic cavity include :
- Sigmoid colon, rectum and anus,
- Some loops of small intestine,
- Urinary bladder, lower parts of the ureters and urethra.
- Some organs of reproductive system.

Upper and lower extremities

The upper and lower extremities or limbs are attached to the trunk.

Upper limbs. There are two upper limbs (right and left). Each upper limb or upper extremity consists of :
- *Arm.* The region of upper limb which extends from the shoulder to elbow.
- *Forearm.* The region between elbow and wrist.
- *Wrist.* The area between forearm and hand.
- *Hand.* It is the distal part of the upper limb which comprises the palm and digits (fingers and thumb).

Lower limbs. There are two lower limbs (right and left). Each lower limb or lower extrimity consists of :
- *Thigh.* The region between hip and knee joint.

- *Leg.* The region between knee joint and ankle.
- *Ankle.* The junction between the leg and foot.
- *Foot.* The distal most part of lower limb which comprises, the sole and digits (toes).

ANATOMICAL TERMS

For precise anatomical description of the mutual relationship of various structures of the body, following special anatomical terms are used :

Body positions

1. *Anatomical position.* To ensure accuracy and consistency all anatomical descriptions are made in relation to the anatomical position. The anatomical position refers to the position of body in which a person is persumed to be standing upright, with the head facing forward, the arms held by the sides of the body with the palms of the hands facing forward and the feet together (Fig.1.1-3).

Fig. 1.1-3. *Anatomical positions of the body.*

2. *Supine position.* Lying down (recumbent) position with the face directed upwards (Fig.1.1-4A).

3. *Prone position.* Lying down (recumbent) position with the face directed downwards. (Fig.1.1-4B).

4. *Lithotomy position.* Lying supine with the buttocks at the edge of the table, the hips and knees fully flexed, and the feet straped in position.

Anatomical planes

Anatomical planes, to describe positions of the body, are (Fig.1.1-5) :

1. *Median plane.* Median or mid sagittal plane refers to the plane which passes longitudinally through midline

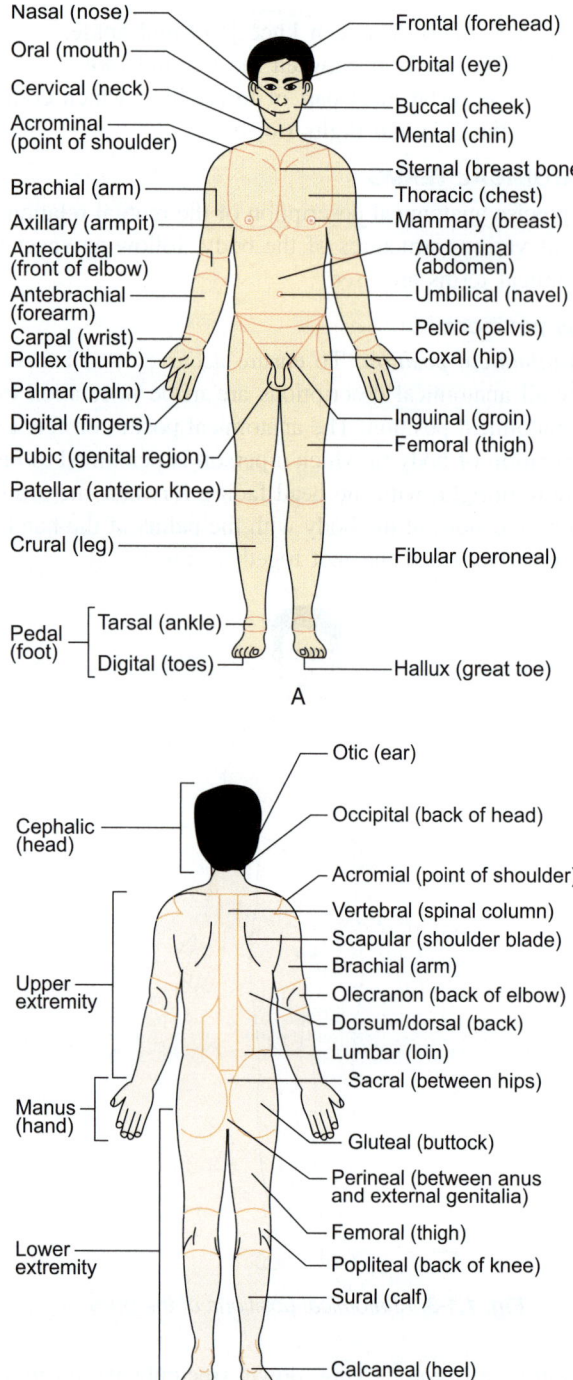

Nasal (nose)
Oral (mouth)
Cervical (neck)
Acromial (point of shoulder)
Brachial (arm)
Axillary (armpit)
Antecubital (front of elbow)
Antebrachial (forearm)
Carpal (wrist)
Pollex (thumb)
Palmar (palm)
Digital (fingers)
Pubic (genital region)
Patellar (anterior knee)
Crural (leg)
Pedal (foot) — Tarsal (ankle), Digital (toes)

Frontal (forehead)
Orbital (eye)
Buccal (cheek)
Mental (chin)
Sternal (breast bone)
Thoracic (chest)
Mammary (breast)
Abdominal (abdomen)
Umbilical (navel)
Pelvic (pelvis)
Coxal (hip)
Inguinal (groin)
Femoral (thigh)
Fibular (peroneal)
Hallux (great toe)

A

Otic (ear)
Cephalic (head)
Occipital (back of head)
Acromial (point of shoulder)
Vertebral (spinal column)
Scapular (shoulder blade)
Brachial (arm)
Olecranon (back of elbow)
Dorsum/dorsal (back)
Upper extremity
Lumbar (loin)
Sacral (between hips)
Gluteal (buttock)
Manus (hand)
Perineal (between anus and external genitalia)
Femoral (thigh)
Popliteal (back of knee)
Lower extremity
Sural (calf)
Calcaneal (heel)
Plantar (sole)

B

Fig. 1.1-4. *Supine (A) and prone (B) positions of the body.*

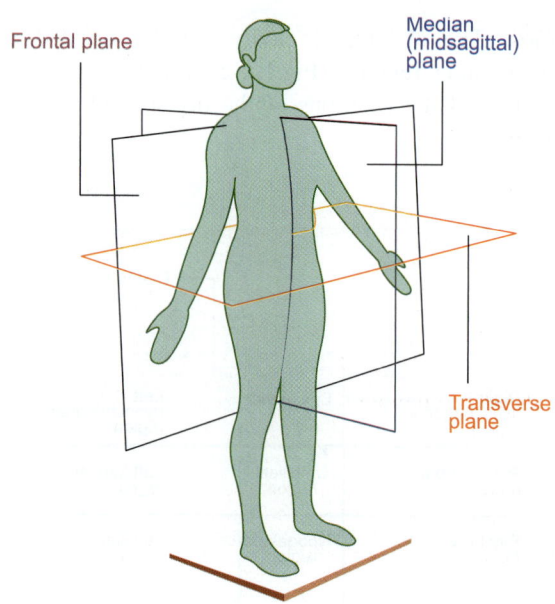

Fig. 1.1-5. *Anatomical planes of reference.*

when the body is in anatomical position. The median plane thus divides the body into two equal right and left halves.

2. *Paramedian or sagittal planes* refer to those planes which pass vertically through the body either to the right or left of the median plane and are parallel to the latter.

3. *Coronal or frontal plane* refers to the plane which is placed at right angle to the median plane and devides the body into anterior (ventral) and posterior (dorsal) parts.

4. *Horizontal plane* refers to the plane which passes horizontally across the body (i.e. at right angles to both the sagittal and coronal planes) and divides the body into upper and lower parts).

5. *Transverse plane.* Transverse plane passes at right angle to the longitudinal axis of the structure concerned. Thus, a transverse section through an artery is not necessarily horizontal. A transverse section through the hand is horizontal, whereas a transverse section through the foot is coronal.

Paired directional terms

Paired directional terms used in anatomy are :

1. *Medial versus lateral.* The term medial is used to describe a structure which is near to the median plane as compared to other structure. For example, the heart is medial to the lung. While the term lateral is used for a structure which is away from the median plane. For example, the lungs are lateral to the heart.

2. *Anterior (ventral) versus posterior (dorsal).* The term anterior or ventral is used to describe the position of a structure which lies near the front of the body. For example the sternum is anterior to heart. While the term posterior or dorsal is used to describe a structure which lies near to back of the body. For example heart is posterior to the sternum.

3. *Superior versus inferior.* Structure located near the head is called superior. For example skull is superior to scapula. While a structure located farther from the head is labelled inferior. For example, scapulae are inferior to the skull. While referring to structures in the trunk the term *cranial* (towards the head) is sometimes used instead of superior; and the term *caudal* (towards the tail) in place of inferior.

4. *Superficial versus deep.* The term superficial is used for the structure which is placed towards the body surface, and the term deep is used for the structure which is placed inner to the surface.

5. *Ipsilateral versus contralateral.* The term ipsilateral is used to denote the structures of the same side and contralateral to denote the structures of the opposite side.

Special terms used for limbs

1. *Promimal versus distal.* The term proximal is used for the attached end of a limb. For example in the upper limb the humerous bone is proximal to radial bone. While the term distal is used for the structure which is away from the attached end of the limb. For example in the lower limb tibia is distal to femur.

2. *Flexor versus extensor surface.* Flexor surface refers to anterior surface of the upper limb and posterior surface of the lower limb. While the term extensor surface is used to describe posterior surface of the upper limbs and anterior surface of the lower limbs.

3. *Palmar or volar versus plantar.* The term palmar pertains to (towards) the palm of the hand and the term plantar pertains to (towards) the sole of the foot.

Terms used for hollow organs

1. *Interior versus exterior.* The term interior is used to describe inner of the hollow organs while the term exterior is used to describe the outer of hollow organs.

2. *Invegination versus evagination.* The term invegination refers to inward protusion while evagination refers to outward protusion.

FUNCTIONAL ORGANIZATION OF THE HUMAN BODY

The human body is actually composed of about 100 trillion cells organized into different functional structures. The cells with similar features constitute different tissues and the tissues combine to form organs and some organs combinedly form a system. For convenience of description, the human body can be considered to be functionally organized into various systems.

1. SKIN AND ITS APPENDAGES

Skin is the outermost covering of the human body. Its appendages include hairs, nails, sebacious glands and sweat glands. In addition to providing mechanical protection to the underlying tissues, the skin performs following important functions:

- It acts as a physical barrier against entry of micro-organisms and other substances.
- It prevents loss of water from the body.
- It is a very important sensory organ, containing receptors for touch and related sensations.
- It plays an important role in regulating body temperature.

2. SKELETAL SYSTEM

The basic framework of the body is provided by a large number of bones that collectively form the *skeleton*. At joints, the bones are united to each other by fibrous bands called *ligaments*. In addition to the bones and joints, the skeletal system also includes the *cartilages* present in the body.

3. MUSCLE SYSTEM

Overlying and usually attached to the bones are various muscles. Muscles are composed of many elongated cells called *muscle fibres* which are able to contract and relax. Three distinct types of muscles can be identified which are skeletal muscles, smooth muscles and cardiac muscles.

4. NERVOUS SYSTEM

The nervous system is made up, predominantly, of tissue that has the special property of being able to conduct impulses rapidly from one part of the body to another. The specialized cells that constitute the functional units of the nervous system are called *neurons*. The nervous system may be divided into: (i) the *central nervous system*, made up of brain and spinal cord, and (ii) the *peripheral nervous system*, consisting of the peripheral nerves and the ganglia associated with them.

5. CARDIOVASCULAR SYSTEM

The cardiovascular system consists of the *heart* and the *blood vessels*. The blood vessels that take blood from the heart to various tissues are called *arteries*. The smallest arteries are called *arterioles*. Arterioles open into a network of *capillaries* that perfuse the tissues. Exchange of various substances between the blood and the tissues take place through the walls of capillaries. In some situations, capillaries are replaced by slightly different vessels called *sinusoids*. Blood from capillaries (or from sinusoids) is collected by small *venules* which join to form *veins*. The veins return blood to the heart.

6. RESPIRATORY SYSTEM

The respiratory system consists of the lungs and the passages through which air reaches them. The passages are nasal cavities, the pharynx, the trachea, the bronchi and their intrapulmonary continuations.

7. DIGESTIVE SYSTEM

The digestive or the so-called alimentary system includes all those structures that are concerned with eating, and with the digestion and absorption of food. The system consists of an alimentary canal which starts at the mouth and ends at the anus. The alimentary canal includes the oral cavity, pharynx, oesophagus, stomach, small intestine and large intestine. Other structures included in the digestive system are the liver, the gall bladder and the pancreas.

8. EXCRETORY SYSTEM

Excretion is the removal of waste products of metabolism from the body. *Egestion* (or defaecation) is the removal of undigested food from the gut and is not regarded as excretion because the material taken into the gut through the mouth is not made by the body itself. The organs forming excretory system are the kidney, the ureters, the bladder and the urethra.

9. REPRODUCTIVE SYSTEM

Reproduction is the production of a new generation of individuals of the same species. It involves the transmission of genetic material from one generation to the next. The *male reproductive organs* are the testis, the epididymis, the ductus deferens, and the seminal vesicles (which are paired), and the prostate, the male urethra and the penis (which are unpaired). *The female reproductive organs* are the right and left ovaries and uterine tubes, the uterus, the vagina, the external genitalia and the mammary glands.

10. ENDOCRINE SYSTEM

Endocrine tissue is made up essentially of cells that produce secretions which are poured directly into blood. The secretions of the endocrine cells are called *hormones*.

Some organs are entirely endocrine in function. They are referred to as *endocrine glands* (or *ductless glands*). Those traditionally included under this heading are the hypophysis cerebri (pituitary gland), the pineal gland, the thyroid gland, the parathyroid glands, and the suprarenal (adrenal) glands. Groups of endocrine cells may be present in the organs that have other functions. These include the *islets of Langerhans of* pancreas, the interstitial cells of the testis, the follicles and corpora lutea of the ovaries. Hormones are also produced by some cells in the kidney, the thymus and the placenta. Some workers describe the liver as being partly an endocrine gland.

11. BLOOD AND IMMUNE SYSTEM

Blood is regarded as a modified connective tissue because the cellular elements in it are separated by a considerable amount of 'intercellular substance' and because some of the cells in it have close affinities to cells in general connective tissue.

Circulating blood normally contains three main types of cells which perform their respective physiologic functions: (i) the red cells (*erythrocytes*) are largely concerned with oxygen transport, (ii) the white cells (*leucocytes*) play various roles in the body defence against infection and tissue injury, and (iii) platelets (*thrombocytes*) which are primarily involved in maintaining integrity of blood vessels and in preventing blood loss. Detailed physiology of each organ system is considered in the relevant chapters.

Composition and Internal Environment of the Human Body

1.2

BODY COMPOSITION

Total body water
- Body fluid compartments

Body electrolytes

INTERNAL ENVIRONMENT AND HOMEOSTASIS

Internal environment
Homeostasis
- Role of different systems of body
- Mode of action of homeostatic control system
- Negative feedback mechanism
- Positive feedback mechanism
- Adaptive control system

BODY COMPOSITION

The normal body in an average adult male is composed of *water* (60%), *minerals* (7%), *protein* and related substances (18%), and *fat* (15%).

TOTAL BODY WATER

Water is the principal and essential constituent of the human body. The total body water is about 10% less in a normal young adult female (average 50%) than that in average adult male (60%) due to relatively greater amount of adipose tissue in the females. In both sexes the value tends to decrease with age.

THE BODY FLUID COMPARTMENTS

The total body water is distributed into two main compartments of the body fluids separated from each other by membranes freely permeable to water (Fig.1.2-1, Table 1.2-1):

1. Intracellular fluid compartment

The intracellular fluid (ICF) compartment comprises about 40% of the body weight, the bulk of which is contained in the muscles.

Table 1.2-1 : Distribution of total body water in a normal 70 kg person

Compartment	Volume (L)	Percentage Body weight	Percentage Body water
Total body water (TBW)	42	60	100
• Intracellular fluid (ICF)	28	40	67
• Extracellular fluid (ECF)	14	20	33
– Plasma (25% of ECF)	3.5	05	08
– Interstitial fluid, transcellular fluid and mesenchymal tissue fluid (75% of ECF).	10.5	15	25

2. Extracellular fluid compartment

The extracellular fluid (ECF) compartment constitutes about 20% of the body weight. The ECF compartment comprises of the following :

i. *Plasma.* It is the fluid portion of the blood (*intravascular fluid*) and comprises about 5% of the body weight (i.e. 25% of the ECF). On an average out of 5 litres of total blood volume 3.5 litres is plasma.

ii. *Interstitial fluid including lymph.* It constitutes the major portion (about 3/4) of the ECF. The composition of interstitial fluid is the same as that of plasma except it has

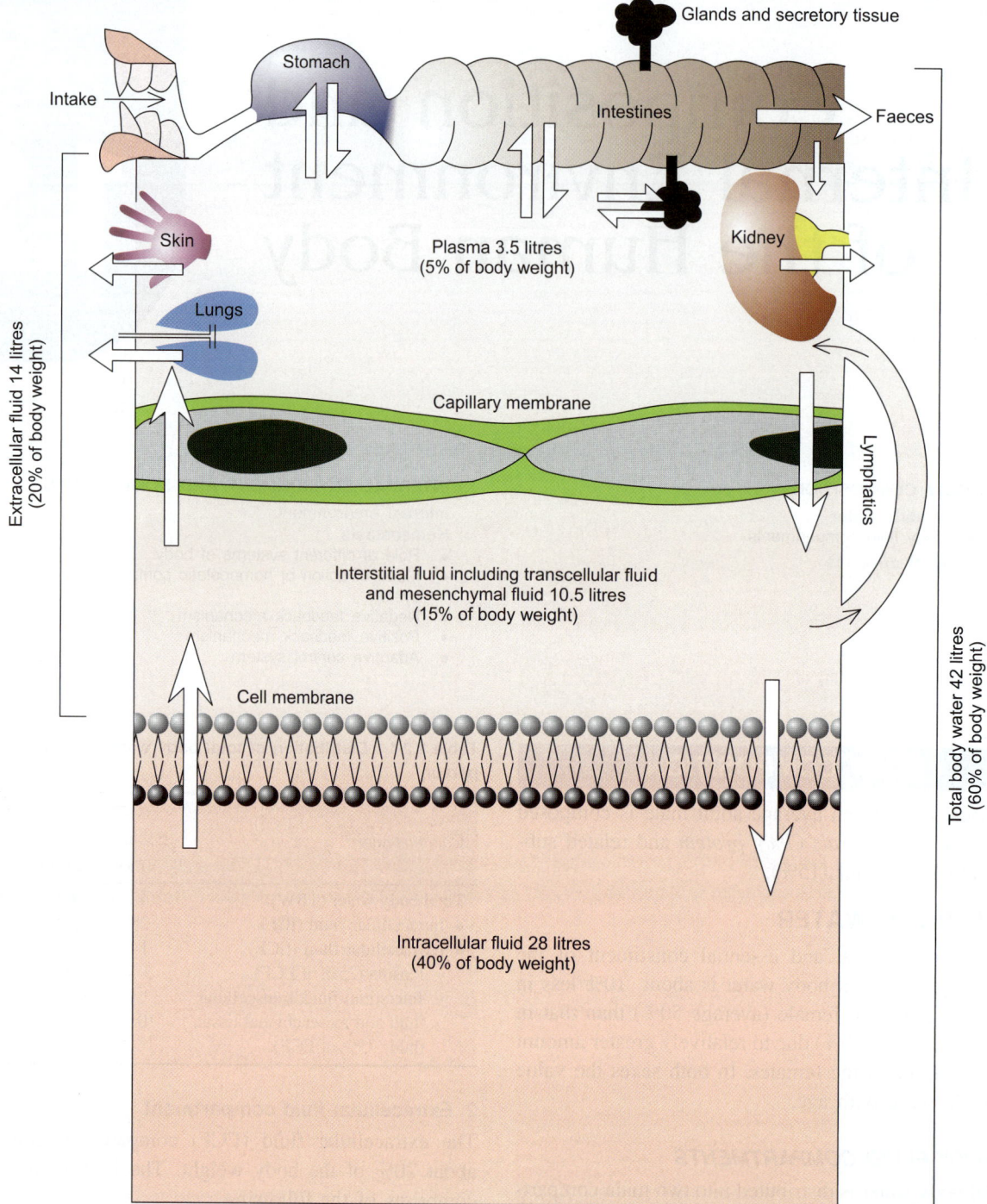

Fig. 1.2-1. *Distribution of total body water in different compartments. Arrows indicate fluid movement.*

little protein. Thus, interstitial fluid is an ultrafiltrate of plasma.

iii. *Transcellular fluid.* It is the fluid contained in the secretions of the secretory cells and cavities of the body e.g. saliva, sweat, bile, cerebrospinal fluid (CSF), intraocular fluids (aqueous humour and vitreous humour), pericardial fluid, fluid present between the layers (pleura,

peritoneum and synovial membrane), lacrimal fluid and luminal fluids of the gut, thyroid and cochlea.

iv. *Mesenchymal tissue fluid.* The mesenchymal tissues such as dense connective tissue, cartilage and bones contain about 6% of the body water.

The interstitial fluid, transcellular fluid and mesenchymal tissue fluid combinedly form the 75% of ECF.

The normal distribution of total body water in the fluid compartments is kept constant by two opposing sets of forces: osmotic and hydrostatic pressure.

BODY ELECTROLYTES

The electrolytes constitute about 7% of the total body weight. The distribution of electrolytes in various compartments differs markedly. Table 1.2-2 shows the distribution of electrolytes in two major compartments of body fluid: the extracellular fluid (ECF), and the intracellular fluid (ICF).

From Table 1.2-2 it may be noted that in the ICF the main cations are K^+ and Mg^{2+}, and the main anions are PO_4^{3-} and proteins. While in ECF, the predominant cation is Na^+ and the principal anions are Cl^- and HCO_3^-. Besides these, a small proportion of non-diffusible proteins, nutrients and metabolites such as glucose and urea are also present in ECF.

Table 1.2.2 : Distribution of ions in the ECF and ICF (Values are in meq/L of H_2O)

Ion	Extracellular fluid	Intracellular fluid
Cations		
Na^+	142	14
K^+	5.5	150
Ca^{2+}	5	< 1
Mg^{2+}	3	58
Anions		
Cl^-	103	4
HCO_3^-	28	10
PO_4^{3-}	4	75
Protein	5	40

It is important to note that :
- Essentially all of the body K^+ is in the exchangeable pool.
- Only 65-70% of the body Na^+ is exchangeable.
- Almost all of the body Ca^{2+} and Mg^{2+} are non-exchangeable.
- Only the exchangeable solutes are osmotically active.

Functions of electrolytes
1. Electrolytes are the main solutes in the body fluids for maintenance of acid-base balance.
2. Electrolytes maintain the proper osmolality and volume of body fluids.
3. The concentration of certain electrolytes determine their specific physiologic functions, e.g. the effect of calcium ions on neuromuscular excitability.

INTERNAL ENVIRONMENT AND HOMEOSTASIS

INTERNAL ENVIRONMENT

Claude Bernarde (1949), the great French physiologist, introduced the term *internal environment* of the body or the *milieu interieur* for the extracellular fluid (ECF) of the body. He said so since all the body cells essentially depend upon the ECF for maintenance of cellular life. Cells are capable of living, growing, and performing their special functions so long as the proper concentration of oxygen, glucose, different ions, amino acids, fatty substances, and other constituents are available in the internal environment.

HOMEOSTASIS

Homeostasis, a term introduced by WB Cannon, refers to the mechanism by which the constancy of the internal environment is maintained and ensured. For this purpose, living membranes with varying permeabilities such as vascular endothelium and cell membrane play important role.

Factors involved in the maintenance of internal environment can be summarized as:
- Maintenance of pH of ECF (acid-base balance),
- Regulation of temperature,
- Maintenance of water and electrolyte balance,
- Supply of nutrients, oxygen, enzymes and hormones, and
- Removal of metabolic and other waste products.

ROLE OF DIFFERENT SYSTEMS OF THE BODY IN HOMEOSTASIS

Almost all the systems of the human body play vital role in the maintenance of internal environment. The details of the role played by each system is described in the relevant chapters.

MODE OF ACTION OF HOMEOSTATIC CONTROL SYSTEM

The homeostasis is a complex phenomenon. The mode of operation of all the systems, which are involved in the homeostasis is through 'feedback' mechanism and the adaptive control system. Feedback mechanism is of two types: the negative feedback mechanism and the positive feedback mechanism.

NEGATIVE FEEDBACK MECHANISM

Most control systems of the body act by negative feedback. That is, in general if the activity of a particular system is increased or decreased, a control system initiates a negative feedback, which consists of a series of changes that return the activity toward normal.

Examples of a feedback mechanism
1. When the blood pressure suddenly rises or lowers, it initiates a series of reactions that tries to bring the blood pressure to normal levels.

2. When thyroxine secretion is more, it inhibits the secretion of thyroid stimulating hormone (TSH) from pituitary so that, thyroxine is not secreted from the thyroid gland.

POSITIVE FEEDBACK MECHANISM

Positive feedback is better known as a vicious circle. Usually it is harmful and in some instances even death can occur due to positive feedback. For example, as shown in Fig. 1.2-2, when a person has suddenly bled 2L of blood, a vicious circle of progressively weakening of the heart is set which ultimately causes death.

Sometimes positive feedback can serve useful purposes, e.g. under following circumstances:

Fig. 1.2-2. Showing how a positive feedback mechanism can cause death.

- *Clot formation* following rupture of vessels is accelerated by vicious cycle of thrombin formation (for details see page 66). This stops the bleeding.
- *Child birth* during labour is facilitated by progressively increasing uterine contractions due to positive feedback from stretching of cervix by head of the baby (for details see page 407).
- *Generation of nerve signals* by the vicious cycle of progressive leakage of Na^+ ions from the channels set up following stimulation of membrane of nerve fibre is due to the positive feedback.

ADAPTIVE CONTROL SYSTEM

Adaptive control system refers to a delayed type of negative feedback mechanism. This is seen in nervous system. For example, when some movements of the body occur very rapidly, there is not enough time for nerve signals to travel from the peripheral parts of the body all the way to the brain and then back to the periphery again in time to control the movements. Under such circumstances brain uses a principle called *feed-forward control* to cause the required muscle contraction which retrospectively is conveyed to the brain by the sensory nerve signals from the moving part. If the movement performed is found incorrect, then the brain corrects the *feed-forward signals* that it sends to the muscle the next time the movement is required. Such a correction made by successive retrospecitive feedback mechanism is called *adaptive control*.

The Cell and the Tissues

THE CELL

CELL STRUCTURE

The cell is the smallest structural and functional unit of the body. The human body contains about 100 trillion cells. Different types of cells of the body possess features which distinguish one type from the other and are specially adapted to form one or few particular functions, e.g. the red blood cells transport oxygen from lungs to the tissues, muscle cell is specialized for the function of contraction, the intestinal mucosal cells specialized for absorption of foodstuffs and so on. However, most mammalian cells have an overall common structure and certain basic characteristics which are described here.

A typical cell, as seen by the light microscope consists of three basic components:

- Cell membrane,
- Cytoplasm, and
- Nucleus.

CELL MEMBRANE

Cell membrane or the plasma membrane is the protective sheath, enveloping the cell body. It separates the contents of cell from the external environment and controls ex-change of materials between the fluid outside the cell (extracellular fluid) and the fluid inside the cell (intracellular fluid). A detailed knowledge of its structure (Fig. 1.3-1) is essential for the understanding of cell functions.

Structure. Electron microscopy has shown that cell membrane/plasma membrane has a *trilayer* structure having total thickness of 7-10 nm (70-100 Å). The three layers consist of *two electron dense layers* separated by an *electron lucent layer* (clear zone). Biochemically the cell membrane is composed of complex mixture of lipids (40%), proteins (55%), and carbohydrates (5%).

Fluid mosaic model of membrane structure

In 1972, Singer and Nicolson put forward the fluid mosaic model of membrane structure (Fig. 1.3-2), which is presently most accepted. According to this model:

1. *Phospholipid bilayer* is the basic continuous structure forming the cell membrane. The phospholipids are present in fluid form. This fluidity makes the membrane quite flexible and thus allows the cells to undergo considerable changes in the shape without disruption of structural integrity.

Each lipid molecule in the lipid bilayer of the cell membrane primarily consists of phospholipid, cholesterol

Globular head

Fig. 1.3-1. Structure of a typical cell (in the centre) showing various organelles: A, mitochondrion; B, endoplasmic reticulum (rough and smooth); C, Golgi apparatus; D, centrosome; E, nucleus; and F, secretory granules.

Nucleolus   Rough   Smooth

and glycolipids. The lipid molecule is of clothespin shape and consists of a *head end* and a *tail end*.

The head end or the globular end is positively charged and quite soluble in water (i.e. *polar* or *hydrophilic*). The tail end is quite insoluble in water (*nonpolar* or *hydrophobic*). These lipid molecules are arranged as bilayer in such a way that their nonpolar hydrophobic tail ends are directed towards the centre of the membrane whereas their polar hydrophilic head ends are directed outwards on either side of the membrane (Fig. 1.3-2). In this way head ends of molecules face the aqueous phase, i.e. extracellular fluid on outside and the intracellular fluid (cytoplasm) on inner side.

2. The protein molecules are present as a discontinuous mosaic of globular proteins which float about in the fluid phospholipid bilayer forming a *fluid mosaic pattern*. Two types of proteins recognised in the cell membrane are:

1. *Peripheral proteins.* These are present peripheral to the lipid bilayer both inside and outside to it.

i. *Intrinsic proteins.* These are located in the inner surface of the lipid bilayer and serve mainly as enzymes.

ii. *Extrinsic or surface proteins.* These are the protiens located on the outer surface of the lipid bilayer. Some of these proteins serve as *cell adhesion molecules* (CAM) that anchor cells to neighbouring cells and to the basal lamina.

2. *Integral proteins or transmembrane proteins.* These are the proteins which extend into the lipid bilayer. The integral proteins, on the basis of functions they serve, are:

• Channel proteins,
• Carrier proteins,
• Receptor proteins,
• Antigens, and
• Pumps.

Phospholipid molecules — Carbohydrate side chain — Peripheral proteins — Head — Tail — Channel protein — Peripheral proteins — Integral proteins

Fig. 1.3-2. *Fluid mosaic model of the structure of cell membrane.*

3. *The carbohydrates* are attached either to the proteins (glycoproteins) or the lipids (glycolipids). Throughout the surface of cell membrane, carbohydrate molecules form a thin loose covering called *glycocalyx.*

- The glycocalyx helps in tight fixation of the cells with one another.
- Some of the carbohydrate molecules also serve as *receptors.*

CYTOPLASM

Cytoplasm is an aqueous substance (cytosol) containing a variety of cell organelles and other structures. The structures dispersed in the cytoplasm can be broadly divided into three groups: organelles, inclusion bodies and cytoskeleton.

A. Organelles

The organelles are the permanent components of the cells which are bounded by limiting membrane and contain enzymes hence participate in the cellular metabolic activity. These include the mitochondria, the endoplasmic reticulum, ribosomes, the Golgi apparatus, peroxisomes, centrosomes and centriole.

1. *Mitochondria.* Mitochondria are the major sites for aerobic respiration. These are oval structures and more numerous in metabolically active cells. The mitochondria consist of two layers of the membrane and the matrix. The outer membrane is smooth and inner is folded into incomplete septa called cristae (Fig. 1.3-1A).

Matrix of the mitochondria contains enzymes required in Krebs' cycle by which products of carbohydrate, fat and protein metabolism are oxidised to produce energy which is stored in the form of ATP.

Functions. In addition to their role as power generating units, the mitochondria may have a role in synthesizing proteins since they also possess DNA and ribosomes.

2. *Endoplasmic reticulum.* Endoplasmic reticulum (ER) is a system of flattened, membrane-bound vesicles and tubules called *cisternae* (Fig. 1.3-1B). It is continuous with the outer membrane of the nuclear envelope and Golgi apparatus. Morphologically, two types of endoplasmic reticulum can be identified: rough or granular and smooth or agranular.

i. *Rough endoplasmic reticulum.* The rough ER is characterized by the presence of a number of ribosomes on its surface. The rough ER is especially well developed in cells active in protein synthesis.

ii. *Smooth endoplasmic reticulum.* Smooth ER is devoid of ribosomes on its surface. It is a site of lipid and steroid synthesis. In the skeletal and cardiac muscles, smooth ER is modified to form sarcoplasmic reticulum which is involved in the release and sequestration of calcium ions during muscular contraction.

3. *Golgi apparatus.* The Golgi apparatus or complex is a collection of membranous vesicles, sacs or tubules which is generally located close to the nucleus. It is continuous with the endoplasmic reticulum. Golgi apparatus is particularly well developed in exocrine glandular cells (Fig. 1.3-1C). Its main functions are:

- Synthesis of carbohydrates and complex proteins.
- Packaging of proteins synthesised in the rough ER into vesicles.

4. *Ribosomes.* Ribosomes are spherical particles which contain 80 to 85% of the cell's RNA. They may be present in the cytosol as free or in bound form. Slightly smaller forms of ribosomes are also found in mitochondria. They are the site of protein synthesis. They synthesize all transmembrane proteins, secreted proteins and most proteins that are stored in Golgi apparatus, lysosomes and endosomes.

5. *Lysosomes.* Lysosomes are rounded to oval membrane-bound organelles containing powerful lysosomal digestive (hydrolytic) enzymes. They are formed by the Golgi apparatus. Lysosomes are particularly abundant in cells involved in phagocytic activity, e.g. neutrophils, and macrophages.

6. *Peroxisomes.* Peroxisomes, also known as microbodies, are spherical structures enclosed by a single layer of unit membrane. These are predominantly present in hepatocytes and tubular epithelial cells. They essentially contain two types of enzymes:

- *Oxidases* which are active in oxidation of lipid; and
- *Catalases* which act on hydrogen peroxide to liberate oxygen.

CHAPTER 1.3

7. Centrosome. The centrosome consists of two short cylindrical structures called centrioles (Fig. 1.3-1D). It is situated near the centre of the cell close to the nucleus. The centrioles are responsible for movement of chromosomes during cell division.

B. Cytoplasmic inclusions

The cytoplasmic inclusions are the temporary components of certain cells. A few examples of cytoplasmic inclusions are:

- Lipid droplets,
- Glycogen,
- Proteins as secretory granules,
- Melanin pigment, and
- Lipofuscin.

C. Cytoskeleton

The cytoskeleton is a complex network of fibres that maintains the structure of the cell and allows it to change shape and move. It primarily consists of microtubules, intermediate filaments and microfilaments along with proteins which anchor and tie them together.

Microtubules. Microtubules are long hollow tubular structures without limiting membrane about 25 nm in diameter.

Intermediate filaments. Intermediate filaments are filamentous structures about 10 nm in diameter. Some of these filaments connect the nuclear membrane to the cell membrane. Their main function is to mechanically integrate the cell organelles within the cytoplasm.

Microfilaments. Microfilaments are long solid filamentous structures having diameter of 6-8 nm. These are made up of contractile proteins, actin and myosin. Actin is the most abundant protein in the mammalian cell. It attaches to various parts of cytoskeleton by other proteins (anchor proteins). In the skeletal muscle, presence of actin and myosin filaments is responsible for their contractile property.

NUCLEUS

Nucleus is present in all the eukaryotic cells. It controls all the cellular activities including reproduction of the cell. The nucleus consists of an outer nuclear membrane enclosing nucleoplasm and nucleoli (Fig. 1.3-1E).

1. Nuclear membrane. The nuclear membrane is double-layered porous structure having a 40-70 nm wide space called *perinuclear cistern* which is continuous with the lumen of endoplasmic reticulum. The outer layer of the nuclear membrane is continuous with endoplasmic reticulum. The exchange of materials between nucleoplasm and cytoplasm occurs through nuclear membrane.

2. Nucleoplasm. The nucleoplasm or the nuclear matrix is a gel-like ground substance containing large quantity of genetic material in the form of deoxyribonucleic acid (DNA). When a cell is not dividing, the nucleoplasm appears as dark-staining thread-like material called nuclear *chromatin.* During cell division, the chromatin material is converted into rod-shaped structures, the chromosomes. There are 46 chromosomes (23 pairs) in all the dividing cells of the body except the gamete (sex cells) which contain only 23 chromosomes (haploid number). Each chromosome is composed of two chromatids connected at the centromere to form 'X' configuratioin having variation of the location of centromere. The chromosomes are composed of three components: DNA, ribonucleic acid (RNA), and other nuclear proteins. The nuclear DNA carries the genetic information which is passed via RNA into the cytoplasm for synthesis of proteins of similar composition.

3. Nucleolus. The nucleus may contain one or more rounded bodies called nucleoli. The nucleoli are the site of synthesis of ribosomal RNA. The nucleoli are more common in growing cells or in cells actively synthesising proteins.

INTERCELLULAR JUNCTIONS

The cell membranes of the neighbouring cells are connected with one another through the *intercellular junctions* or the junctional complexes, which are of three types.

1. Tight junction. This is also called *zona occludens* or the *occluding zone* (Fig. 1.3-3A). In this type of intercellular junction, the outer layer of the cell membrane of the neighbouring cells fuse with each other, thus obliterating the space between the cells. Such junctions form a barrier to the movement of ions and other solutes from one cell to another.

2. Adherens junction. This is also called *zonula adherens*. In this type of junction, cell membrane of the adjacent cells are separated by a 15-20 nm wide space which is at focal places obliterated by the dense accumulation of the proteins at the cell surface. Bundles of intermediate filaments project from the intercellular junctional areas and radiate into the cytoplasm. This holds the adjacent cells at these focal places. These are of two types:

- *Desmosomes* are the adherens junctions where thickened focal areas are formed on both the apposing cell membranes (Fig. 1.3-3B).
- *Hemidesmosomes* are the adherens junctions where focal thickening is seen only on the membrane of one of the two adjacent cells.

3. Gap junction. Gap junctions or the nexus are the channels on the lateral surfaces of the two adjacent cells through which the molecules are exchanged between the cells (Fig. 1.3-3C). Gap junctions serve the following functions:

Fig. 1.3-3. *Schematic diagram of a cell to show various intercellular junctions: A, tight junction; B, adherens junction; and C, gap junction.*

- These permit the intercellular passage of glucose, amino acids, ions and other substances which have a molecular weight of about 1000.
- These permit rapid propagation of electrical potential changes from one cell to another as seen in cardiac muscle and other smooth muscle cells.
- These help in the exchange of chemical messengers between the cells.

THE TISSUES

DEFINITION AND CLASSIFICATION

Body organs are made of many tissues. Tissues are collections of cells performing the same function and having almost similar structure.

Adult tissues are classified into four major groups (each having subdivisions):
- Epithelial tissue or epithelium,
- Connective tissue,
- Muscle tissue, and
- Nervous tissue.

EPITHELIAL TISSUE

Epithelial tissue or epithelium consists of a single layer or multiple layers of cells which are closely packed without any intercellular space. The cells usually lie on a basement membrane which is an inert connective tissue. Epithelial tissue does not have blood supply of its own and depends upon the diffusion from the underlying vascularized tissues for their nutrition.

Location. Epithelium lines or covers the external and internal surfaces of the human body organs as below:
- Lines outer surface of the body i.e. skin.
- Forms the mucosa of the luminal surfaces of the cavities within the body such as in gastrointestinal tract (GIT), urinary tract, blood vessels, heart chambers, uterus etc.
- Epithelial tissue also lines the ducts and secretory elements of glands (which develop as outgrowths from epithelium-lined surfaces).

Functions of epithelium include:
- *Protection* against injuries, bacteria and chemical agents.
- *Secretion.* The epithelium lining the glandular tissue secretes different juices and enzymes.
- *Excretion.* Epithelium performs excretory function in kidneys and skin.
- *Absorption.* The intestinal epithelium plays role in absorption of digested food.
- *Lubrication.* The mesothelial cells lining the serous cavities help in lubrication, e.g. in pleural cavity.
- *Sensory function* e.g., as taste buds and organ of Corti (neuroepithelium).

Classification. Epithelium is of following types:
I. *Simple epithelium*
  - Simple squamous epithelium
  - Simple cuboidal epithelium
  - Simple columnar epithelium
  - Simple columnar ciliated epithelium
  - Pseudostratified columnar epithelium
II. *Compound or stratified epithelium*
  - Stratified squamous epithelium
  - Stratified columnar epithelium
  - Stratified columnar ciliated epithelium
  - Transitional epithelium

I. SIMPLE EPITHELIUM

Simple epithelium refers to a cellular sheet formed of single layer of cells. According to the shape of constituting cells the different types of simple epithelium are described below.

1. Squamous epithelium

Structure. Squamous epithelium is composed of single layer of flat cells resting on the basement membrane with flattened nuclei. The cells are closely packed like flat stones, so also called as pavement epithelium (Fig. 1.3-4A).

Functions and location. Squamous epithelium forms thin smooth surface for easy diffusion of fluid and gases of the following structures:

- Endothelium of heart, blood vessels and lymph vessels,
- Alveoli of the lung,
- Bowman's capsule of kidney,
- Endothelium of cornea, and
- Mesothelium of serous membranes such as pleura, pericardium and peritonium which facilitate the movement of viscera.

2. Cuboidal epithelium

Structure. Simple cuboidal epithelium is composed of a single layer of cubical cells resting on the basement membrane. Nucleus in the cuboidal cells is rounded and centrally placed (Fig. 1.3-4B).

Functions and location. Cuboidal epithelium is actively involved in secretion, absorption and excretion, and also provides limited protection to the organ as a covering. It is present in the following locations:

- Lining the thyroid follicles.
- Lining the tubules of the kidneys.
- Lining the acini and small ducts of glands.
- Germinal epithelium of ovary.

3. Columnar epithelium

Structure. Columnar epithelium is composed of a single layer of tall columnar cells resting on basement membrane. Nucleus of columnar cells is oval and is placed centrally or towards base (Fig. 1.3-4C).

Functions and location. Columnar epithelium is mainly concerned with secretion, absorption and protection. It is present in following areas:

- Gastrointestinal tract and its glands.
- Gall bladder, common bile duct and pancreatic duct.

4. Columnar ciliated epithelium

Structure. The columnar ciliated epithelium is composed of simple columnar cells, the free surfaces of which bear large number of cilia. Nucleus in these cells is oval and placed towards base.

Functions and location. These cells are protective in function. The wave-like movement of the cilia push the contents of the tubes, which they line, in one direction. Ciliated epithelium is found lining the:

Fig. 1.3-4. Types of simple epithelium: A, squamous; B, cuboidal; C, columnar; and D, pseudostratified.

- Respiratory passages i.e. trachea and its branches
- Uterine tubes
- Outer or bony part of eustachian tube
- Central canal of spinal cord and brain ventricles.

5. Pseudostratified columnar epithelium

Structure. Pseudostratified columnar epithelium consists of single layer of tall columnar cells of different heights. All the cells rest on the basement membrane but some cells are small in size and do not reach the surface. Thus, their nuclei appear at different levels forming false rows, hence the name pseudostratified epithelium (Fig. 1.3-4D).

Functions and location. Pseudostratified columnar epithelium is protective and secretory in function. Three different types of pseudostratified columnar epithelia are located as below:

1. *Pseudostratified columnar ciliated epithelium with goblet cells (with motile cilia)* is found lining the:
- Upper respiratory passages such as nasal air sinuses, nasopharynx, part of larynx, trachea and bronchi;
- Inner or cartilagenous part of eustachian tube; and
- Lacrimal sac
2. *Pseudostratified columnar ciliated epithelium* (with microvilli or stereocilia) is only present in the epididymis.

3. *Pseudostratified columnar non-ciliated epithelium* is present in:
- Upper part of ductus deferens;
- Large ducts of salivary glands; and
- Male urethra (penile part).

II. COMPOUND OR STRATIFIED EPITHELIUM

Compound or stratified epithelium refers to the cellular sheet formed of several layers of cells of various shapes. The superficial layers of stratified epithelium grow up from the basal layer. Differnt types of stratified epithelia are described below:

1. Stratified squamous epithelium

Structure. Stratified squamous epithelium consists of multiple layers of cells of different shapes arranged as below (Fig. 1.3-5A).
- *Basal cells* or the deepest cells are columnar in shape and rest on a clear wavy basement membrane.
- *Intermediate layers* are formed of polygonal cells with desmosomes anchoring them to each other between their cell boundaries.
- *Superficial layers* are of flat squamous cells which may be nucleated or non-nucleated.

Types. Stratified squamous epithelium is of two types:

1. *Non-keratinised squamous epithelium.* In this epithelium all cells are living and have nuclei up to the surface. This is found on following wet surfaces that may be subject to wear and tear but are protected from drying:
- *Eye.* Cornea and exposed part of conjunctiva.
- *GIT.* Oral cavity i.e., inner surface of lips, tongue, gums, palatine tonsils, oropharynx, oesophagus and middle part of anal canal.
- *Genitourinary tract.* Vagina, and terminal parts of male and female urethra.

2. *Keratinised squamous epithelium.* The surface layer of this epithelium consists of dead cells which have lost their nuclei and the protein keratin has been added to them (Fig. 1.3-5B). This tough layer of dead cells protects and prevents drying of underlying cells. This is found in following areas:
- Epidermis of skin.
- Tip of filliform papillae of tongue
- Hair and nails.

2. Stratified columnar epithelium

Structure. It is formed of multiple layers (less in number than stratified squamous epithelium). Superficial cells are columnar in type (Fig. 1.3-5B).

Location and function. Stratified columnar epithelium is rare epithelium seen in the ducts of some glands.

3. Transitional epithelium

Structure. Transitional epithelium is composed of several layers of cells arranged classically in three strata (Fig. 1.3-5C):

- *Superficial layer* is formed by large polyhedral um-brella-like cells.
- *Intermediate layers* are made up of pear-shaped cells; the tip is directed towards membrane.
- *Basal cell layer* is formed of high cuboidal cells.

Location and function. Transitional epithelium is found in the renal pelvis and calyces, the ureter, the urinary bladder, and part of the urethra. Because of this distribution it is also called *urothelium.*

In the urinary bladder the transitional epithelium allows for stretching when the bladder fills with urine. When stretched it is not damaged and appears to be thinner with cells becoming flattened and rounded (Fig. 1.3-5C).

Squamous cells

Columnar cells

A

B

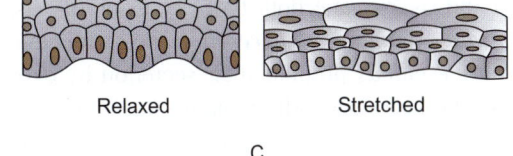

Relaxed   Stretched

C

Fig. 1.3-5. *Types of compound or stratified epithelium: A, squamous; B, columnar; and C, transitional (relaxed and stretched).*

GLANDS OR GLANDULAR EPITHELIUM

Epithelial cells which are specialized to produce secretion constitute the glandular epithelium or the so-called glands.

Types of glands

Glands can be classified in different ways:

A. *According to number of constituting cells* the glands may be:

- *Unicellular glands* i.e. made of a single cell. These glands are interspersed amongst other (non-secretory) epithelial cells. For example *goblet cells* found in the epithelium lining the intestine and respiratory tract.
- *Multicellular glands.* Most glands in the body are made up of multiple cells. For example sweat glands and mammary glands.

B. *According to the nature of secretion* the glands may be:

- *Mucus-secreting glands,* e.g. goblet cells and sublingual salivary gland.
- *Serous glands,* e.g., parotid gland.
- *Mixed or seromucous glands,* e.g., submandibular gland.
- *Watery secretion glands,* e.g., sweat glands.
- *Waxy secretion glands,* e.g., ceruminous glands of ear.
- *Fatty secretion glands,* e.g. sebaceous glands.
- *Cellular secretory glands,* e.g., testis and ovary.

C. *According to mode of pouring the secretion* the glands may be:

- *Endocrine or ductless glands* pour their secretion directly into the blood. Examples of endocrine glands are thyroid, parathyroid, pituitary, suprarenal, pineal body, and islets of Langerhans of pancreas.
  Endocrine glands are usually arranged in cords or in clumps that are intimately related to a rich network of blood capillaries or sinusoids. In some cases (for example, thyroid gland) the cells may form rounded follicles. Endocrine cells and their blood vessels are supported by delicate connective tissue, and are usually surrounded by a capsule.
- *Exocrine glands.* These glands pour their secretion onto the epithelial surface directly or through the ducts. Examples of exocrine glands are salivary glands, sweat glands and sebaceous glands.
- *Mixed glands.* These glands have features of both endocrine and exocrine glands. For example, pancreas, testis and ovary have both types of glandular tissues.

D. *According to manner of secretion* the glands may be:

- *Merocrine glands* produce their secretion by exocytosis i.e. the secretory cells remain intact. Most glands such as pituitary, pancreas etc are merocrine glands.
- *Apocrine glands* lose apical portion of the secretory cells along with the secretory product, as in axillary sweat glands and mammary glands.
- *Holocrine glands* discharge the entire cell with secretion, e.g., sebaceous glands of skin.

Classification of exocrine glands

Depending upon the shape of secretory part and their ducts the multicellular exocrine glands can be classified as below:

A. *Simple glands.* These have a single duct in which all the secretory cells pour their secretion. Depending upon the arrangement of secretory cells the simple glands may be tubular, alveolar or tubuloalveolar:

1. *Simple tubular glands.* The tube-shaped simple glands may be (Fig. 1.3-6):

- Straight, e.g., intestinal glands (crypts of Lieberkuhn).
- Coiled, e.g., sweat glands of skin.
- Branched, e.g., glands of stomach and uterus.

2. *Simple alveolar glands.* These glands have a single duct and the secretory cells are arranged in the form of flask-shaped structures called alveoli (Fig. 1.3-6). For example sebaceous glands and tarsal glands.

3. *Simple tubuloalveolar glands.* These glands have tubular as well as alveolar arrangement of secretory cells.

B. *Compound glands.* These glands are composed of a number of groups of secretory cells, each group discharging into its own duct. The ducts from each group of

Fig. 1.3-6. Types of exocrine glands.

secretory cells unite to form large ducts that ultimately drain on the epithelial surface. Depending upon the arrangement of secretory cells (like that of simple glands) the compound glands may also be (Fig. 1.3-6):

1. *Compound tubular glands,* e.g., kidney and testis.
2. *Compound alveolar glands,* e.g., mammary glands.
3. *Compound tubuloalveolar glands,* e.g., pancreas, prostate, and salivary glands.

CONNECTIVE TISSUE

GENERAL CONSIDERATIONS

The term connective tissue is applied to a tissue which connects one tissue or organ with other tissues or organs.

Structure of connective tissue in general

Connective tissue, in general, is formed of cells and matrix.

Cells. The cells forming the connective tissue differ in different types of connective tissues. The peculiar feature of all connective tissues is that the cells are more widely separated from each other than those forming the epithelium.

Matrix. The matrix refers to the intercellular substance. The matrix is present in considerably large amount in all the connective tissues. The structure of matrix varies in different types of connective tissues.

Note. The specific types of cells and the structure of matrix is described with the different types of connective tissues.

Types of connective tissues.

Depending upon the type of cells and nature of matrix the connective tissue is of following types:

- Connective tissue proper (described below)
- Skeletal (supporting) connective tissue i.e. bone and cartilage (for details see page 93).
- Fluid connective tissue i.e. blood and lymph (for details see page 35).

CONNECTIVE TISSUE PROPER

Definition and functions

Connective tissue proper is in fact the connective tissue in real sense which serves following functions:

- *Connects* the various tissues and organs of the body with each other. Thus the connective tissue fills the interstices between more specialized elements and serves to hold them together.
- *Supports* the tissues and organs of the body by providing a framework.
- *Protects* the tissues and organs by withstanding internal as well as external mechanical stresses. It also defends the body from invasion by micro-organisms.

Structure of connective tissue proper

Depending upon the structure the connective tissue proper is of various types (which are described later). In general, the connective tissue proper is composed of:

- Cells,
- Matrix i.e. intercellular substance which includes fibres and ground substance.

A. Cells of connective tissue proper

As mentioned earlier the connective tissue proper is found in all organs supporting the specialized tissues. The different types of cells of connective tissue proper are:

- Fibroblasts and fibrocytes,
- Fat cells,
- Plasma cells,
- Mast cells,
- Macrophages (histiocytes),
- Leukocytes,
- Pigment cells, and
- Mesenchyme cells.

1. *Fibroblasts and fibrocytes.* Fibroblasts on maturation change to fibrocytes.

- *Structure.* Fibroblasts are flat, branched (irregular) cells with multiple processes (Fig. 1.3-7A). Cytoplasm of these cells is deeply basophilic and rich in RNA, granular endoplasmic reticulum and Golgi apparatus.
- *Function.* Fibroblasts are responsible for formation of both the collagen and elastic fibres as well as ground substance of the matrix. These cells are particularly active in tissue repair (wound healing) where they may bind together the cut surfaces of wounds to form granulation tissue.

2. *Fat cells* also known as *adipocytes* may be found singly or in groups.

- *Structure.* Fat cells are large ovoid with peripheral nucleus (signet ring appearance) (Fig. 1.3-7B). They vary in size and shape depending upon the amount of fat they contain.
- *Function.* They store fat and are especially abundant in adipose tissue.

3. *Plasma cells.* these are ovoid or rounded in shape. Chromatin in the nucleus is arranged in radiating manner giving the appearance of *cartwheel shape* (Fig. 1.3-7C). Their cytoplasm contains *Russel bodies* (immunoglobulin granules). These cells play role in defence mechanism.

4. *Mast cells.* These cells are present in loose connective tissue. They are usually present in groups around the blood vessels.

- *Structure.* Mast cells are oval or rounded in shape similar to basophil leukocytes. Their cytoplasm is filled with large basophilic granules which are precursor of histamine (Fig. 1.3-7D).
- *Functions.* These cells produce histamine and heparin which are released when the cells are damaged by disease or injury. Histamine is involved in local and general inflammatory reactions.

5. *Macrophages* or histiocytes form the part of macrophage system of the body.

- *Structure.* Macrophages are irregular, usually branched with multiple processes (Fig. 1.3-7E), but may be elongated or spindle-shaped. Their cytoplasm is basophilic and may be granular or vacuolated.
- *Function.* They form important part of body's defence mechanism as they are actively phagocytic, engulfing worn-out leucocytes (which die in the process of destroying bacteria), bacteria and foreign bodies.

6. *Leukocytes* i.e. white blood cells, particularly lymphocytes, are normally found in small number in healthy connective tissue. Their number increases in chronic infections when they play an important role in tissue defence.

7. *Pigment cells.* They are particularly found in the connective tissue of skin, and uveal tissue of eye.

- *Structure.* They are small stellate-shaped cells with many branching processes. Their cytoplasm contains numerous pigment granules (Fig. 1.3-7F).
- *Function.* These cells protect the skin against the harmful effects of sun rays.

8. *Mesenchyme cells.* These are undifferentiated cells and can give rise to all varieties of connective tissue cells.

- *Structure.* They are small stellate-shaped cells with large oval nucleus (Fig. 1.3-7G).
- In adult connective tissue, they are arranged along blood vessels. They develop into endothelial cells lining the blood capillaries.

B. Connective tissue fibres

The adult connective tissue contains three types of fibres:
- Collagen fibres,
- Elastic fibres, and
- Reticular fibres.

1. *Collagen fibres.* Their characteristic features are:
- Colourless, strong fibres arranged in bundles (Fig. 1.3-8A).
- Flexible but non-extensible.
- Formed of a protein tropocollagen which can be transformed into gelatin on boiling.
- Found in all types of connective tissue but are specially abundant in skin, dense connective tissue, tendons, ligaments, aponeurosis and meninges of the brain.
- Abnormal conditions include deficient formation in scurvy due to vitamin C deficiency and excessive production and abnormal organization in rheumatoid arthiritis.

2. *Elastic fibres.* Characteristic features are:
- Very elastic, yellowish branched fibres which run singly and not in bundles (Fig. 1.3-8B)
- Formed of the protein tropoelastin which is resistant to boiling.

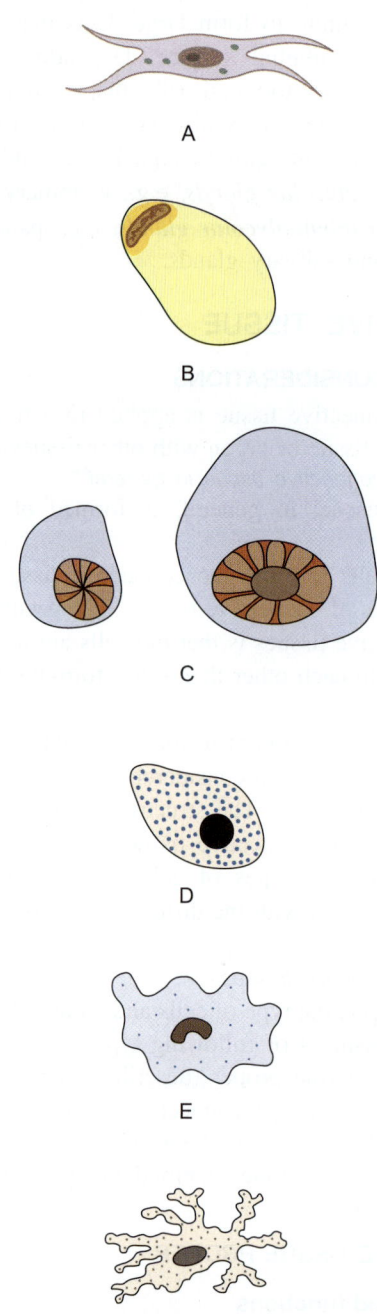

Fig. 1.3-7. *Cells of connective tissue proper: A, fibroblast; B, fat cell; C, plasma cell; D, mast cell; E, macrophage; and F, pigment cell.*

- Found in ligamentum nuchae, ligamentum flavus, walls of large arteries and lining of nerve cells.

3. *Reticular fibres* are type of collagen fibres having following features (Fig. 1.3-8C):
- Thin branching fibres arranged in a net-like framework called reticulum.
- Found in glandular organs, lymphoid tissue, spleen and liver.

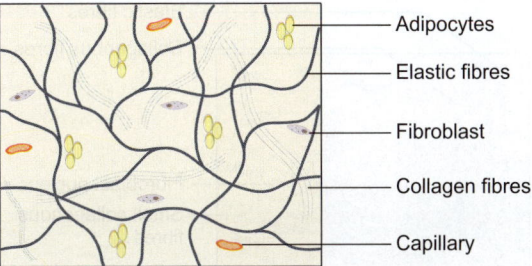

Fig. 1.3-9. Loose (areolar) connective tissue.

Fig. 1.3-8. Fibres of connective tissue proper: A, collagen fibres; B, elastic fibres; and C, reticular fibres.

C. Ground substance of matrix of connective tissue

- It is an amorphous material in which are embedded the cells and fibres of connective tissue.
- It contains a number of proteoglycans which are composed of glycosaminoglycans (GAGs) linked to specific polypeptide chains. The proteoglycans bind water and provide resilience to connective tissue.
- It is synthesized by fibroblasts, osteoblasts, chondroblasts, and smooth muscle cells.

Types of connective tissue proper
Depending upon the relative amount of fibres, cells and matrix the connective tissue proper is of following types:
- Loose (or areolar) connective tissue,
- Dense connective tissue,
- Reticular connective tissue,
- Adipose connective tissue, and
- Pigmented connective tissue.

1. Loose (areolar) connective tissue
Structural characteristics of loose (areolar) connective tissue include (Fig. 1.3-9):
- *Matrix* is semisolid and contains loose, irregularly arranged collagen and elastic fibres in the amorphous ground substance.
- *Cells* embedded in the matrix include fibroblasts, some fat cells, mast cells and macrophages. Cells are widely separated by the fibres.

Location. Areolar connective tissue is widely distributed all over the body. It is present mainly:

- Under the skin,
- In between the muscles,
- In stroma of most of the organs,
- Below the mucous membranes,
- Around the vessels and nerves,
- In serous membranes,
- In glands supporting secretory cells.

Functions. Areolar connective tissue provides elasticity and tensile strength to almost every part of the body.

2. Dense (white fibrous) connective tissue
Structure. It is formed mainly by closely packed bundles of collagen tissue with very little ground substance. Cells (fibrocytes) are few in number and are found lying in rows between the bundles of fibres.

Location. Dense connective tissue is of two types, regular and irregular. The dense regular (Fig. 1.3-10) (white fibrous) connective tissue is present in tendons, ligaments and aponeurosis. The dense irregular connective tissue is present in dermis, periosteum, perichondrium and capsule and stroma of some organs and glands, dura mater and sclera of the eyeball.

Fig. 1.3-10. Dense connective tissue.

Functions. Dense connective tissue connects (supports) and forms tough covering to the various organs.

3. Reticular connective tissue
Structure. It is made up mainly of stellate-shaped reticular cells and fibrillar network of reticular fibres (Fig. 1.3-11). The reticular fibres are thin immature collagen fibres.

Location. Reticular connective tissue is present in the

Fig. 1.3-11. *Reticular connective tissue.*

Fig. 1.3-12. *White adipose tissue.*

stroma of bone marrow, spleen, lymph nodes, thymus, liver, testis, ovary, and endocrine glands.

Function. The reticular connective tissue forms a network in the background of organs and glands.

4. Adipose connective tissue

Adipose connective tissue is of two types: white and brown.

i. *White adipose connective tissue*

Structure. It is mainly composed of large fat cells (more than 100 microns in diameter), each containing a single large globule of non-pigmented fat, in a matrix of areolar tissue (Fig. 1.3-12).

Location and functions. In well-nourished adults it makes up 20-25% of the body weight. It is present:

- Between muscle fibres and under the skin in superficial fascia where it acts as thermal insulator.
- Around the kidneys and eyeballs where it provides a supporting cushion.

- In the abdominal wall, mesentery and abdomen as fat storage.

ii. *Brown adipose tissue*

Structure. It is made up of small fat cells which are filled with many droplets of pigmented fat. It appears brown because it is rich in cytochrome pigments. It has more extensive capillary network than white adipose tissue.

Location and function. Brown adipose tissue is mainly present in the newborn and persists for few months after birth. It acts as *heat generator* and protects the infant from cold after birth. It is located in interscapular region, axillary region, and mediastinal region.

Note. It is impotant to note that adipose connective tissue is not present in the eyelids, penis, labia minora, clitoris, nipples and scrotum.

5. Pigmented connective tissue

Structure. It is similar to loose areolar connective tissue with a large number of pigment cells.

Location. It is present in the vascular layer of the eyeballs (iris, ciliarly body and choroid) and in the skin.

Transport Through Cell Membrane and Membrane Potential

PASSIVE TRANSPORT

Diffusion
- Simple diffusion
- Facilitated diffusion
- Factors affecting diffusion

Osmosis
- Osmotic pressure
- Osmole, osmolality and osmolarity
- Tonicity of fluids

ACTIVE TRANSPORT

Primary active transport
- Sodium-potassium pump
- Calcium pump
- Potassium-hydrogen pump

Secondary active transport
- Sodium co-transport
- Sodium counter-transport

VESICULAR TRANSPORT

Endocytosis

Exocytosis

Transcytosis

OTHER TRANSPORT PROCESSES
- Transport across epithelial membrane
- Ultrafiltration

MEMBRANE POTENTIAL

Genesis of membrane potential
- Selective permeability of the cell membrane
- Gibbs-Donnan equilibrium
- Nernst equation
- Sodium-potassium ATPase pump

The physiological activities of a cell depend upon the substances like nutrients, oxygen and water, which must be transported into the cell, and at the same time metabolic waste must be transported out of the cell. Various processes involved in the transport of substances across the cell membrane may be grouped as under:
- Passive transport
- Active transport
- Vesicular transport.

PASSIVE TRANSPORT

Passive transport refers to the mechanism of transport of substances along the gradient without expenditure of any energy. This process is also called *downhill movement*. It depends upon the physical factors like concentration gradient, electrical gradient and pressure gradient. The passive transport mechanisms operating at the cell membrane level are diffusion and osmosis.

DIFFUSION

Diffusion refers to passive transport of molecules from areas of higher concentration to areas of lower concentration. Diffusion through cell membrane is of two subtypes, called simple diffusion and facilitated diffu-sion.

SIMPLE DIFFUSION

In simple diffusion transport of atoms or molecules occurs from one place to another due to their random movement. Due to constant random movement, the molecules collide with each other and also strike with the cell membrane.

The frequency of collision and the probability of striking to the cell membrane will be higher on the side of the membrane having higher concentration of that particular molecule. In this process there occurs a net flux of the molecules from the areas of high concentration to areas of low concentration. The net movement of the molecules ceases when the concentration of molecules equals, and there occurs a condition of *diffusional equilibrium.* Quantitatively the net movement of the molecules across a permeable membrane, where only simple diffusion is occurring, is expressed by *Fick's law of diffusion,* which states that rate of diffusion (J) is directly proportional to the difference in the concentration of the substance in two regions (concentration gradient, i.e. $C_1 - C_2$) and cross-sectional area (A) and inversely proportional to the distance to be travelled (thickness of the membrane, i.e. T).

$$\text{Thus:} \quad J = D\,\frac{A\,(C_1 - C_2)}{T}$$

where D is the diffusion coefficient.

The diffusion of molecules across the biological membranes differs depending upon the lipid solubility, water solubility, type of electrical charge and size of the molecules. Further, selective permeability of the semipermeable cell membrane also affects the diffusion of different molecules. How the different molecules diffuse across a cell membrane is discussed below.

Simple diffusion of lipid soluble substances through the cell membrane

The rate of diffusion through the lipid bilayer of the cell membrane is directly proportional to the solubility of a substance in lipids. Therefore, molecules of oxygen, nitrogen, carbon dioxide, alcohol, steroid hormones and weak organic acids and bases, being lipid soluble, diffuse very rapidly through the lipid bilayer of the cell membrane.

Simple diffusion of water and other lipid insoluble molecules through the cell membrane

Astonishingly, water and other lipid insoluble substances can also pass easily through the cell membrane. It has been shown that it is possible due to the presence of the so-called *protein channels.*

DIFFUSION THROUGH PROTEIN CHANNELS

The protein channels are tube-shaped channels which extend in the cell membrane from the extracellular to the intracellular ends (Fig. 1.4-1).

The protein channels have been equipped with following characteristics:
- Selective permeability and
- Gating mechanism.

Fig. 1.4-1. *Simple diffusion.*

Selective permeability of protein channels

The protein channels are highly selective, i.e. each channel can permit only one type of ion to pass through it. Examples of some selective channels are:
- *Sodium channels* and
- *Potassium channels*

Gating mechanism in protein channels

Some protein channels are continuously open, whereas most others are 'gated'. This gating mechanism is a means of controlling the permeability of the channels. The opening and closing of gates are controlled by three principal ways:

1. Voltage-gated channels. These respond to the electrical potential across the cell membrane. Sodium and potassium channels are voltage-gated channels. In the case of sodium channels the gates are located at the outer end of the channels (Fig. 1.4-2A) and these remain tightly closed. When the inside of cell membrane loses its negative charge, the sodium channel gates open and there occurs a tremendous inflow of sodium ions. This is the basis of occurrence of action potentials in nerves that are responsible for nerve signals.

In the case of potassium channels, the gates are located at inner end of the channel (Fig. 1.4-2B) and they too open when inside of the cell membrane loses its negative charge. The opening of potassium channel gates is partly responsible for terminating the action potential.

2. Ligand-gated channels. Gates of these channels open when some other chemical molecule binds with the gate proteins. That is why this is also called *chemical gating.*
- One of the most important examples of ligand channel gating is the effect of acetylcholine on the so-called *acetylcholine channels.* This gate plays an important role in transmission of nerve signals from one nerve cell to another and from nerve cells to muscle cells.

3. Mechanical-gated channels. Some protein channels are opened by mechanical stretch. These mechano-sensitive channels play an important role in cell movements.

FACILITATED DIFFUSION

The water-soluble substances having larger molecules such as glucose cannot diffuse through the protein chan-

Fig. 1.4-2. *Voltage-gated sodium channels (A); and potassium channels (B).*

nels by simple diffusion. Such substances diffuse through the cell membrane with the help of some carrier proteins. Therefore, this type of diffusion is called *facilitated* or the *carrier-mediated diffusion*. There are many types of carrier proteins in the cell membrane, each type having binding sites that are specific for a particular substance. Among the most important substances that cross cell membranes by facilitated diffusion are *glucose* and most of the *amino acids*.

Types of carrier protein systems

Three types of carrier protein systems are known (Fig. 1.4-3):

1. Uniport. In this system the carrier proteins transport only one type of molecules.

2. Symport. In this system transport of one substance is linked with transfer of another substance. For example, facilitated diffusion of glucose in the renal tubular cells is linked with the transport of sodium.

3. Antiport. In this system the carrier proteins exchange one substance for another. For example, Na^+-K^+ exchange or Na^+-H^+ exchange in the renal tubules.

Differences between simple and facilitated diffusion

1. Specificity. The carrier proteins are highly specific for different molecules.

2. Saturation. As shown in Fig. 1.4-4, in simple diffusion the rate of diffusion increases proportionately with the increase in the concentration of the substance and there is no limit to it. However, in facilitated diffusion the rate of diffusion reaches a limit. This is called *saturation* point and here all the binding sites on the carrier proteins are occupied and the system operates at its maximum capacity.

Fig. 1.4-4. *Effect of concentration of substance on rate of diffusion in: A, simple diffusion; and B, facilitated diffusion.*

OSMOSIS

Osmosis refers to diffusion of water or any other solvent molecules through a semipermeable membrane, (i.e.

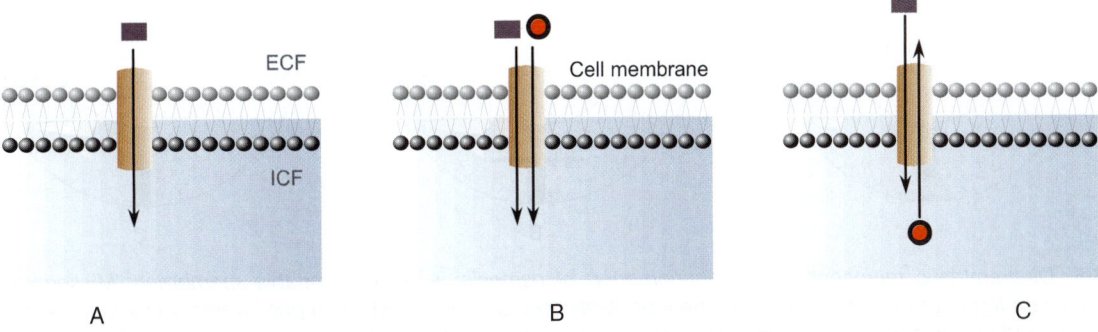

Fig. 1.4-3. *Various types of carrier protein systems: A, uniport; B, symport; and C, antiport.*

CHAPTER 1.4

membrane permeable to solvent but not to the solute) from a solution containing lower concentration of solutes towards the solution containing higher concentration of solutes. Fig. 1.4-5 shows osmosis across a selective permeable membrane. When a sodium chloride solution is placed on one side of the membrane and water on the other side (Fig. 1.4-5A), net movement of water occurs from the pure water into the sodium chloride solution (Fig. 1.4-5B).

OSMOTIC PRESSURE

Osmotic pressure refers to the minimum pressure which when applied on the side of higher solute concentration prevents the osmosis. Fig. 1.4-5C shows that when appropriate pressure is applied the net diffusion of water into the sodium chloride solution is prevented.

The osmotic pressure in the body fluids refers to the pressure exerted by the solutes dissolved in water or other solvents. The osmotic pressure exerted by the colloidal substances in the body is called *colloidal osmotic pressure.* The colloidal osmotic pressure due to plasma colloids (proteins) is called *oncotic pressure.* The osmotic pressure depends upon the number of molecules or ions dissolved in a solution.

Osmole, osmolality and osmolarity

Osmole is the unit used in place of grams to express the concentration in terms of number of osmotically active particles in a given solution. One osmole is equal to the molecular weight of a substance in grams divided by the number of freely moving particles liberated in solution by each molecule. Thus:

- a molar solution of glucose contains 1 mole and exerts osmotic pressure of 1 atmosphere,
- a molar solution of NaCl contains 2 osmoles (1 mole of Na+ and 1 mole of Cl−) and exerts osmotic pressure of 2 atmospheres, and
- a molar solution of $CaCl_2$ contains 3 osmoles (1 mole of Ca^{2+} and 2 moles of Cl−) and thus exerts osmotic pressure of 3 atmospheres.
- One milliosmole (mOsm) is 1/1000 of an osmole.

Osmolality of a solution refers to the number of osmotically active particles (osmoles) per kilogram (kg) of a solution, while *osmolarity* refers to the number of osmoles per litre (L) of a solution. Therefore, osmolarity is affected by the volume of the various solutes in the solution and the temperature, while the osmolality is not. The osmotic pressure is determined by the osmolality and not the osmolarity.

Normal plasma osmolality. The normal osmolality of the extracellular and intracellular fluids is 290 milliosmoles per kilogram (mOsm/kg).

Tonicity of fluids

In clinical practice the word tonicity always refers to tonicity of a solution with respect to that of plasma (290 mOsm). In other words, it is the red blood cell (RBC) membrane across which the tonicity is tested. Thus:

- *Isotonic fluids* are those which have osmolality similar to plasma. RBCs neither shrink nor swell in such solution (Fig. 1.4-6A). A solution of 0.9% NaCl is isotonic with plasma.

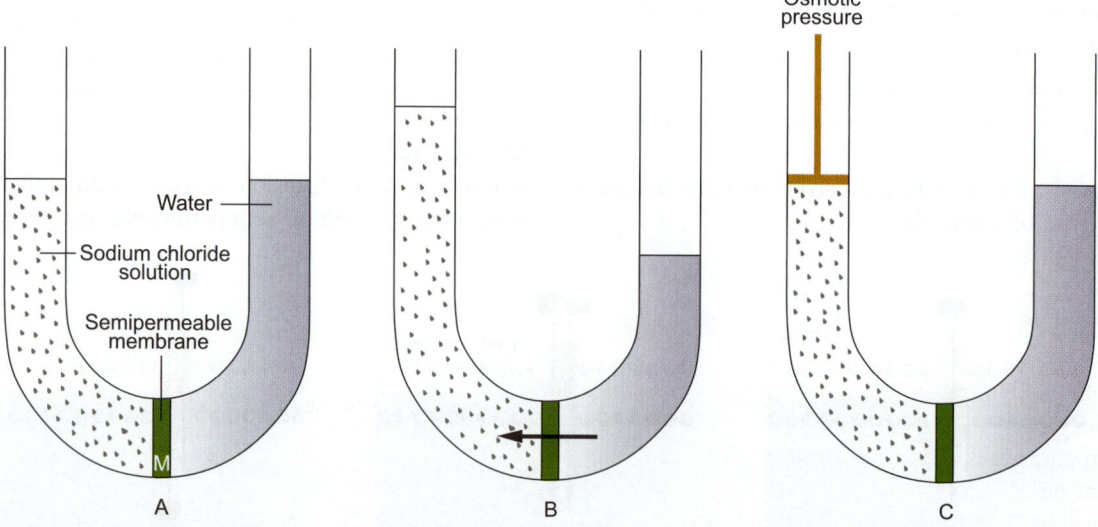

Fig. 1.4-5. *Diagrammatic representation of phenomenon of osmosis: A, semipermeable membrane 'M' separates sodium chloride solution from pure water; B, net movement of water occurs through (M) from pure water side into the sodium chloride solution side; and C, demonstration of osmotic pressure (net movement of water from pure water side to sodium chloride solution is prevented by applying appropriate pressure on the solution side).*

- *Hypertonic fluids* have osmolality higher than the plasma. The RBCs shrink in such solutions by losing water by osmosis (Fig. 1.4-6B).
- *Hypotonic fluids* are those whose osmolality is lower than that of plasma. The RBCs swell up in hypotonic solutions by gaining water by osmosis (Fig. 1.4-6C).

Clinically applied aspects

The total plasma osmolality may increase in patients having severe dehydration, severe diabetes and renal diseases.

Structure of Na⁺-K⁺ pump (Fig. 1.4-7)

The carrier protein involved in Na^+-K^+ pump is a complex consisting of two separate protein units, a larger, the α subunit, and a smaller, β subunit. The α subunit is mainly concerned with Na^+-K^+ transport. It has got following binding sites:

- Three intracellular sites, one each for binding sodium ions ($3Na^+$) and ATP, and one phosphorylation site.
- Two extracellular sites, one each for binding potassium ions ($2K^+$) and ouabain.

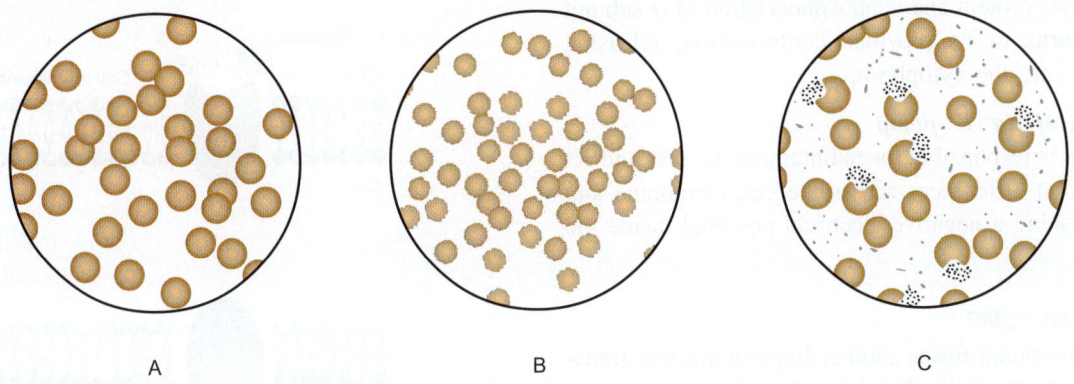

Fig. 1.4-6. *Tonicity of fluids: A, isotonic fluid (0.9% NaCl) has osmolarity similar to plasma, RBCs neither shrink nor swell in it; B, hypertonic fluid (2% NaCl) has osmolarity higher than plasma, RBCs shrink in it; and C, hypotonic fluid (0.3% NaCl) has osmolarity lower than plasma, RBCs swell in it.*

ACTIVE TRANSPORT

Active transport refers to the mechanism of transport of substances against the chemical and/or electrical gradient. Active transport involves expenditure of energy which is liberated by breakdown of high energy compounds like ATP. This process is also called *uphill movement*.

TYPES OF ACTIVE TRANSPORT

The active transport is of two types:
- Primary active transport, and
- Secondary active transport.

A. PRIMARY ACTIVE TRANSPORT PROCESSES

In primary active transport process, the energy is derived directly from the breakdown of adenosine triphosphate (ATP) or some other high-energy phosphate compound. Some of the important pumps involved in the primary active transport processes are:
- Sodium-potassium pump,
- Calcium pump, and
- Potassium hydrogen pump.

1. SODIUM-POTASSIUM PUMP

Sodium-potassium (Na^+-K^+) pump is present in all the cells of the body.

Fig. 1.4-7. *Sodium-potassium ATPase pump: A, structure; and B, mechanism of operation.*

Mechanism of operation of Na⁺–K⁺ pump (Fig. 1.4-7B)
The functioning of Na⁺–K⁺ pump involves the use of enzyme ATPase. The enzyme ATPase is activated when three sodium ions and one ATP molecule bind to their respective binding sites. The activated ATPase catalyzes the hydrolysis of ATP to ADP and liberates a high-energy phosphate bond of energy (phosphorylation). The energy so liberated is believed to cause a conformational change in the carrier protein molecule extruding sodium into the extracellular fluid. This is followed by binding of two potassium ions to the receptor site on extracellular surface of the carrier protein and dephosphorylation of α subunit which returns to its previous conformation, releasing potassium into the cytoplasm.

Functions of Na⁺-K⁺ pump

This pump is responsible for maintaining the Na⁺ and K⁺ concentration differences across the cell membrane and for establishing a negative electrical potential inside the cells.

2. CALCIUM PUMP

The calcium pump forms another important active transport mechanism. Like Na⁺-K⁺ pump it also operates through a carrier protein which has ATPase activity. The calcium pump helps in maintaining extremely low concentration of calcium in the intracellular fluid (10,000 times less than the ECF).

3. POTASSIUM-HYDROGEN PUMP

The primary active transport system of hydrogen ion also operates through ATPase (K⁺-H⁺ ATPase) activity. These are present at following two places in the human body:

- *Parietal cells of gastric glands*, and
- *Renal tubules*.

B. SECONDARY ACTIVE TRANSPORT

In secondary active transport processes, the energy is derived secondarily from the energy which has been stored in the form of ionic concentration differences between the two sides of a membrane, created in the first place by primary active transport. The secondary active transport of substance may occur in the form of sodium co-transport or sodium counter-transport.

Sodium co-transport

The carrier protein here acts as symport, i.e. transports some other substance along with the sodium. Substances carried by sodium co-transport include glucose, amino acids, chloride and iodine.

1. *Sodium co-transport of glucose.* The glucose is transported into most cells against large concentration gradient. As shown in Fig. 1.4-8A, the carrier protein has two

receptor sites on the outer surface, one for sodium and other for glucose. The special feature of the carrier protein is that the conformational change in it occurs only when both the sodium and glucose molecules are attached to it. Due to conformational change in the carrier protein both the sodium and the glucose are transported simultaneously inside the cell (Fig. 1.4-8B). The co-transport of glucose occurs during its absorption from the intestine into the blood and during the reabsorption of glucose from renal tubule in the blood.

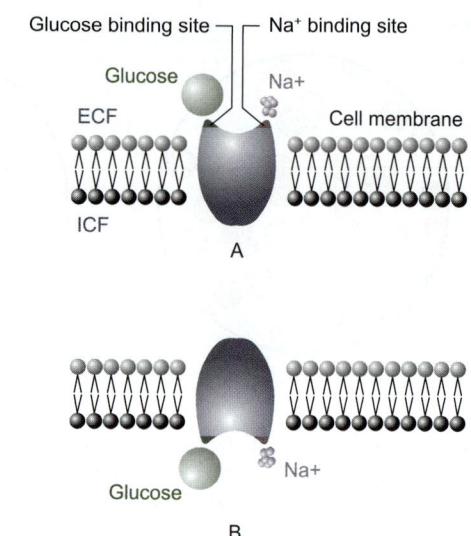

Fig. 1.4-8. *Postulated mechanism of sodium co-transport of glucose (secondary active transport): A, carrier protein has two receptor sites, one for sodium and one for glucose; and B, conformational change in carrier proteins causes transport of both glucose and sodium inside the cell simultaneously.*

2. *Sodium co-transport of amino acids.* Occurs especially in the epithelial cells of intestinal tract and renal tubules during absorption of the amino acids into the blood.

Sodium counter-transport

The carrier protein involved here acts as *antiport*, i.e. sodium ion is exchanged for some other substance. Some of the sodium counter-transport mechanisms occurring in the body are:
1. Sodium-calcium counter-transport
2. Sodium-hydrogen counter-transport

VESICULAR TRANSPORT

Vesicular transport mechanisms are involved in the transport of macromolecules such as large protein molecules which can neither pass through the cell membrane by diffusion nor by active transport mechanisms. The vesicular transport mechanisms include endocytosis, exocytosis and transcytosis.

ENDOCYTOSIS

Endocytosis is the process in which the substance is transported into the cell by infolding of the cell membrane around the substance and internalising it (Fig. 1.4-9).

Fig. 1.4-9. Endocytosis.

EXOCYTOSIS

Exocytosis (Fig. 1.4-10) is reverse of endocytosis, i.e. by this process the substances are expelled from the cell without passing through the cell membrane. In this process, the substances which are to be extruded are collected in the form of granules or vesicles which move towards the cell membrane. Their membranes then fuse to the cell membrane. The area of fusion breaks down releasing the contents to the exterior and leaving the cell membrane intact. Release of hormones and enzymes by secretory cells of the body occurs by exocytosis.

Fig. 1.4-10. Exocytosis.

TRANSCYTOSIS

Vesicular transport within the cell is called transcytosis or cytopemisis. It is quite similar to exocytosis and endocytosis. Three basic steps involved in this process are: (i) vesicle formation, (ii) vesicle transportation, and (iii) docking in the cell.

OTHER TRANSPORT PROCESSES

Some of these processes discussed briefly are:
- Transport across epithelia, and
- Ultrafiltration.

TRANSPORT ACROSS EPITHELIA

Transport across epithelia involves movement of the substances from one side of the epithelium to the other. The transepithelial transport occurs in body cavities lined by continuous sheet of cells such as in gastrointestinal tract, renal tubules, pulmonary airways and other structures. Transport across epithelia may occur in two ways:

- Transport through the cells proper.
- Transport across the tight junction.

ULTRAFILTRATION

When a solution of protein and salt is separated from plain water or a less concentrated salt solution by a membrane permeable to salt and water and not to the protein, there will be a net movement of water on the protein side by diffusion and a movement of salt away from the protein side. This process is called *dialysis*.

Ultrafiltration. Refers to occurrence of dialysis under hydrostatic pressure (Fig. 6.3-10). Ultrafiltration is occurring at the capillary level in the body. The capillary blood is under hydrostatic pressure. The pressure is 35 mm Hg near the arteriolar end and gradually declines to 12 mm Hg near the venous end of the capillary. Through the capillaries there occurs ultrafiltration of all the constituents of the plasma except the proteins into the interstitial spaces. Ultrafiltration plays important role in the formation of body fluids (see page 191) (Fig. 6.3-10).

MEMBRANE POTENTIAL

There exists a potential difference across the membrane of all living cells with the inside being negative in relation to the outside. This potential difference is named *membrane potential,* because the cations and anions arrange themselves along the outer and inner surfaces of the cell membrane. The magnitude of membrane potential varies from cell to cell and in a particular cell varies according to its functional status. For example, a nerve cell has a membrane potential of –70 mV (inside negative) at rest, but when it gets excited the membrane potential becomes about +30 mV (inside positive). The membrane potential at rest is called *resting membrane potential* or resting transmembrane potential or simply resting potential. The term rest does not imply that cell is metabolically quiescent but that it is not undergoing any electrical change. The membrane potential measured during excited state of the cell is called *action potential.*

GENESIS OF MEMBRANE POTENTIAL

Membrane potential is basically due to unequal distribution of ions across the cell membrane, which in turn results due to the combined effect of various forces acting

CHAPTER 1.4

on the ions. The factors involved in genesis of membrane potential which need elaboration are:

- Selective permeability of the cell membrane,
- Gibbs-Donnan equilibrium,
- Nernst equation, and
- Sodium-potassium ATPase pump.

SELECTIVE PERMEABILITY OF THE CELL MEMBRANE

The cell membrane is selectively permeable, that is, to some ions it is freely permeable, to others impermeable and to some others it has variable permeability as:

- Ions like Na^+, K^+, Cl^- and HCO_3^- are diffusible ions. The cell membrane is freely permeable to K^+ and Cl^- and moderately permeable to Na^+.
- The cell membrane is practically impermeable to intracellular proteins and organic phosphate which are negatively charged ions.
- Presence of gated channels in the cell membrane is responsible for the variable permeability of certain ions in different circumstances.

GIBBS-DONNAN MEMBRANE EQUILIBRIUM

According to Gibbs-Donnan membrane equilibrium, when two ionized solutions are separated by a semipermeable membrane, at equilibrium:

- Each solution shall be electrically neutral, i.e. total charges on cations will be equal to total charges on anions.
- The product of diffusible ions on one side of the membrane will be equal to product of diffusible ions on the other side of the membrane.

Since the intracellular fluid (ICF) contains non-diffusible anions like proteins and organic phosphate, so, according to Gibbs-Donnan equilibrium there should be an asymmetrical distribution of diffusible ions across the cell membrane.

NERNST EQUATION

The asymmetrical distribution of diffusible ions across the cell membrane in the form of excess diffusible cation inside due to Gibbs-Donnan equilibrium (as explained above) results in concentration gradient. As a result of this diffusible cations (K^+) will try to diffuse back into the ECF from ICF, but it is counteracted by the electrical gradient, which will be created due to the presence of non-diffusible anions inside the cell. Thus an equilibrium will be reached between the concentration gradient and the electrical gradient resulting in diffusion potential (equilibrium potential) across the cell membrane. The magnitude of this equilibrium potential can be determined by Nernst equation as:

$$E_{(m)} = \pm 61 \ \log \frac{(Conc)_i}{(Conc)_o}$$

The equilibrium potential (E_m) for some of the important ions in the mammalian spinal motor neuron calculated from the simplified Nernst equation is shown in Table 1.4-1.

Table 1.4-1. Equilibrium potential (E_m) for important ions in a mammalian spinal motor neuron

Ion	Concentration (in mmol/L of H_2O)		Equilibrium potential (in mV)
	outside the cell	inside the cell	
Na^+	150	15	+60
K^+	5.5	150	–90
Cl^-	125	9	–70

ROLE OF NA^+-K^+ ATPase PUMP

The role of Na^+-K^+ ATPase lies in building the concentration gradient. It serves to pump back the Na^+ that diffuses into the cell and K^+ that diffuses out of the cell. The Na^+-K^+ pump is potentially electrogenic, since it pumps out $3Na^+$ ions for $2K^+$ ions.

Blood and Immune System

Blood Composition, Plasma and Plasma Proteins

BLOOD

Blood is a fluid connective tissue which transports substances from one part of the body to another. It provides nutrients and hormones to the tissues and removes their waste products. Blood, confined in the cardiovascular system, constitutes a major part of the extracellular fluid of the body. Some of the important physical characteristics of blood are:

- *Colour* of the blood is opaque red due to the pigment haemoglobin in the RBCs. The arterial blood is bright red and venous blood is dark red in colour.
- *Volume* of blood in an average adult is about 5 to 6 L (8% of the body weight or 80 ml/kg body weight).
- *Viscosity* of blood is five times more than that of water.
- *Specific gravity* of blood is 1.050–1.060. Specific gravity of RBC is greater (1.090) than that of plasma (1.030).
- *pH of blood* is about 7.4 (ranges from 7.38 to 7.42), i.e. it is alkaline in nature. In acidosis pH of blood falls below 7.38 and in alkalosis pH is more than 7.42.

Composition

Blood is composed of two main components, plasma and cellular elements.

Plasma constitutes about 55% of the blood volume. It is a clear straw-coloured fluid portion of blood. *Plasma proteins,* an important constituent of plasma, form about 7% of its volume.

Cellular elements of blood are about 45% of the total blood volume and constitute the so-called packed cell volume (PCV). Blood cells are:

- Erythrocytes or red blood cells (5 million/mm³) see page 39.
- Leucocytes or white blood cells (4000–11000/mm³) see page 48.
- Platelets or thrombocytes (1.5–4 lac/mm³) see page 63.

Functions of blood

1. *Nutritive function.* Blood carries the nutritive substances like glucose, amino acids, fatty acids, vitamins, electrolytes and others from the gut to the tissues where they are utilized.

2. *Respiratory functions.* Blood picks up oxygen from the lungs and delivers it to the various tissues. Most important function of the blood is the uninterrupted delivery of O_2 to heart and brain. It also carries away CO_2 from the tissues to the lungs from where it is expelled out in the expired air.

3. *Excretory function.* Blood transports various metabolic waste products such as urea, uric acid and creatinine to excretory organs (kidney, skin, intestine and lungs) for their disposal.

4. *Transport function.* The various hormones produced by endocrine glands, the biological enzymes and antibodies are transported by the blood to the target tissue to modulate metabolic process.

5. Protective function. Blood plays an important role in the defence mechanism of the body:

- Neutrophils and monocytes engulf the micro-organisms entering the body by phagocytosis.
- Lymphocytes and gamma globulins initiate immune response.
- Eosinophils accomplish detoxification, disintegration and removal of foreign proteins.

6. Homeostatic function. Blood plays an important role in maintaining the internal environment of the body (homeostatic function):

- The water content of blood is freely interchangeable with the interstitial fluid and helps in maintaining the water and electrolyte balance of the body.
- Plasma proteins and haemoglobin act as buffers and help in maintaining the acid-base balance and pH of the body fluids.

7. Maintenance of body temperature. Blood plays an important role in regulation of the body temperature.

8. Storage function. Blood serves as a ready-made source of substances stored in it (such as glucose, water, proteins, and electrolytes for use in emergency conditions like starvation, fluid loss and electrolyte loss).

PLASMA

Plasma is the clear straw-coloured fluid (with dissolved solid substances) portion of the blood minus its cellular elements. It constitutes about 55% of the blood volume.

Composition

Plasma contains the following constituents:

Water. Water is the main constituent of plasma forming 91% of it.

Solids. The solids dissolved in the plasma constitute a total of 9% of the plasma. The solid constituents of plasma are given below :

- *Plasma proteins* form 7% of the solids in plasma.
- *Other organic molecules* which form 1% of the solids include Carbohydrates, Fats, Non-protein nitrogenous (NPN) substances, Hormones, enzymes and antibodies.
- *Inorganic substances* which constitute 1% of the solids in plasma include sodium, potassium, calcium, magnesium, chloride, iodide, iron, phosphates and copper.

Gases present in the plasma are oxygen, carbon dioxide and nitrogen.

SERUM

Plasma from which fibrinogen and clotting factors (II, V and VIII) have been removed is called serum. Serum is formed when the blood is allowed to clot in a test tube

and clot is retracted. Serum has a higher serotonin (5HT) content because of the breakdown of platelets during clotting.

PLASMA PROTEINS

CLASSIFICATION OF PLASMA PROTEINS

Plasma proteins form the major solid constituent of the plasma. The total plasma protein concentration is 7.4 gm% (ranges from 6.4 to 8.3 gm%). The major forms of plasma proteins are (Fig. 2.1-1):

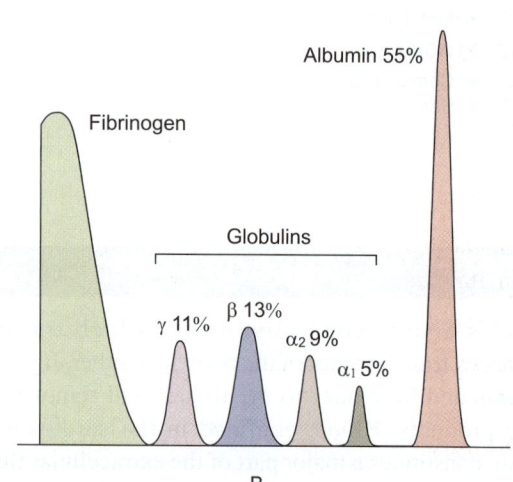

Fig. 2.1-1. *Paper electrophoresis showing: A, bands of different plasma proteins; and B, relative amount of plasma proteins.*

- Albumin (4.8 gm%),
- Globulins (2.3 gm%) include :
  - Alpha 1 (α_1) globulin,
  - Alpha 2 (α_2) globulin,
  - Beta (β) globulin, and
  - Gamma (γ) globulin
- Fibrinogen (0.3 gm%).

FEATURES OF INDIVIDUAL FRACTION OF PLASMA PROTEINS

1. Albumin

Plasma levels are 4.8 gm% (range 3–5 gm%).

Molecular weight of albumin is 69,000.

Synthesized in liver.

Half-life is about 10 days.

2. Globulins

Plasma levels are 2.3 gm% (range 2 to 3 gm%).

Molecular weight varies from 90,000 to 15,600.

Types include alpha 1, alpha 2, beta 1, beta 2 and gamma globulins.

Forms of globulins are described below.

(i) *Glycoproteins* consist of carbohydrates and protein

(ii) *Lipoproteins* consist of alpha 2 globulin and lipids. It has got the following subtypes:

- High density lipoproteins (HDL).
- Low density lipoproteins (LDL).
- Very low density lipoproteins (VLDL).
- Chylomicron (CM).

(iii) *Transferrin* has the specific property of iron binding and thus helps in its transport and storage.

(iv) *Haptoglobin* forms stable complexes with free haemoglobin.

(v) *Ceruloplasmin* binds with copper and helps in its transport and storage.

(vi) *Fetunin* is a growth promoting protein seen in infants and newborn.

(vii) *Immunoglobulins* are gamma globulins which play role in immunity.

(viii) *Angiotensinogen* is alpha 2 globulin.

(ix) *Haemagglutinins* are antibodies against the red blood cell antigens.

3. Fibrinogen

- *Plasma levels* are 0.3 gm%.
- *Molecular weight* varies from 4,00,000 to 5,00,000.
- *Synthesized* in the liver.
- *Functions* as a clotting protein.

4. Prothrombin

- *Plasma levels* are 40 mg%.
- *Molecular weight* is 68,000.
- *Synthesized* in the liver. Synthesis is promoted by vitamin K.

FUNCTIONS OF PLASMA PROTEINS

1. *Exert osmotic pressure.* The protein molecules are unable to pass across the capillary membrane and consequently exert colloid osmotic pressure of about 25 mmHg on the capillary membrane. About 70 to 80% of the osmotic pressure is contributed by the albumin fraction. The colloid osmotic pressure plays an important role in exchange of water between the blood and tissue fluid (see page 190).

2. *Contribution to blood viscosity.* Fibrinogen and globulins are significant contributors to blood viscosity because of their asymmetrical shape.

3. *Role in coagulation of blood.* The fibrinogen, prothrombin and other coagulation proteins present in the plasma play an important role in the coagulation of blood.

4. *Role in defence mechanism of the body.* The gamma globulins are antibodies which play an important role in the immune system meant for defence of the body against the microorganisms.

5. *Role in maintaining acid-base balance of the body.* Plasma proteins act as buffers and contribute for about 15% of the buffering capacity of blood. Because of their amphoteric nature plasma proteins can combine with acids and bases.

6. *Transport function.* Plasma proteins combine easily with many substances and play an essential role in their transport. The substances transported by plasma proteins are carbon dioxide, thyroxine, cortisol, vitamin A, D and E, vitamin B_{12}, bilirubin, drugs, calcium, copper, and free haemoglobin.

7. *Role as reserve proteins.* Plasma proteins serve as reserve proteins and are utilized by the body tissues during conditions like fasting, inadequate protein intake.

8. *Role in suspension stability of red blood cells.* Suspension stability refers to the property of red blood cells by virtue of which they remain uniformly suspended in the blood. Globulins and fibrinogen accelerate this property.

9. *Fibrinolytic function.* The enzymes of fibrinolytic system digest the intravascular clot (thrombus) and thus save from the disastrous effects of thrombosis.

10. *Role in genetic information.* Many plasma proteins exhibit *polymorphism*. Polymorphism is a Mendelian trait that exists in the population with differing prevalence. They serve as valuable tool for the studies of population genetics. Plasma proteins that show polymorphism are haptoglobin, transferrin, ceruloplasmin and immunoglobulins.

SYNTHESIS OF PLASMA PROTEINS

Site of synthesis

In adults plasma proteins are synthesized as described below:

- The albumin and fibrinogen are synthesized mostly by reticuloendothelial cells of the liver.
- Alpha and beta globulins are synthesized by the liver, spleen, and bone marrow.
- Gamma globulins are synthesized by B lymphocytes. Dietary proteins play an important role in synthesis of plasma proteins.

CHAPTER 2.1

CHANGES IN PLASMA PROTEINS IN HEALTH AND DISEASE

Physiological variations

- *In infants*, the total protein level is low (about 5.5 gm%) due to low gamma globulins.

- *In old age*, there is a tendency for the albumin level to fall and the total globulin level to rise.

- *In pregnancy*, during first six months, the albumin and globulin levels decrease while the fibrinogen level increases.

Abnormalities of plasma protein levels

Hypoproteinaemia refers to generalized decrease in the levels of plasma proteins.

Causes of hypoproteinaemia include the following:

- Dietary deficiency
- Malabsorption syndrome
- Liver diseases
- Renal diseases
- Haemorrhage and extensive burns
- Hereditary analbuminaemia
- Congenital afibrinogenaemia

Effects of hypoproteinaemia

Low levels of plasma proteins are associated with a decrease in the plasma osmotic pressure which causes water retention and oedema of the body tissue.

Hyperproteinaemia, i.e. increase in the plasma protein levels is seen in following conditions:

- *Acute inflammatory conditions* are associated with increased synthesis of the so-called *acute phase proteins* which include C-reactive proteins.

- *Acute tissue destruction* as in myocardial infarction is also associated with raised levels of acute phase proteins.

- *Chronic inflammation and malignancies* are also associated with raised levels of C-reactive proteins.

- *Multiple myeloma* is associated with increased levels of the so-called *Bence Jones* proteins and myeloma globulin due to their abnormal formation in the bone marrow.

Reversal of normal A/G ratio. The normal albumin: globulin (A/G) ratio (1.7:1) is reversed in the following conditions:

- When albumin synthesis is decreased as occurs in liver diseases (globulin levels being normal because many globulins are synthesized by B lymphocytes).

- When globulin levels are increased (as occurs in most of the conditions associated with hyperproteinaemia).

Red Blood Cells and Anaemias

2.2

CHARACTERISTIC FEATURES OF RBCs

Functional morphology
- Normal size, shape and counts
- Variations in counts
- Packed cell volume
- Rouleaux formation and erythrocyte sedimentation rate

Formation of red blood cells
- Sites of haemopoiesis
- Blood cell precursors
- Control of haemopoiesis
- Stages of erythropoiesis
- Regulation of erythropoiesis
- Factors necessary for erythropoiesis

Haemoglobin
- Normal blood haemoglobin
- Structure of haemoglobin
- Functions of haemoglobin
- Varieties of haemoglobin
- Derivatives of haemoglobin
- Synthesis of haemoglobin

Life span and fate of red blood cells
- Life span of red blood cells
- Fate of red blood cells

Bilibrubin and Jaundice
- Bilirubin
- Jaundice

ANAEMIAS
- Definition and classification
- General clinical features

CHARACTERISTIC FEATURES OF RED BLOOD CELLS

FUNCTIONAL MORPHOLOGY

The red blood cells (mature erythrocytes) form one of the important constituents of the cellular elements of the blood. Each red blood cell (RBC) like any other cell in the body is bounded by a *cell membrane* but is *non-nucleated* and lacks the usual cell organelles. The cytoplasm of the RBC contains a special pigmented protein called the *haemoglobin* which forms 90 per cent of the weight of erythrocyte. The red colour of the RBCs and thus of the blood is due to the presence of haemoglobin.

NORMAL SIZE, SHAPE AND COUNTS OF RBCs

Normal size

- *Diameter* of each RBC is 7.2 μm (range 6.9–7.4 μm),
- *Thickness* in the periphery is 2 μm and in the centre 1 μm,
- *Surface area* of each RBC is about 120–140 μm², and
- *Volume* is about 80 μm³ (range 78–86 μm³).

Normal shape

The red blood cells are circular, biconcave discs (Fig. 2.2-1).

Advantages of biconcave shape are:

- It renders the red cells quite flexible so that they can pass through capillaries whose minimum diameter is 3.5 μm (Fig. 2.2-2).

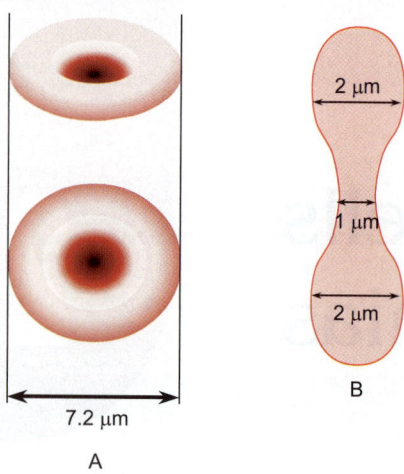

Fig. 2.2-1. *Size and shape of a normal red blood cell: A, biconcave disc (diameter 7.2 μm); and B, thickness (2 μm at the periphery and 1 μm in the centre).*

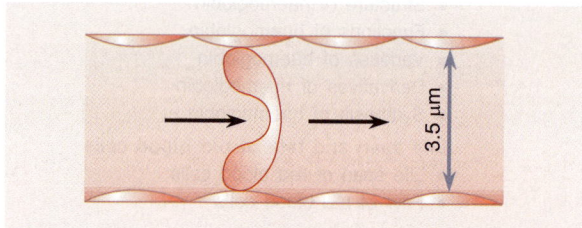

Fig. 2.2-2. *Showing how flexibility of red blood cell allows it to pass through smaller capillaries (diameter 3.5 μm).*

- The biconcavity provides greater surface area as compared to volume which allows considerable alterations in the cell volume. Thus, the RBC can withstand considerable changes of osmotic pressure. In this way the RBCs can resist haemolysis to certain extent when placed in hypotonic solution.
- Greater surface area allows easy exchange of O_2 and CO_2 and rapid diffusion of other substances.

Normal counts
- *At birth*, normal RBC count is 6–7 million/mm³.
- *In adult males,* the normal count varies from 5 to 6.5 million/mm³ (average 5.5 million/mm³).
- *In females* it varies from 4.5 to 5.5 million/mm³ (average 4.8 million/mm³).
- *Clinically,* a count of 5 million/mm³ is considered as 100%.

ABNORMALITIES IN COUNTS OF RBCs
Polycythaemia or pathological increase in RBC count (above 7 million/mm³) is seen in malignancies of bone marrow and conditions associated with chronic hypoxia.
Anaemia. In anaemia there may occur marked reduction in the RBC count or the haemoglobin level or both (see page 46).

PACKED CELL VOLUME
Packed cell volume (PCV) refers to the percentage of the cellular elements (RBCs, WBCs and platelets) in the whole blood. Since the volume of WBCs and platelets is very less, so for all practical purposes the PCV is considered equivalent to the volume of packed red cells (VPRC) or the so-called *haematocrit value.* The normal values of PCV in males is about 45% and in females about 42%. The PCV is increased in polycythaemia and decreased in anaemia.

ROULEAUX FORMATION AND ERYTHROCYTE SEDIMENTATION RATE

Rouleaux formation
- Rouleaux formation refers to the tendency of RBCs to pile one over the other like a pile of coins (Fig. 2.2-3). The discoid shape and protein coating of red cells play major role in rouleaux formation. Rouleaux formation does not occur in normal circulation under physiological conditions, as the moving cells show little or no tendency to adhere.

Fig. 2.2-3. *Rouleaux formation.*

- This is a reversible phenomenon, but it promotes sedimentation of RBCs. It should not be confused with agglutination where the cells are irreversibly clumped.
- Albumin decreases the rouleaux formation, while fibrinogen, globulin and other products of tissue destruction increase rouleaux formation.

Erythrocyte sedimentation rate
Erythrocyte sedimentation rate (ESR) is the rate at which the red blood cells sediment (settle down) when the blood containing an anticoagulant is allowed to stand in a vertically placed tube. It is expressed in millimetre at the end of first hour.

Clinical significance of ESR
- *Normal values* of ESR by Westergren's method in males vary from 3 to 7 mm and in females from 5 to 9 mm in first hour.
- Values of ESR are raised in a large number of pathological conditions, so it has got no specific diagnostic value. However, raised levels of ESR do suggest

presence of some chronic inflammatory condition in the body.

- Estimation of ESR is more useful as a *prognostic test,* i.e., to judge the progress of the disease in patients under treatment.

FORMATION OF RED BLOOD CELLS

Formation of red blood cells is a part of the process of development of blood cells (RBCs, WBCs and platelets) called *haemopoiesis* which includes:

- Erythropoiesis, i.e. development of RBCs,
- Leucopoiesis, i.e. development of WBCs, and
- Thrombopoiesis or megakaryocytopoiesis, i.e. development of platelets.

SITES OF HAEMOPOIESIS

- In the first two months of gestation, the *yolk sac* is the main site of haemopoiesis.
- *From third month of gestation,* liver and spleen become the main sites of blood formation.
- *From 20th week of gestation,* haemopoiesis begins in the bone marrow.
- *At birth* (in normal full-term), almost whole of the haemopoiesis occurs in the bone marrow.
- *In young children,* active haemopoietic bone marrow is found in both axial skeleton and bones of extremities. The active haemopoietic bone marrow is red in colour due to marked cellularity and hence is called *red bone marrow.* However, during this period, there occurs a progressive fatty replacement throughout the long bones converting red bone marrow into the so-called *yellow bone marrow.*
- *In adults,* haemopoietic (red) bone marrow is confined to *axial skeleton* (skull, vertebrae, sternum, ribs, sacrum and pelvis) and *proximal ends of long bones* (humerus, femur and tibia). Even in these haemopoietic areas, about 50% the bone marrow consists of fat.

BLOOD CELL PRECURSORS

The stem cells

The *monophyletic theory* of haemopoiesis is now widely accepted, according to which all blood cells originate from *pluripotent multipotent stem cell.* Stem cells possess two *fundamental properties:*

- *Self-replication,* i.e. stem cells are capable of cell division to give rise to more stem cells, and
- *Differentiation and commitment,* i.e. the stem cells have ability to differentiate into specialized cells called progenitor cells.

Progenitor cells

The stem cells, after a series of divisions, differentiate into progenitor cells (Fig. 2.2-4):

Pluripotent progenitor cells which can give rise to any type of blood cells,

Lymphoid (immune system) stem cells which ultimately develop into lymphocytes, and

Myeloid (trilineage) stem cells which later differentiate into three types of cell lines:

- *Granulocyte-monocyte progenitors* which produce all leucocytes except the lymphocytes,
- *Erythroid progenitors* which produce red blood cells, and
- *Megakaryocyte progenitors* which produce platelets.

Progenitor cells possess ability to give rise to *clones* (group of cells), so they are also called *colony-forming cells* (CFC) or *colony-forming units* (CFU).

The broad outlines of haemopoiesis discussed above are summarized in Fig. 2.2-4. Further details of erythropoiesis are discussed in this chapter and details of development of other blood cells are discussed in the relevant chapters.

STAGES OF ERYTHROPOIESIS

The red blood cells develop from the burst-forming unit – erythrocyte (BFU-E) and colony-forming unit – erythrocyte (CFU-E) which are derived from the committed progenitor cells.

The different stages of erythropoiesis (Fig. 2.2-5) are as under:

1. **Pronormoblast** or proerythroblast is the earliest recognisable cell of the erythroid series seen in the red bone marrow.

2. **Early (basophilic) normoblast** (basophilic early erythroblast). The pronormoblast progresses into the early normoblast.

3. **Intermediate (polychromatic) normoblast** (poly-chromatic erythroblast) is the next maturation stage in erythroid series. *Haemoglobin* appears in this stage.

4. **Late (orthochromatic) normoblast** (orthochromatic erythroblast) is the last nucleated cell of erythroid series.

5. **Reticulocyte** is the last stage in the formation of erythrocytes, that is why it is also called young red cell. Its features are :

- *Size and shape.* The reticulocyte is a flat, disc- shaped, slightly larger (7–7.5 µm) than the mature erythrocytes.
- *Cytoplasm* still contains small amounts of RNA. With supervital stain such as brilliant cresyl blue, the RNA appears in the form of a reticulum (net-like structure). Because of this character the cell is called reticulocyte.
- *Nucleus* is absent.

Summary of changes occurring in cells of erythroid series during maturation

It takes 7 days for the formation and maturation of red blood cells. Various changes which occur during matura-

Fig. 2.2-4. *Schematic broad outline of haemopoiesis.*

Fig. 2.2-5. *Stages of erythropoiesis.*

tion from the stage of pronormoblast to erythrocyte are summarized below:

Size of the cell (from 15–20 μm of pronormoblast) goes on decreasing with subsequent stages till it reaches about 7 μm.

Nucleus first condenses, then becomes pyknotic and finally disappears at the stage of reticulocyte formation.

Haemoglobin synthesis starts at the stage of intermediate normoblast and then its content increases progressively.

Cytoplasm staining. Initially, before the appearance of haemoglobin the cytoplasm is basophilic. When haemoglobin starts appearing cytoplasm becomes polychromatic, i.e. stained both by acidic and basic dyes. In the stage of late normoblast when haemoglobin synthesis is almost completed, cytoplasm is stained by acidic dye.

Mitosis is seen up to the stage of intermediate normoblast. During these stages 3–5 cell divisions occur. In this way, each pronormoblast gives rise to 8–320 late normoblasts. From the stage of late normoblast onwards the mitosis ceases and cell only matures.

REGULATION OF ERYTHROPOIESIS

Erythropoietin

Erythropoietin is a hormone which regulates the process of erythropoeisis.

Site of formation. Erythropoietin is mainly produced by the juxtaglomerular apparatus of kidney.

Stimulus for secretion. A certain basal level of the hormone is necessary for the normal rate of erythropoiesis. Whenever, there is hypoxia or decrease in the number of red blood cells (e.g. after haemorrhage or in haemolytic anaemia), there occurs a release of renal erythropoietic factor from juxtaglomerular cells of kidney. Renal erythropoietic factor acts on the plasma alpha globulin called erythropoietinogen to form the erythropoietin. Thus the levels of erythropoietin vary with degree of hypoxia or number of circulating red blood cells.

FACTORS NECESSARY FOR ERYTHROPOIESIS

Factors other than erythropoiesis necessary for erythropoiesis include:

Vitamin B₁₂ and intrinsic factor of Castle

Vitamin B_{12} (cyanocobalamin), also known as extrinsic factor is essential for maturation of red cells.

Role of vitamin B_{12}. It is required for the synthesis of DNA and maturation of nucleus and cell. Deficiency of vitamin B_{12} leads to:

- Failure of maturation of nucleus.
- Cells remain large (megaloblasts) and become more fragile.

Folic acid

Folic acid (pteroylglutamic acid) and related compounds known as folates play an important role in the synthesis of DNA.

Folate deficiency causes megaloblastic anaemia (see page 47).

III. Factors necessay for haemoglobinization

Various factors necessary for haemoglobin formation in the red blood cells are described on page 44.

HAEMOGLOBIN

The cytoplasm of erythrocytes (red blood cells) contain an *oxygen-binding protein* called haemoglobin. Erythrocyte precursors synthesize haemoglobin, while the mature erythrocytes lose the property of synthesizing haemoglobin.

NORMAL BLOOD HAEMOGLOBIN

The normal blood haemoglobin concentration ranges from 16.5 to 18.5 gm/dl.

- *At birth,* the haemoglobin concentration is 23 gm/dl.
- *In adult males* the mean blood haemoglobin (Hb) concentration is 15.5 gm/dl (range 14–18 gm/dl).

- *In adult females* the mean Hb concentration is 14 gm/dl (range 12–15.5 gm/dl).

STRUCTURE OF HAEMOGLOBIN (Fig. 2.2-6)

Haemoglobin is a globular molecule which consists of the protein *globin* combined with iron-containing pigment called *haem.*

Structure of globin

The protein globin, present in the haemoglobin, is made of four polypeptide chains. HbA consists of the following four polypeptide chains:

- *Two α chains,* each containing 141 amino acid residues, and
- *Two β chains,* each containing 146 amino acid residues.

  Therefore, the normal adult haemoglobin A is written as HbA ($\alpha_2\beta_2$).

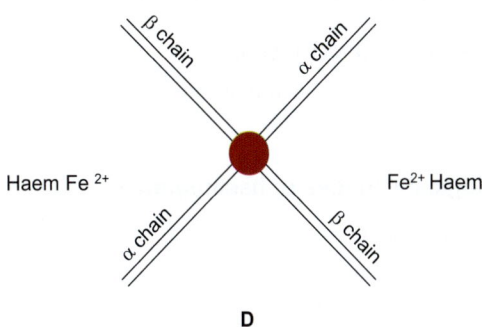

Fig. 2.2-6. *Chemistry of haemoglobin: A, structure of a pyrrole ring; B, conventional outline of a pyrrole ring; C, arrangement of pyrrole rings in one unit of haem (iron protoporphyrin X); and D, arrangement of four units of haem in one molecule of haemoglobin.*

Structure of haem

The haem is a iron-porphyrin complex called *iron-proto-porphyrin IX,* i.e., it consists of a porphyrin nucleus and the iron.

- The iron in the haem is in *ferrous* (Fe^{2+}) form.

One molecule of haemoglobin contains four units of haem, each attached to one of the four polypeptide chains constituting globin (Fig. 2.2-6D). As there are four units of haem in one molecule of haemoglobin, so there are four iron atoms in one molecule of Hb which can carry four molecules (eight atoms) of oxygen.

FUNCTIONS OF HAEMOGLOBIN

1. Transport of O_2 from lungs to tissues

- *In the lungs,* one molecule of O_2 is attached loosely and reversibly at the sixth covalent bond of each iron atom of the haemoglobin to form *oxyhaemoglobin* represented as HbO_2:

$$\begin{array}{ccccc} \text{Hb} & + & O_2 & \rightarrow & HbO_2 \\ \text{Deoxygenated} & & & & \text{Oxygenated} \\ \text{(reduced) haemoglobin} & & & & \text{haemoglobin} \end{array}$$

2. Transport of CO_2 from the tissues to the lungs

Haemoglobin also transports CO_2 from the tissues to the lungs.

- It is important to note that CO_2 from the tissues is transported by combining with amino acids of the globin part as shown below and not in combination with Fe^{2+} atom like O_2.

$$\begin{array}{ccc} \overset{\displaystyle H}{\underset{\displaystyle H}{R-N}} + CO_2 & \rightarrow & \overset{\displaystyle H}{\underset{\displaystyle COOH}{R-N}} \\ \text{Haemoglobin} & & \text{Carbamino-haemoglobin} \end{array}$$

3. Control of pH of the blood

The haemoglobin constitutes the most important acid-base buffer system of blood. Hb has six times the buffering capacity as compared to plasma proteins.

VARIETIES OF HAEMOGLOBIN

Various varieties of haemoglobin can be grouped as under:

Physiological varieties of haemoglobin

Adult haemoglobin

Adult haemoglobin is of two types.

i. Haemoglobin A [HbA ($\alpha_2\beta_2$)]. It is the main form of normal adult haemoglobin. As described on page 43, its globin part consists of two alpha and two beta polypeptide chains.

ii. Haemoglobin A$_2$ [HbA$_2$ ($\alpha_2\delta_2$)]. It is a minor component (about 2.5% of the total Hb) in normal adults. Its globin part consists of two alpha and two delta polypeptide chains.

Fetal haemoglobin

Fetal haemoglobin, or haemoglobin F [HbF $\alpha_2\gamma_2$] as the name indicates refers to the haemoglobin present in the fetal RBCs and gradually disappears 2–3 months after birth. In HbF globin part consists of two alpha and two gamma polypeptide chains (in place of beta chains of HbF). Special features of HbF are given below :

- *Affinity for oxygen* in case of HbF more than that of HbA, i.e., it can take more oxygen than HbA at low oxygen pressure.
- *Resistance to action of alkalies* is more in HbF than HbA. This property is used in a photoelectric calorimetric method to estimate HbF in the presence of HbA.

Haemoglobinopathies

Haemoglobinopathies, i.e., abnormal formation of haemoglobin occurs due to disorders of globin synthesis; haem synthesis being normal. Disorders of globin synthesis are of two main types:

- *Formation of abnormal polypeptide chains.* Example of such a disorder is haemoglobin S.
- *Suppression* of synthesis of polypeptide chain of globin as seen in thalassaemia.

SYNTHESIS OF HAEMOGLOBIN

Haemoglobin is synthesized in the cytoplasm of intermediate normoblasts.

Synthesis of haem

Haem is synthesized in the mitochondria. Succinyl-CoA (derived from the citric acid cycle in mitochondria) and glycine are the starting substances in the synthesis of haem.

Synthesis of globin

Globin, the protein part of the haemoglobin, is synthesized in ribosomes.

Factors controlling haemoglobin formation

1. Role of proteins. First class proteins provide amino acids required for synthesis of globin part of the haemoglobin. A low protein intake retards haemoglobin regeneration even in the presence of excess iron.

2. Role of iron. Iron is necessary for formation of haem part of haemoglobin. In addition to dietary iron, the iron released by degradation of RBCs is also reused for synthesis of haemoglobin.

3. Role of other metals

- *Copper.* Copper is essential for haemoglobin synthesis, as it promotes the absorption, mobilization and utilization of iron.

- *Cobalt.* In some species cobalt increases the production of erythropoietin which in turn stimulates RBC formation.
- *Calcium.* Calcium is reported to help indirectly by conserving iron and its subsequent utilization.

4. *Role of vitamins.* Vitamin B$_{12}$, folic acid, and vitamin C help in synthesis of nucleic acid which in turn is required for the development of RBCs. Vitamin C also helps in absorption of iron from the gut.

5. *Role of bile salts.* Presence of bile salts in the intestine is necessary for proper absorption of metals like copper and nickel which in turn are essential factors for synthesis of haemoglobin.

LIFE SPAN AND FATE OF RED BLOOD CELLS

LIFE SPAN OF RED BLOOD CELLS

Normally, the average life span of red blood cells is 120 days.

FATE OF RED BLOOD CELLS

The cell membrane of old RBCs (after about 120 days) becomes more fragile due to decreased NADPH acitivity. The destruction of red cells occurs mostly in the capillaries of spleen because they have very thin lumen. Because of this spleen is also called the graveyard of red blood cells. The haemoglobin released after haemolysis of red cells is taken up by the tissue macrophages.

The tissue macrophage system (reticuloendothelial system) includes the following phagocytic cells:

- *In the bone marrow* these cells form part of the lining of the blood sinuses (littoral cells);
- *In the liver* they lie at intervals along the vascular capillaries (Kupffer cells),
- *In the spleen* they are found in the pulp, and
- *In the lymph nodes* they line the lymphatic paths.

Fate of haemoglobin (Fig. 2.2-7)

- In the macrophages the haem part of the haemoglobin molecule is altered by oxidation of one of its methine (=CH) bridges. As a result of chemical changes, the globin, iron and biliverdin (tetrapyrrole straight chain free from globin and iron) are formed.
- *Globin* is degraded into amino acids and joins the amino acid pool of plasma and is released.
- *Iron* released into the circulation is:
  – carried into the bone marrow for reutilization, and
  – in the other tissues it combines with apoferritin to form the ferritin (storage form of iron).
- *Biliverdin* (tetrapyrrole straight chain free from globin and iron) is converted into bilirubin (by the enzyme biliverdin reductase) and is released into the blood.

Fig. 2.2-7. *Fate of haemoglobin.*

BILIRUBIN AND JAUNDICE

BILIRUBIN FORMATION AND ITS FATE

As discussed above the bilirubin is formed in the macrophages. It undergoes the following changes:

1. *Uptake of bilirubin.* Macrophages release the bilirubin into circulation. This bilirubin is called free or *unconjugated bilirubin.* It is lipid-soluble which prevents its excretion by the kidneys.

2. *Conjugation of bilirubin.* The unconjugated bilirubin (bound to albumin) from the circulation is taken up by the liver. In the hepatic cells it is conjugated with uridine diphosphate glucuronic acid (UDP-glucuronic acid) making it a water-soluble conjugated *bilirubin.*

3. *Excretion of bilirubin.* The conjugated bilirubin from the hepatic cells is excreted into the bile and enters the intestine. Some of it escapes into general circulation and is excreted by the kidneys in urine as *urine bilirubin.*

4. *Formation and excretion of urobilinogen.* The conjugated bilirubin which enters the intestine with the bile is degraded by the intestinal bacteria and bilirubin is converted into the *urobilinogen* (stercobilinogen) which is a colourless compound.

- Some urobilinogen (20%) from the intestine is reabsorbed and goes via the portal system to the liver. From the liver some urobilinogen escapes into general circulation and some is re-excreted into the bile (enterohepatic circulation).
- From general circulation the urobilinogen is filtered off by the kidney and is excreted in the urine.

Bilirubin

The normal serum bilirubin level ranges from 0.3 mg – 1.0 mg/100 ml.

JAUNDICE

Jaundice (icterus) refers to the yellow appearance of the skin, sclera and mucous membranes resulting from an increased bilirubin concentration (*hyperbilirubinaemia*) in the body fluids. Clinically jaundice is detectable when the plasma bilirubin exceeds 2-3 mg/100 ml.

Types

Hyperbilirubinaemia can result from following mechanisms :

i. *Excessive breakdown* of red blood cells (Haemolysis) produces *haemolytic jaundice* or *prehepatic jaundice.*
ii. *Damage to liver cells* produces hepatic or hepatocellular jaundice.
iii.*Obstruction to bile duct* produces posthepatic or obstructive jaundice.

Physiological jaundice of newborn

Physiological jaundice of newborn is also called neonatal jaundice.

Mechanism of production

A hyperbilirubinaemia-producing jaundice may be seen normally in the newborn. It appears within 2-5 days of birth and usually disappears in 2 weeks. Its mechanism of production includes:

- *Excessive destruction of RBCs* occurs in first few days after birth causing increase in serum bilirubin.
- *Hepatic immaturity* in the first few (7-10) days after birth also contributes to increased serum bilirubin.

Prevention and treatment

- *Prevention.* Neonatal jaundice can be prevented by administration of hepatic microsomal enzyme inducers (e.g. phenobarbital) to the pregnant mother or newborn. The microsomal enzyme inducers increase the activity of glucuronyl transferase in liver.
- *Treatment.* Normal jaundice can be effectively treated by *phototherapy.* Exposure of the skin to white light causes photoisomerization of bilirubin to water-soluble *lumirubin* which can be rapidly excreted in bile without requiring any conjugation.

ANAEMIAS

DEFINITION AND CLASSIFICATION

DEFINITION

Anaemia is not a single disease but a group of disorders in which haemoglobin concentration of blood is below the normal range for the age and sex of the subject. Therefore anaemia is labelled when haemoglobin concentration is less than:

- 13 gm/dl in adult males,
- 11.5 gm/dl in adult females,
- 15 gm/dl in newborn, and
- 9.5 gm/dl at 3 month of age.

Low RBC count (less than 4 million/mm^3) is usually, but not always, associated with low haemoglobin levels in anaemia.

Grading of anaemia, depending upon the level of haemoglobin, has somewhat arbitrarily been made as:

- Mild anaemia — Hb 8 to 10 gm%
- Moderate anaemia — Hb 6 to 8 gm%, and
- Severe anaemia — Hb below 6 gm%.

CLASSIFICATION

Aetiological (Whitby's) classification

Types of anaemia depending upon the causative mechanism are:

A. *Deficiency anaemias*

- Iron-deficiency anaemia
- Megaloblastic anaemia (pernicious anaemia) due to deficiency of vitamin B$_{12}$
- Megaloblastic anaemia due to deficiency of folic acid
- Protein and vitamin C deficiency can also cause anaemia.

B. *Blood loss anaemias* or haemorrhagic anaemias are commonly known and can be:

- *Acute post-haemorrhagic anaemia* as in accidents, and
- *Chronic post-haemorrhagic anaemia*

C. *Haemolytic anaemias.* These are relatively uncommon and occur in conditions associated with increased destruction of red blood cells.

D. *Aplastic anaemia.* It occurs due to failure of bone marrow to produce RBCs.

E. *Anaemia due to chronic diseases.* It is seen in tuberculosis, chronic infections, malignancies, chronic lung diseases, etc.

IRON DEFICIENCY ANAEMIA

Iron deficiency anaemia is the commonest nutritional deficiency disorder present throughout the world, but its prevalence is higher in the developing countries. In India, iron deficiency is the commonest cause of anaemia. Iron deficiency anaemia is much more common:

- In women between 20-45 years than in men.
- At periods of active growth in infancy, childhood and adolescence.

Daily requirement and dietary sources of iron

Daily requirement. Only 10% of the dietary intake of iron is absorbed. Therefore, daily requirement in adult males is 5-10 mg/day and in females is 20 mg/day (to compensate the menstural loss). Pregnant and lactating women require about 40 mg of iron per day.

Dietary sources. Foodstuffs vary both in their iron content and availability of iron for absorption into the body. The dietary sources of iron are meat, liver, egg, leafy vegetables, whole wheat and jaggery. The iron in foods of animal origin is better absorbed than iron in foods of vegetable origin.

Causes of iron deficiency anaemia

Causes of iron deficiency vary with age, sex and country of residence of patient. In general, the causes of iron deficiency anaemia can be grouped as:

1. *Inadequate dietary intake of iron* as in:
- Milk-fed infants
- Poor economic status individuals,
- Anorexia, e.g. in pregnancy
- Elderly individuals due to atrophy and poor dentition.

2. *Increased loss of iron* (as blood loss) from the body, e.g.
- Uterine bleeding in females in the form of excessive menstruation, repeated miscarriages, postmenopausal bleeding, etc.
- Gastrointestinal bleeding due to peptic ulcer, haemorrhoids, ulcerative colitis, etc.
- Renal tract bleeding, e.g. haematuria
- Nasal bleeding, i.e. repeated epistaxis.
- Bleeding from lungs as haemoptysis.

3. *Increased demand of iron* as in:
- Infancy, childhood and adolescence,
- Menstruating females, and
- Pregnant females.

4. *Decreased absorption* of iron, as seen in:
- Partial or total gastrectomy,
- Achlorhydria, and
- Intestinal malabsorption diseases.

MEGALOBLASTIC ANAEMIA

Megaloblastic anaemias are characterized by abnormally large cells of erythrocyte series. These are caused by defective DNA synthesis due to deficiency of vitamin B_{12} and/or folic acid (folate).

GENERAL CLINICAL FEATURES OF ANAEMIA

General clinical manifestations of anaemia which occur either due to tissue hypoxia or due to compensatory mechanisms are:

- Generalized muscular weakness
- Pallorness of skin and mucous membranes
- Breathlessness
- Palpitation
- Visual disturbances
- Anorexia, atrophy of papillae on tongue.
- In females, menstrual disturbances occur such as amenorrhoea and menorrhagia.

White Blood Cells and Immune System

WHITE BLOOD CELLS

Types of white blood cells (WBCs) and their counts
- Types of WBCs
- Normal WBC counts
  - Total leucocyte count
  - Differential leucocyte count
- Variations in WBC count
  - Leucocytosis
  - Leucopenia

Formation of WBCs
- Formation of granulocytes and monocytes
  - Myeloid series
  - Monocyte-macrophage series
- Formation of lymphocytes
  - Lymphoid series
- Regulation of leucopoiesis

Morphology, life span, functions and variations in counts of WBCs
- Neutrophils
- Eosinophils
- Basophils
- Lymphocytes
- Monocytes

Applied aspects
- Leukaemias

IMMUNE SYSTEM

Architecture of immune system
- Mononuclear–phagocytic system
- Lymphoid organs
  - Central lymphoid organs
  - Peripheral lymphoid organs

Immunity
- Innate
- Acquired
  - Active
  - Passive

Antigens
- Definition
- Some facts about antigenicity
- Histocompatibility antigens

Antibodies
- Structure of antibody
- Types of immunoglobulins

Development of immune response
- Humoral immune response
- Cellular immune response
- Cytokines

Other immune mechanism related aspects
- Immune tolerance
- Autoimmunity
- Hypersensitivity
- Immunodeficiency diseases

WHITE BLOOD CELLS

TYPES OF WHITE BLOOD CELLS AND THEIR COUNTS

TYPES OF WHITE BLOOD CELLS

The white blood cells (WBCs) or leucocytes are so named since they are colourless in contrast to red colour of RBCs.

These are nucleated cells and play important role in defence mechanism of the body. The leucocytes of the peripheral blood are of two main varieties: granulocytes and non-granulocytes.

Granulocytes

The white blood cells with granules in their cytoplasm are called granulocytes. Depending upon the colour of granules, granulocytes are further divided into three types:

- Neutrophils
- Eosinophils
- Basophils

Agranulocytes

White blood cells which do not contain granules in their cytoplasm are called agranulocytes. These are of two types:

- Lymphocytes, and
- Monocytes.

NORMAL WBC COUNTS

Total leucocyte count

Total leucocyte count (TLC) varies with age as:

Adults : 4000-11000/mm³ of blood.

At birth, in full-term infant : 10000–25000/mm³ of blood.

Infants upto 1 year of age : 6000 – 16000/mm³ of blood.

Differential and absolute leucocyte count

Differential leucocyte count (DLC) and absolute count in normal adults is shown in Table 2.3-1.

Table 2.3-1. Differential leucocyte count and absolute count in normal adults

WBCs	Differential count (%)	Absolute count (per mm³)
Granulocytes		
• Neutrophils	40–75	2000–7500
• Eosinophils	1–6	40–440
• Basophils	0–1	0–100
Agranulocytes		
• Lymphocytes	20–40	1500–4000
• Monocytes	2–10	500–800

Clinical significance of differential and absolute counts

The differential leucocyte count (DLC) tells us if there is an increase or decrease in a particular type of leucocyte, because in different diseases one or the other type of cells show an increase or decrease in its numbers. The differential count is done in 100 or 200 cells and tells only a relative increase or decrease in particular variety of cells. DLC alone is not of much importance and so never done as an isolated test, but always it is part of full blood counts including TLC and then calculating absolute count.

VARIATIONS IN WBC COUNT

Leucocytosis

Leucocytosis refers to increase in total WBC count above 11000/mm³.

Physiological causes of leucocytosis

1. *Age.* In newborn babies upto the age of one year WBC count is higher. At birth WBC count is about 18,000/mm³ which drops gradually to adult level.

2. *Exercise.* The WBC count is increased after exercise.

3. *After food intake* the WBC count is raised.

4. *Mental stress* and emotional conditions like anxiety are associated with raised WBC count.

5. *Pregnancy.* At full-term pregnancy WBC count is 12000-15000 mm³.

6. *Exposure to low temperature* also causes leucocytosis.

Pathological causes of leucocytosis :

- Acute bacterial infections especially by pyogenic organisms,
- Acute haemorrhage,
- Burns,
- Postoperative period, and
- Tuberculosis.

Leucopenia

Leucopenia refers to decrease in the total WBC count below 4000/mm³.

Causes of leucopenia :

1. Infections by non-pyogenic bacteria especially typhoid fever and paratyphoid fever.
2. Viral infections such as influenza, smallpox, mumps, etc.
3. Protozoal infections.
4. Starvation and malnutrition.
5. Aplasia of bone marrow.
6. Bone marrow depression due to:
   - Drugs such as chloromycetin and cytotoxic drugs used in malignant diseases.
   - Repeated exposure to X-rays or radiations.
   - Chemical poisons like arsenic, dinitrophenol, and antimony.

FORMATION OF WHITE BLOOD CELLS

The process of development and maturation of white blood cells (leucocytes) called *leucopoiesis* is a part of haemopoiesis (formation of blood cells). All the blood cells develop from the so-called pluripotent *haemopoietic stem cells (PHSCs)*. The stem cells after a series of divisions differentiate into *progenitor cells* which are also called colony-forming units (CFU) (for details see page 41).

The leucopoiesis can be discussed under two headings:

- Formation of granulocytes (granulopoiesis) and monocytes, and
- Formation of lymphocytes (lymphopoiesis).

FORMATION OF GRANULOCYTES AND MONOCYTES

The granulocytes and monocytes are formed in the bone marrow from the colony-forming unit called CFU-GM (colony-forming unit granulocytes and monocytes): The progenitor cells (CFU-GM) forming different cells are further named as:

- CFU-G are neutrophil forming units,
- CFU-EO refers to eosinophil forming units,
- CFU-Ba are basophil forming units, and
- CFU-M refers to monocyte forming units.

The development of granulocytes through various stages is called *myeloid series* and development of monocytes through various stages is called *monocyte-macrophage series*.

Myeloid series

Some facts about granulopoiesis.

- The cells of myeloid series include myeloblast (most primitive precursor), promyelocytes, myelocytes, meta-myelocytes, band forms and segmented granulocyte (mature form).
- The process of granulopoiesis takes about 12 days.
- Granulocytes are formed and stored in the bone marrow. When need arises they are released in circulation. Normally about three times or many granulocytes are stored in the bone marrow as these circulate in the peripheral blood.

Monocyte-Macrophage series (Fig. 2.3-1)

Monocyte macrophage series include monoblast, promonocytes and monocyte.

From the bone marrow, the monocytes migrate into spleen and lymphoid tissues in considerable numbers. The transformed stages of these cells in various tissues are called *tissue macrophages* and form a part of *tissue-macrophage system,* which was previously known as *reticuloendothelial system.*

FORMATION OF LYMPHOCYTES

The lymphocytes are formed from the *lymphocyte stem cells* which are formed from the pluripotent haemopoietic stem cells (PHSC) in the bone marrow (Fig. 2.3-2). The lymphocyte stem cells migrate into thymus and peripheral lymphoid tissues where they proliferate and mature into lymphocytes. The tissues which actively produce lympho-cytes from the germinal centres of lymphoid follicles as a response to antigenic stimulation constitute the so-called *secondary* or *reactive lymphoid tissue.* It is comprised by the:

- Lymph nodes,
- Spleen, and
- Gut-associated lymphoid tissue (GALT).

Lymphoid series

The maturation stages of lymphoid series are lymphoblast, prolymphocytes and lymphocyte. (Fig. 2.3-2)

Prolymphocytes mature successively into large lym-phocyte and small lymphocyte, both of which are found in circulation.

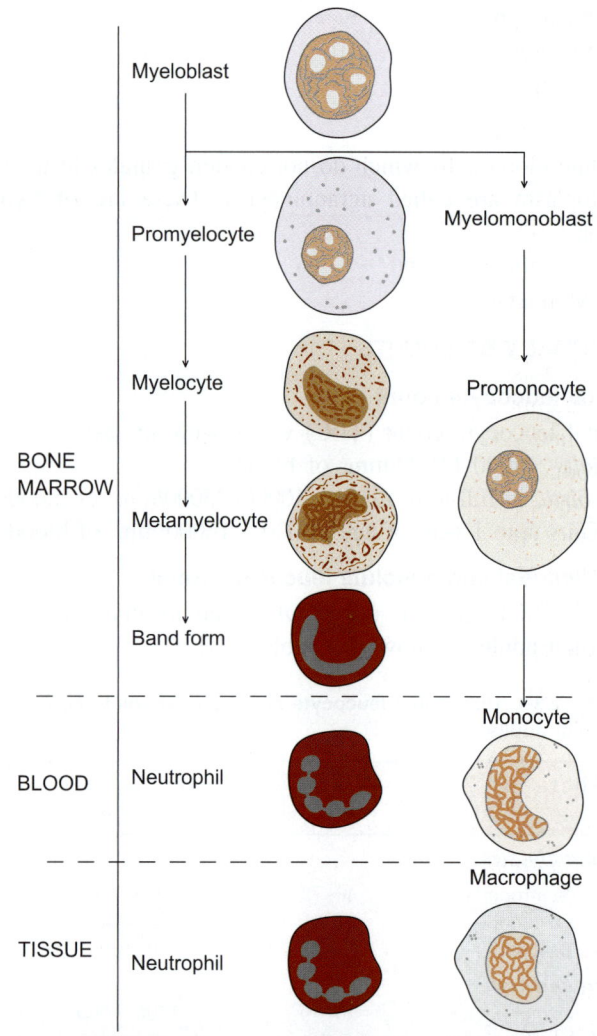

Fig. 2.3-1. *Granulopoiesis and features of the cells of myeloid series and monocyte-macrophage series.*

Fig. 2.3-2. *Formation of lymphoid series cells.*

- Then some lymphocytes enter thymus where they are processed and come out as T lymphocytes.
- Some lymphocytes are processed in liver (in fetal life) and bone marrow (after birth). These come out as B *lymphocytes.* The word B comes from 'bursa of Fabricius which is the site of B cell processing in birds. Morphological features of large and small lymphocytes are described on page 52.

REGULATION OF LEUCOPOIESIS

The constancy of leucocyte count suggests a feedback mechanism to control their production and release. During tissue injury and inflammation, bacterial toxins, products of injury, etc. cause a great increase in the rate of production and release of leucocytes. Thus, unlike erythropoiesis, the products of dead and dying white cells themselves control leucopoiesis. The substances which stimulate or inhibit the process of leucopoiesis are complex and include the following:

Role of cytokines

The cytokines which control the formation of different types of granulocytes are called *colony stimulating factors (CSFs).* The CSFs are glycoproteins formed by monocytes and T-lymphocytes.

Role of prostaglandins

Prostaglandins formed by monocytes, and possibly some other agents also play role in control of leucopoiesis.

MORPHOLOGY, FUNCTIONS AND VARIATIONS IN COUNTS OF WBCs

Morphological features of various types of WBCs as studied under microscope with Leishman's staining and haematoxylineosin stain (Fig. 2.3-3) are summarized below along with their functions and variations in their counts.

NEUTROPHILS

Morphological features

The polymorphonuclear neutrophils commonly called polymorphs or neutrophils have following morphological features (Fig. 2.3-3A):

Diameter. Diameter of a neutrophil varies from 10-14 µm.

Nucleus. Nucleus of a mature neutrophil is purple in colour and multilobed (2-6 lobes).

Cytoplasm. Cytoplasm of neutrophil is pale bluish in colour and full of fine (pinpoint) granules.

- Granules take both acidic and basic stain and look violet-pink in colour.

Functions

The neutrophils along with monocytes constitute the first line of defence against the microorganisms, viruses and

Fig. 2.3-3. *Morphological features of white blood cells : A, Neutrophil; B, Eosinophil; C, Basophil; D, Small lymphocyte; E, Large lymphocyte; and F, Monocyte.*

other injurious agents that enter the body. Neutrophils subserve this role by following mechanisms:

1. *Phagocytosis.* The neutrophils engulf the foreign particles or bacteria and digest them and ultimately may kill them by a process called phagocytosis.

2. *Reaction of inflammation.* The neutrophils also release leucotrienes, prostaglandins, thromboxanes, etc. that bring about the reactions of inflammation like vasodilatation and oedema.

3. *Febrile response.* The neutrophils contain a fever-producing substance called *endogenous pyrogen* which is an important mediator of febrile response to the bacterial pyrogens.

Variations in counts

Neutrophilia refers to increase in the circulating neutrophil counts (absolute count > 10000/mm³). It is the commonest cause of leucocytosis.

Physiological causes of neutrophilia are :

- Newborn babies
- After exercise
- After meals
- Pregnancy, menstruation, parturition and lactation

- Mental stress and emotional stress
- After injection of epinephrine.

Pathological causes of neutrophilia are:

- Acute pyogenic bacterial infections
- Non-infective inflammatory conditions like gout, acute rheumatic fever

Neutropenia. Decrease in neutrophil count is known as neutropenia (absolute count < 2500/mm³).

Common causes :

- Typhoid and paratyphoid fever, and
- Malaria

EOSINOPHILS

Morphological features

Morphological features of eosinophils (Fig. 2.3-3B) are:

Diameter of eosinophils is similar to neutrophils, i.e. 10-14 μm.

Nucleus is purple in colour and is bilobed *spectacle-shaped.*

Cytoplasm is acidophilic and appears bright pink in colour.

- It contains coarse, deep red staining granules which do not cover the nucleus.
- The granules contain histamine, lysosomal enzymes and eosinophil chemotactic factor of anaphylaxis (ECF-A).

Functions of eosinophils

1. Mild phagocytosis. Eosinophils are not very motile and thus have very mild phagocytic activity.

2. Role in parasitic infestations. They play important role in the defence mechanism of body especially in *parasitic infestations.*

3. Role in allergic reaction. The eosinophils increase in number in allergic conditions like bronchial asthma and hay fever.

4. Role in immunity. The eosinophils are present in abundance in the mucosa of respiratory tract, gastro-intestinal tract and urinary tract, where they probably provide mucosal immunity.

Variation in counts

Eosinophilia refers to increase in the eosinophil count (absolute count > 500/mm³).

Causes of eosinophilia are:

- Bronchial asthma, and hay fever.
- Parasitic infestation, e.g. intestinal worms like hookworm, roundworm and tapeworm.
- Skin diseases like urticaria.

Eosinopenia is the decrease in eosinophil count (absolute count < 50/mm³). It occurs in stressful conditions.

BASOPHILS

Morphological features (Fig. 2.3-3C)

Diameter of a basophil is similar to neutrophil and eosinophil, i.e. 10-14 μm.

Nucleus of basophil is irregular, may be bilobed or trilobed, and its boundary is not clearly defined because of overcrowding with coarse granules.

Cytoplasm of basophils is slightly basophilic and appears blue. It is full of granules.

- Granules of basophils are very coarse and stain deep purple or blue with basic (methylene) dye.
- They contain heparin, histamine and 5-HT.

Functions

1. Mild phagocytosis. Basophils have very mild phago-cytic function.

2. Role in allergic reaction. Basophils release histamine, bradykinin, slow reacting substances of anaphylaxis (SRS-A) and serotonin (5HT). These substances, in turn, cause many allergic manifestations.

3. Role in preventing spread of allergic inflammatory process. Basophils also release eosinophil chemotactic factor that causes eosinophils to migrate toward the inflamed allergic tissue. Eosinophils then phagocytose and destroy antigen-antibody complexes and prevent spread of local inflammatory process.

4. Release of heparin. Basophils release heparin in the blood which prevents clotting of the blood.

Variation in counts

Basophilia refers to increase in the basophil count (absolute count > 100/mm³)

Causes of basophilia are:

- Viral infections, e.g. influenza, smallpox and chicken-pox,
- Allergic diseases, and
- Chronic myeloid leukaemia.

Basopenia. Decrease in basophil count is called basopenia.

LYMPHOCYTES

Morphological features

There are two types of lymphocytes large and small having almost similar structure. Morphological features of lymphocytes are:

Diameter. Diameter of large lymphocytes varies from 12-16 μm and that of small lymphocytes from 7-10 μm. (Fig. 2.3-3D and E).

Nucleus. Lymphocytes have a large round, single nucleus which almost completely fills the cell. It stains blue very deeply giving *ink-spot appearance.* Nuclear chromatin is coarsely clumped and shapeless.

Cytoplasm. The cytoplasm is scanty, i.e. its amount is always less than that of nucleus. It is seen as crescent of clear light blue colour around the nucleus. Cytoplasm does not contain visible granules.

Functional subtypes

Based on their developmental background, lifespan and functions, the small lymphocytes have been broadly classified into 3 subtypes (Fig. 3.3-6):

1. *B lymphocytes* which are processed in the bone marrow are concerned with the humoral immunity.

2. *T lymphocytes* which are processed in the thymus are concerned with cellular immunity.

3. *Natural killer (NK) cells* are lymphocyte-like cells that nonspecifically kill any cell that is coated with immunoglobulin IgG. This phenomenon is called *antigen-dependent cell-mediated cytotoxicity (ADCC)*. Thus NK cells provide *innate immunity*.

Functions

Lymphocytes play important role in immunity. B lymphocytes are responsible for the development of *humoral immunity* also called antibody-mediated immunity (AMI) (see page 57).

   T lymphocytes are responsible for the development of *cellular immunity,* also called cell-mediated immunity (CMI) or T cell immunity (see page 59).

Variations in count

Lymphocytosis refers to increase in the lymphocyte count (absolute count > 4000/mm^3).

   In healthy infants and young children the lymphocyte count is usually high (about 60% in DLC) while the TLC is normal (relative lymphocytosis).

Pathological causes of lymphocytosis are:

- Chronic infections like tuberculosis, hepatitis and whooping cough.
- Viral infections like chickenpox, and
- Lymphatic leukaemia (most common cause of lymphocytes > 10,000/mm^3).

Lymphopenia or lymphocytopenia refers to decrease in lymphocyte count (absolute count below 1500/mm^3).

Causes of lymphopenia are:

- Patients on corticosteroid and immunosuppressive therapy,
- Hypoplastic bone marrow, and
- Acquired immunodeficiency syndrome (AIDS).

MONOCYTES

Morphological features (Fig. 2.3-3F)

Diameter. The monocyte is the largest mature leucocyte in the peripheral blood measuring some 12-20 µm in diameter.

Nucleus. The nucleus of monocyte is large, single and eccentric in position, i.e. present on one side of the cell.

It may be notched, or indented, i.e. horseshoe- or kidney-shaped.

Cytoplasm. The cytoplasm is abundant, pale-blue and usually clear (no granules). Sometimes, it may contain fine purple, dust-like granules called *azur granules.*

Functions

1. *Role in defence mechanism.* Monocytes along with neutrophils play important role in the body's defence mechanism. Their main function is *phagocytosis.* Monocytes after entering in the tissue get converted to macrophages. They also have ability to engulf large particles such as red blood cells and malarial parasites.

2. *Role in tumour immunity.* Monocytes may also kill tumour cells after sensitization by lymphocytes.

3. *Synthesis of biological substances.* Monocytes synthesize complement and other biologically important substances.

Variations in count

Monocytosis. A rise in the blood monocytes above 800/mm^3 is termed monocytosis.

Causes of monocytosis are:

1. Certain bacterial infections such as tuberculosis, syphilis and subacute bacterial endocarditis.

2. Infectious mononucleosis or the so-called glandular fever.

3. Viral infections

4. Protozoal and rickettsial infections, e.g. malaria and kala-azar.

Monocytopenia refers to decrease in the monocyte count. It may be seen in hypo-plastic bone marrow.

APPLIED ASPECT: LEUKAEMIAS

Leukaemias constitute a group of malignant diseases of the blood in which there occurs an increase in the total WBC count associated with presence of immature WBCs in the peripheral blood. The total WBC count is usually above 50000/mm^3 and may be as high as 100,000 to 300,000/mm^3.

- The proliferation of leukaemic cells takes place primarily in the bone marrow and in certain form in the lymphoid tissues.

Types of leukaemias

Leukaemias account for 4% of all cancer deaths. Leukaemias are classified on the basis of cell types predominantly into *myeloid* (involving cells derived from the myeloid stem cells) and *lymphoid* (involving the cells derived from lymphoid stem cells) The main types of leukaemias are:

1. Acute myeloblastic leukaemia (AML),

2. Acute lymphoblastic leukaemia (ALL),

3. Chronic myeloid leukaemia (CML),

4. Chronic lymphoid leukaemia (CLL).

IMMUNE SYSTEM

The immune system which constitutes the body's defence system consists of lymphoid organs, reticulo-endothelial components and the various types of immunological cells distributed throughout the body.

Immune response. The immune system of the body responds to an antigen by two ways:

- *Humoral* or antibody-mediated immunity (AMI) which is mediated by antibodies produced by plasma cells; and
- *Cell-mediated immunity* (CMI) which is mediated directly by the sensitized lymphocytes.

ARCHITECTURE OF IMMUNE SYSTEM

The immune system consists of immunological cells distributed in two main components:

1. Mononuclear-phagocytic system, and

2. Lymphoid component.

MONONUCLEAR-PHAGOCYTIC SYSTEM

Mononuclear-phagocytic system (MPS) also known as *tissue-macrophage system* is the new name given to the system previously called as *reticuloendothelial system (RES).*

Constituent cells of mononuclear-phagocytic system

The mononuclear-phagocytic system include the following constituents:

- Precursor cells of the monocyte series,
- Promonocytes, and
- Monocytes from the bone marrow and blood.

Functions of mononuclear-phagocytic system

The mononuclear-phagocytic system (MPS) plays following roles in the body :

- Role in inflammation and healing.
- Role in defence against the bacteria invading the body tissues.
- Role in the immune response.
- Role in removal of old RBCs, WBCs and platelets.

LYMPHOID ORGANS

The lymphoid component of the immune system consists of a network of lymphoid organs, tissues and cells and the product of these cells. Lymphoid organs can be classified into:

A. *Central or primary lymphoid organs*, which include

I. Thymus, and

II. Bursa equivalent (fetal liver and bone marrow); and

B. *Peripheral lymphoid organs* which include:

I. Lymph nodes,

II. Spleen, and

III. Mucosa associated lymphoid tissues (MALT).

A. PRIMARY (CENTRAL) LYMPHOID TISSUES

I. Thymus

The thymus gland is located in mediastinum just above the heart. It consists of many lobules. Histologically each lobule consists of outer *cortex* and inner *medulla.* Both cortex and medulla contain *epithelial cells* and *thymocytes.* The main function of the thymus is development of cell-mediated immunity.

II. Bursa equivalent

In the human being the fetal liver and bone marrow appear to be the equivalent of avian bursa of Fabricius. *Bursa of Fabricius* in birds is also a site of lymphocytic proliferation and differentiation. Immunocompetent lymphocytes produced in the bursa are called bursa lymphocytes or B lymphocytes or B cells. The mature B cells migrate from the bursa into outer or superficial cortex of the germinal follicles and medullary cords of lymph nodes and lymphoid follicles of spleen. These sites are known as *bursa-dependent* or *thymus-independent* areas.

B. PERIPHERAL LYMPHOID ORGANS

I. Lymph nodes

The lymph nodes are small bean-shaped or oval structures which form part of lymphatic network distributed throughout the body.

Structural characteristics of lymph node (Fig. 2.3-4)

- *Capsule* of connective tissue covers each lymph node. From the capsule trabeculae penetrate into the lymph node.
- *Afferent lymphatics* enter into each lymph node at its convex surface and drain into the peripheral subcapsular sinus.
- *Efferent lymphatics* leave the lymph node at the concavity (hilum) as a single large lymph vessel.

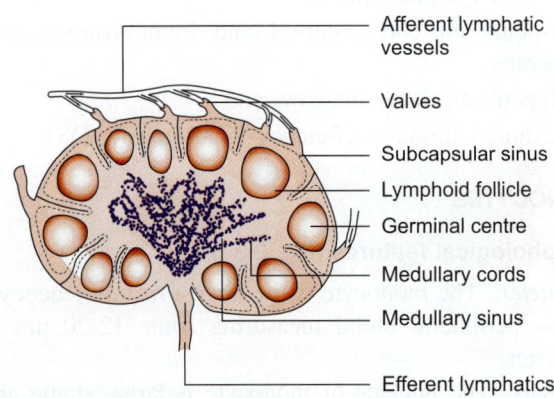

Afferent lymphatic vessels

Valves

Subcapsular sinus

Lymphoid follicle

Germinal centre

Medullary cords

Medullary sinus

Efferent lymphatics

Fig. 2.3-4. Structure of a lymph node.

- *Microscopically,* the lymph node consists of two parts – peripheral cortex and central medulla.
- *Cortex* of the lymph node consists of several rounded aggregates of lymphocytes called *lymphoid follicles,* representing B cell area of the node.
- *Paracortex* is deeper part of cortex, i.e. the zone between the peripheral cortex and the inner medulla and represents the *T-cell area* (the *bursa-independent area).*
- *Medulla* is predominantly composed of cords of plasma cells and some lymphocytes *(medullary cords).*

Functions of lymph nodes

1. *To mount immune response in the body.* Processing of antigens and antibody production occurs in the lymphoid follicles.

2. *The lymph nodes act as inline filters*. Lymph must pass through at least one lymph node before mixing with the blood stream. Over 99% of the lymph passes through the lymph sinuses and only 1% penetrates the lymphoid follicles.

II. Spleen

The spleen is the largest lymphoid organ of the body. The average weight of the spleen is about 150 gm.

Structural characteristics (Fig. 2.3-5)

Capsule of connective tissue surrounds the spleen. From the capsule connective tissue *trabeculae* extend into the pulp of the organ and serve as supportive network. The spleen consists of homogeneous, soft, dark red mass called *red pulp.* In the red pulp are seen scattered white nodules called *white pulp* (malpighian bodies).

Microscopically, the structural characteristics are:
- *Red pulp* consists of the thin-walled *blood sinuses* with *splenic cords* between them.
- *White pulp* consists of lymphocytes surrounding an eccentrically placed central artery.

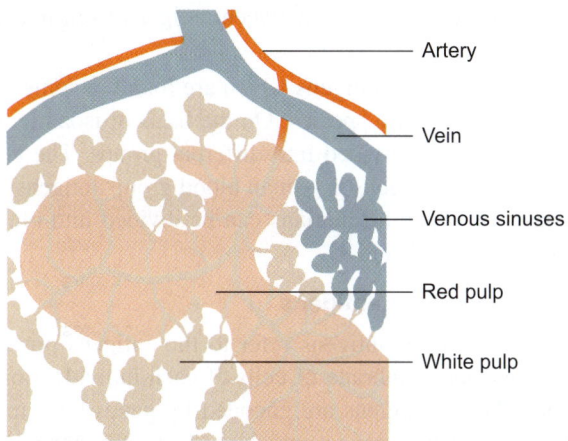

Artery

Vein

Venous sinuses

Red pulp

White pulp

Fig. 2.3-5. *Structure of spleen.*

Functions of spleen

1. *Role in immune response.* The spleen is an active site for production of T and B lymphocytes and antibodies.

2. *Role in removal of old RBCs, WBCs and platelets.* Tissue macrophages present in the spleen play important role in removal of old RBCs, WBCs and platelets.

3. *Role in haematopoiesis.* During 4th and 5th month of fetal life erythropoiesis occurs in spleen.

4. *Role in iron metabolism.* Spleen macrophages recycle the iron liberated from the phagocytozed RBCs, for synthesis of fresh haemoglobin in the bone marrow.

5. *Role as a reservoir.* Spleen serves as a reservoir for mobilization of RBCs in some animals like cat and dog. In human being spleen serves as reservoir for *platelets.*

III. Mucosa associated lymphoid tissue

Mucosa associated lymphoid tissue (MALT) include : Tonsils, adenoids and Peyer's patches of small intestine also known as gut associated lymphoid tissue (GALT). GALT plays a primary role in defence against infectious organisms entering via the gastrointestinal tract (GIT).

IMMUNITY

Immunity refers to resistance of the body to pathogens and their toxic products. It can be classified as:

I. *Innate immunity*
   1. Non-specific
   2. Specific innate immunity

II. *Acquired immunity*
   1. Active acquired immunity
   2. Passive acquired immunity

INNATE IMMUNITY

- *Innate or natural immunity* is the inborn capacity of the body to offer resistance to pathogens and their toxic products. It is due to genetic and constitutional make up of an individual.
- It may be *specific* (against a particular organism) or *non-specific.*

Mechanisms of innate immunity

1. *Mechanical barrier* The intact skin and mucosa in the body act as barrier against invading microorganism.

2. *Surface secretions* constitute one of the important mechanisms of innate immunity. These include:
- *Secretions* from the sebacious glands of skin kill many bacteria and fungi.
- *Saliva,*
- *Gastric juice*
- *Tears*

3. *Humoral defence mechanisms* provide innate immunity by the non-specific microbicidal substances present in the body fluids, e.g. *lysozyme, basic polypeptides, complements and interferons* (antiviral substances).

4. Cellular mechanisms of defence which provide non-specific innate immunity are:

- *Phagocytes,* i.e. neutrophils and the monocyte-macrophage system cells constitute the most important non-specific cellular defence against the invading microorganisms.
- *Natural killer (NK) cells* refer to a subpopulation of lymphocytes which provide non-specific cellular defence against viruses, tumour cells and other infected cells.
- *Eosinophil* granules contain enzymes and toxic molecules that act against larvae of helminths.

ACQUIRED IMMUNITY

The resistance that an individual acquires during his lifetime is known as acquired immunity. It is antigen-specific and may be antibody-mediated or cell-mediated. It is of two types: active and passive.

1. Active immunity

Active immunity is acquired by the synthesis of antibodies (humoral immunity) and production of immunocompetent cells (cell-mediated immunity) by the individual's own immune system in response to antigenic stimulation. Active immunity can be induced naturally or artificially.

i. Natural active immunity. Natural active immunity results either from a subclinical or clinical infection. For example, natural active immunity to poliomyelitis.

ii. Artificial active immunity. Artificially the active immunity is induced by introducing antigens in the body in the form of vaccines and this process is called *active immunisation.* The vaccines are preparations of live or killed microorganisms or their products. Examples of vaccines are:

- Bacterial vaccines
  - Live: BCG vaccine for tuberculosis
  - Killed: TAB vaccine for typhoid
- Bacterial product vaccines
  - Tetanus toxoid
  - Diphtheria toxoid
- Viral vaccines
  - Live: Sabin vaccine for poliomyelitis, MMR vaccine for measles, mumps and rubella, and
  - Killed: Salk vaccine for poliomyelitis, neural and non-neural vaccines for rabies.

2. Passive Immunity

Passive immunity refers to the immunity that is transferred to a recipient in a ready-made form. Here the individual's immune system does not play active role.

Natural and artificial passive immunity

i. Natural passive immunity is transfer of ready-made antibodies from the mother as:

- *In fetus* the IgG antibodies are transferred from the mother through the placenta.
- *After birth,* immunoglobulins are passed to the newborn through the breast milk. Human colostrum is rich in IgA antibodies which are resistant to digestion in stomach and small intestine.

Immunization of pregnant women with tetanus toxoid is recommended in countries where neonatal tetanus is common.

ii. Artificial passive immunity. Artificially, passive immunity can be transferred to the recipients by injecting ready-made antibodies. This is done by administration of hyperimmune sera.

Examples of artificial passive immunity include injection of:

- Anti-tetanus serum (ATS),
- Anti-diphtheric serum (ADS), and
- Anti-gas gangrene serum (AGS).

The passively administered antibodies are removed by metabolism. Therefore, immunity conferred is short-lived.

ANTIGENS

Definition

Antigen. Antigens are substances that can stimulate an immune response in the body. Most antigens are proteins, but some are carbohydrates, lipids and nucleic acids. The specificity of an antigen is due to specific areas of its molecule called *determinant sites* or *epitopes.*

Some facts about antigenicity

Immunogenicity, i.e. ability of a antigen to stimulate an immune response.

Antigen specificity is determined by chemical grouping and acid radicals.

Species specificity. Tissues of all individuals in a species contain species-specific antigens. However, some degree of cross-reactivity is seen between antigens from related species.

Isoantigens are the antigens which are found in some but not all members of a species. On the basis of isoantigens a species may be divided into different groups. The best example of isoantigens is human blood group antigens on the basis of which all humans can be divided into blood groups A, B, AB and O.

Histocompatibility antigens

Histocompatibility antigens refer to the antigens present on the plasma membrane of cells of each individual of a species. These antigens are encoded by genes known as histocompatibility genes which collectively constitute major histocompatibility complex (MHC). These are present on the surface of leucocytes known as human leucocyte associated antigens (HLA). No two persons except identical twins have the same MHC proteins. There are two subclasses of MHC genes :

MHC class I molecules are found on the surface of virtually all the cells of the body excluding red blood cells.

MHC class II. In man, MHC class II antigens are only found on immunologically reactive cells such as B lymphocytes, macrophages, monocytes and activated T lymphocytes.

ANTIBODIES

Antibodies or immunoglobulins (Igs) are gamma globulins which are produced in response to antigenic stimulation. These react specifically with the antigens which stimulated their production. All antibodies are immunoglobulins but all immunoglobulins are not antibodies. Immunoglobulins (Igs) have been divided into five distinct classes or isotypes namely IgG, IgA, IgM, IgD and IgE.

Structure of antibody

IgG has been studied extensively and serves as a model of basic structural unit of all Igs. An immunoglobulin is a Y-shaped molecule made of four polypeptide chains: 2 heavy (H) and 2 light (L). These are held together by disulphide bonds (Fig. 2.3-6).

Fig. 2.3-6. *Basic structure of an antibody showing the arrangement of heavy and light chains and its variable and constant domains.*

Functions. The specific functions of various immunoglobulins appear as:

- *IgG* protects the body fluids,
- *IgA* protects the body surfaces,
- *IgM* protects the blood stream,
- *IgE* mediates type I hypersensitivity, and
- *IgD's* role is not clearly known.

DEVELOPMENT OF IMMUNE RESPONSE

Development of immune response implies *development of acquired active immunity* in the body. The immune system of the body responds to an antigen by two ways:

1. Humoral or antibody-mediated immunity (AMI), and

2. Cell-mediated immunity (CMI).

DEVELOPMENT OF HUMORAL IMMUNITY

The humoral immunity is mediated by antibodies and so is also called antibody-mediated immunity (AMI). The antibodies are produced by plasma cells which in turn are produced by B lymphocytes.

Role of humoral immunity

1. The humoral immunity provides defence against most extracellular bacterial pathogens and viruses that infect through the respiratory and intestinal tract.

2. It participates in immediate hypersensitivity reactions of type I, II and III

3. Humoral immunity is also associated with certain autoimmune diseases.

Types of humoral immune responses

The antibody response to stimulation by antigen is of two types (Fig. 2.3-7):

- Primary humoral response, and
- Secondary humoral response.

Fig. 2.3-7. *Response of body immune system to an antigen.*

1. *Primary response* refers to the response of the body's immune system to an antigen which is introduced into the body for the first time. Always there is a latent period varying from 4 days to 4 weeks before the primary response in the form of a rise in the serum antibodies titre can be detected.

2. *Secondary response* refers to the response of the body's immune system to an antigen which is introduced into the body on a second occasion. Such a response occurs more

quickly and more abundantly. This is because of the fact that the immune system is liable to retain the memory of a prior antigenic exposure for long periods (immunological memory) and produce enhanced response when encountered with the same antigen for the second time.

Stages of humoral immune response (Fig. 2.3-8)

1. Antigen processing and presentation

Once the antigen enters the body, it is phagocytosed by the macrophages (non-specific response), broken down into polypeptide fragments. The fragments of the processed antigen are then presented to immunocompetent lymphocytes by the macrophages. So, the macrophages are also called *antigen presenting cells.*

2. Recognition of antigen by lymphocytes

Processed antigen then bind to specific receptors that present on the surface of lymphocytes is called *recogni-*

tion of antigen by lymphocytes. Thus many million different T and B lymphocytes, each with the ability to respond to particular antigen, are present in the body.

3. Lymphocyte activation

The lymphocytes that have combined with antigen are activated, i.e. the lymphocytes become larger and look like a lymphoblast. This is known as *blast transformation.* Activated B lymphocytes and helper T cells (CD$_4$ cells) play major role in humoral immunity. The B lymphocytes proliferate and transform into:

- Plasma cells, and
- Memory B cells.

Role of plasma cells. The plasma cells secrete antibodies.

Role of memory B cells. Memory B cells have a long lifespan and remain inactive. When the body is exposed to the same antigen for the second time, they are able to

Fig. 2.3-8. *Broad outline of development of humoral immune response: 1, antigen processing and presentation to immunocompetent cell; 2, recognition of antigen by the lymphocytes; and 3, activation of lymphocytes (blast transformation).*

recognize it, become active, i.e. they are responsible for secondary response of antibodies.

4. Production of antibodies

The plasma cells so formed secrete antibodies which are also called immunoglobulins (Igs). Each plasma cell produces about 2000 molecules of antibodies per second. A plasma cell secretes an antibody of a single specificity.

5. Inactivation of antigen or attack phase or effector phase of immune response

Antibodies act on the invading antigen in two ways:

i. Direct attack on the invading agents

Antibodies can inactivate the invading agent by following reactions:

Agglutination. By this reaction, large number of particles (bacteria or red cells) with antigens on their surface are bound together to form a clump. Clumping increases the susceptibility to phagocytosis.

Precipitation. In this reaction antigen-antibody complex forms insoluble precipitate.

Neutralization. Antibodies cover the toxic sites of antigen and neutralize them.

Cytolysis. Antibodies attack the membranes of cellular agents thereby causing rupture of cells.

ii. Attack on the antigen through complement system

The complement system includes 11 enzymatic proteins which are named as C1 to C9, B and D. All these are present in the blood as plasma proteins. These are also present in the tissue fluid.

DEVELOPMENT OF CELLULAR IMMUNE RESPONSE

The cellular immunity refers to specific acquired immunity which is accomplished by effector T cells and macrophages (Fig. 2.3-9). It is also called cell-mediated immunity (CMI).

Role of cellular immunity

1. Cellular immunity protects the host against fungi, most of the viruses and intracellular bacterial pathogens like *Mycobacterium tuberculosis, M. leprae* and *Brucella.*

2. It participates in allograft rejection and graft versus host reaction.

3. CMI participates in delayed hypersensitivity reaction.

4. CMI is also associated with certain autoimmune diseases.

5. It provides immunological surveillance and immunity against cancer (tumour immunity).

Types of cellular immune response

Like humoral immune response, the cellular immune response is also of two types:

1. *Primary cellular response* which is produced by initial contact with a foreign antigen, and

2. *Secondary cellular response* which is produced when the host is subsequently exposed to the same antigen. The secondary cell-mediated immune response is usually more pronounced and occurs more rapidly.

Stages of cellular immune response

1. Antigen processing and presentation

Antigen entering the host body is phagocytosed and degraded into polypeptide fragments by the antigen processing cells (APCs) which include macrophages and dendritic cells present in the peripheral lymphoid tissue. The antigen polypeptide fragments then become associated with MHC antigen and are expressed on the surface of APC.

2. Recognition of antigen by lymphocytes

T lymphocytes possess the antigenic recognition receptors known as *T cell receptors* (TCRs). Further, the mature T lymphocytes can be differentiated into 2 antigenic subtypes CD4+ cells and CD8+ cells.

- CD8+ cells recognize the combination of foreign antigen and class I MHC antigen, and
- CD4+ cells recognize the combination of foreign antigen and class II MHC antigen.

3. T lymphocyte differentiation (activation)

The CD8+ type of T lymphocytes after combining with foreign antigen MHC I complex are activated and differentiate into:

- Cytotoxic T cells (Tc cells), and
- Suppressor T cells (Ts cells).

CD4+ type of T lymphocytes after combining with foreign antigen MHC-II complex are activated and differentiate into:

- Helper T cells (TH cells), and
- Delayed type hypersensitivity T cells (TD cells).

T-T cooperation. The differentiation of T lymphocytes into T_H, T_C, T_S and T_D cells is interdependent. This interdependence is called T-T cooperation.

Release of differentiated T cells. The differentiated T lymphocytes so formed are released into the lymph and then enter the blood and are distributed throughout the body. The T lymphocytes circulate again and again throughout the body sometimes lasting for months or years.

T lymphocyte memory cells are also formed. These spread throughout the lymphoid tissues of entire body of T cells occurs far more rapidly and much more powerfully than in first response (secondary response).

4. Attack phase of cell-mediated immunity

Role of cytotoxic T cells

Cytotoxic T cells (Tc cells) and natural killer cells (NK cells) are responsible for the attack phase of cell-mediated immunity.

1. Antigen processing and presentation

Antigen(Bacterium)

Antigen

Nucleus

Lysosome — **MHC II**

MHC I

Antigen presenting cell having MHC II on its surface

Antigen accomplished with MHC II

Antigen accomplished with MHC I

2. Recognition of antigen by lymphocytes

TCRs on T lymphocyte

CD$_4$+ lymphocyte

CD$_8$+ lymphocyte

3. T lymphocyte activation

Delayed T cells(T$_D$)

Helper T cell(T$_H$)

Suppressor T cell(T$_S$)

Cytotoxic T cell(T$_C$)

T$_{H1}$ — Activate CD$_8$ T cells

T$_{H2}$ — Induce antibody production

Fig. 2.3-9. *Broad outline of development of cellular immune response.*

Role of Helper T cells (T$_H$ cells)

Helper T cells are of two types: T$_{H1}$ and T$_{H2}$.

i. Helper T$_1$ (T$_{H1}$) cells play their roles by secreting 3 cytokines:

- *Interleukin 2 (IL-2)*
- *γ interferon (IFN-γ)* has the direct ability to kill antigen bearing cells.
- *Tumour necrosis factor-B (TNF-B)* can induce apoptosis in antigen-bearing cells.

ii. Helper T$_2$ (T$_{H2}$) cells secrete interleukins 4, 5, 6, 10 and 13 and are primarily with activation of B lymphocytes to produce antibodies (T-B cooperation) (Fig. 2.3-10).

Role of suppressor T lymphocytes (T$_S$ cells)

- Suppressor T cells regulate the activity of cytotoxic T cells also suppress the activities of helper T cells.

CYTOKINES

Cytokines are small protein molecules which act like hormones to regulate immune response.

The cytokines are secreted not only by lymphocytes and macrophages but also by endothelial cells, neuroglial cells, and other types of cells. Broadly, cytokines can be grouped as:

Interleukins (IL). These are the principal cytokines and include IL-1 to IL-13.

Fig. 2.3-10. *Summary of immune response.*

Other cytokines include:

- Chemokines,
- Growth factors,
- Colony stimulating factors (CSF),
- Tumour necrotic factors (TNF α and TNF β),
- Interferons (IFN).

OTHER IMMUNE MECHANISM RELATED ASPECTS

IMMUNE TOLERANCE

Immune tolerance may be defined as a state of unresponsiveness to an antigen. It occurs in two forms: natural and acquired.

1. *Natural tolerance* refers to nonresponsiveness to a self-antigen. During embryonic development, when immune system is immature, any antigen which comes in contact with immature immune system is recognised as self-antigen. Therefore, it does not evoke any response in later life when body is exposed to the same antigen.

2. *Acquired tolerance* means unresponsiveness to a potential antigen. It results due to impairment of immune system; hence there is lack of responsiveness to potential antigens.

AUTOIMMUNITY

During fetal life, when many antigens are presented to immune system, they are recognised as self-antigens and antibodies and cytotoxic T cells are not produced.

Therefore, tolerance to self-antigen is produced. However, sometimes body starts producing antibodies or T cells against self-antigen (own cells or tissue) leading to an autoimmune disease. Therefore, auto-immunity may be defined as immune response to self-antigen.

Autoimmune diseases

Common autoimmune diseases include:

1. *Autoimmune anaemia.* For example:
   - Haemolytic anaemia: Antibodies react with own RBCs.
   - Pernicious anaemia: Antibodies react against gastric mucosa.
2. *Thrombocytopenic purpura.* Autoantibodies react with self-platelets.
3. *Graves' disease.* Autoantibodies bind to thyroid cells and stimulate them.
4. *Hashimoto's disease.* T cells react against antigen on the thyroid cells.
5. *Insulin-dependent diabetes mellitus.* Antibodies damage the β cells (insulin-producing cells) of the pancreas.
6. *Rheumatoid arthritis.* Antibodies damage the joints.

7. *Rheumatic fever.* Antibodies cross-react with valves of the heart.

HYPERSENSITIVITY

Hypersensitivity is an abnormal response which produces physiological or histopathological damage in the host. There are four types of hypersensitivity reactions:

- Type I (Anaphylaxis or IgE-mediated)
- Type II (Antibody-mediated cytotoxicity),
- Type III (Immune complex-mediated disorders), and
- Type IV (Delayed type or T cell-mediated hypersensitivity).

IMMUNODEFICIENCY DISEASES

Immunodeficiency diseases occur when body defence mechanisms are impaired.

Immunodeficiency diseases may be classified as primary or secondary.

Primary immunodeficiency

Primary immunodeficiency occurs due to defect in the development of the immune system.

Secondary immunodeficiency disease

Acquired deficiencies of immunological response mechanisms can occur secondarily to number of diseases. Secondary immunodeficiency is more common than the primary immunodeficiency. Acquired immune deficiency syndrome (AIDS) is the most important.

Acquired immune deficiency syndrome

AIDS, i.e. acquired immune deficiency syndrome is characterised by reduction in the number of helper T cells because of infection by human immunodeficiency virus (HIV). AIDS was first of all detected in USA in 1981.

Spread of disease. AIDS is a major worldwide life-threatening disease spreading rapidly. Daily about 8500 persons get infected with HIV. The high-risk groups include sex workers, drug addicts, homosexual males, persons with extramarital relations and recipients of unscreened blood transfusion.

Transmission. There are mainly three routes of transmission:

1. *Parenteral route* is through blood contact involving:
- Unscreened blood transfusion,
- Tattooing,
- Use of infected razors, syringes and needles, etc.
- Use of poorly sterilized dental instruments, and
- Organ transplants.

2. *Sexual route* accounts for about 85% of HIV infection due to multiple sex partners, sex workers, homosexuality and artificial insemination. The virus is present in sufficient concentration in the semen and vaginal secretions of the infected person.

3. *Transplacental route.* Infection can be transmitted from infected mother to her fetus (vertical transmission) across the placenta and also to infant through breast milk (perinatal transmission).

AIDS does not spread through mosquito bites, hugging, kissing and sharing meals.

Prevention. Preventive measures against HIV infection include:

- *Education.* National AIDS control organisation (NACO) has been set up under Ministry of Health and Family Welfare. Awareness is being imparted through all means of publicity and by NGOs in schools, colleges, factories, farms, etc.

- *Screening* is compulsarily carried out in case of blood donors, organ donors, semen donors, foreigners, and sex workers.

- *AIDS-positive* persons are advised to prevent sexual contacts and pregnancy.

- Ban on prostitution.

- *Safer sex* with single partner, use of condoms and barrier creams.

- Use of disposable syringes, needles, blood bags and I/V sets.

- Proper sterilization of razors, blades and dental equipment by using 70% alcohol, 35% sodium hypochloride, 5% formaldehyde, boiling for 15 minutes or autoclaving.

Platelets, Haemostasis, and Blood Coagulation

PLATELETS

STRUCTURE AND COMPOSITION

Platelets (small plates) also known as thrombocytes (thrombo = clot; cytes = cells) have following features:

- *Size.* Platelets are the smallest blood cells varying in diameter from 2 to 4 μm, with an average volume of 5.8 μm³.

- *Shape and colour.* Platelets are colourless, spherical or oval discoid structures.

- *Leishman staining* shows a platelet to consist of faint bluish cytoplasm containing reddish purple granules.

- *Nucleus* is absent in the platelets and therefore these cannot reproduce.

Electron microscopic structure

Under electron microscope, a platelet shows following structural and compositional characteristics (Fig. 2.4-1):

Fig. 2.4-1. *Structure of a platelet.*

1. **Cell membrane.** It consists of lipids (phospholipids, cholesterol and glycolipids), carbohydrates, proteins and glycoproteins.

2. **Microtubules.** Microtubules are made up of proteins called tubulins. These form a compact bundle which is present immediately beneath the platelet membrane. These

are responsible for maintenance of discoid shape of circulating platelets.

3. Cytoplasm. Cytoplasm of the platelets contains:

- *Endoplasmic reticulum and Golgi apparatus.* These structures synthesize various enzymes and store large quantities of calcium.
- *Mitochondria.* These are capable of forming ATP and ADP.
- *Contractile proteins* include actin, myosin and thrombosthenin. Contractile proteins can cause the platelet to contract and are thus responsibile for the clot retraction.
- *Other proteins* present in the cytoplasm are:
  - Fibrin-stabilizing factor
  - Platelet-derived growth factor
  - Von Willebrand factor
- *Granules* present in the cytoplasm of platelets.
  - Contain substances (like phospholipids, trigly-cerides, cholesterol) ATP, ADP and serotonin (5HT).
  - Clotting factors, and platelet-derived growth factor (PDGF).
- *Enzymes* present in the cytoplasm of platelets include adenosine triphosphatase and the enzyme necessary for synthesis of prostaglandins.

PROPERTIES AND FUNCTIONS

Properties of platelets (Fig. 2.4-2)

1. Adhesiveness. Platelets possess the property of adhesiveness, i.e. when they come in contact with any wet surface or rough surface, these are activated and stick to the surface. Factors responsible for adhesiveness are collagen, thrombin, ADP, thromboxane A_2, calcium ions and von Willebrand factor.

2. Aggregation. Platelets have the property to aggregate, i.e. they stick to each other. This is due to ADP and thromboxane A_2.

3. Agglutination. Clumping together of platelets is called agglutination. This occurs due to the actions of some platelet agglutinins.

Functions of platelets

When activated, platelets perform following functions:

1. Role in haemostasis. Haemostasis refers to spontaneous arrest of bleeding from an injured blood vessel (see page 65).

2. Role in clot formation. Platelets play an important role in the formation of the intrinsic prothrombin activator which is responsible for onset of blood clotting (see page 66).

3. Role in clot retraction. Contraction of contractile proteins (actin, myosin and thrombosthenin) present in the platelets play an important role in clot retraction (see page 68).

4. Role in repair of injured blood vessels. The platelet-derived growth factor (PDGF) present in the cytoplasm plays an important role in the repair of endothelium of the injured/damaged blood vessels.

5. Role in defence mechanism. Platelets, due to their property of agglutination, are capable of phagocytosis.

6. Transport and storage function. The 5HT is stored in the platelets and transported to the site of injury where it is released.

NORMAL COUNT AND VARIATIONS

Normal count

Normal platelet count ranges from 1,50,000 to 4,50,000/ mm^3 with an average count of 2.5 lac/mm^3.

Physiological variations

1. Age. Platelet count is less in infants (1 lac to 2 lac/ mm^3). Adult levels are reached by 3rd month of age.

2. Sex. Normally there is no difference in the platelet counts of males and females. However, during menstruation the count is reduced in females.

3. After meals the platelet count is slightly increased.

4. After severe muscular exercise platelets may increase.

5. At high altitude platelet count is increased.

Pathological variations

A. Thrombocytosis. An increase in the number of platelets (more than 4.5 lac/mm^3) is called thrombocytosis. *Causes of thrombocytosis.* Platelet count is increased:

1. After splenectomy,
2. After haemorrhage, severe injury, major surgical operation, and parturition.

Fig. 2.4-2. *Properties of platelets : A, adhesiveness; B, aggregation; and C, formation of harmostatic plug.*

3. In myeloproliferative disorders such as:
   - Chronic myeloid leukaemia,
   - Polycythemia vera,
   - Myelofibrosis.

B. *Thrombocytopenia.* Decrease in the number of platelets below 1.5 lac/mm^3 is called thrombocytopenia. *Causes of thrombocytopenia* are:

1. Idiopathic thrombocytopenic purpura
2. Bone marrow depression due to:
   - Effects of various cytotoxic drugs,
   - Whole body irradiation,
   - Hypoplastic and aplastic anaemia.
3. Acute leukaemia or secondary deposits of malignancy in the bone marrow.
4. In infections like smallpox, chickenpox, typhoid and dengue fever.
5. In hypersplenism
6. In toxaemia, septicaemia and uraemia.

FORMATION OF PLATELETS

Formation or development of platelets is called *thrombopoiesis*. The platelets are produced in the bone marrow. The pluripotent stem cell destined to form platelets is converted into colony forming units called Meg-CFU which develop into platelets after passing through various stages (Fig. 2.4-3).

Platelets are formed from pseudopodia of mega-karyocyte cytoplasm which get detached into the blood stream. Each megakaryocyte may form upto 4000 platelets. The formation of platelets from the stem cell takes about 10 days.

Control of thrombopoiesis

Thrombopoiesis seems to be regulated by following humoral factors:
- Thrombopoietin, and
- Megakaryocyte - colony stimulating activity (Meg CSA).

The factors stimulating the synthesis and release of these agents are not yet known.

LIFESPAN AND FATE OF PLATELETS

Lifespan of platelets varies from 8 to 12 days with an average of 10 days. Platelets are destroyed by tissue macrophage system in spleen. Therefore:
- *Splenomegaly* causes reduction in the platelet count, and
- *Splenectomy* is followed by an increase in platelet count.

HAEMOSTASIS

Haemostasis refers to spontaneous arrest or prevention of bleeding from the injured/damaged vessels by the physiological process. It involves three main steps (Fig. 2.4-4):

Fig. 2.4-3. Stages of thrombopoiesis.

PLURIPOTENT STEM CELL

PROGENITOR CELL (MEGAKARYOBLAST)

Endoreduplication

PROMEGAKARYOCYTE

MEGAKARYOCYTE

PLATELETS

Fig. 2.4-4. Steps of haemostasis.

1. Vasoconstriction

Initial vasoconstriction is caused by direct effect of injury on the vascular smooth muscles following injury to the vessels and due to release 5 HT and other vasconstrictors.

2. Formation of temporary haemostatic plug

Formation of a temporary haemostatic plug by the plate-lets at the site of injury involves following steps:

- Platelet adhesion.
- Platelet activation.
- Platelet aggregation.

The platelet adherence and aggregation ultimately lead to the formation of platelet plug. At first it is a fairly loose plug but is successful in blocking the blood loss if the vascular opening is small.

3. Formation of definitive haemostatic plug

The temporary platelet plug is converted into the defini-tive haemostatic plug by the process of clot formation (blood coagulation). Platelets play an important role in the formation of the intrinsic prothrombin activator which is responsible for initiating the process of clot formation (see page 67).

BLOOD COAGULATION

Blood remains in fluid condition within the blood vessels throughout life. But, when the blood is shed from the blood vessels or collected in a container, it looses its fluidity within a few minutes and gets converted into a jelly-like mass, which is called *clot*. This phenomenon is called *coagulation* or clotting of blood.

CLOTTING FACTORS

The process of coagulation essentially involves a stepwise activation of certain substances mostly proteins present in the blood and/or tissue fluids. These substances are called clotting factors and have been given Roman numerals:

- Factor I (Fibrinogen),
- Factor II (Prothrombin),
- Factor III (Thromboplastin),
- Factor IV (Calcium),
- Factor V (Labile factor or proaccelrin or accelerator globulin),
- Factor VI (non-existent),
- Factor VII (Stable factor or proconvertin),
- Factor VIII (Antihaemophilic factor A (AHF) or antihaemophilic globulin (AHG)),

- Factor IX (Christmas factor or plasma thromboplastic component (PTC or antihaemophilic factor B),
- Factor X (Stuart-Prower factor),
- Factor XI (Plasma thromboplastin antecedent, i.e. PTA or antihaemophilic factor C),
- Factor XII (Hageman factor or glass factor or contact factor),
- Factor XIII (Fibrin stabilizing factor or fibrinase or Laki-Lorand factor),
- HMW-K (High molecular weight kininogen or Fitzgerald factor),
- Pre-Ka (Prekallikrein or Fletcher factor),
- Ka (Kallikrein), and
- PL (Platelet phospholipid).

MECHANISM OF COAGULATION

Normally, blood circulates in the blood vessels and does not clot spontaneously. Clot formation is initiated under following situations:

- Trauma to the vascular wall and adjacent tissues,
- Trauma to blood,
- Contact of blood with damaged endothelial cells or collagen or other tissue elements outside the vessel.

The process of coagulation involves a *cascade* of reactions in which activation of one factor leads to activation of next clotting factor (Fig. 2.4-5). This enzyme cascade reaction is also called water fall *sequence*. The process of coagulation can be divided into three main steps:

A. Formation of prothrombin activator,

B. Conversion of prothrombin to thrombin, and

C. Conversion of fibrinogen into fibrin.

A. Formation of prothrombin activator

Two different mechanisms involved in the formation of prothrombin activator are:

1. Extrinsic pathway, and
2. Intrinsic pathway.

1. Extrinsic pathway

The extrinsic pathway of formation of prothrombin acti-vator begins with trauma to the vascular wall or the tissues outside the blood vessel. It includes following three basic steps (Fig. 2.4-5) :

1. *Release of tissue thromboplastins.* The traumatized tissues release several substances which are together known as *tissue thomboplastin (factor III).*

2. *Activation of factor X to form activated factor X.* Tissue thromboplastin combines with factor VII (stable

Fig. 2.4-5. *Mechanism of blood coagulation.*

factor) to form the tissue thromboplastin-factor VII complex which in the presence of Ca²⁺ activates factor X to form activated factor X (Xa).

3. *Effect of activated factor X to form prothrombin activator.* The activated factor X along with tissue phospholipids or phospholipids released from platelets, factor V (Labile factor) and Ca²⁺ forms a complex which is called prothrombin activator.

2. Intrinsic pathway

The intrinsic pathway of formation of prothrombin activator begins in the blood itself following trauma to blood itself or exposure of blood to collagen in a traumatized vascular wall. The steps of intrinsic pathway are summarized in Fig. 2.4-5:

Activation of factor XII. Trauma to blood or exposure to collagen fibres underlying damaged vascular endothelium (or electronegatively charged wettable surface such as glass, in vitro) activates plasma factor XII to form XIIa and initiates the intrinsic pathway. Platelets are also activated.

Activation of factor XI to form XIa is caused by the activated factor XII.

Activation of factor IX to form IXa is in turn caused by the activated factor XI in the presence of Ca²⁺.

Activation of factor X. Factor IXa in the presence of activated factor VIII, Ca²⁺ and phospholipids (released by activated platelets) activate factor X to form Xa.

Formation of prothrombin activator. The activated factor X along with the phospholipids released by activated platelets, activated factor V and Ca²⁺ forms a complex which is called prothrombin activator.

B. Conversion of prothrombin to thrombin

Conversion of prothrombin to thrombin is caused by the prothrombin activator in the presence of Ca²⁺. This occurs at the surface of platelets which form the platelet plug at the site of injury.

Thrombin

Thrombin so formed acts as proteolytic enzyme. It has been estimated that the amount of thrombin produced during clotting of only 1 ml of blood is sufficient to coagulate 3 litres of blood.

Roles played by thrombin :

- *Conversion of fibrinogen to fibrin* (discussed below).
- *Positive feedback role of thrombin*: It accelerates the rate of formation of prothrombin activator by activating factor VIII, V and XIII.
- *It also activates protein-C* (which is an anticoagulant).

C. Conversion of fibrinogen to fibrin

Conversion of fibrinogen into fibrin involves three reactions (Fig. 2.4-6):

1. *Proteolysis.* Thrombin acting as proteolytic enzyme removes four low molecular weight peptide chains from

Fig. 2.4-6. *Types of reactions involved in conversion of soluble fibrinogen into insoluble fibrin clot.*

each molecule of fibrinogen to convert it into fibrin monomer.

2. Polymerization. Fibrin monomer polymerizes with another monomer to form *long fibrin* threads which form reticulum of the clot.

3. Stabilization of fibrin polymers. Fibrin stabilising factor (factor XIII) which is activated by the thrombin to form XIIIa but XIIIa in the presence of Ca^{2+} causes formation of covalent crosslinkages between fibrin threads, thus adding tremendous strength to the fibrin meshwork. The fibrin meshwork traps the remaining components of plasma and blood cells to form a solid mass called clot.

The fibrin threads of the clot adhere to damaged surface of blood vessels.

At this juncture, it is important to note that *coagulation is the property of plasma alone*. The RBCs and WBCs do not take part in it. They only become caught up in the meshwork of the clot.

Blood clot retraction

Within a few minutes after a clot is formed, it begins to contract and usually squeezes out most of the fluid called *serum* (plasma without fibrinogen and other clotting factors) within 30-60 minutes.

- *Platelets are essential* for clot retraction. The contractile proteins (platelet thrombosthenin, actin and myosin) present in the cytoplasm of platelets cause strong contraction of platelet spicules attached to fibrin fibres.

Role of calcium in blood coagulation

From the study of mechanism of blood coagulation, it is quite clear that except for the first two steps in the intrinsic pathway, calcium ions are required for promotion of all the reactions. Therefore in the absence of calcium ions blood clotting will not occur.

Role of vitamin K, liver and vascular wall in haemostasis and coagulation

Role of vitamin K. In the liver, synthesis of following coagulation factors is dependent upon vitamin K:

- Prothrombin,
- Factor VII, IX and X, and

- Circulatory anticoagulant protein.

Vitamin K deficiency. In the deficiency of vitamin K prothrombin time and blood clotting time is prolonged and serious haemorrhages may occur.

Role of liver. Liver plays following significant role in the coagulation mechanism:

1. *Synthesis of procoagulants.* It is the site of synthesis of factor V, VII, IX, X, prothrombin and fibrinogen.

2. *Removal of activated procoagulants.* Liver also removes the activated procoagulants from the blood.

3. *Synthesis of anticoagulants.* Liver also synthesizes anticoagulants like heparin, antithrombin III and protein C.

Liver failure can cause both:

- *Bleeding disorders* due to hypocoagulability of the blood; and

- *Uncontrolled extensive clotting* inside the blood vessels where clotting is not only unwanted but dangerous as well.

Role of blood vessels. Endothelium, subendothelial tissue and smooth muscles of the media of the blood vessels in coagulation and haemostasis mechanisms:

- Endothelium secretes von Willebrand's factor (VWF). The plasma VWF initiates platelet aggregation and haemostasis.

- Tissue factor (TF) released by endothelial cells following trauma initiates the process of extrinsic pathway of clotting mechanism.

Thrombosis

We have studied that physiologically under normal conditions the circulating blood does not clot and that clotting of blood occurs only extravascularly when a vessel has been injured and bleeding has occurred. However, under certain pathological conditions the intravascular clotting may occur. The intravascular clotting is called *thrombosis* and the clot so formed is called thrombus.

Predisposing factors. Virchow described three primary events which predispose to thrombus formation (*Virchow's triad*). These are:

1. *Endothelial injury* may occur in atherosclerosis, haemodynamic stress in hypertension, arterial disease, diabetes mellitus and hypercholesterolaemia.

2. *Alterations in flow of blood.* Both in turbulence as well as stasis of blood normal axial flow of blood is disturbed and platelets come in contact with endothelium initiating thrombus formation.

3. *Hypercoagulability of blood* which may occur due to:

- Increase in fibrinogen, prothrombin, factors VIa, VIIa and Xa.

- Increase in platelet count and their adhesiveness, and

- Decreased levels of coagulation inhibitors such as antithrombin III and fibrinogen degradation products.

Effects of thrombi. Intravascular thrombi may cause:

1. *Ischaemia and infarction.* Thrombi may decrease or stop the blood supply to part of an organ and cause ischaemia which may subsequently result in infarction. For example, thrombus formation in coronary arteries may cause myocardial ischaemia and infarction.

2. *Thromboembolism.* The thrombus or its part may get dislodged and be carried along in the blood stream as *embolus* to lodge in a distant vessel. Examples of emboli formation are:

- Pulmonary embolism,
- Cerebral embolism

ANTIHAEMOSTATIC MECHANISMS AND ANTICOAGULANTS

The factors which balance the tendency of the blood to clot in vivo constitute the *antihaemostatic factors.* These can be grouped as:

A. Factors preventing platelet aggregation

Prostacyclin is an endogenous factor which prevents platelet aggregation by inhibiting the thromboxane A_2 formation (which promotes platelet aggregation).

B. Circulatory anticoagulants

The natural anticoagulants circulating in the blood constitute the anticoagulant mechanism of the body. These include:

1. *Heparin.* Heparin is a powerful naturally acting anticoagulant. Heparin is secreted by the basophils and mast cells (present in various tissues such as liver, lungs and tissues rich in connective tissue).

2. *Antithrombin III* is present in plasma as well as vascular endothelium. It inactivates a number of coagulation factors including thrombin.

3. *Protein C.* Protein C is a plasma protein synthesized in liver. It, along with *thrombomodulin* and *protein S,* constitutes an important negative feedback pathway that keeps the coagulatory process under control.

C. Fibrinolytic mechanism

Fibrinolysis refers to the process that brings about the dissolution of fibrin. The important component of the fibrinolytic system is *plasmin* or fibrinolysin which is present in the blood in an inactive form called *plasminogen* or profibrinolysin.

ANTICOAGULANTS

Anticoagulants refer to the substances which delay or prevent the process of coagulation of blood. Anticoagulants may be divided into endogenous and exogenous anticoagulants.

A. *Endogenous anticoagulants.* Endogenous anticoagulants are those which are present inside the blood naturally:

- Heparin,
- Antithrombin III, and
- Protein C.

B. *Exogenous anticoagulants.* Exogenous anticoagulants are administered from outside or are used in vitro. These include:

1. *Heparin.* Heparin, a naturally acting anticoagulant, can also be synthesized. It inhibits blood coagulation both in vivo and in vitro.

2. *Calcium sequesters or decalcifying agents.* In vitro, blood clotting can be prevented by substances which sequester (remove) calcium from the blood such as sodium citrate and sodium oxalate, and calcium chelators which bind calcium e.g. ethylene diaminetetraacetic acid (EDTA).

3. *Vitamin K antagonists.* These are used orally and thus can prevent coagulation in vivo effectively e.g. dicoumarol, and warfarin,

4. *Defibrination substances.* Defibrination substances are those which cause destruction of fibrinogen e.g., *Arvin or ancord.* It is purified preparation of snake venom. It is glycoprotein in nature and is administered by injection.

5. *Cold.* Keeping blood cold (at 5 to 10°C) can retard the process of coagulation but cannot absolutely prevent it. Because of this reason blood is stored in blood banks at low temperature.

BLEEDING DISORDERS

Bleeding disorders are characterized by spontaneous escape of blood from blood vessels (in the tissues, inside the body cavities or on few surfaces like skin and mucous membrane or persistent and/or excessive bleeding following minor injuries like tooth extraction etc.

Classification of bleeding disorders

I. Platelet disorders
II. Coagulation disorder or defective coagulation mechanism
III. Vascular disorders. Damage of capillary endothelium (non-thrombocytopenic purpura)

Only a few important bleeding disorders, purpura and haemophilia, are described briefly.

Purpura

Purpura is a group of bleeding disorders occurring due to various causes. The term purpura is derived from purple-coloured petechial haemorrhages and bruises in the skin. The blood that leaks out changes colour from red to blue to dark blue and green over a period of time.

Causes and types of purpura

1. *Deficiency of platelets* (thrombocytopenic purpura). Decrease in the platelet count below 1.5 lac/mm³ is called thrombocytopenia. Thrombocytopenic purpura may be:

- *Primary thrombocytopenic purpura* (idiopathic). In this the cause is not known. In many of the idiopathic cases antibodies develop against platelets (immune thrombocytopenic purpura, ITP).

- *Secondary causes of platelet deficiency* (secondary thrombocytopenic purpura) are:

  - Bone marrow depression due to effects of various cytotoxic drugs, whole body irradiations and hypoplastic and aplastic anaemia.

  - Leukaemia and secondary deposits of malignancies in the bone marrow,

  - Hypersplenism.

2. Von Willebrand's disease. It is inherited as autosomal dominant trait. This condition is associated with a deficiency of factor VIII related antigen (VIII R:Ag) also called as Von Willebrand factor (VWF). This factor acts as carrier of factor VIII, so its deficiency results in diminished adherence of platelets to collagen fibres in a damaged vessel.

3. Vascular disorders. Bleeding tendencies seen in patients with vascular disorders (damage to capillary endothelium) are referred to as *non-thrombocytopenic purpura*. In all cases of purpura due to vessel wall defects the platelet counts are normal, but bleeding time is prolonged and capillary fragility test is positive.

Hemophilia

Hemophilia is the name given to a group of disorders occurring due to *hereditary deficiency of coagulation* and characterised by bleeding tendencies associated with increased clotting time (CT). The hemophilia includes:

- Hemophilia A (83% cases),

- Hemophilia B (15% cases), and

- Hemophilia C (2% cases).

1. Hemophilia A. Hemophilia A, also known as true or classical hemophilia, occurs due to *deficiency of factor VIII, i.e.* antihemophilic globulin (AHG).

- Being sex-linked recessive disease it affects males exclusively and females act as carriers (Fig. 2.4-7). The carrier female shows no symptoms.

2. Hemophilia B also known as *Christmas disease,* occurs due to deficiency of factor IX (Christmas factor or plasma thromboplastin component, PTC). It was discovered in a family with surname Christmas.

Like hemophilia A, hemophilia B is also a recessive X-linked disease that occurs in males and is transmitted by females.

Hemophilia C. Hemophilia C refers to deficiency of PTA (factor XI).

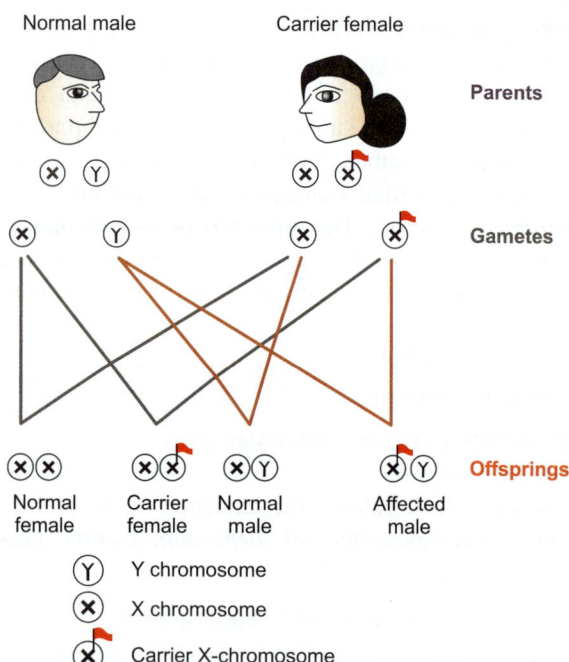

Fig. 2.4-7. Sex linked inheritance of haemophilia.

Disseminated intravascular coagulation

Disseminated intravascular coagulation (DIC), as the name indicates, refers to the condition when clotting mechanism becomes activated in widespread areas of the circulation.

Due to widespread intravascular coagulation there occurs plugging of small vessels with clots resulting into decreased O_2 and nutrient supply to its tissues causing multiple organ damage.

Laboratory tests in bleeding disorders

Bleeding time (BT). Bleeding occurs from the skin when it is pricked with a needle, which normally stops of its own within a few minutes. The time lapse between the skin prick and the arrest of bleeding is called *bleeding time* (BT).

Normal BT by Duke's method varies from 1 to 6 minutes. Normal BT indicates that platelet count and their function as well as health of capillaries are normal.

Prolonged BT occurs in purpura, while it is normal in hemophilia.

Platelet count varies from 1.5 lac to 4.5 lac/mm³ with an average 2.5 lac/mm³. Platelet count is decreased in primary and secondary thrombocytopenic purpura.

Coagulation time (CT). Coagulation time (CT) refers to the time taken by the fresh fluid blood to get coagulated demonstrated by formation of fibrin threads. It is an insensitive measure in the assessment of coagulation defects and is abnormally prolonged when the coagulation factors are seriously deficient. The CT is prolonged in hemophilia and other clotting disorders.

Blood Groups and Blood Transfusion

BLOOD GROUPS

INTRODUCTION

Agglutinogens and agglutinins

Agglutinogens refer to the antigens present on the cell membranes of RBCs. A variety of antigens are present on the cell membrane, but only a few of them are of practical significance.

Agglutinins refer to the antibodies against the agglutinogens. These are present in the plasma.

Agglutination of RBCs can be caused by the antigens present on their cell membranes in the presence of suitable agglutinins (antibodies). That is why, these antigens are called agglutinogens.

Blood grouping systems

Depending upon the type of agglutinogen present or absent on the red cell membranes various blood grouping systems are known, which can be classified as:
- The classical ABO blood grouping system, and
- Rh (CDE) blood grouping system.

Landsteiner law

Karl Landsteiner in 1900 framed a law in relation to agglutinogens and agglutinins, which states that:

1. *If an agglutinogen is present* on the red cell membrane of an individual, the corresponding agglutinin must be absent in the plasma; and

2. *If an agglutinogen is absent* from the cell membrane of RBCs of an individual, the corresponding agglutinin must be present in the plasma.

It is important to note that:
- The Landsteiner law is applicable to ABO blood group system only
- The law is not applicable to other blood group systems, because there are no naturally occurring agglutinins in these systems.

CLASSICAL ABO BLOOD GROUPING SYSTEM

A and B agglutinogens

- The classical ABO blood grouping system is based on the presence of A and B agglutinogens on the cell membrane of RBCs. These are complex oligosaccharides differing in their terminal sugars.

- The A and B antigens present on the membranes of RBCs are also present in many other tissues like salivary glands, pancreas, kidney, liver, lungs and testis; and also in body fluids like saliva, semen, and amniotic fluid. The antigens on RBCs membrane are glycolipids, while in the tissues and body fluids they are soluble glycoproteins.

Anti-A and anti-B agglutinins

- Anti-A (or α) agglutinin and anti-B (or β) agglutinin refer to the antibody, i.e. which reacts with or acts on the antigen A, and antigen B, respectively.
- The α and β agglutinins are globulins of IgM type and cannot cross the placenta.
- The α and β agglutinins act best at low temperature (5°C to 20°C) and are therefore also called as cold antibodies.
- There are two types of α agglutinins: the α_1 and α proper.

Types of ABO blood groups

Depending upon the presence or absence of A and B agglutinogens and α and β agglutinins there are four types of blood groups :

Blood group A is characterized by:

- Presence of A agglutinogen and absence of B agglutinogen on the cell membrane of RBC.
- Presence of anti-B (or β) agglutinin and absence of anti-A (or α) agglutinin from the plasma.
- Group A has two subgroups: A_1 and A_2. The α_1-agglutinin agglutinates with subgroup A_1 only, while α-proper agglutinin agglutinates with both A_1 and A_2 subgroups.

  Blood group B is characterized by:

- Presence of B agglutinogen and absence of A agglutinogen on the membrane of RBCs, and
- Presence of anti-A (or α) agglutinin and absence of anti-B (or β) agglutinin from the plasma.

Blood group AB is characterized by:

- Presence of both A and B agglutinogens on the cell membrane of RBCs, and
- Absence of both anti-A (or α) and anti-B or (β) agglutinins from the plasma.
- Blood group AB has two subgroups namely A_1B and A_2B.

Blood group O is characterized by:

- Absence of both A and B agglutinogens on the red cell membrane, and
- Presence of both anti-A and anti-B agglutinins in the plasma.

Determination of ABO blood groups

The ABO blood group of an individual can be determined by mixing one drop of suspension of his red cells (in isotonic saline) with a drop each of anti-serum A (containing α agglutinins) and anti-serum B (containing β agglutinins) separately on a glass slide. The anti-serum A will cause agglutination (clumping of RBCs having A antigens and anti-serum B will cause agglutination of RBCs having B antigens). The blood group of the individual will be shown by the presence of agglutination with one, both or none of the sera (Table 2.5-1 and Fig. 2.5-1).

Note : The antisera A and B are available commercially. For a quick identification, the anti-A serum is tinted blue and anti-B serum is tinted yellow.

Rh (RHESUS) BLOOD GROUPING SYSTEM

Rh antigens

- The antigens responsible for this blood grouping system are called Rh antigens or Rh agglutinogens or Rh factor because these were first discovered in the RBCs of rhesus monkeys. Based on the presence of Rh antigen, two types of blood groups are described:

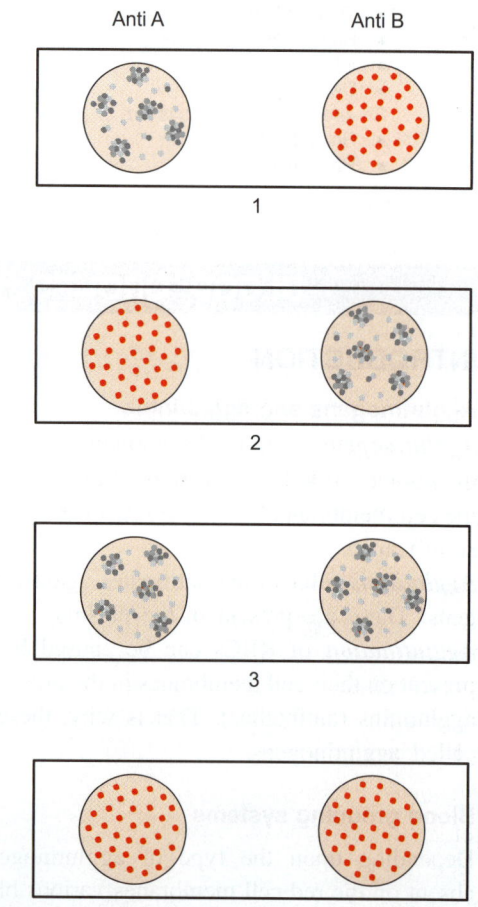

Fig. 2.5-1. Determination of blood groups—the RBCs showing agglutination with antisera are: 1, of blood group 'A' with antisera A; 2, of blood group B with antisera B; 3, of blood group 'AB' with antisera A and B (both); and 4, of blood group 'O' with none.

Table 2.5.1. Determination of blood group of an individual

Blood group of RBC suspension	Agglutination with	
	anti-serum A (containing α agglutinins)	anti-serum B (containing β agglutinins)
A	+	–
B	–	+
AB	+	+
O	–	–

– Rh positive blood group, and

– Rh negative blood group.

- Three types of Rh antigens, viz. C, D and E have been recognised. However, D antigen is commonest and produces worst transfusion reactions. Therefore, for all practical purposes, the term Rh antigen refers to D antigen.
- Rh antigens are integral membrane proteins. These are *not found* in tissues other than RBCs.

Rh antibodies

- There are no natural antibodies of Rh antigens.
- Rh antibodies (also called anti-D) are produced only when a Rh –ve individual is transfused with Rh+ blood or when a Rh –ve mother gives birth to Rh +ve baby (Rh +ve RBCs of fetus enter into the maternal circulation). Rh antibodies are of IgG type and can cross the placenta. Since these react best at body temperature so these are also called warm antibodies.
- Once produced, the Rh antibodies persist in the blood for years and can produce serious reactions during the second transfusion.

Inheritance of Rh antigens

- The Rh antigen (D antigen) is inherited as dominant gene D. When gene D is absent from a chromosome, its place is occupied by the alternate form (allelomorph) called 'd' Rh gene is inherited from both the parents (father and the mother).
- Rh-positive individual may have two genotypes. DD (homozygous) or Dd (heterozygous). Of 85% Rh +ve individuals about 35% have DD genotype and 50% have Dd genotype.
- The genotype of Rh –ve individual is dd.
- Therefore the genotype (gene composition) of offspring will be:
  - DD, when gene D is carried by both sperm and ovum
  - Dd, when one gamete carries D and other d; and
  - dd, when both the gametes carry gene d.

Inheritance of Rh antigen is summarized in Fig. 2.5-2.

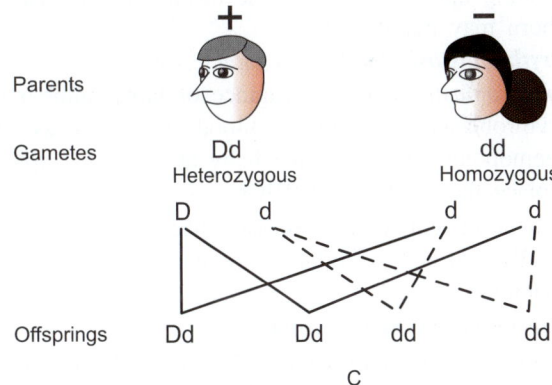

Fig. 2.5-2. *Inheritance of Rh antigen: A, when father is homozygous Rh +ve and mother is homozygous Rh –ve; then all the offsprings are heterozygous Rh +ve; B, when father and mother both are homozygous Rh –ve then all the offsprings are homozygous Rh –ve; and C, when father is heterozygous Rh +ve and mother is homozygous Rh –ve, then 50% of offsprings are Rh +ve (heterozygous) and other 50% are Rh –ve (homozygous).*

Haemolytic disease of newborn

Haemolytic disease of newborn occurs as a result of incompatibility of Rh blood groups between the mother and fetus.

Mechanism of haemolytic disease of newborn in Rh incompatibility

Mechanism of development of haemolytic disease of the newborn can be described under following steps:

1. *Entrance of Rh +ve fetal RBCs into Rh –ve mother's circulation during first pregnancy.* When a Rh –ve mother (genotypes dd) bears a Rh +ve child (genotype Dd) with father being Rh +ve (genotype DD or Dd) at the time of delivery the fetal RBCs enter maternal circulation because of severance of umbilical cord. Before delivery, usually the fetal and maternal circulation do not mix. Since no Rh +ve RBCs enter maternal circulation during delivery, so the first child is usually normal.

2. *Production of Rh antibodies (anti-D) in mother.* During postpartum period, i.e. within a month after delivery, the mother develops Rh antibodies in her blood. As mentioned earlier the Rh antibodies are of IgG type and are able to cross the placental barrier. Once formed the Rh antibodies persist for a long period in mother's blood.

3. *Rh incompatibility reaction during second pregnancy.* When the Rh –ve mother in the second pregnancy also bears a Rh +ve child, the Rh antibodies present in the mother's blood enter the fetal circulation by crossing the placental barrier and cause agglutination of fetal RBCs leading to haemolytic disease of newborn.

Manifestations of haemolytic disease of newborn

Depending upon the severity the haemolytic disease of newborn may manifest as:

1. *Erythoblastosis fetalis* is characterized by:
- *Erythroblastosis,* i.e. appearance of large number of erythroblasts in peripheral blood. It occurs as the haemopoietic tissue of the baby attempts to rapidly replace the haemolysed RBCs.
- *Anaemia* occurs due to excessive haemolysis of RBCs by Rh antibodies. Infant may even die of severe anaemia.

2. *Icterus gravis neonatorum*
- *Jaundice* may occur within 24 hours of birth due to excessive formation of bilirubin as a result of excessive haemolysis of RBCs.
- *Liver and spleen* are enlarged.

3. *Kernicterus.* It is a neurological syndrome occurring in newborns with severe haemolysis. The excessive bilirubin formed may enter the brain tissue as the blood-brain barrier is not well developed in infants and cause damage. The bilirubin mostly affects the basal ganglia producing disturbance of motor activities. It usually develops when serum bilirubin level exceeds 18 mg%.

4. *Hydrops fetalis,* i.e. the fetus is grossly oedematous. It occurs when haemolysis is very severe. Usually there occurs intrauterine death of fetus or if born prematurely or even at term, the infant dies within a few hours.

Prevention and treatment

Prevention of haemolytic disease of newborn. The haemolytic disease in the newborn during second pregnancy can be prevented by injecting single dose of Rh antibodies (anti-D) in the form of Rh-immunoglobulin to mother soon after first childbirth. These antibodies will destroy the Rh +ve RBCs of the fetus which have gained access to maternal circulation. In this way active antibodies will not be formed by the mother.

Treatment of haemolytic disease of newborn. Treatment of haemolytic disease of the newborn is replacement of baby's Rh +ve blood with Rh –ve blood exchange transfusion.

CLINICAL APPLICATIONS OF BLOOD GROUPING

1. *In blood transfusion.* Before blood transfusion always crossmatching is done (see page 75).

2. *In preventing haemolytic disease* in newborn due to Rh incompatibility (as discussed above).

3. *In paternity disputes.* The ABO, Rh and MNS blood grouping is helpful in settling cases of disputed paternity.

4. *In medicolegal cases.* Any red stain on a clothing may be claimed to be blood by a supposed victim. Therefore, it is first confirmed that it really is blood by preparing hemin crystals from the stain extract.

5. *In knowing susceptibility to diseases.* The incidence of certain diseases is related to blood groups, e.g.
- Individuals with blood group O (non-secretors) are said to be more susceptible to duodenal ulcer (peptic ulcer) than the individuals with blood group A and B (secretors).
- Individuals with blood group A are more susceptible to carcinoma of stomach, pancreas and salivary glands.
- To some extent incidence of diabetes mellitus is more in individuals with blood group A.

BLOOD TRANSFUSION

Indications

Blood transfusion is a life-saving measure and should be carried out when it is absolutely essential. Common situations in which blood transfusion is indicated are:

1. *Blood loss.* Severe blood loss is the most important indication for blood transfusion.

2. *For quick restoration of haemoglobin* in patients with severe anaemia is required in situations like pregnancy and emergency surgery.

3. *Exchange transfusion* is required in haemolytic disease of newborn.

4. *Blood diseases* like aplastic anaemia, agranulocytosis, leukaemias, hemophilia, purpura and clotting defects may require blood transfusion.

5. *Acute poisoning,* e.g. carbon monoxide poisoning.

Donor and recipient

Donor refers to a person who donates the blood and the person who receives blood is a recipient.

Universal donor. Blood of the individuals with blood group O does not contain any agglutinogen. So when this blood is transfused to a person with any blood group (A, B, AB or O), theoretically its RBCs will not be agglutinated. Because of this fact an individual with blood group O is called universal donor. However, practically this term is no longer valid, as it ignores the complications produced by existence of Rh factor and other blood group systems.

Universal recipient. Blood of an individual with blood group AB does not contain any agglutinins. So, theoretically when such an individual receives blood from the individual with any blood group (A, B, AB or O), there should be no transfusion reaction. Because of this fact an individual with AB blood group is called universal recipient. However, practically this term is no more valid because it ignores the complications produced by the existence of Rh factor and other blood group systems.

Precautions to be observed during blood transfusion

1. *Absolute indication* should always be there for the transfusion of blood.

2. *Crossmatching* should always be done before the blood transfusion. For it blood is collected from donor as well as recipient. Plasma and RBCs are separated in each. The crossmatching involves two steps: major and minor crossmatching.

- *Major crossmatching involves mixing of donor's cells with recipient's plasma.* This is called major crossmatching because of the fact that when mismatched blood is transfused in a recipient, the donor's cells get agglutinated as against their agglutinogen there is sufficiently high concentration of agglutinins in the recipient's plasma.

- *Minor crossmatching involves mixing of recipient's cells with donor's plasma.* This is called minor crossmatch due of the fact that reaction of donor's plasma and recipient's cells usually does not occur or is very very mild on giving mismatched blood transfusion because:

  - Firstly, the donor's plasma in the transfusion (about 250 ml) is usually so diluted by the much larger volume of recipient's blood (about 5 L) that it rarely causes agglutination even when the titre of agglutinins against the recipient's cell is high, and

  - Secondly, donor's agglutinins are also neutralized by soluble agglutinogen which are found free in the recipient's body fluid.

3. *Rh +ve blood should never be transfused to Rh −ve person.* It is particularly must for females at any age before menopause, because once she is sensitized by the Rh antigen, the anti-D antibodies are formed and she will not be able to bear a Rh +ve fetus. In other words, Rh+ transfusion may make a woman permanently childless.

4. *Donor's blood should always be screened* for diseases which are spread through blood such as AIDS, hepatitis-B, malaria and syphilis.

5. *Blood bag/bottle should be checked* for the name of recipient and blood group on the label before starting the blood transfusion.

6. *Blood transfusion should be given at slow rate.* If rapid transfusion is given, citrate present in stored blood may cause chelation of calcium ions leading to decreased serum calcium level and tetany.

7. *Proper aseptic measures* must be taken during transfusion of blood.

8. *Careful watch on recipient's condition* is must for the first 10-15 minutes of starting the transfusion, and from time to time later.

CHAPTER 2.5

Integumentary System

The Skin

3.1

GENERAL CONSIDERATIONS
- Definition
- Surface area and thickness
- Colour of skin
- Skin surface ridges and grooves

STRUCTURE OF THE SKIN
- Epidermis
- Dermis

APPENDAGES OF SKIN
- Nails
- Hairs

- Sebaceous glands
- Sweat glands

FUNCTIONS OF SKIN

CLINICALLY APPLIED ASPECTS
- Skin burns
- Wound healing
- Pressure sores
- Skin infections
- Malignant tumours of skin

GENERAL CONSIDERATIONS

Definition

Skin refers to the outer or external covering of the body. In addition to providing complete covering to the body, the skin performs many other important functions, and therefore it is regarded as an important organ of the body. At the orifices the skin is continuous with the mucous membranes of the body.

Thickness and surface area of skin

Skin accounts for seven percent of the body weight. Its thickness varies from about 0.5 to 3 mm. The surface area of skin is about 1.5 to 2 (1.7) square metres in an adult. *Distribution of surface area.* For distribution of the surface area of the skin rule of nine can be followed. It is particularly used to assess the area of skin involved in burns. The rule of nine is as below (Fig. 3.1-1) :

- Head and neck : 9%
- Each upper limb : 9% (two limbs 18%)
- Front of trunk : 18%
- Back of trunk including buttocks : 18%

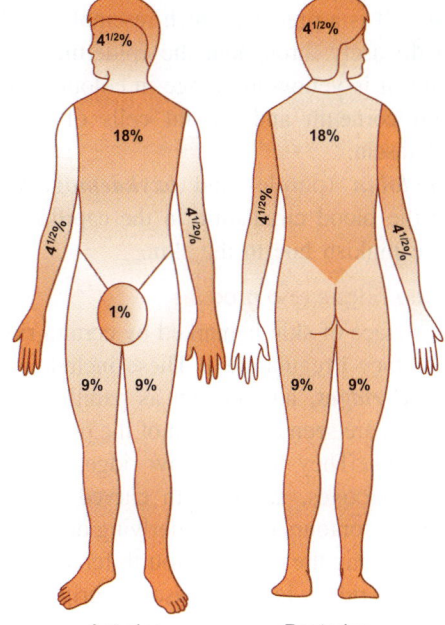

Anterior   Posterior

***Fig. 3.1-1.** Distribution of surface area.*

- Each lower limb : 18% (two limbs 36%)
- Perineum : 1%

Calculation of surface area. The surface area of an individual can be calculated by *Du Bois formula,* which is :

$$a = w \times h \times 71.84$$

where :

a = Surface area in square centimetres,

w = Weight in kilograms, and

h = Height in centimetres

Colour of skin

The colour of skin varies with the race, age, part of the body and exposure to sunlight. The determinants of skin colour are the pigments present at different levels and places in the skin. These include :

1. *Melanin.* The pigment melanin is brown in colour and present in the germinative zone of the epidermis. It is synthesized in cells called *melanocytes* located in the deep germinative layer.

The melanocytes synthesize melanin from the amino acid tyrosine in the presence of an enzyme called tyrosinase. On exposure to sunlight (ultraviolet radiations) both the amount and darkness of melanin produced is increased.

An inherited inability of an individual in any race to produce melanin results in the condition called *albinism.* In this condition the pigment is absent in skin, hairs and uveal tissue of the eyes.

2. *Melanoid.* It is a pigment which resembles melanin. It is present diffusely throughout the epidermis.

3. *Carotene.* It is yellow to orange in colour; is found in the stratum corneum and the fat cells of dermis and superficial fascia.

4. *Haemoglobin* (purple) and ***oxyhaemoglobin*** (red) present in the blood circulating in the capillaries of the dermis give pinkish hue to the skin.

Skin surface ridges and grooves

The outer surface of skin is marked by certain ridges and grooves (surface irregularities). These include :

1. *Epidermal ridges,* also known as papillary ridges or friction ridges, are seen on the skin of the palms and soles and their digits. They form narrow ridges separated by fine parallel grooves, arranged in curved arrays. They conform to the contours of the underlying dermal papillae and develop during the third and fourth fetal months. The function of the ridges is to increase the grip of the hand or foot by increasing friction.

The study of ridge pattern constitutes a branch of science, called *dermatographics.* The ridge pattern, which is determined genetically by multifactorial inheritance, is unique for each individual. It does not change throughout life, except to enlarge and this can serve as the basis for identification through fingerprints or footprints. The major patterns in the human finger-prints include loops, whorls and arches.

2. *Tension lines* are the epidermal grooves which form a network of linear furrows which divide the surface into polygonal or diamond-shaped area. These lines to some extent correspond to variations in the pattern of fibres in the dermis. These can be seen conspicuously on the dorsum of hand as an example.

3. *Flexor lines,* also known as *skin creases* or *skin joints,* are certain permanent epidermal grooves along which the skin folds during habitual movements (chiefly flexion) of the joints. The skin along these lines is thin and firmly bound to the deep fascia. The lines are prominent opposite the flexure of the joints, particularly on the palms, soles and digits.

STRUCTURE OF THE SKIN

The skin consists of two distinct layers (Fig. 3.1-2):

- Epidermis, and
- Dermis.

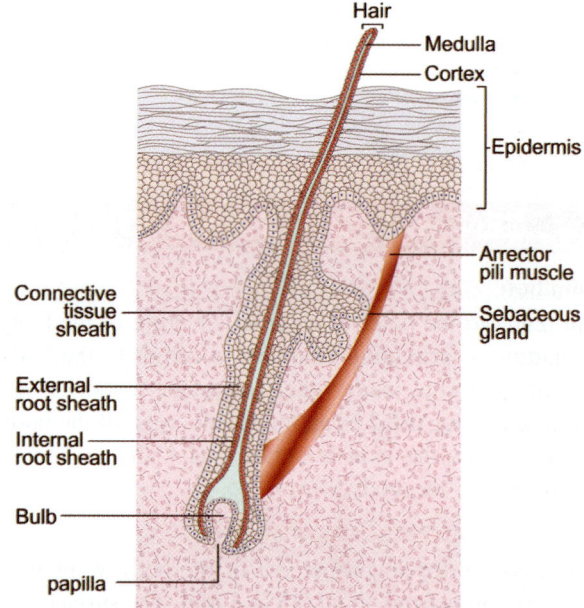

Fig. 3.1-2. *Structure of skin.*

EPIDERMIS

Epidermis is the most superficial avascular part of skin. It is composed of keratinized stratified squamous epithelium. It is ectodermal in origin and gives rise to appendages of the skin.

Thickness of epidermis

Thickness of epidermis varies in different parts of the body. It is thickest in the palms of hands and soles of the feet.

Layers of epidermis

The keratinized stratified squamous epithelium forming the epidermis is organized in four (in thin skin) or five (in thick skin) layers of cells. From the deepest to the most superficial these layer are :

1. Stratum basale or basal layer, also called as stratum germinativum or germinal layer or Malpighian layer is the deepest layer formed of single layer of cuboidal to columnar cells. These cells are capable of continued cell division. Thus, these cells proliferate and pass towards the surface to replace cornified cells lost due to wear and tear. As the cells migrate superficially, they become more and more flattened, and lose their nuclei.

The stratum basale also contains *melanocytes* (melanoblasts, dendritic cells, or clear cells) of neural crest origin, which synthesize melanin.

2. Stratum spinosum. This layer is formed of 4-8 layers of polyhedral cells (*kerationocytes)* with rounded central nucleus. Cells of this layer are connected to those of neighbouring cells by spine-like processes which are actually desmosomes, linking the adjacent cells tightly.

The stratum spinosum and stratum basale collective form the so-called *germinative zone* (the zone where new cells are germinated).

3. Stratum granulosum or granular cell layer consists of 2-4 layers of flattened, diamond-shaped cells with flat nuclei. The cytoplasm of these cells contains darkly stained keratohyalin granules, which give an overall darker appearance to this cell layer.

4. Stratum lucidum. This layer is well formed in thick non-hairy skin of palms and soles and is usually absent in thin hairy skin. When well formed it appears as a thin, clear, homogenous band between the stratum granulosum and stratum corneum. It consists of several rows of clear or flat, dead cells that contain droplets of a substance called eleidin This layer is named because eleidin is translucent (lucidum = clear). Eleidin is formed from keratohyalin and is eventually transformed to keratin.

5. Stratum corneum, also known as horny layer, is made up of several non-nucleated dead cells called squames in which the cytoplasm has been replaced by the fibrous protein keration. The squames are held together by a material containing lipids and carbohydrates. These cells are continuously shed and replaced. The stratum corneum is waterproof and serves as an effective barrier against light and heat waves, bacteria, and many chemicals.

Note : The stratum corneum, stratum lucidum, and stratum granulosum combinedly form the so-called *cornified zone.*

Cells in the epidermis

The cells present in the epidermis are :

1. Keratinocytes form about 85% of the cells and are responsible for regeneration of epidermal cells.

2. Melanocytes are present in the stratum basale and stratum spinosum of the epidermis. They produce melanin pigment which gives colour to the skin.

3. Langerhans cells. These are phagocytic macrophage cells present in the stratum spinosum layer of the epidermis. These play important role in protecting the skin against viral and other infections.

4. Merkel's cells. These are modified sensory receptor cells present mainly in the stratum basale.

Maintenance of epidermis

The healthy epidermis is maintained as a result of three synchronised processes :

- *Desquamation* (shedding) of the keratinised cells from the surface.
- *Effective keratinisation* of the cells approaching the surface.
- *Continual cell division* in the germinative zone with newly formed cells being pushed to the surface.

Source of nutrition

There are no blood vessels or nerve endings in the epidermis. The deeper layers of epidermis are bathed in interstitial fluid from the dermis which provides oxygen and nutrients, and is drained away as lymph.

DERMIS

Dermis or corium is the deep vascular layer of the skin. It is made up of connective tissue containing collagenous and elastic fibers mixed with blood vessels, lymphatics and nerves. It varies in thickness in different parts of the body, but is generally thicker than epidermis. The connective tissue forming dermis is arranged into a superficial papillary layer and a deep reticular layer (Fig. 3.1-2) :

1. Papillary layer of dermis is formed of loose areolar connective tissue containing fine collagenous, reticular and elastic tissue. This layer of connective tissue projects as dermal papillae which fit into the concavities on the undersurface of epidermis. Some dermal papillae contain *Meissner's tactile corpuscles* which are touch receptors.

2. Reticular layer of dermis is composed chiefly of dense connective tissue containing bundles of collagen and elastic fibres which form a network. Fibroblasts, macrophages and mast cells are the main cells found in dermis. Spaces between the fibres are occupied by a small quantity of adipose tissue, hair follicles, nerves, sebaceous glands, and ducts of the sweat glands. Varying thickness of reticular layer is responsible for differences in the thickness of skin.

The toughness and elasticity of the skin is due to combination of collagenous and elastic fibres in the reticular layer. Rupture of the elastic fibres occurs when the skin is overstretched, resulting in permanent *striae* or stretch marks, that may be found in pregnancy and obesity.

CHAPTER 3.1

Appendages of the skin refer to the structures developed from the embryonic epidermis. These include :
- Nails,
- Hairs,
- Sebaceous glands, and
- Sweat glands.

NAILS

Nails are hardened keratin plates (cornified zone) which make solid covering over the dorsal surfaces of the terminal portions of the fingers and toes.

Parts. Each nail has following parts (Fig. 3.1-3) :

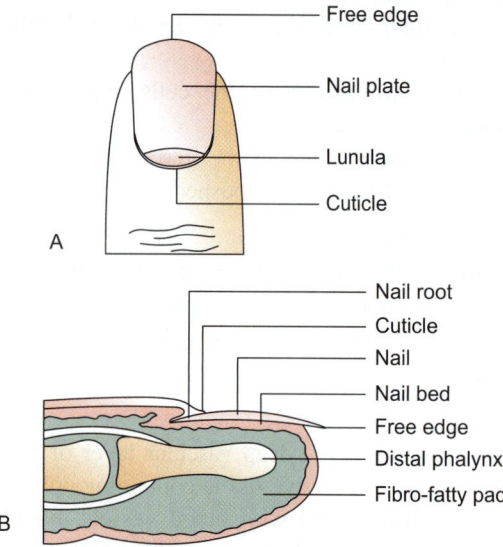

Fig. 3.1-3. *Structure of a nail : A, finger nail viewed from above; and B, cross-section of the finger nail and nail bed.*

- *Nail root* is the proximal hidden part which is buried into the nail groove and is overlapped by the nail fold of skin.
- *Free edge* is the part of the nail that projects beyond the distal end of digit.
- *Nail body* is the visible part of nail which is adherent to the underlying skin. The whitish crescentric area at the proximal end of the nail body is called *lunule*.

Skin surrounding the nail is named as below :
- *Nail fold* or nail wall refers to the fold of skin overlapping the proximal and lateral borders of the nail.
- *Nail bed* refers to the epidermis lying beneath the nail root and nail body. The germinative zone of the nail bed beneath the root and lunula is thick and proliferative (germinal matrix), and is responsible for the growth of the nail. The rest of nail bed is thin (sterile matrix) over which the growing nail glides.
- *Nail groove* refers to the furrow between the nail fold and nail bed.

Important facts about nails are :

- *Pinkish colour* of the nails is due to very vascular corium below the translucent nail bed. In anaemia the nails are pale and white.
- *Nail growth* is faster in summer than in winter, in the fingers than in toes, and in the longer fingers than in the shorter ones. It takes about 90-120 days for the whole nail (body) to grow.

HAIRS

Definition, distribution and development of hair

Definition and distribution. Hairs are keratinous filaments distributed all over the body except for the palms, soles, dorsal surface of distal phalanges, umbilicus, glans penis, inner surface of prepuce, the labia minora and inner surface of labia majora. The length, thickness and colour of the hairs vary in different parts of the body and in different individuals.

Development. The invaginations of the germinative layer of epidermis into the dermis occur by 3rd and 4th month of fetal life to form the *hair follicles* from which the hairs are derived.
- *Lanugo* (primary hairs) refer to the delicate hairs which cover the fetal skin by the 5th and 6th month. The lanugo are mostly shed by birth.
- *Vellus* (secondary hairs) are fine hairs which replace the lanugo during infancy. These are retained in most parts of the body except in hairy areas.
- *Terminal hair* are thick and dark hair which replace the vellus in the area of scalp, eyebrows and other hairy areas of adult skin.

Parts and structure of the hair proper

Parts of hair. Each hair consists of following parts:
- *Shaft* refers to the superficial portion, most of which projects above the surface of skin.
- *Root* is the embedded part of the hair that penetrates into the dermis and even into the subcutaneous tissue.

Microscopic structure of hair. Microscopically each hair consists of three layers :
- *Medulla* is the innermost part composed of rows of polyhedral cells containing granules of eleidin and air spaces.
- *Cortex* is the middle part which forms the major part of hair and consists of elongated cells that contain pigment granules in dark hairs, but mostly air in white hair.
- *Cuticle* is the outermost part which consists of a single layer of thin flat scale-like cells that are the most heavily keratinized.

Structures surrounding the hair

Hair follicle is the downgrowth of the epidermal cells into the dermis which surrounds the hair. The wall of hair follicle consists of three layers the inner root sheath, outer root sheath and connective tissue sheath. The hair follicle is expanded at its proximal end to form the *hair bulb.* Each hair bulb is invaginated at its end by the *hair papilla* (vascular connective tissue) which forms the neurovascular hilum of hair and its sheath. Hair grows at the hair bulb by proliferation of its cells capping the papilla.

Arrector pili is a smooth muscle supplied by sympathetic nerves that connects the undersurface of the follicles to the superficial papillary layer of the dermis. Contraction of this muscle erects the hair, depresses the adjacent skin forming goose skin and compresses the sebaceous glands, so as to expel its secretion.

SEBACEOUS GLANDS

Distribution. Sebaceous glands are widely distributed all over the dermis of skin except for the palms and soles. They are especially abundant in the scalp and face and are also very numerous around the apertures of nose, ear, mouth and anus.

Locations. Sebaceous glands associated with hair are situated in the angle between the hair follicle and the arrector pili muscle (Fig 3.1-2).

Structure. The sebaceous glands are simple or branched *alveolar glands* formed of secretory parts and excretory ducts.

- *Secretory part* of each gland is made up of a cluster of about 2-5 piriform alveoli.
- *Ducts* of the sebaceous glands open into the hair follicles, with the exception of lips, glans penis, inner surface of prepuce, labia minora, nipple and areola of the breast and tarsal glands of eyelids, where the ducts open on surface of skin.

Secretion of subaceous glands, known as *sebum,* is oily in nature. It keeps the hair soft and pliable and gives it a shiny appearance. On the skin it provides some waterproofing and acts as a bactericidal and fungicidal agent preventing the successful invasion of microbes. It also prevents drying and cracking of the skin. The secretion is under hormonal control especially the androgens.

SWEAT GLANDS

Sudreferous or sweat glands are distinguished into two principal types on the basis of structure and location. These are :
- Eccrine sweat glands, and
- Apocrine sweat glands.

Eccrine sweat glands

Distribution. Eccrine sweat glands are more abundant and distributed in almost every part of the skin except for the margins of lips, nail beds of fingers and toes, glans penis, glans clitoris, and ear drums. These glands are most numerous in the skin of palms and soles.

Structure. Each gland is a single tube having two parts:

- *Body* of the gland is highly coiled secretory part which lies in the deeper part of corium or in the subcutaneous tissue.
- *Duct* is the straight part of the gland which traverses the dermis and epidermis and opens on the surface of skin.

Nervous control. The eccrine sweat glands are supplied and controlled by cholinergic sympathetic nerves.

Secretion. The eccrine sweat glands are *merocrine* in nature i.e. they produce their thin watery secretion without any disintegration of epithelial cells.

Function. The glands help in regulation of the body temperature by evaporation of sweat and also help in excreting the body salt.

Apocrine glands

Distribution. Apocrine glands are distributed primarily to the skin of the axilla, eyelids (Moll's glands), pubic region, and areola of the breasts. Ceruminous glands of the external auditory meatus are modified apocrine sweat glands.

Structure. These are simple branched tubular glands. The secretory portion of the glands is located in the dermis and excretory duct opens into the hair follicle.

Secretion. Apocrine glands begin to function at puberty and produce a more viscous secretion having a characteristic odour.

Nervous control. The apocrine glands are also merocrine in nature, but are regulated by a dual autonomic control.

Function. They do not respond sufficiently to temperature changes as do eccrine glands. Therefore, some workers are not inclined to call them sweat glands. In animals they produce chemical signals pheromones, which are important in courtship and social behaviour.

FUNCTIONS OF SKIN

1. *Protective function.* Skin performs protective function for the body structures by following mech-anisms:
- *Mechanical protection.* The skin provides mechanical protection to underlying tissues. For this function skin is thickest over area exposed to greatest friction.
- *Physical barrier.* Due to keratinized stratum corneum the skin forms a relatively waterproof layer and acts as barrier against microbial invasion, chemicals (acids and alkalies), wet and draught, hot and cold and mechanical injuries.
- *Immune mechanism.* Specialised immune cells called Langerhans cells are present in the dermis. These cells phagocytose the antigen entering the skin and present it to the T-lymphocytes in the lymphoid tissue. In this way an immune response is stimulated.
- *Reflex action.* The sensory nerve endings present in the skin initiate the reflex action against any unpleasant or

painful stimuli. As a result the body protects itself from further damage.

- *Absorption of ultraviolet rays.* The melanin and thick first layer of epidermis absorb ultraviolet rays of the sun and thus prevent the skin from getting ultraviolet radiation injury.

2. Regulation of body temperature is an important function performed by the skin. Heat is lost through evaporation of sweat; and heat is conserved by the fat and hair.

3. Sensory function. Skin contains nerve endings and receptors sensitive to touch, pain and temperature which play an important role in the sensory perception.

4. Absorptive function. Though skin forms a relatively waterproof barrier, the oily substances are freely absorbed by the skin. Some drugs are administrated as transdermal patches e.g. hormones used as replacement therapy in postmenopausal women, anti-inflammatory drugs such as diclophenac sodium patch, and nicotine patch as an aid to stopping smoking.

5. Secretory functions. Skin secretes sweat and sebum.

6. Excretory function. Skin also acts as an excretory organ or it helps in eliminating excess of water, salts and waste products like urea (especially when kidney function is impaired) through sweat.

7. Synthesis. In the skin vitamin D is synthesized from ergosterol by the action of ultraviolet rays of sun.

8. Regulation of pH. Skin plays a role in the regulation of body pH. A good amount of acid is excreted through the sweat.

9. Role in maintaining water balance. The epidermis is such a membrane that it does not allow water to pass in and out. The importance of this function is seen in persons who have lost extensive areas of skin through burns. One important cause of death in such cases is water loss from the body.

CLINICALLY APPLIED ASPECTS

WOUND HEALING

The most frequently injured tissue of the body is skin. The skin wounds heal well, as it has got an excellent power of regeneration.

Factors affecting wound healing

1. Systemic factors which reduce the rate of wound healing are :
- Impaired immunity,
- Poor nutritional status,
- Anaemias,
- Chronic debilitating diseases,
- Diabetes mellitus,

- Systemic infections, and
- Old age.

2. Local factors which delay wound healing are :
- Uneven wounds,
- Contaminated wounds,
- Infected wounds, and
- Poor blood supply to the region.

Types of wound healing

Depending upon the type of wound and prevailing local and systemic factors wound healing is of two types :
- Primary wound healing, and
- Secondary wound healing.

1. Primary wound healing

Factors favouring primary wound healing. The primary wound healing, also known as healing by first intention, occurs under following circumstances:
- When cut edges are sharp and clean and can be brought together,
- Wound is not contaminated by foreign bodies or toxic materials,
- Wound is not infected,
- Immunity is not impaired, and
- Blood supply to the area is good.

Stages of primary healing :

1. *Stage of inflammation.* Immediately after injury the gap between the cut edges is filled with blood clot and the cut surface of skin become inflamed.
- Phagocytes (from the blood and connective tissue) migrate into the wound and start engulfing and removing the dead tissue including the clot.
- Fibroblasts also migrate to the wound and start multiplying rapidly. These cells secrete collagen fibres which begin to bind the cut surfaces together.
2. *Stage of proliferation* or stage of granulation tissue formation involves following events :
- Proliferation of new capillaries, fibroblasts, and connective tissue leads to formation of granulation tissue which fills the gap.
- Proliferation of epithelial cells covers the surface of wound.
- Clot above the new tissue becomes scab and separates after 3 to 10 days.
3. *Stage of maturation.* In this stage the collagen laid down by fibroblasts matures with tissue and firmly binds the tissues. The granulation time is slowly replaced by the fibrous tissue scar. Over the time the scar becomes less vascular and the area is restored to a more or less normal condition with fine clean scar left behind.

2. Secondary wound healing

Factors responsible for secondary wound healing. The

secondary wound healing or healing by second intention occurs under following situations :

- When distruction is much and some tissue is lost.
- When the cut surfaces cannot be brought together.
- When the wound is infected.

Stages of wound healing by second intention :

1. *Stage of inflammation.* The wound area shows dead and necrotic tissue (slough). Inflammatory process sets in on the surface of healthy tissue below the necrotic tissue. Slowly the dead tissue is removed by the phagocytes. This stage lasts long.
2. *Stage of proliferation* or stage of granulation tissue formation involves following events :

- Proliferation of new capillaries, fibroblasts and connective tissue leads to formation of granulation tissue at the base of cavity.
- Slowly the granulation starts filling the cavity and grows towards the surface over the time.
- Contraction of collagen tissue laid down by fibroblasts reduces the wound size.
- When the wound is filled with granulation upto the level of dermis, epithelial cells at the edges proliferate and cover the surface restoring continuity.

3. *Stage of maturation.* Gradually the granulation tissue is replaced by thick fibrous tissue over several months. The scar formed in healing by second intention is very thick, dense, shiny and does not contain sweat glands, hair follicles or sebaceous gland.

SKIN BURNS

Burns refer to the injury caused to skin and other body tissue by heat, electricity, ionizing radiations, strong chemicals. Thus skin burns may be :

- Thermal burns,
- Electric burns,
- Radiational burns, and
- Chemical burns (caused by acids and alkalies).

Scalds refer to the burns caused by hot fluids.

Types of burns. Depending upon the depth of burnt area, the burns may be :

- *First-degree burns or partial thickness or superficial burns,* when only the epidermis is involved. Symptoms include localized redness, swelling and pain.
- *Second-degree burns,* when epidermis and upper region of dermis is also involved. Symptoms mimic first-degree burns, but blisters also appear.
- *Third-degree or full thickness (deep) burns* involve entire thickness of skin. Burned area appears grey-white, cherry red or black. There is no initial oedema. These burns are relatively less painful as the sensory nerve endings in the dermis are destroyed. After a few days, the damaged tissue coagulates and forms in eschar, or thick scab, which sloughs off after 2 to 3 weeks.

Estimation of extent of burns in adults is made following the 'rule-of-nine' as described earlier (see page 79, Fig. 3.1-1).

Estimation of severity of burns. Burns are *considered critical* if :

- Over 25% of the body has second-degree burns, or
- Over 10% of the body has third-degree burns, or
- Third-degree burns involve face, hands and feet.

Hypovolamic shock usually develops in adults when 15% of the surface area is burnt.

Fatality is likely in adults with full thickness burns when the total of patient's age and the surface area affected is greater than 80.

PRESSURE SORES

Pressure sores or bed sores, also known as decubitus ulcer, refer to the area of sloughing of skin which occur over the pressure areas where the skin is compressed for long periods between the bony prominences and a hard surface.

Predisposing factors for pressure sores. Pressures sores occur when the patient lies over the bed for a prolonged period without moving the body parts as occurs is :

- Paralysed patients,
- Patients having multiple limb fractures,
- Old debilitated patients, and
- Comatosed patients.

Occurrence of bed sores in such patients is precipitated by moisture, infection, poor nutritional status, sensory impairment and poor circulation.

SKIN INFECTIONS

Common skin infections are :

1. **Viral infections.** These include :

- *Warts and veruccas* are caused by human papilloma virus (HPV). These present as small firm growths on the hands, face and soles of the feet.
- *Chickenpox and shingles* are caused by zoster virus.
- *Cold sores (herpes labialis) and genital herpes* are caused by herpes simplex virus type I and type II, respectively.

2. **Bacterial infections** of skin of common occurrence are:

- *Impetigo* is a highly infectious condition manifesting as superficial skin pustules usually around the nose and mouth. Common causative bacteria are *Staphylococcus aureus* and *Streptococcus pyogenes*.
- *Cellulitis* is a diffuse infection of the skin and subcutaneous tissue. The causative bacteria enter the body through a break in the skin and these include *Streptococcus pyogenes* or *Clostridium perfringens*. If untreated, it may be complicated by necrotising fascitis or even septicaemia.
- *Acne vulgaris* is characterized by pustule formation on the face in adolescents. Basically it occurs due to

infection in the blocked sebaceous glands in hair follicle. Increased level of male sex hormones during puberty are implicated in the etiology.

3. *Fungal infections* of skin which need to be mentioned here are :

- *Candidiasis* is an intertriginous infection affecting submammary folds, axillae and digital clefts. It is a common cause of vulvovaginitis in females.
- *Pityriasis versicolor.* It is characterised by small confluent scaly depigmented patches.
- *Dermatophytosis* (ringworm infection). The lesions are red, scaly and itchy. The groin and feet (tinea pedis) are common sites.

MALIGNANT TUMOURS OF SKIN

Common malignant tumours of the skin are :

1. *Basal cell carcinoma.* It is the commonest malignant tumour of skin. It is locally invasive but seldom metastasises. It most commonly involves skin of face and head and neck area, i.e., the most sun-exposed sites. It starts as small nodule which undergoes central ulceration with pearly rolled margins. The tumour grows by burrowing and destroying the tissues locally like a rodent and hence the name rodent ulcer.

2. *Squamous cell carcinoma.* It commonly arises from the mucocutaneous junctions in the body such as lid margin, lips, penis, etc. Its incidence is much less than the basal cell carcinoma. It commonly presents as an ulcerated growth with elevated and indurated margins. It metastasises in the lymph nodes.

3. *Malignant melanoma.* It is a rare tumour that may arise from a pre-existing naevus, or denovo from the melanocytes present in the skin.

Clinically, it often appears as a flat or slightly elevated naevus which has varigated pigmentation and irregular borders. It may ulcerate and bleed.

Metastasis. The tumour spreads locally as well as to distant sites by lymphatics and blood stream.

4. *Sebaceous gland carcinoma.* It is a rare tumour arising from the sebaceous glands of skin. In the eyelids it arises from the meibomian glands (modified sebaceous glands). Clinically it presents on a nodular swelling.

INTRODUCTION

Fascia has been described along with skin in this section, because like skin it also forms a covering around the body structures. Fascia is a sheet/band of fibrofatty tissue that lies deep to the skin and invests muscles and other deep structures. In reality, it is a packing material; a connective tissue that remains between areas of more specialized tissue. It varies widely in structure and thickness according to the functional requirements. The fascia is classified into:

- Superficial fascia, and
- Deep fascia

SUPERFICIAL FASCIA

Superficial fascia is also known as hypodermis or subcutaneous tissue or tela subcutanea. It is a general coating of the body beneath the skin, comprising of loose areolar tissue with varying amount of fat.

Distribution and special features

Superficial fascia is widely distributed below the skin in the body (Fig. 3.2-1). It has some special features in different regions of the body.

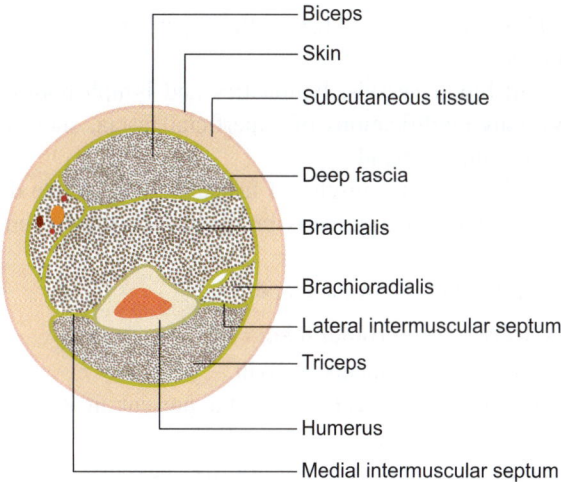

Biceps
Skin
Subcutaneous tissue
Deep fascia
Brachialis
Brachioradialis
Lateral intermuscular septum
Triceps
Humerus
Medial intermuscular septum

Fig. 3.2-1. *Cross-section of an arm showing the arrangement of superficial and deep fascia.*

- *Most distinct areas.* Superficial fascia is most distinct in the lower part of the anterior abdominal wall, perineum, and the limbs.
- *Very thin* superficial fascia is seen over dorsal aspect of hands and feet, sides of neck and around the anus.

- *Very dense* superficial fascia is seen in the scalp, palms and soles.
- *Stratification* of superficial fascia (into two layers) occurs in the lower part of anterior abdominal wall, perineum and uppermost small part of the thighs.

Fat of superficial fascia

Fat is most important constituent of the superficial fascia. The subcutaneous layer of fat is called *panniculus adiposus.* This acts as a barrier to the heat loss from the body and is responsible for the shape and contours of the body. Some features of the distribution of fat in the body are as below :

Males versus females. In females, fat is more abundant, more evenly distributed and forms a thicker layer than in males. In females fat is in the superficial fascia of lower abdomen and upper thighs, whereas in males it is inside the abdominal cavity.

Areas of the body with excessive fat. Fat is abundant in the gluteal region (buttocks), lumbar region (flanks), front of thighs, anterior abdominal wall below the umbilicus, mammary gland, postdeltoid region, and the cervicothoracic region.

Area of the body with no fat. Fat is absent from the eyelids, external ear, penis, scrotum, labia minora, clitoris and nipples.

Contents of superficial fascia

In addition to fibrofatty tissue, the superficial fascia also contains :

- Small blood vessels, lymphatics and lymph nodes.
- Various modifications of superficial fascia, such as:
  - Mammary gland
  - Subcutaneous muscles of fascia, which include dartos, platysma, palmaris brevis and corrugator cutis ani.
- Deeply situated sweat glands.

Functions of superficial fascia

- Facilitates movements of skin.
- Conserves body heat, as the fat present in it is bad conductor of heat.
- Serves as a soft medium for the passage of blood vessels and nerves to the skin.

DEEP FASCIA

Deep fascia is a fibrous sheet which invests the body beneath the superficial fascia. In other words, it is dense, inelastic and tough membrane which separates superficial fascia from the underlying deeper structures. It is devoid of fat.

Distribution and arrangement

Deep fascia is widely distributed in the body. Some features about distribution and arrangement of deep fascia in the body are as below :

Best versus ill-defined areas of deep fascia :

- It is *best defined* in the limbs where it forms tough and tight sleeves. In the iliotibial tract of fascia lata it is specially well developed.
- In the neck the deep fascia is *well developed* and forms a collar.
- Over rectus sheath and external oblique aponeurosis of abdominal wall it is *quite thin* and barely demonstrable.
- It is *absent* in the area of face and ischiorectal region.

Extensions (prolongations) from deep fascia run along various body structures such as muscles, nerves, vessels. These are described in detail under modifications of deep fascia.

Arrangement of deep fascia vis-a-vis superficial fascia in the body is depicted in a cross-section of an arm (Fig. 3.2-1).

Modification of deep fascia

Deep fascia is modified in different areas to serve special functions. Some of the important modifications of deep fascia are summarized below :

Modifications of deep fascia in relation to muscles are (Figs. 3.2-1 and 3.2-2) :

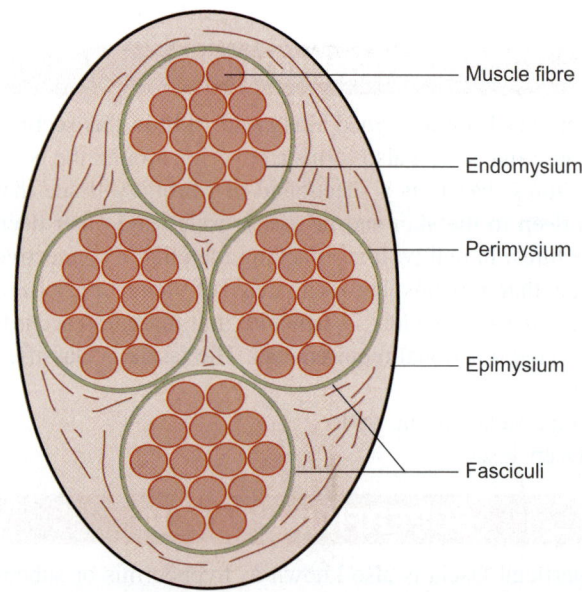

	Muscle fibre
	Endomysium
	Perimysium
	Epimysium
	Fasciculi

Fig. 3.2-2. *Transverse section of skeletal muscle showing arrangement of epimysium, perimysium and endomysium.*

- *Intermuscular septa* are the extensions from the deep fascia which envelop the functionally different group of muscles into separate compartments (Fig. 3.2-1).
- *Epimysium* refers to the extension of deep fascia which arises from the intermuscular septum and surrounds the single muscle belly (Fig. 3.2-2).

- *Perimysium* refers to sheath of connective tissue which extends from the epimysium which encloses each muscle fasciculus. Fasciculi are bundles of muscle fibres which form a muscle (Fig. 3.2-2).
- *Endomysium* is the extension from the perimysium which surrounds each muscle fibres (Fig. 3.2-2).

Modification of deep fascia in relation to blood vessels. Deep fascia forms *perivascular sheaths* around large arteries and veins. Examples include carotid sheath, axillary sheath and femoral sheath. The perivascular sheath around the arteries is dense and rather loose around the veins to give an allowance for the vein to distend.

Modifications of deep fascia in relation to nerves are as follows :
- *Epineurium* refers to deep fascia covering around each nerve.
- *Perineurium* is the covering around each nerve fasciculus.
- *Endoneurium* refers to the fascial covering around each nerve fibre.

These connective tissue coverings support the nerve fibres and carry capillaries and lymphatics.

Modifications in deep fascia in relation to joints include:
- *Synovial membrane, capsule and bursa* are modified forms of deep fascia in relation to most of the joints.
- *Tendon sheaths and associated bursae* are the modifications of deep fascia which prevent wear and tear of the tendons and minimize friction.
- *Retinaculae* refer to thickened bands of deep fascia in relation to some joints, e.g., wrist and ankle (Fig. 3.2-3). The retinacula act as pulley during the movements of joints and also keep tendons in position.

Modification in relation to palms and soles. In the region of palm and sole deep fascia is modified to form *aponeurosis*, e.g., palmar and plantar aponeurosis which

protect the underlying structures, e.g., nerves, blood vessels and delicate tendons.

Modifications in relation to bones are :
- Deep fascia becomes continuous with the *periosteum in bare bones.*
- *Interosseous membrane* refers to the modified deep fascia present in between the two bones of forearms and legs. This membrane keeps the two bones at optimum distance and increases surface area for attachment of muscles.

Modification in relation to neck. In the neck area the deep fascia is very well developed and forms an investing layer called collar which gives the neck a proper shape.

Functions of deep fascia

- *Keeps in position* the underlying structures.
- *Preserves* the characteristic surface contour of the limbs.
- *Provides extra surface* for attachment of muscles.
- *Helps in venous and lymphatic return.* The contraction of calf muscles in the tight sleeve of deep fascia helps in pushing the venous blood and lymph towards heart.
- *Assists muscles in their action* by the degree of tension and pressure it exerts upon their surfaces.
- *Prevents the loss of power.* Modification of deep fascia in the form of retinacula (as mentioned earlier) act as pulley and serves to prevent the loss of power. In such situations the friction is minimized by the synovial sheaths of the tendons.

CLINICALLY APPLIED ASPECTS

- *Surgical plane to drain pus from the deeper tissues* is helped by knowledge of applied anatomy. A deeply accumulated pus often tends to track down from its primary site to a more dependent part of the body. The course taken by the pus is determined by the fascial planes and neurovascular bundles.
- *Oedema* or collection of fluid in the legs can develop following damage to fascia of leg, as it can affect the venous return leading to accumulation of blood and fluid.
- *Dupuytren's contracture* refers to the contraction of palmar fascia leading to flexion deformity of fingers. The condition is most frequent in middle-aged males. The exact cause of this condition is not known. It is characterized by painless progressive thickening of palmar aponeurosis leading to bending of 4th and 5th fingers into the palm. Extension of the involved finger becomes difficult. The condition begins unilateraly but soon becomes bilateral.

Extensor tendons and their synovial sheaths

Extensor retinaculum

Fig. 3.2-3. *Extensor retinaculum of wrist.*

Skeletal System

The Human Skeleton

4.1

INTRODUCTION

The skeleton forms the main supporting framework of the body, and is primarily designed for a more effective production of movements by the attached muscles. A familiarity with the names, shapes and positions of individual bones will be very useful in understanding the regional anatomy of the body and functioning of the other organ systems.

Divisions of human skeleton

The human skeleton can be grouped into two principal divisions :
- Axial skeleton, and
- Appendicular skeleton.

A total of 206 bones constitute the adult human skeleton, of these 80 bones form the axial skeleton and 126 bones form the appendicular skeleton (Table 4.1-1 and Fig. 4.1-1).

AXIAL SKELETON

The axial skeleton consists of the bones that lie around the axis of body (a straight line that runs vertically along the body's centre of gravity). These include (Fig. 4.1-1) :
- The skull,
- The hyoid bone,
- The vertebral column,
- Sternum or breast bone, and
- Ribs.

Anterior view

Cranium
Clavicle
Scapula
Sternum
Humerus
Ribs
Pelvis
Ulna
Radius
Carpal bones
Metacarpal bones
Phalanges
Femur
Patella
Tibia
Fibula
Tarsal bones
Metatarsal bones
Phalanges

Lateral view

Cranium
Cervical vertebrae
Scapula
Ribs
Thoracic vertebrae
Lumbar vertebrae
Pelvis
Sacrum
Coccyx
Femur
Patella
Tibia
Fibula
Calcaneus
Metatarsal bones
Phalanges

Fig. 4.1-1. *The human skeleton.*

THE SKULL

The skull, including the mandible, is a highly modified region of the axial skeleton. The skull is composed of a large number of separate bones which are united by sutures (fibrous immovable joints). The skull can be divided into two parts : cranium and facial skeleton.

CRANIUM

The cranium is the upper bowl-shaped part of the skull which contains the brain. The cranium consists of eight bones (two parietal, two temporal, and one each the occipital, frontal, sphenoid, and ethmoid bone) which are described briefly (Figs. 4.1-2 and 4.1-3) :

Parietal bones

The paired parietal bones form the roof and sides of the cranium (Fig. 4.1-2). They articulate with each other at the midline in the sagittal suture, with the occipital bone posteriorly in the lambdoid suture, and with the frontal bone anteriorly at the coronal suture. The parietal bone articulates inferiorly with the temporal bone and the greater wing of the sphenoid bone.

Table 4.1-1. Bones forming the axial and appendicular divisions of skeleton system

Regions of skeleton	Number of bones
AXIAL SKELETON	
Skull	
Cranium	8
Face	14
Hyoid	1
Auditory ossicles (3 in each ear)	6
Vertebral column	26
Thorax	
Sternum	1
Ribs	24
Total	**80**
APPENDICULAR SKELETON	
Pectoral (shoulder) girdles	
Clavicle	2
Scapula	2
Upper extremities	
Humerus	2
Ulna	2
Radius	2
Carpals	16
Metacarpals	10
Phalanges	28
Pelvic (hip) girdle	
Coxal, pelvic, or hip bone	2
Lower extremities	
Femur	2
Fibula	2
Tibia	2
Patella	2
Tarsals	14
Metatarsals	10
Phalanges	28
Total	**126**
Total bones in human skeleton : 80 + 126 = 206	

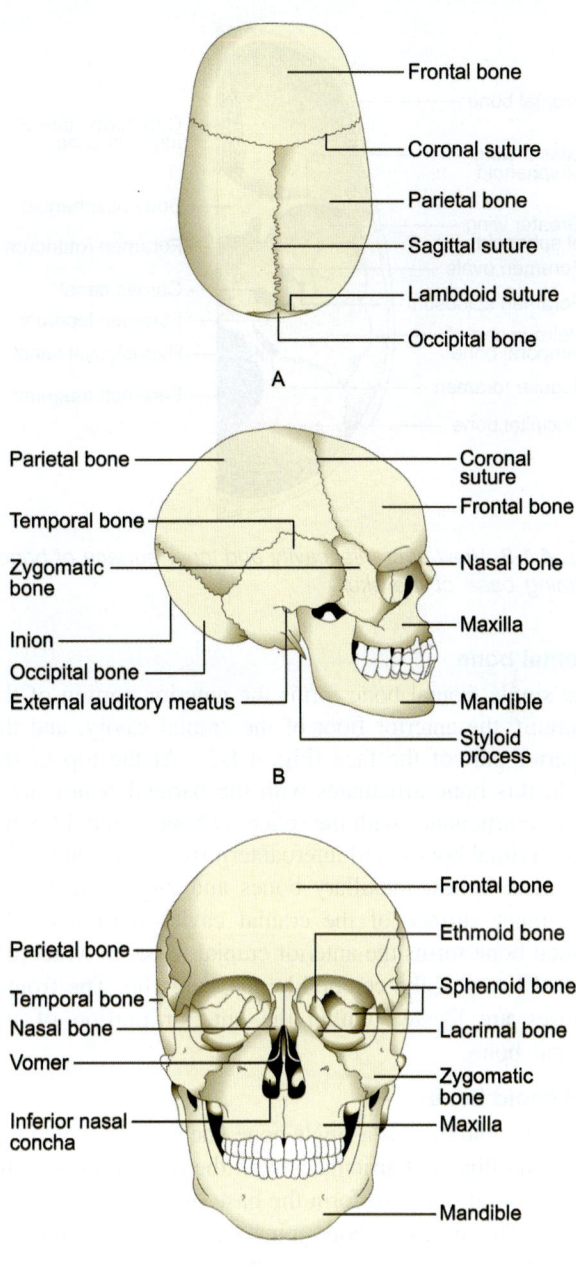

Fig. 4.1-2. *Bones of skull : A, superior view of cranium; B, lateral view of skull; and C, anterior view.*

Occipital bone

The occipital bone forms the posterior aspect of the skull and the posterior floor of the cranial cavity. A prominence, the external occipital protuberance, or inion, is found on the external surface at the posterior midline (Fig. 4.1-2). The large foramen magnum is found in the inferior aspect of the occipital bone. The inner surface of the bone forms the posterior cranial fossa in which there are depressions in which the cerebellum, pons, and medulla oblongata lie. Fig. 4.1-3 shows the inner aspect of the cranial floor. The occipital bone articulates with the temporal bones, the parietal bones, and the sphenoid bone.

Temporal bones

Each of the temporal bones is composed of two portions: a large, flat plate, the squamous portion; and a thickened, wedge-shaped area, the petrous portion. The squamous portion forms the side of cranium and articulates with the parietal bone and the sphenoid bone. An anterior projection, the zygomatic process, articulates with the zygomatic bone (Fig. 4.1-2). The petrous portion extends within the cranium and houses the midline and inner ear structures. The mastoid process and styloid process project from the inferior aspect, and between these two is located the stylomastoid foramen, through which the facial nerve exits the skull. The petrous portion articulates with the occipital bone in the floor of the skull. The carotid canal runs superiorly and anteriorly through the petrous portion and provides entrance for the internal carotid artery into the cranial cavity.

CHAPTER 4.1

SECTION 4

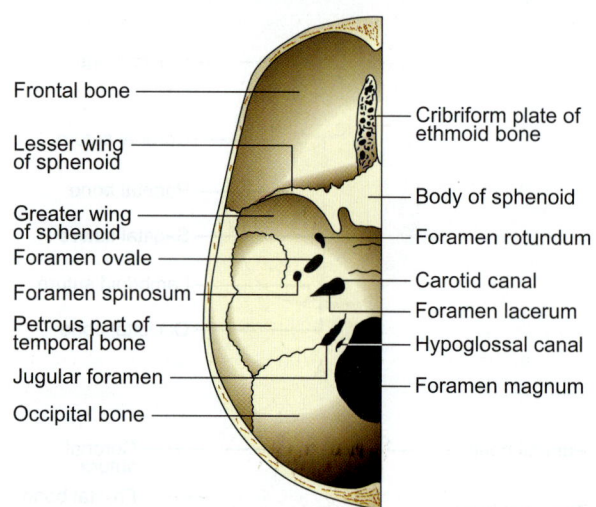

Frontal bone

Lesser wing
of sphenoid

Greater wing
of sphenoid

Foramen ovale

Foramen spinosum

Petrous part of
temporal bone

Jugular foramen

Occipital bone

Cribriform plate of
ethmoid bone

Body of sphenoid

Foramen rotundum

Carotid canal

Foramen lacerum

Hypoglossal canal

Foramen magnum

Fig. 4.1-3. *View of cranial cavity and inner surface of bones forming base of the skull.*

Frontal bone

The single frontal bone forms the anterior portion of the cranium, the anterior floor of the cranial cavity, and the superior part of the face (Fig. 4.1-2). At the top of the skull, this bone articulates with the parietal bones; inferiorly it articulates with the sphenoid bone, ethmoid bone, and lacrimal bones; and inferoanteriorly it articulates with the nasal bones, maxillary bones and zygomatic bones. The inner surface of the cranial cavity portion of the frontal bone forms the anterior cranial fossa, in which the frontal lobes of the cerebral hemispheres lie. The frontal sinuses are located within the anterior portion of the frontal bone.

Sphenoid bone

The sphenoid bone is a single bone, the body of which lies in the midline and articulates with the occipital bone and the temporal bones to form the base of the cranium (Fig. 4.1-3). The sphenoid bone joins the zygomatic bones to form the lateral walls of the orbits. Anteriorly and inferiorly, the sphenoid bone articulates with the maxillary and the palatine bones, superiorly with the parietal bones, and anteriorly and superiorly with the ethmoid and frontal bones. The depression on the superior cranial surface of the body of the sphenoid bone, the hypophyseal fossa (or the sella turcica), houses the pituitary gland; a portion of the body is hollow, forming the sphenoid sinus cavity.

Two pairs of wings project from the body of the sphenoid bone. The lesser wings project from the anterior aspect of the body and are more superior and smaller than the greater wings (Fig. 4.1-3). They are attached to the body by two small roots, and it is the gap between the two roots that forms the optic foramen or canal through which the optic nerve exits the orbit. The lesser wings articulate with the frontal and ethmoid bones.

The greater wings project from the lateral aspects of the body and articulate with the frontal bone, the parietal bones, the squamous portions of the temporal bones, and the zygomatic bones. The pterygoid process projects from the base of the greater wing and articulates with the vertical stem of the palatine bones; each contributes to a shallow depression, the pterygopalatine fossa. Three important foramina are located in the greater wing (Fig. 4.1-3) : the foramen rotundum, through which the maxillary nerve passes; the foramen ovale, through which the mandibular nerve passes; and the foramen spinosum, through which the middle meningeal artery passes.

Ethmoid bone

The single ethmoid bone resembles a rectangular box that contains a midline perpendicular plate. This plate bisects the top of the box, the horizontal cribriform plate, which is perforated for the passage of the olfactory nerves. The sides of the box parallel to the perpendicular plate are the orbital plates and are separated from the perpendicular plate by the ethmoid air cells. The ethmoid bone articulates with the sphenoid and frontal bones superiorly and with the vomer inferiorly; the orbital plates also articulate with the maxillary and lacrimal bones.

FACIAL SKELETON

The lower part of the skull is described as the facial skeleton or the *viscerocranium*. It concists of 14 bones, of which only two are single (Fig. 4.1-2.

The single frontal bone forms the forehead and articulates with the nasal bones, the maxillae, and the zygomatic bones in the formation of the face. The sutures joining adjacent bones of the face are generally named according to the names of the two bones that are connected (e.g. the suture between the frontal arches—Fig. 4.1-2). They also articulate with the maxillary bones and with the greater wings of the sphenoid bone.

Mandible

The mandible forms the movable lower jaw. It is a horseshoe-shaped bone consisting of a curved horizontal body and two perpendicular processes, the rami.

CAVITIES OF THE SKULL

The skull contains multiple cavities which reflect its multiple functions :

- *Cranial cavity.* It houses, supports and protects the brain.
- *Nasal cavity.* It is concerned with respiration and olfaction.
- *Oral cavity.* It is the first part of the gastrointestinal tract responsible for mastication and initial food processing, and houses taste receptors.
- *Orbits.* The orbits contain the eyes and other related structures and are described in detail later.

CRANIAL CAVITY

The cranial cavity houses the brain and its meninges and their associated vessels in addition to the intracranial portions of the cranial nerves. The base of the cranial cavity can be subdivided into three fossae : anterior, middle, and posterior (Fig. 4.1-3).

Anterior cranial fossa

The anterior cranial fossa is limited in front and laterally by the frontal bone and posteriorly by the lesser wing of the sphenoid. Its floor is formed by the orbital plate of the frontal bone, the cribriform plate of the ethmoid (with a median crest-like ridge, the crista galli which forms the anterior attachment of falx cerebri), and the lesser wings and anterior part of the body (jugum) of the sphenoid.

Middle cranial fossa

The middle cranial fossa lies at a lower plane than the anterior cranial fossa but is higher than the posterior cranial fossa. Its floor is shaped like a butterfly, namely it consists of a narrow central or median part and expanded lateral parts (wings). It is bound anteriorly by the posterior free edge of the lesser wing of the sphenoid, the anterior clinoid processes and the anterior margin of the sulcus chiasmatis. Posteriorly, it extends to the superior borders of the petrous temporal bones and dorsum sellae of the sphenoid and laterally it is bound by the squamous part of the temporal bone, part of the parietal bones, and the greater wings of the sphenoid.

Posterior cranial fossa

This is the deepest of the three cranial fossae, its floor lying below the level of the middle fossa. Its roof is formed by the tentorium cerebelli. It lodges the hindbrain, the cerebellum, pons, and medulla oblongata. The fossa is bound anteriorly by the superior border of the petrous temporal bone and the dorsum sella, and surrounds the foramen magnum, the cerebellum being housed in the cerebellar fossae on the squamous part of the occipital bone.

Pituitary fossa

The pituitary fossa (hypophyseal fossa) is an indentation in the roof of the body of the sphenoid bone in the middle cranial fossa. It is bound anteriorly by the tuberculum sellae, in front of which lies the sulcus chiasmatica, and posteriorly by the dorsum sellae, a ridge of the bone at either end of which lie the posterior clinoid processes. The pituitary fossa houses the pituitary gland or hypophysis cerebri.

ORBITS

The bony orbits are quadrangular truncated pyramids situated between the anterior cranial fossa above and the maxillary sinuses below (Fig. 4.1-4). Each orbit is formed by portions of seven bones : (1) frontal, (2) maxilla, (3) zygomatic, (4) sphenoid, (5) palatine, (6) ethmoid, and (7) lacrimal. It has four walls (medial, lateral, superior and inferior), base and an apex.

The medial walls of two orbits are parallel to each other and, being thinnest, are frequently fractured during injuries.

The inferior orbital wall (floor) is triangular in shape and is quite thin.

Frontal bone

Greater wing of sphenoid

Zygomatic bone

Maxillary sinus

Vomer

Maxilla

Crista galli

Cribriform plate

Cavity of orbit

Superior nasal concha

Middle nasal concha

Perpendicular plate

Inferior nasal concha

Palate

***Fig. 4.1-4.** Schematic coronal section through orbit and nasal cavity.*

The lateral wall of the orbit is triangular in shape. It covers only posterior half of the eyeball.

The roof is triangular in shape and is formed mainly by the orbital plate of frontal bone.

Base of the orbit is the anterior open end of the orbit. It is bounded by thick orbital margins.

The orbital apex. It is the posterior end of orbit. Here the four orbital walls converge. It has two orifices, the *optic canal* which transmits optic nerve and ophthalmic artery and the *superior orbital fissure* which transmits a number of nerves, arteries and veins.

Contents of the orbit

The *volume* of each orbit is about 30 cc. Approximately one-fifth of it is occupied by the eyeball. Other contents of the orbit include part of optic nerve, extraocular muscles, lacrimal gland, lacrimal sac, ophthalmic artery and its branches, third, fourth and sixth cranial nerves and ophthalmic and maxillary divisions of the fifth cranial nerve, sympathetic nerve, orbital fat and fascia.

PARANASAL SINUSES

Anatomically, the orbital cavity is bounded on three sides by the air-containing cavities - the paranasal sinuses also called paraorbital sinuses (Figs. 4.1-5A and 4.1-5B). The paranasal sinuses are four on each side. These are :

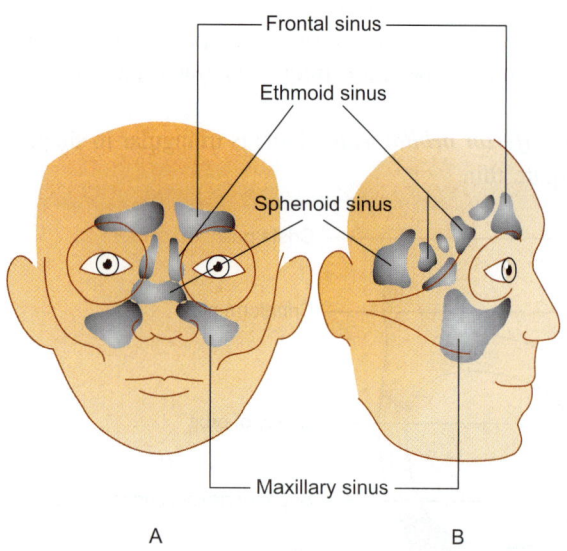

Frontal sinus
Ethmoid sinus
Sphenoid sinus
Maxillary sinus

A   B

Fig. 4.1-5. *Relations of paranasal sinuses to the orbits: A, frontal view; and B, lateral view.*

Maxillary sinus

Maxillary sinus is the largest of paranasal sinuses and occupies the body of maxilla (Fig. 4.1-5).

On an average, maxillary sinus has a capacity of 15 ml in adults. It is pyramidal in shape with following features:

Base of the maxillary sinus forms part of the lateral wall of the nose.

Apex of this pyramidal cavity is directed laterally into the zygomatic process.

Anterolateral wall is formed by facial surface of the maxilla and is related to soft tissue of cheek.

Posterior wall is related to infratemporal and pterygopalatine fossae.

Floor is formed by maxillary alveolar process and is situated about 1.25 cm below the floor of the nose. Roots of the molars and premolars are in close relation to the floor separated from it by a thin lamina of bone. With advancing age, the floor undergoes absorption, which may expose the roots, especially of the first molar. Orodental fistulae can result from extraction of teeth.

Roof of the maxillary sinus is formed by the orbital plate of the maxilla, which also forms the floor of the orbit. Growths of the maxillary sinus may push the roof upward causing proptosis with upward displacement of the eyeball.

Osteum of the maxillary sinus is situated high up in its medial wall and opens in the posterior part of ethmoidal infundibulum into the middle meatus. It is unfavourably situated for natural drainage.

Frontal sinuses

Frontal sinuses are situated between the inner and outer tables of frontal bone and are separated by a thin septum. On an average the height of the frontal sinus is 3 cm, the breadth 2.5 cm and depth 2 cm. Its anatomical features are as follows :

Anterior wall of the sinus is related to the skin over the forehead.

Inferior wall or floor of the sinus is related to the orbit and its contents.

Posterior wall of the sinus is related to meninges and frontal lobe of the brain.

Opening of the frontal sinus is situated in its floor and leads into the middle meatus directly or through a canal called *frontonasal duct.*

Ethmoidal sinuses

Ethmoidal sinuses are thin-walled air cavities mostly situated in the lateral mass of the ethmoid. These are completed by the adjoining bones viz, frontal palatine, sphenoid, maxillary and lacrimal. Collectively, they form an *ethmoid labyrinth.*

The ethmoidal sinuses vary from 3-18 in number and occupy the space between upper third of lateral nasal wall and the medial wall of the orbit.

The sinuses are divided by irregular septa into anterior, middle and posterior groups (Fig. 4.1-5). The *anterior and middle sinuses* open into the middle meatus and the posterior sinuses open into the superior meatus. Relations of ethmoid labyrinth are as follows :

Roof of the ethmoidal sinuses is formed by anterior cranial fossa lateral to cribriform plate. Meninges of brain form important relations here.

Lateral wall of these sinuses is related to the orbit.

Sphenoid sinuses

The sphenoidal sinuses situated in the body of sphenoid bones are separated by a thin bony septum which is often obliquely placed and thus the right and left sinuses are rarely symmetrical. Some important anatomical relations of the sphenoid sinuses are as follows :

Roof of the sinus in anterior part is related to the olfactory tract, optic chiasma and frontal lobe. In the posterior part, roof is related to pituitary gland in the sella turcica.

Lateral wall of the sinus in the anterior part is related to internal carotid artery, maxillary nerve and optic nerve anterosuperiorly (which often ridge each sinus). In the posterior part, each lateral wall is related to cavernous sinus, internal carotid artery and cranial nerves - 3rd, 4th, 6th and all the divisions of 5th.

Floor of the sinus lies above the nasal cavity and houses pterygoid canal, which may ridge it.

Anterior wall of the sphenoidal sinus is related to the posterior ethmoidal sinus which may in fact be bulging in it (Fig. 4.1-5).

Osteum of the sphenoid sinus is situated in the upper part of its anterior wall and drains into sphenoethmoidal recess.

THE HYOID BONE

The hyoid bone is a unique component of the axial skeleton because it does not articulate with any other bone.

Location. The hyoid bone is located in the neck between the mandible and larynx.

It is suspended from the styloid process of the temporal bone by ligaments and muscles.

Features. The hyoid bone consists of a horizontal body and paired projections called the *lesser cornu* and the *greater cornu* (Fig. 4.1-6). Muscles and ligaments attach to these paired projections.

Functions. It supports the tongue and provides attachment for some of the muscles.

VERTEBRAL COLUMN

The vertebral column, also known as backbone, is a strong, flexible column formed by vertebrae piled one upon another.

CURVES OF VERTEBRAL COLUMN

When viewed from the side the vertebral column presents four curves (2 primary and 2 secondary) which are alternatelly convex and concave (Fig. 4.1-7A).

Primary curves. The two concave curves (*thoracic and*

Fig. 4.1-6. Hyoid bone : A, anterior view; and B, lateral view.

pelvic) are called primary curves because they exist in fetal life and are designed for the accommodation of viscera.

Secondary curves. The two convex curves (*cervical* and *lumbar*) are called secondary or compensatory curves because they are developed after birth.

STRUCTURE OF VERTEBRAL COLUMN

The vertebral column is made up of :
- Vertebrae (a series of small bones),
- Intervertebral discs, and
- Ligaments.

A. VERTEBRAE

The vertebral column is formed of 33 vertebrae in all. These include (Fig. 4.1-7) :
- Cervical vertebrae (in the neck) : 7 (Movable)
- Thoracic or dorsal vertebrae (in the thorax) : 12 (Movable)
- Lumbar vertebrae (in the loin) : 5 (Movable)
- Sacral vertebrae (in the pelvis) : 5 (Fused)
- Coccygeal vertebrae (in the pelvis) : 4 (Fused)

From the above it is clear that in terms of separate bones, the vertebral column consists of 26 bones (24 separate movable vertebrae, one sacrum (made of 5 fused vertebrae) and one coccyx (made of 4 fused vertebrae).

General anatomical features of a typical vertebra

The movable vertebrae though differ in size, shape and have some distinguishing features, but all have many similar structural characteristics. A typical vertebra has the following parts (Fig. 4.1-8):

Body of a vertebra forms the anterior, solid cylindrical mass of bone. The size varies with the site. They are

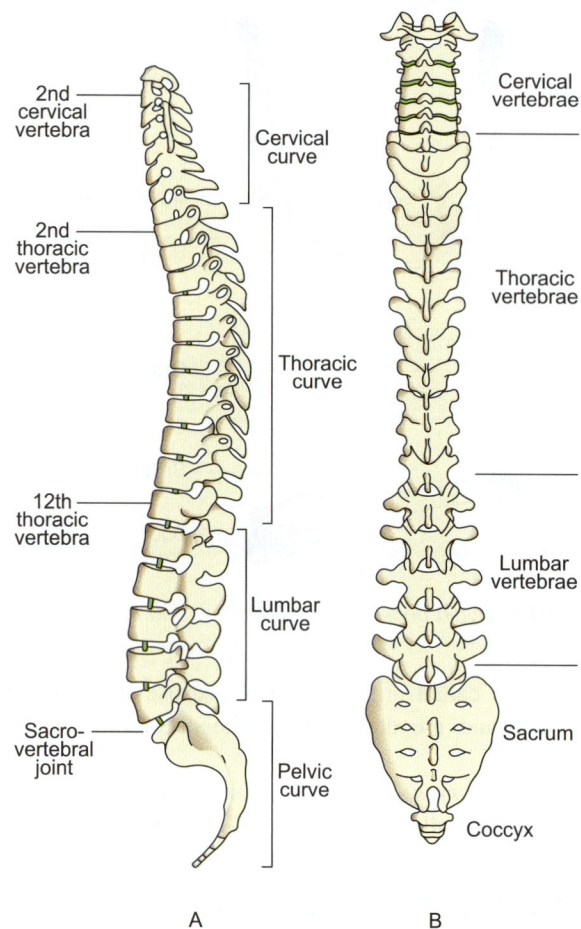

Fig. 4.1-7. *The vertebral column : A, lateral view; and B, dorsal view.*

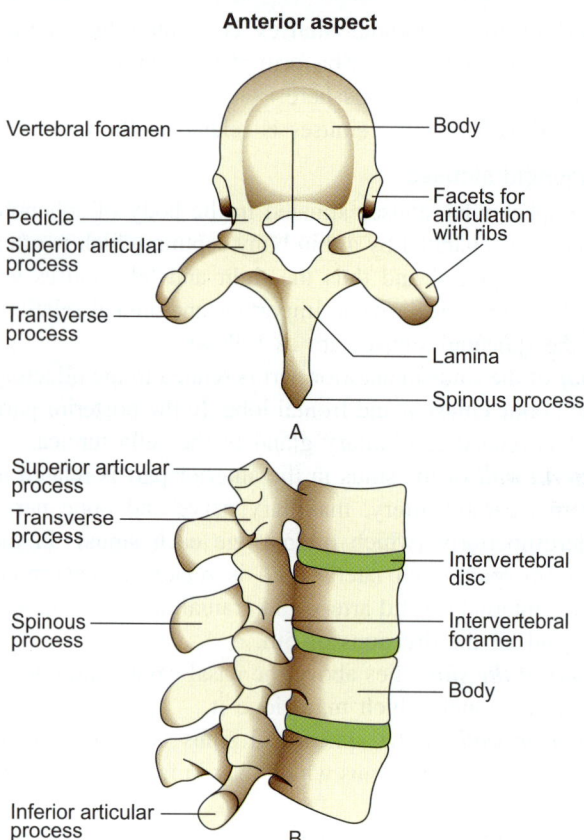

Fig. 4.1-8. *Structure of a typical vertebra: A, viewed from above; B, lateral view of several vertebrae with intervertebral discs.*

smallest in the cervical region and become larger towards the lumbar region. The bodies of adjoining vertebrae are firmly united to one another through intervertebral discs (Fig. 4.1.8B).

Pedicles and laminae. Pedicles (right and left) are two short, thick processes which project backward from the body, one on each side, to join with the *laminae.* The two laminae (right and left) join posteriorly with each other in the midline. The pedicles and laminae together constitute the *vertebral neural arch.* This arch encloses the *vertebral foramen.* Collectively the vertebral foramina form the *vertebral canal* which houses the spinal cord and its meninges.

Processes. Each vertebra has several processes :

- *Articular processes* are four in number, two to connect with bone above, and two to connect with the bone below.
- *Transverse processes* are two in number, one at each side where the pedicle and lamina join.
- *Spinous process,* one from each vertebra, projects backward from the junction of the laminae in midline.

Special anatomical features of different vertebrae

Typical cervical vertebrae

Typical cervical vertebrae (C_3 to C_7) have following special features :

- Their *transverse processes* have a foramen through which a vertebral artery passes towards brain.
- The spinous processes are short.
- Bodies of the cervical vertebrae are smaller than the thoracic but the arches are larger.

Atypical cervical vertebrae

First and second cervical vertebrae are atypical and need special description.

- *First cervical vertebra,* also called as *atlas,* looks very different from a typical cervical vertebrae, as it has no body and no spine. It simply consists of a ring of bone with two short transverse processes (Fig. 4.1-9).
- *Second cervical vertebra,* also called as *axis,* is characterized by the presence of the dens or odontoid process (a thick finger-like projection arising from the upper part of body) (Fig. 4.1-10). The odontoid process fits into the space between the anterior arch of the atlas and its transverse ligament to form the *median atlanto-*

Anterior aspect

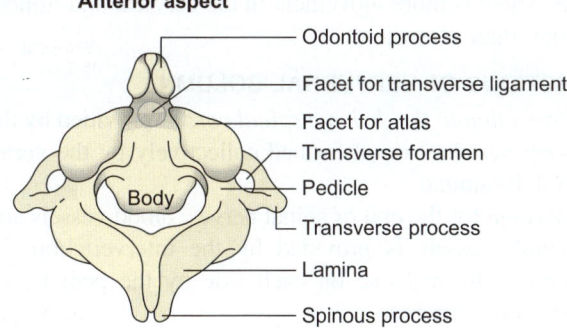

Fig. 4.1-9. The first cervical (atlas) vertebra viewed from above.

Anterior aspect

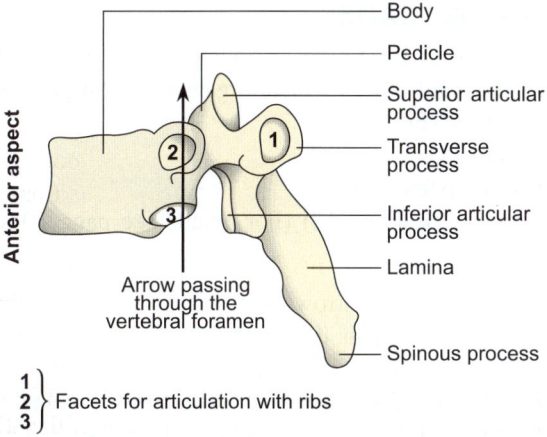

Fig. 4.1-10. The second cervical (axis) vertebra viewed from above.

occipital joint. The movement at this joint is turning the head from side to side.

Thoracic vertebrae

Thoracic vertebrae have following distinguishing features (Fig. 4.1-11) :

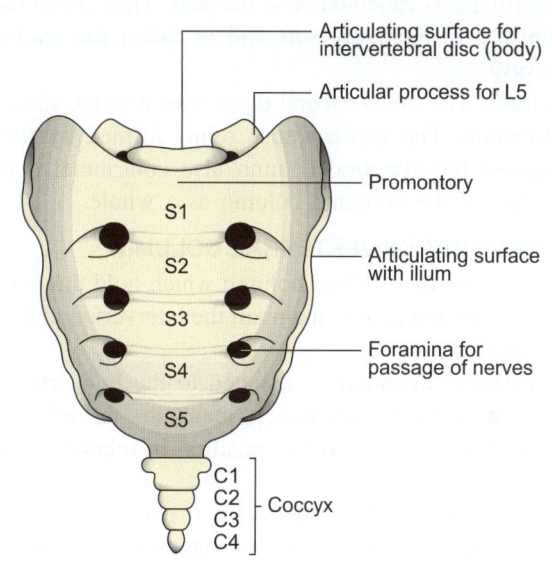

Anterior aspect

Arrow passing through the vertebral foramen

1
2 } Facets for articulation with ribs
3

Fig. 4.1-11. Side view of a typical thoracic vertebra.

- *Costal facets* for articulation with ribs are present on the sides of the bodies and on the transverse process.
- *Size* of these vertebrae is larger than those of cervical vertebrae.
- *Spinous processes* are long and are directed downward.

Lumbar vertebrae

Lumbar vertebrae can be distinguished from cervical vertebrae by the absence of foramina transversaria and from the thoracic vertebrae by the absence of costal facets for attachment of the ribs. Further, the bodies of these vertebrae are the largest and heaviest in the spine. The processes are short, heavy and thick.

Sacrum

It is a large triangular or wedge-shaped bone formed by the union of five sacral vertebrae. Its features are (Fig. 4.1-12) :

Fig. 4.1-12. The sacrum and coccyx bones viewed from the anterior surface.

- *Pelvic surface* is concave, comparatively smooth and marked by four transverse ridges. At the ends of ridges are four pairs of pelvic sacral foramina.
- *Dorsal surface* is convex and irregular.
- *Base* or upper part of the sacrum articulates with the 5th lumbar vertebra.
- *At sides,* this bone articulates with the ilium to form sacroiliac joint.
- *Its inferior tip* articulates with the coccyx.

Coccyx

It is a small triangular bone formed by fusion of coccygeal vertebrae (Fig. 4.1-12). It is the most rudimentary part of the vertebral column. At the base it articulates with the tip of sacrum.

CHAPTER 4.1

Intervertebral foramina

Intervertebral foramina are formed one on each side between the pedicles of two adjacent vertebrae. Thus half boundary of each foramen is formed by the vertebra above and half by the one below. Through these foramina pass the spinal nerves, blood vessels and lymph vessels on each side between every pair of vertebrae throughout the length of the vertebral column.

B. INTERVERTEBRAL DISCS

As mentioned above in between the bodies of adjoining vertebrae from the axis to the sacrum are present fibro-cartilagenous plates called the intervertebral discs. These discs are thinnest in the cervical region and become progressively thick towards the lumbar region. They are kept in place by the posterior longitudinal ligament of the vertebral canal.

Parts. The *peripheral part* of the disc, a rim made of fibrocartilage, is called *annulus fibrosus*. The *central part* of the disc is relatively soft and is called the *nucleus pulposus*.

Functions. The intervertebral discs have a shock absorbing function. The cartilagenous joints formed by them throughout the vertebral column also contribute to the flexibility of the vertebral column as a whole.

C. LIGAMENTS OF VERTEBRAL COLUMN

The ligaments of vertebral column which hold the vertebrae together and help to maintain the intervertebral discs in position are :

1. **Transverse ligament** is attached to the bony ring of atlas (first cervical vertebra). It maintains the odontoid process of the axis in correct position in relation to the atlas.

2. **Anterior longitudinal ligament.** It extends along the anterior surfaces of the bodies of vertebrae from axis to the sacrum. It connects the bodies of the vertebrae to each other anteriorly.

3. **Posterior longitudinal ligament.** It lies inside the vertebral canal and extends along the posterior surface of the bodies from the axis to sacrum. Thus, it binds the bodies of vertebrae together posteriorly.

4. **Ligamenta flava.** These are broad thin ligaments that connect the laminae of adjacent vertebrae.

5. **Ligamentum nuchae.** It extends from the protuberance of the occiput to the spinous process of 7th cervical vertebra. It connects apices of the spinous processes of cervical vertebrae.

6. **Supraspinous ligament.** It is the downward continuation of ligamentum nuchae. It extends from the 7th cervical vertebra to the sacrum and connects spinous processes of these vertebrae.

7. **Interspinal ligaments.** Adjacent spinous processes are connected by interspinal ligaments which extend from the root to the apex of each process and meet the ligamenta flava in front and supraspinal ligament behind.

8. **Intertransverse ligaments.** These connect the transverse processes and are placed between them.

MOVEMENTS OF VERTEBRAL COLUMN

The spinal curves confer springiness and strength upon the vertebral column, and the elasticity is further increased by ligamenta flava and the discs of fibrocartilage. As a result the vertebral column as a whole is movable, being capable of :

- *Flexion,* i.e., bending forward freely,
- *Extension,* i.e., bending backward (less freely),
- *Lateral flexion,* i.e., bending from side to side (less freely), and
- *Rotation* of limited amount is possible in cervical and thoracic regions.

Note. There is more movement in the cervical and lumbar regions than elsewhere.

FUNCTIONS OF VERTEBRAL COLUMN

- *Protection to the delicate spinal cord* is provided by the bony vertebral canal formed collectively by the vertebral foramina.
- *Passage* for the exit of spinal nerves, blood vessels and lymph vessels is provided by the intervertebral foramina, formed one on each side by the pedicles of adjacent vertebrae.
- *Movability to the trunk* is provided by the elasticity and flexibility of the vertebral column as a whole.
- *Support* to the cranium and trunk is provided by the vertebral column.
- *Shock absorption* is possible due to the pads formed by intervertebral discs. These pads mitigate the effects of contusion arising from falls or blows, protecting the brain.
- *Axis of the trunk* giving attachment to the ribs, shoulder girdle and upper limbs, and the pelvic girdle and lower limbs, is formed by the vertebral column.

THORACIC CAGE

The skeleton of the thorax or thoracic cage protects the heart, lungs and other thoracic organs. The thoracic cage is formed by (Fig. 4.1-13):

- Sternum (1)
- Ribs (12 pairs), and
- Thoracic vertebrae (12) (For details see page 101)

STERNUM

Sternum is a flat, narrow bone about 6 inches long, situated in the median line in the front of the chest. It consists of three parts (Fig. 4.1-14) :

1. **Manubrium,** the uppermost part, bears notches for attachment with the clavicles and costal cartilages of first two pairs of ribs.

Fig. 4.1-13. Anterior view of thoracic cage.

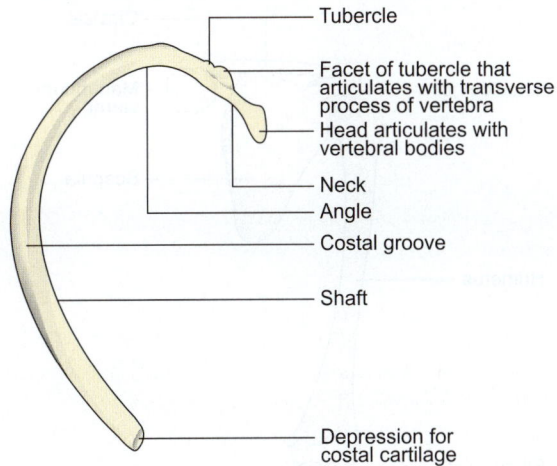

Fig. 4.1-15. A typical rib viewed from below.

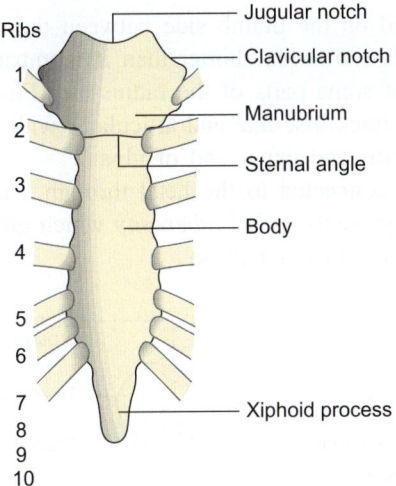

Fig. 4.1-14. The sternum and its attachments.

2. Body, the middle part, possesses notches for attachment with costal cartilages of ribs.

3. Xiphoid process, the lower part, has no ribs attached to it but gives attachment to some of the abdominal muscles.

RIBS

The twelve pairs of ribs form the side walls of thorax (Fig. 4.1-13). Each rib is a long curved bone having a posterior end and an anterior end (Fig. 4.1-15). Posterior ends of all the twelve ribs are attached to the vertebral column. Depending upon the attachment of anterior end, the ribs have been classified into three groups :

True ribs. The anterior end of the upper seven pairs of ribs is attached to the sternum through a bar of costal cartilage. These are called true ribs.

False ribs. The costal cartilages of 8th, 9th and 10th ribs are not attached to the sternum directly, but end by getting attached to the next higher cartilage. That is, they are attached indirectly to the sternum and are called false ribs. *Floating ribs* refer to 11th and 12th ribs, the anterior ends of which are free (floating).

APPENDICULAR SKELETON

The appendicular skeleton consists of a total of 126 bones. The appendages are :
* Upper limbs and shoulder girdle, and
* Lower limbs and pelvic girdle.

SHOULDER GIRDLE AND UPPER LIMBS

Each shoulder girdle consists of two bones, 1 clavicle and 1 scapula; and each upper limb is formed by 30 bones (1 humerus, 1 radius, 1 ulna, 8 carpal bones, 5 metacarpal bones and 14 phalanges (Fig. 4.1-16).

Clavicle or collar bone

The clavicle is a long bone with a double curvature (Fig. 4.1-17). It is placed horizontally at the upper and anterior part of thorax above the first rib. The inner or *sternal end* of the clavicle articulates with the sternum and the outer or *acromial end* articulates with the scapula. The clavicle forms the only bony link between upper limb and axial skeleton.

Scapula

The scapula, also called as shoulder blade, is a flat triangular bone placed behind the upper part of thorax. The scapula presents following important features (Fig. 4.1-18) :
* *Glenoid cavity* is a shallow socket present at the lateral angle. It receives the head of humerus forming the shoulder joint.
* *Spine* forms a prominent ridge on the posterior surface of scapula and terminates in a triangular, the *acromian process,* which articulates with clavicle.

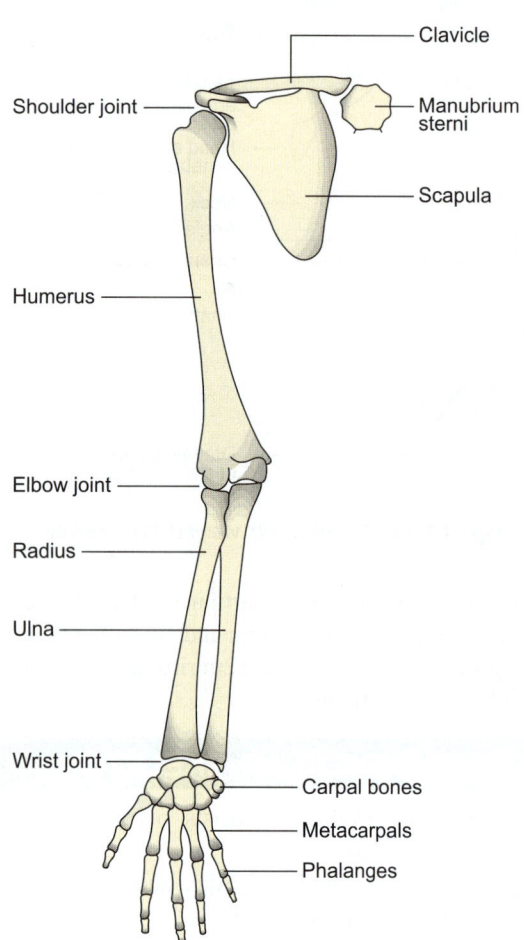

Fig. 4.1-16. Skeleton of right shoulder girdle and upper limb.

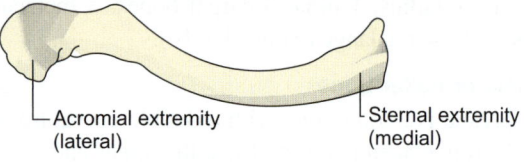

Fig. 4.1-17. The right clavicle seen from above.

Humerus or arm bone

Humerus is the largest and longest bone of the upper limb. It presents following parts (Fig. 4.1-16):

- *Rounded head* at the upper end which articulates with the glenoid cavity of the scapula to form the shoulder joint.
- *Shaft* of the humerus is connected above to the head through a narrow part neck and below to the condyle.
- *Condyle* is the lower end of humerus which presents two surfaces that articulate with the radius and ulna to form the elbow joint.

Radius

The radius along with ulna forms the bones of the forearm.

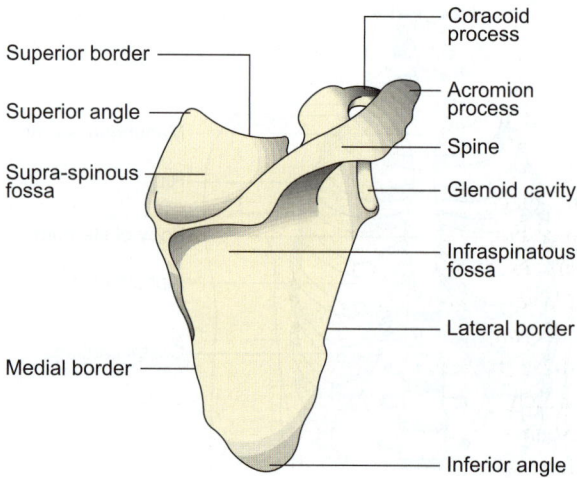

Fig. 4.1-18. The right scapula (posterior view).

It is located on the thumb side between the elbow and wrist and is somewhat shorter than its companion.

Features of some parts of the radius are (Fig. 4.1-19):

- *Head* is thick disc-like and articulates with lower end of humerus and upper end of ulna.
- *Shaft* is connected to the head through a constricted neck. It presents *radial tuberosity* which gives attachment to the biceps muscle.

Fig. 4.1-19. Anterior view of right radius and ulna with interosseus membrane.

- *Lower end* of radius articulates with scaphoid and lunate bones of the wrist and the ulna. The lateral *styloid process* present at the lower end gives attachment to the ligaments of the wrist.

Ulna

Ulna, placed on the medial side of radius, is comparatively longer bone of the forearm.

Features of some parts of ulna are (Fig. 4.1-19) :

- *Upper end* of ulna presents two processes—the *olecranun process* and *coronoid process.* In between these two processes is present the *trochlear notch* which articulates with the trochlea of humerus.
- *Shaft* of ulna is attached to that of radius with interosseous membrane.
- *Lower end* presents knob-like *head* which articulates with a notch of the radius (ulnar notch) laterally and with a disc of fibrocartilage inferiorly which separates it from the wrist. The *medial styloid process* present at the lower end of ulna gives attachment to ligaments of wrist.

Bones of the hand

Hand is composed of a wrist, a palm and five fingers. Bones of the hand include (Fig. 4.1-20) :

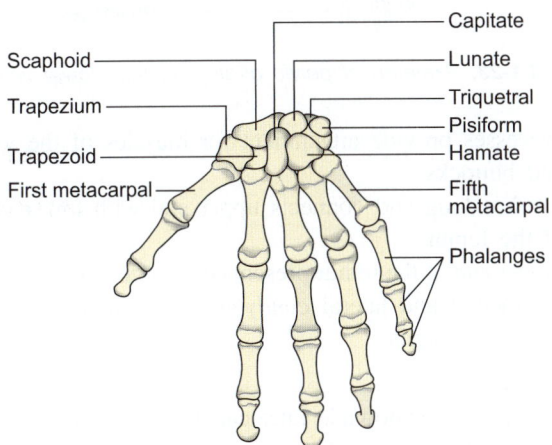

Scaphoid — Capitate — Lunate — Trapezium — Triquetral — Pisiform — Trapezoid — Hamate — First metacarpal — Fifth metacarpal — Phalanges

Fig. 4.1-20. Bones of hand.

Carpal bones, eight in number, bonded together in two rows of four bones each, form the bones of wrist. The compact mass of eight bones is called *carpus.* The carpus at its proximal surface articulates with the lower end of radius and ulna and at its distal surface articulates with the metacarpal bones.

Metacarpal bones, five in number (one in line with each finger) form the skeleton of the palm of hand (Fig. 4.1-20). These bones are cylindrical, with rounded distal ends that make the knuckles on a clenched fist. Proximally the metacarpal bones articulate with the carpus and distally with the phalanages.

Phalanges form the bones of fingers. Each finger consists of three phalanges - a proximal, a middle and a distal. The thumb has two phalanges.

PELVIC GIRDLE AND LOWER LIMBS

Pelvic girdle

Pelvic girdle is formed by two hip bones also known as innominate bones or ossa coxae.

Innominate or hip bones

Each hip bone consists of three parts (bones)—the ileum, ischium and pubis—which are fused together in the region of *acetabulum* (a socket into which the head of femur fits and forms the hip joint). Features of three fused bones forming hip bone are (Fig. 4.1-21) :

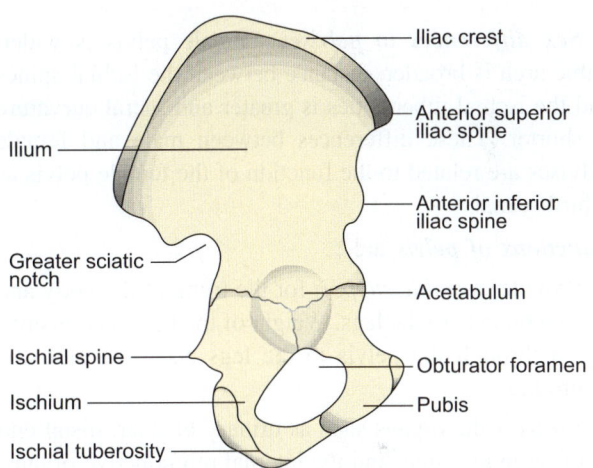

Ilium — Greater sciatic notch — Ischial spine — Ischium — Ischial tuberosity — Iliac crest — Anterior superior iliac spine — Anterior inferior iliac spine — Acetabulum — Obturator foramen — Pubis

Fig. 4.1-21. The hip bone showing the union of ilium, ischium and pubis in the acetabulum.

1. Ileum, the upper expanded part of hip bone forms the prominence of hip. Posteriorly it joins the sacrum at sacroiliac joint. It bears an *iliac crest* and *anterior superior iliac spine.*

2. Ischium forms the inferior and posterior part of hip bone. It bears *ischial tuberosity* and ischial spine. The largest foramen in the skeleton, called the *obturator foramen,* is situated between the ischium and pubis.

3. Pubis, the anterior part of the hip bone, the two pubis bones are fused anteriorly at *symphysis pubis.*

The pelvis

Pelvic girdle, together with sacrum and coccyx forms the ring-like structure of pelvis which resembles a basin (Fig. 4.1-22).

Parts. The pelvis is divided into two parts by the brim of pelvis :

- *Greater or false pelvis* is above the pelvic brim, and
- *Lower or true pelvis* is below the pelvic brim.

Fig. 4.1-22. *The pelvis formed by two hip bones along with sacrum and coccyx.*

Sex differences in pelvises. Female pelvis is wider, pubic arch is broader, distance between the ischial spines and the ischial tuberosities is greater and sacral curvature is shorter. These differences between male and female pelvises are related to the function of the female pelvis as a birth canal.

Functions of pelvis are :

- Provides a *stable support* for the trunk of the body and attachments to the legs. Weight of the body is transmitted through the pelvis to the legs and then onto the ground.
- *Protects* the organs such as urinary bladder, distal end of large intestine, and the internal reproductive organs.
- *True pelvis* in females functions as a birth canal.

Skeleton of free lower limbs

The bones of each free lower limb is formed by following 30 bones (Fig. 4.1-23) :

Femur	1
Patella	1
Tibia	1
Fibula	1
Tarsal bones	7
Metatarsals	5
Phalanges	14

The femur

The femur or thigh bone, the longest and strongest bone of the body, extends from hip to the knee.

Parts of femur bone are (Fig. 4.1-23) :

- *Head* of femur is almost spherical and fits into the acetabulum of the hip bone to form hip joint. Fovea capitis is a pit on the head which marks the attachment of a ligament that holds the femur into acetabulum.
- *Neck* and two processes *(greater trochanter* and *lower trochanter)* are present just below the head. These

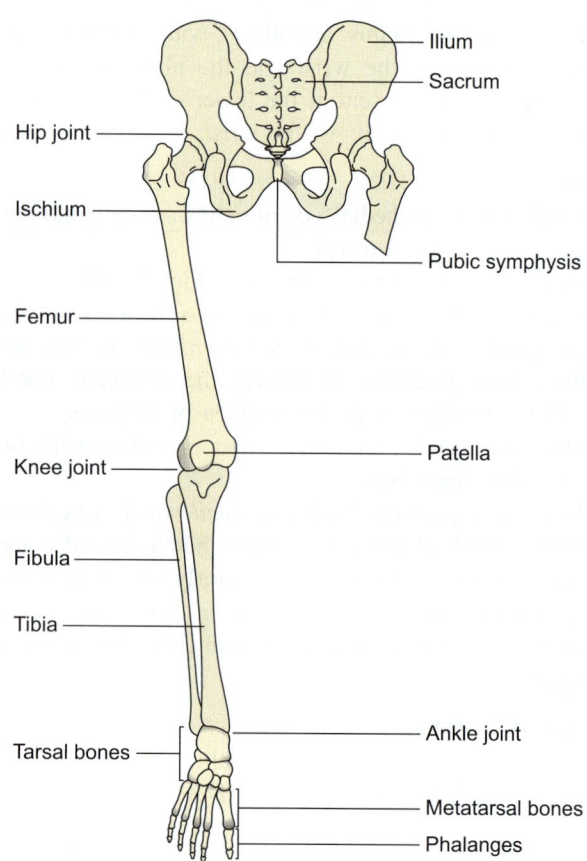

Fig. 4.1-23. *Skeleton of pelvic girdle and right lower limb.*

processes provide attachment for muscles of the legs and buttocks.
- *Shaft* is long and connects upper end with lower end of the femur.
- *Lower end* of the femur presents two large eminences—the medial and lateral *condyles*—and articulates with tibia and patella.

The patella

The patella, also known as knee cap, is a flat sesmoid bone placed in the tendon of quadriceps femoris muscle. Its posterior surface articulates with the patellar surface of lower end of femur.

The tibia

The tibia, or shin bone, is the larger of the two lower leg bones and is located on the medial side. Salient features of tibia are (Fig. 4.1-24):

- *Upper end* is expanded into two condyles, lateral and medial. Superior surfaces of condyles are concave and receive the convex condyles of fenur to form the knee joint. Head of fibula articulates with the inferior aspect of lateral condyle.
- *Shaft* of the tibia presents tibial tuberosity on its anterior surface below the condyles. Tibial tuberosity provides an attachment for the patellar ligament.

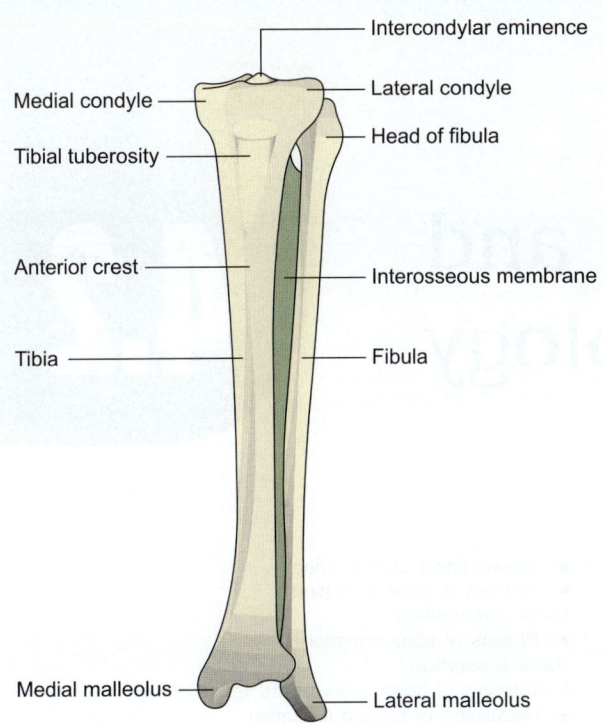

Fig. 4.1-24. *Anterior view of left tibia and fibula with interosseus membrane.*

- *Lower end* of tibia articulates with talus and fibula to form the ankle joint. A downward projection of lower end of tibia medial to the ankle joint is called *medial malleolus.*

The fibula

Fibula is a long, slender bone located on the lateral side of fibula. Its saliant features are (Fig. 4.1.24):
- *Upper end* is slightly enlarged to form the irregular head which articulates with tibia but does not enter the knee joint. Thus, fibula does not bear any of the body weight.
- *Shaft* of fibula is attached with shaft of the tibia through an interosseous membrane.
- *Lower end* is enlarged to form lateral malleolus which articulates with the ankle and can be felt as a prominence on the lateral side.

Bones of foot

The foot consists of an ankle, instep and five toes. Bones of the foot include (Fig. 4.1-25) :
Tarsal bones, seven in number, form the posterior part of the foot. Of these :
- *Talus* articulates with the lower end of tibia and fibula at the ankle joint.
- *Remaining 6 tarsal bones* are bound firmly together, forming a mass on which talus rests.

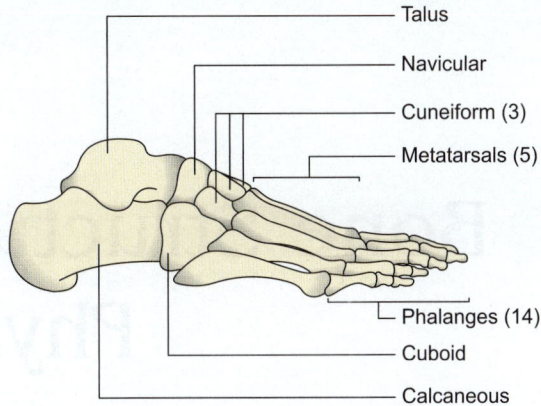

Fig. 4.1-25. *Bones of foot (superolateral view).*

- *Calcaneous,* or heel bone, is the largest tarsal bone. It is located below the talus where it projects backward to form the base of heel.

Metatarsal bones, five in number (one in line with each toe), form the skeleton of instep (Fig. 4.1-25). These bones are elongated and articulate posteriorly with the tarsus and anteriorly with the phalanges.

Phalanges. There are three phalanges in each toe, except the great toe which has only two.

Arches of foot

The tarsal and metatarsal bones of the foot are arranged and bound by ligaments in such a way that arches of the foot are formed (Fig. 4.1-26) :
- *The longitudinal arch* is highest on the medial side and extends from the heel to the toe.
- *The transverse arches* run across the foot in the metatarsal region.

Functions of arches of foot. The arches of feet provide a stable, springy base for the body. Sometimes, however, the tissues that bind the metatarsals together become weakened, producing a condition called 'fallen-arches' or flatfoot.

Fig. 4.1-26. *Arches of the foot.*

Bone Structure and Physiology

4.2

BONE : TYPES, PARTS AND COMPOSITION

TYPES OF BONES

Bone is a specialized tough connective tissue that forms skeleton of the body. Depending upon the size and shape the bones have been classified as:

- Long bones, e.g. limb bones
- Short bones, e.g. wrist and ankle bones.
- Flat bones, e.g. scapula, skull bones and mandible.
- Irregular bones, e.g. vertebrae.
- Sesamoid bones, e.g. patella.

PARTS

Parts of a typical long bone are (Fig. 4.2-1.) :

- Diaphysis (shaft) is the mid portion of the long bone.
- Epiphysis is the widened part on either end of the bone.
- Metaphysis is the portion between the diaphysis and epiphysis.
- Epiphyseal cartilage or growth plate refers to a layer of cartilage that is present between the epiphysis and metaphysis during growing age.

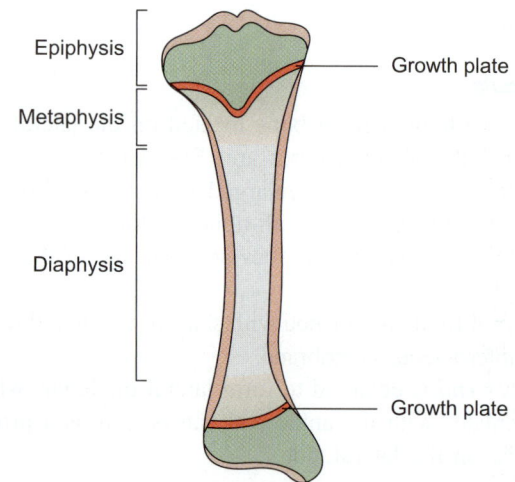

Fig. 4.2-1. *Parts and gross structure of long bone as seen in longitudinal cut section.*

COMPOSITION OF BONE

Bone is composed of a collagenous framework (matrix) impregnated with bone salts. The dry, fat-free bone

108

consists of one-third organic bone matrix, and two-thirds minerals (inorganic).

Bone matrix

Bone matrix, also called osteoid, consists of collagen fibres embedded in the gelatinous ground substance.

Collagen fibres are arranged in lamellae. The fibres of one lamellus run parallel to each other. Over 90% of the organic matrix is type I collagen.

Ground substance is formed by the extracellular fluid and proteoglycans (which include chondroitin sulphate and hyaluronic acid). These substances are concerned with the regulation and deposition of bone salts.

Bone salts

The bone salts constitute the inorganic component of bone which is comprised primarily of calcium and phosphate in the form of hydroxyapatite crystals $[Ca_{10}(PO_4)_6(OH)_2]$. Adsorbed on the surface of hydroxyapatite crystals are present small amounts of other salts such as sodium, potassium, magnesium and carbonate. The bone salts strengthen the bone matrix.

BONE STRUCTURE

Structurally, two types of bones are known: *compact* or *cortical bone*, and *trabecular* or *spongy* or *cancellous* bone. In most of the bones, both compact and cancellous forms are present, but thickness of each type varies in different regions of the bone (Fig. 4.2-1).

Structure of compact bone

The compact bone makes the outer layer of most bones and accounts for the 80% of the bone in the body.

Histologically, the compact bony tissue is made up of several minute cylindrical structures called *osteons* or *Haversian system* (Fig. 4.2-2). Each osteon is formed by several layers of collagen lamellae (Haversian lamellae) arranged concentrically around a centrally placed canal called the *Haversian canal* which contains the blood vessels, lymph vessels and nerve fibres. In between the concentric layers of collagen tissue are present many *lacunae* (small cavities) which contain *osteocytes*. The osteocytes send long process called canaliculi all around.

— Interstitial lamellae
— Haversian canal

Fig. 4.2-2. *Structure of compact bone.*

The compact bone is lined externally by periosteum and internally by endosteum. Both periosteum and endosteum of the long bones contain osteoprogenitor cells which can differentiate into osteoblasts or osteoclasts.

Structure of trabecular or spongy bone

The trabecular or spongy or cancellous bone is present inside the compact bone and makes up the 20% of bone in the body. It is made up of spicules or plates or trabeculae which are separated by wide spaces that are filled in by bone marrow.

The trabeculae are thin and consist of irregular lamellae of bone with lacunae containing osteocytes. The trabeculae are covered by a thin layer of connective tissue called *endosteum* which contains osteoblasts, osteoclasts and osteoprogenitor (stem) cells (Fig. 4.2-3).

— Marrow cavity
— Bony trabeculae
— Bony lamellae

Fig. 4.2-3. *Structure of trabecular bone.*

Cells of bone

1. *Osteoprogenitor cells.* These are stem cells of mesenchymal origin that can proliferate and convert themselves into osteoblasts whenever there is need for bone formation. They resemble fibroblasts in appearance (see page 21).

2. Osteoblasts. *Bone forming cells* are called osteoblasts. These are situated in the outer surface of bone, the marrow cavity and epiphyseal plate cells.

Functions of osteoblast cells include:

i. *Role in laying down of the organic matrix of bone.* Osteoblasts are responsible for synthesis of bone matrix by secreting type I collagen and a protein called *matrix gla protein* (MGP).

ii. *Role in calcification.* Enzyme alkaline phosphatase present in the cell membranes of osteoblasts plays important role in the calcification of bone matrix.

3. Osteocytes. Cells of mature (or developed) bone are called osteocytes. As mentioned above they represent osteoblasts, which during bone formation are 'imprisoned' in the lacunae between the bone lamellae. The cytoplasmic processes from the osteocytes run into canaliculi and ramify throughout the bone matrix. The processes from neighbouring cells have contact with each other forming tight junction.

Functions

Osteocytes play an important role in maintaining the exchange of calcium between the bone and extracellular fluid.

4. Osteoclasts. Bone removing cells are called osteoclasts. These are giant multinucleated cells found in relation to surfaces where bone removal is taking place.

Functions

Osteoclasts are responsible for bone resorption during bone remodelling.

5. Bone lining cells. Bone lining cells are flattened cells which form a continuous epithelium-like layer on bony surfaces. They are present on the periosteal surface as well as endosteal surface.

BONE DEVELOPMENT, GROWTH AND REMODELLING

BONE DEVELOPMENT AND GROWTH

All bone is of mesenchymal origin. The process of bone formation is called ossification. Development of bone tissue starts before birth and completed by 21 years of life. There are two mechanisms of bone formation: endochondral bone formation and intramembranous bone formation.

Endochondral bone formation. During fetal development, formation of most of the bones is preceded by the formation of a cartilaginous model which is subsequently replaced by bone. This kind of ossification is called endochondral bone formation.

Intramembranous bone formation. Formation of some bones, e.g. clavicle, vault of skull and mandibles is not preceded by formation of a cartilage model, but they are formed directly in a fibrous membrane. This kind of ossification is called intramembranous bone formation.

Development of long bones

The steps of formation of long bone are :

1. Formation of a cartilage model. In the region, where a long bone is to be formed, the mesenchyme first lays down a cartilaginous model of bone.

2. Ossification and calcification. The ossification is carried out by osteoblasts which enter the central part of the cartilaginous model. This area is called *primary centre of ossification* (Fig. 4.2-4). Gradually bone formation extends from the primary centre towards the ends of shaft.

3. Growth in length and girth. After birth *secondary centres* of endochondral ossification appear in the cartilages forming the ends of bones. These centres

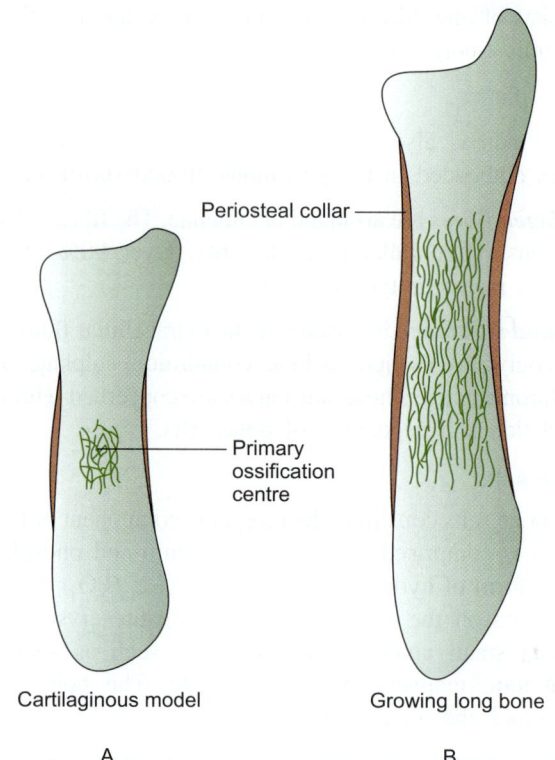

Fig. 4.2-4. *Cartilage model with primary centre for ossification (A) and extension of primary centre for ossification (B).*

enlarge and convert the cartilaginous ends into bone. The portion of the bone formed from one secondary centre is called *epiphysis*. During growth, the bone of diaphysis and the bone of epiphysis are separated by a plate of actively proliferating cartilage, the *epiphyseal plate*. The portion of the diaphysis adjoining the epiphyseal plate is called metaphysis. It is highly vascular and region of active bone formation. The bone increases in length as this plate lays down new bone on the end of shaft. The growth of the bone stops when the epiphysis fuses with the diaphysis *(epiphyseal closure)*. The normal age at which the epiphysis closes in different bones of the body is well known.

Even after bone growth has ceased, the calcium turnover function of bone is most active in the metaphysis which acts as a storehouse of calcium.

Process of bone formation

During growth bone formation is carried out by active osteoblasts. Bone is continuously deposited by these cells. The process of bone formation includes osteoid formation and mineralization of bone matrix (Fig. 4.2-5).

1. Osteoid formation. The osteoblasts synthesize and lay down the type I procollagen molecules into the adjacent extracellular space. These cells also secrete a gelatinous matrix in which the fibres get embedded.

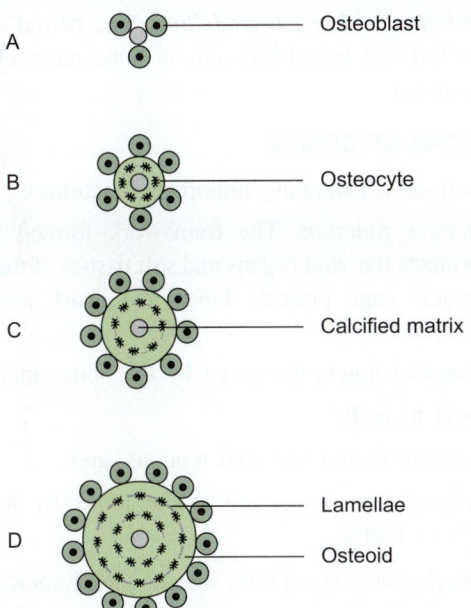

Fig. 4.2-5. *Schematic depiction of process of formation of bone lamella.*

2. Bone matrix mineralization. Soon after formation of osteoid the process of bone matrix mineralization starts. It occurs in two phases: an initial slow process of initiation of mineralization followed by rapid mineralization process.

The process of mineralization greatly depends upon the *calcium × phosphate* ion product in extracellular fluid. This product must be above 30/dl for this process to occur. Most of the calcium phosphate is deposited within 6 to 12 hours. After the process of mineralization of bone matrix is completed, the osteoid is converted into a bone lamella (Fig. 4.2-5). After the formation of one bone lamella (as described above) another layer of osteoid is laid down by osteoblast. The osteoblasts move away from the bone lamella to line the new layer of osteoid. However, some osteoblasts are caught between the lamella and the osteoid (Fig. 4.2-5).

Conversion of trabecular bone to compact bone. All newly formed bone is cancellous. It is converted into compact bone (Fig. 4.2-6):

• Each space between the trabeculae of cancellous bone comes to be lined by osteoblasts (Fig. 4.2-6A and B).

• The osteoblasts lay down lamellae of bone as already described. The first lamella is formed over the inner wall of the original space and is, therefore, shaped like a ring (Fig. 4.2-6C).

• Subsequently, concentric lamellae are laid down inside this ring thus forming an *osteon*. The original space becomes smaller and smaller and persists as a *Haversian canal* (Fig. 4.2-6D).

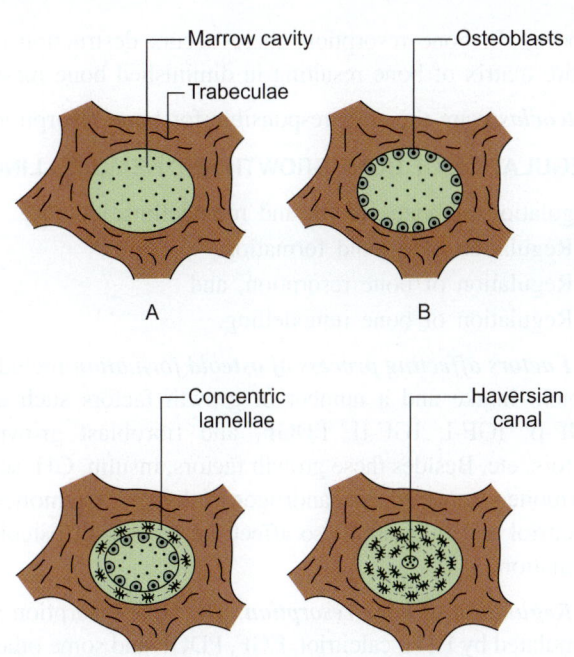

Fig. 4.2-6. *Steps of conversion of trabecular bone into compact bone.*

BONE REMODELLING

Definition. Bone remodelling refers to a process of bone resorption followed by bone formation which keeps on occurring throughout life in a cyclic manner.

Phases of bone remodelling cycle. A bone remodelling cycle takes about 100 days and consists of two phases: the resorption phase and the succeeding formation phase.

1. *Resorption phase* lasts for initial 10 days. In this phase mineralized bone is reabsorbed by osteoclasts releasing calcium and phosphate.

2. *Formation phase* lasts for next 90 days and is characterized by reformation of bone by osteoblasts (assimilating calcium and phosphate).

Physiological significance of continuous bone remodelling include:

• *Bone adjusts its strength* in proportion to the degree of bone stress. For example, in athletes, soldiers and others in whom the bone stress is more, the bones become heavy and strong.

• *Shape of bone can be rearranged* for proper support of mechanical force in accordance with the stress.

• *Old bone becomes relatively weak and brittle.* The development of new bone matrix maintains the toughness of bone.

BONE RESORPTION

Bone resorption, like bone formation, is a continuous

C H A P T E R 4 . 2

process. In bone resorption, there occurs destruction of entire matrix of bone resulting in diminished bone mass.

Osteoclasts are the cells responsible for bone resorption.

REGULATION OF BONE GROWTH AND REMODELLING

Regulation of bone growth and remodelling include:
- Regulation of osteoid formation,
- Regulation of bone resorption, and
- Regulation of bone remodelling.

A. *Factors affecting process of osteoid formation* include protein intake and a number of growth factors such as TGF-β, IGF-I, IGF-II, PDGF, and fibroblast growth factors, etc. Besides these growth factors, insulin, GH, sex hormones (oestrogens, androgen), thyroid hormones, calcitriol and calcitonin also affect the process of osteoid formation.

B. *Regulation of bone resorption.* The bone resorption is stimulated by PTH, calcitriol, EGF, PDGF and some other growth factors. The response is mediated through release of prostaglandins. Thyroxine and vitamin A also increase bone resorption.

C. *Regulation of bone remodelling.* The paired activity of osteoclast and osteoblast cells in bone remodelling is well regulated.

FUNCTIONS OF BONES

Bones subserve following important functions :

1. *Protective function.* The framework formed by the bones protects the vital organs and soft tissues of the body, e.g. thoracic cage protects lungs and heart, and skull protects brain.

2. *Mechanical functions* served by the bones include:
- *Support* to body,
- *Attachment* to muscles and tendons, and
- *Movements* are performed at the joints by leverage effects of bones.

3. *Metabolic functions* of bone include their important role in homeostasis of calcium and phosphate metabolism.

4. *Haemopoietic function* includes the formation of blood cells in the red bone marrow.

SECTION 4

The Joints

4.3

DEFINITION AND CLASSIFICATION

Joints or articulations are junctions between two or more bones or cartilages. The joints can be classified according to their structual composition and according to the amount of movement of which they are capable.

A. *Structural classification.* On the basis of intervening tissue :
- Fibrous joints
- Cartilaginous joints
- Synovial joints

B. *Functional classification.* According to the degree of movement permitted :
- Immovable joints (synarthroses)
- Slightly movable joints (amphiarthroses)
- Freely movable joints (diathroses)

C. *Regional classification* (on the basis of location).
- Skull type
- Vertebral type
- Limb type

GENERAL DESCRIPTION OF JOINTS

For the purpose of description of structure and general features of various joints, following mixed classification is considered :
- Fibrous (or immovable or skull type) joints.
- Cartilaginous (or slightly movable or vertebral type) joints.
- Synovial (or freely movable or limb type) joints.

A. FIBROUS JOINTS

Fibrous or immovable joints (synarthroses) are also called skull type joints, since they are generally limited to skull. These joints have fibrous tissue between the two articulating surfaces. These are of following types:

113

- Sutures,
- Syndesmosis, and
- Gomphosis.

1. *Sutures.* Sutures refer to the immovable joints found between the bones. For example, between skull bones.

Salient features of sutures or sutural joints are :

- A thin layer of fibrous tissue may be present between the two bones (Fig. 4.3-1A).
- According to the shape of bony margins, the sutures can be plane, serrate, *denticulate* dentate, squamous or limbus type.
- Periosteum on the outer and inner surfaces of these bones bridge the gaps between them and form the primary bond at the suture.
- No active movement takes place at an immovable joint.

2. *Syndesmosis.* It is a type of fibrous joint in which two bones are connected by an interosseous ligament. This usually allows slight but occasionally more extensive movement between them (Fig. 4.3-1B). For example, *inferior tibiofibular joint.*

3. *Gomphosis* are also known as *'peg and socket joint'*. These are typically seen as a joint between tooth and jaw *(articulation dentoalveolus).* The cavity in jaw and root of tooth is connected by some fibrous tissue (Fig. 4.3-1C).

4. *Schindylesis* refers to a wedge and groove type joint between two bones. For example, rostrum of sphenoid and ala of vomer.

B. CARTILAGINOUS JOINTS

Cartilaginous or slightly movable joints (amphiarthroses) are also called vertebral type of joints. As the name indicates, in such joints the two bones are joined by cartilage. Cartilaginous joints are of two varieties :

- Primary cartilaginous joints, and
- Secondary cartilaginous joints.

1. *Primary cartilaginous joints (synchondorses).* These are temporary joints seen in childhood during develop- ment of the bones. For example, the shaft *(diaphysis)* of a long bone is joined to the bone end *(epiphysis)* by a plate of hyaline cartilage *(epiphysial plate)* (Fig. 4.3-2A). After the growth of the bone is completed the plate of hyaline cartilage is changed to bone before adult life.

2. *Secondary cartilaginous joints (symphyses).* In such joints the articular surfaces of the two bones are covered by a thin layer of hyaline cartilage, and united by a disc of fibrocartilage (Fig. 4.3-2B).

Salient features of such joints are :

- These joints are permanent and persist throughout life.
- Typically such joints occur in the median plane of the body.

A

B

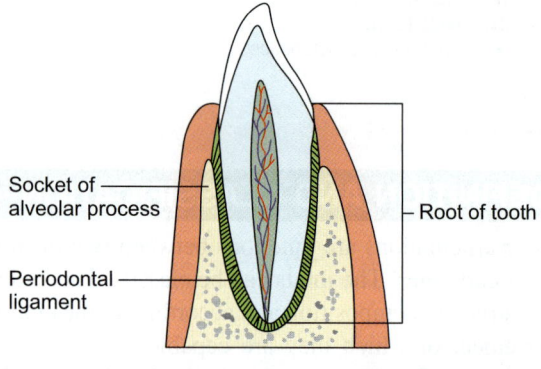

C

Fig. 4.3-1. *The fibrous joints : A, suture; B, syndesmosis; and C, gomphosis.*

- These permit limited movements due to compressible pad of fibrocartilage.

Examples of secondary cartilaginous joints include:

- Pubic symphysis, and
- Joints between bodies of vertebrae.

C. SYNOVIAL JOINTS

Synovial or freely movable joints (diarthroses) are also called limb joints.

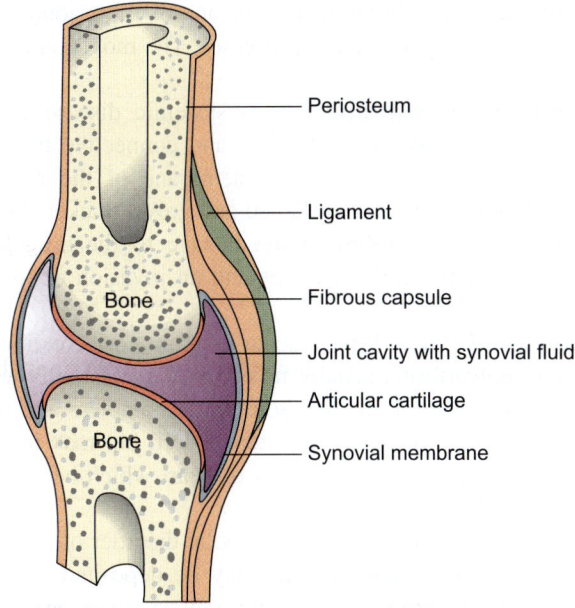

Fig. 4.3-2. The cartilaginous joints : A, primary; B, secondary.

Structural characteristics

Structural characteristics of synovial joints are (Fig. 4.3-3):

Articular or hyaline cartilage caps the ends of two bones taking part in the joint. This cartilage has neither blood vessels nor lymphatics (nor has it any nerves). It receives nourishment from the synovial fluid.

Articular capsule made up of fibrous tissue encloses the ends of two bones making the joint. The fibrous capsule is sufficiently loose to allow free movements at the joint but is strong enough to protect it from injury.

Fig. 4.3-3. The synovial joint.

Synovial membrane, a thin sheet of connective tissue and epithelial cells, lines the inside of fibrous capsule. Synovial membrane also covers all intracapsular structures that do not bear weight. It secretes synovial fluid.

Synovial fluid, slippery like egg white, is a dialysate of blood plasma plus a mucin called hyaluronic acid (which provides viscidity and lubricating properties to the synovial fluid). Synovial fluid serves following *functions:*

- *Lubricates* the intracapsular joint structures.
- *Nourishes* the structures within the joint cavity.
- Maintains joint stability.
- Phagocytes present in it remove microbes and cellular debris from the joint cavity.

Other intracapsular structures which are present in some joints (not all) include :

- *Fat pads and menisci* (semilunar cartilage) are present in knee joints.
- *Bursae,* the closed fluid filled sacs, are also present in some joints e.g. knee joint. They act as cushion to prevent friction.

Extracapsular structures which support the joints from outside the capsule include :

- *Ligaments,* made of dense fibrous tissue, blend with the capsule in the form of thick cords and bands and provide additional stability to most synovial joints.
- *Muscles or their tendons* which are attached on the bones forming joints also provide stability to the joints during movements.

Types of synovial joints

Depending upon the shape of the articulating part of the bone and/or the range of movement permitted, the synovial joints are of various types :

1. *Plane joints or gliding joints* are characterized by flat articulating surfaces which allow only gliding movement, e.g., carpal joints and joints of small tarsal bones.

2. *Hinge joints.* In such joints one articulating surface is concave and other convex. These are *uniaxial joints* which allow movements in one direction (flexion and extension) like a door on its hinges. Examples of hinge joints include elbow joint, knee joint, and interphalyngeal joints of the fingers and toes.

3. *Pivot joints.* In such joints one bone end is rod shaped, that fits into a ring made up partly of bone and partly of ligament. Thus, pivot joints are uniaxial joints in which movements in such joints is limited to rotation about a central axis as with a neck in a collar. Examples of such a joint are joint between first and second cervical vertebrae and the superior radio-ulnar joint.

4. *Condolyoid joints.* In such joints an oval-shaped condyle of one bone fits into an eliptical cavity of another bone as in the case of the joints between the metacarpals and phalanges. These joints are *biaxial* i.e. allow a variety of movements in two planes e.g. flexion and extension, and adduction and abduction; however, rotational movements are not allowed.

5. Ellipsoid joints. In such joints the convex articulating surface is elliptical rather than round and the other a socket, e.g., the radiocarpal (wrist) joint. Such joints are *biaxial* and allow movements in various planes but no rotations.

6. Ball and socket joint. In such joints a ball-shaped head of one bone fits into a cup-shaped socket of another bone. These joints are *multiaxial* and thus allow movements in all planes, as well as rotational movement around a central axis. Examples of such joints are shoulder joint and hip joint.

7. Saddle joints. In such joints articulating surfaces have both concave and convex regions; surface of one bone fits into complementary surface of another. In other words, the surfaces are reciprocally saddle-shaped. Being *multiaxial* such joints allow a variety of movements. Example includes joint between carpal and metacarpal bones of thumb.

Movements of synovial joints

As mentioned above a variety of movements are possible depending upon the type of synovial joint. These can be grouped as below:

1. Gliding movement, i.e., one surface moves over another without any angular or rotatory movement. Such a movement occurs in gliding joints between carpal bones of the wrist and tarsal bones of the foot.

2. Angular movement leads to either increase or decrease in the angle between two articulatory long bones. These are of two types :

- *Flexion and extension,* i.e. bending and straightening, respectively (for example movements of elbow joint, knee joint).

- *Abduction and adduction* i.e. movement away and towards the median plane of the body, respectively. For example lifting the arm away from or at right angle to the body (abduction) and bringing arm to the side of body (adduction).

3. Circumduction i.e. a movement in which a long bone circumscribes a conical space by rotation around an imaginary axis, e.g., swinging the arms or legs.

4. Rotation, i.e. a movement in which a bone moves around a central axis without undergoing any displacement from this axis. For example, rotation of the atlas (first cervical vertebra) around the odontoid process of axis (second cervical vertebra). Examples of rotation are:

- *Supination and pronation.* When the forearm is rotatated so that palm comes to face forwards, the movement is

called *supination.* The opposite rotatory movement is called *pronation.*

- *Inversion and eversion.* A movement at the ankle in which the sole of foot turns inwards is called inversion, and the movement in which the sole turns outwards is called eversion.

CLINICALLY APPLIED ASPECTS

Some common disorders of joints with which a student should become familiar are mentioned here briefly.

TRAUMATIC LESIONS OF JOINTS

Joints are subjected to considerable stress and are commonly injured during strenuous physical activity resulting in dislocations and sprain.

1. Dislocation of joint. This is a condition in which the articular surfaces of a joint are separated and displaced in such a way that one surface loses its contact completely from the other. If a partial contact is still retained, it is better called *subluxation.* Dislocation usually occurs from a fall or other form of trauma and is characterized by pain, deformity, and loss of function. X-ray is confirmatory. The joints of shoulders, knee, elbows, fingers and mandible are common sites for dislocation.

2. Sprains are the result of stretching or tearing of the ligaments or tendons at a joint, i.e. soft tissue injury without dislocating the bones. They are usually caused by wrenching or twisting of joint excessively.

3. Penetrating injuries. May be caused by a compound fracture of one of the articulating bones, or trauma caused by gun shot.

ARTHRITIS

Arthritis refers to inflammation of one or more joints. It can be caused by a variety of diseases. The most common types are :

1. Rheumatoid arthritis. This is systemic disease with widespread involvement of joints and connective tissue. In this condition the synovial membrane of the freely movable joints becomes inflamed and grows thicker. This change is usually followed by damage to the articular cartilages on the ends of bones and an invasion of joint by fibrous tissue.

2. Rheumatic fever. It is an acute inflammatory condition causing polyarthritis usually involving the wrist, elbows, knees and ankles. Usually resolution is complete and no residual change in articular system is left; but may leave permanent damage to the valves of heart which becomes evident in later life.

3. Gouty arthritis. Gout is a metabolic disorder of purine metabolism. Uric acid crystals may be deposited in the joints. The joint most frequently involved is the metatarsophalangeal of the great toe.

DEGENERATIVE DISORDERS

Osteoarthritis. This is a common degenerative non-inflammatory condition which occurs in joints that are subject to a great deal of wear and tear. It usually occurs in individuals after the age of 45 years. The articular cartilage of involved joint shows degenerative change in the centre (fibrillation of cartilage) and proliferative change around the edges (osteophages). The spine and joints of the lower extremity are most frequently involved causing pain and restricted movement of affected joints.

Muscular System

The Skeletal Muscles of Human Body

5.1

GENERAL DESCRIPTION OF SKELETAL MUSCLES
- Gross anatomy
- Nerve supply, muscle mechanics, and lever system
- Group actions of muscles
- Nomenclature of muscles

MAIN SKELETAL MUSCLES OF HUMAN BODY

Muscles of head, face and neck
- Muscles of scalp and facial expression
- Muscles of mastication
- Muscles that move the head
- Muscles of eyes
- Muscles of ears

Muscles of shoulder girdle and upper limb
- Muscles that move the pectoral girdle
- Muscles that move the upper arm
- Muscles that move the forearm
- Muscles that move the wrist, hand and fingers

Muscles of trunk
- Muscles of thorax
- Muscles of abdominal wall

Muscles of back
- Muscles of upper back
- Muscles of lower back

Muscles of pelvis and perineum
- Muscles of pelvis
- Muscles of perineum

Muscles of pelvic girdle and lower limb
- Muscles that move the thigh
- Muscles that move the leg
- Muscles that move the ankle, foot and toes

GENERAL DESCRIPTION OF SKELETAL MUSCLES

Motion is one of the most important aspects of human body. This function is accomplished by the concerted role of bony skeleton, joints and the skeletal muscles of the body. In addition to the motion, the skeletal muscles also serve some other functions.

Gross anatomy

Muscle belly, origin and insertion. The main mass of a skeletal muscle is termed the muscle belly. The fibrous ends of the muscle taper into tendons. Skeletal muscles produce movements by exerting force on tendons, which in turn pull on bones. For producing a movement at any joint the muscle has to be attached on both the bones forming the joint. Ordinarily, the attachment of a muscle tendon to the stationary bone is called the *origin* and to the movable bone is called *insertion*. This can be compared to a door spring on a door. The part of spring fixed on the immovable frame can be considered analogous to the origin of muscle, and the part of spring attached on movable door can be considered analogous to the insertion of a muscle.

Tendons. These are the fibrous ends of the muscles by which they are attached to the bones. Tendons vary considerably :
- They may be hardly noticeable, so that muscles appear to be directly attached to bone both at its origin and insertion.
- More usually, the tendons are well developed at the insertion of muscle.

- Frequently, tendons are long, round, or flattened bands, usually surrounded by sheaths of synovial membrane, especially in the neighbourhood of joints.
- Sometimes, the tendons form a broad, flat expansion termed as *aponeurosis*, e.g. the lumbar aponeurosis.

Nerve supply, muscle mechanics and lever system

Nerve supply. The skeletal muscles being voluntary muscles are controlled by somatomotor and somato-sensory parts of the central nervous system. The nerve controlling the muscle action is called *motor nerve.* Each muscle gets the motor as well as sensory nerve supply either through a mixed nerve or through two separate nerves – one motor and other sensory.

Mechanics of muscle. When a muscle contracts, the force of contraction is said to have three components:

- *Swing,* which is transaxial. For example, this component is maximum during the contraction of brachialis muscle while flexing the elbow.
- *Shunt,* which is transarticular. This component is maximum when the origin of the muscle is close to a joint while insertion is at a distance, e.g., brachio- radialis muscle.
- *Spin,* which is rotatory along its axis. For example, the spin component is predominant in the pronator quadratus muscle, wrapped on the anterior surfaces of lower ends of radius and ulna bones.

Lever systems. In producing a body movement, bones act as levers and joints function as fulcrums of these levers.

Group actions of muscles

Each movement at a joint is coordinated by several skeletal muscles acting in group rather than individually. According to their group actions the muscles are named and classified as below :

1. Agonist (prime mover) refers to the muscle which produces the desired action. For example, biceps brachi which produces flexion at the elbow is considered agonst for this movement. Similarly, triceps brachi, which produces extension at elbow is considered agonist for this movement.

2. Antagonist (opponent). The term antagonist is used for a muscle producing opposite movement than the primary mover at the same joint. For example, triceps which produces extension at elbow joint is antagonist of biceps which produces flexion at the elbow. Similarly for extension movement the triceps is agonist and biceps is antagonist.

It is important to note that a particular movement is brought about by coordinated movement of both agonists and antagonists. For example, for producing flexion movement at elbow the agonist (i.e. biceps muscle) contracts and the antagonist (i.e. triceps) relaxes. Thus, in other words, the antagonist having opposite action coop-

erates for a movement with the agonists by relaxing. This is due to reciprocal innervation of the opposite group of muscles, regulated by the spinal cord through stretch reflex. Reciprocal innervation is goverened by the *Sherrington's law* which states that when the agonist muscles get full innervation from the brain, simultaneously the antagonist gets zero innervation.

3. Fixators refer to a group of muscles which stabilize the proximal joints of a limb, so that the desired movement at the distal joint may occur. For example, for flexion at elbow the deltoid and pectoris major muscles act as fixator, as they stabilize and fix the arm and shoulder in a suitable position so that flexion at elbow can be produced by contraction of agonist (biceps) and relaxation of antagonist (triceps).

4. Synergists refer to the group of muscles which while contracting produce same movement at the particular joint. For example, brachialis and brachioradialis muscles also produce flexion at elbow by their contraction. So, they act as synergists to the biceps brachi muscle.

Nomenclature of skeletal muscles

The human body contains about 700 skeletal muscles, each of which bears a name. The muscles have been named in a number of way :

1. According to the shape of the muscle, e.g. :

- *Deltoid,* a triangular-shaped muscle, is named after the Greek letter delta which is triangular in shape.
- *Trapezoid muscle* is trapezoid in shape.

2. According to the number of heads of origin. For example, biceps (2 heads of origin), triceps (3 heads of origin, quadriceps (4 heads of origin) muscles.

3. According to the function of muscle. For example:

- *Flexor carpiradialis* produces flexion at the wrist.
- *Extensor carpiradialis* produces extension at the wrist joint.
- *Adductor longus* produces adduction.
- *Abductor hallucis longus* produces abduction.
- *Levator scapulae* produces upward movement of scapula.

4. Based on the region in which muscle is located. For example :

- *Pectoralis major* and *pectoralis minor* are named because they are located in pectoral region (front of the chest).
- *Gluteus maximus, gluteus medius* and *gluteus minimus* muscles are named so because they are located in the gluteal region (region of buttock) and are large, medium and small in size, respectively.
- *Temporalis muscle* is located in temple region.
- *Intercostal muscles* are located in between the ribs.

5. According to the direction of muscle fibres, e.g. :

- *Rectus abdominis,* because of straight fibres (rectus = straight) :

- *Oblique abdominis,* because of oblique fibres.
- *Transversus,* because of transverse fibres.

6. *According to attachment,* e.g., sternomastoid, stylohyoid, cricothyroid.

7. *According to gross appearance,* e.g., semitendinous, semimembranous etc.

MAIN SKELETAL MUSCLES OF HUMAN BODY

Muscles of the human body are too numerous to be considered in any detail. They can, however, be divided into several main groups and subgroups, and salient features of some of the muscles may be considered as below :

- Muscles of head and neck.
- Muscles of shoulder girdle and upper limb.
- Muscles of trunk.
- Muscles of back.
- Muscles of pelvis.
- Muscles of pelvic girdle and lower limb.

MUSCLES OF HEAD, FACE AND NECK

These can be divided into following subgroups :

- Muscles of scalp and facial expression
- Muscles of mastication
- Muscles that move the head
- Muscles of eyes (see page 485)
- Muscles of ears (see page 494)
- Muscles of pharynx (see pages 220 and 267)
- Muscles of larynx (see page 221)

Muscles of scalp and facial expression

Muscles of facial expression connect the bones of the skull to various regions of the overlying skin. Because of their attachment to skin they enable us to express our feelings as surprise, sadness, anger, fear, pain, happiness, disgust, etc.

Common muscles of scalp and facial expression include (Fig. 5.1-1) :

- Epicranius,

- Orbicularis oculi,
- Orbicularis oris,
- Buccinator,
- Zygomaticus, and
- Platysma

Nerve supply. These muscles are supplied by branches of the 7th cranial (facial) nerve.

Origin, insertion and action of these muscles are summarized in Table 5.1-1.

Muscles of mastication

Muscles of mastication produce chewing movements which include closure of jaw (for biting), side-to-side grinding motions, movements of opening, closing and protuding the jaw. Four pairs of muscles of mastication, that are attached to the mandible, include (Fig. 5.1-1):

- Masseter,
- Temporalis,
- Internal pterygoid, and
- External pterygoid.

Nerve supply. Muscles of mastication are supplied by branches of 5th cranial (trigeminal) nerve.

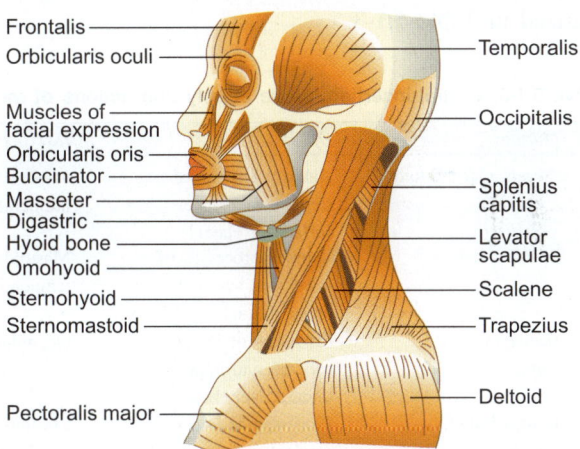

Fig. 5.1-1. *The skeletal muscles of facial expression, muscles of mastication and muscles of neck which move the head.*

Table 5.1-1. Origin, insertion, nerve supply and actions of muscles of facial expression

Muscle	Origin	Insertion	Nerve supply	Actions
1. Occipitofrontalis (frontal belly)	Epicranial aponeurosis	Skin superior to supraorbital margin	Facial (VII) nerve	Raises eyebrow
2. Orbicularis oculi	Maxillary and frontal bones	Skin around eye	Facial (VII) nerve	Closes eye
3. Orbicularis oris	Muscles near the mouth	Skin of central lip	Facial (VII) nerve	Closes lips, protrudes lips
4. Buccinator	Outer surfaces of maxilla and mandible	Upper and lower lips	Facial (VII) nerve	Compresses cheeks inward
5. Zygomaticus	Zygomatic bone	Skin arowned the mouth	Facial (VII) nerve	Raises corner of mouth
6. Platysma	Fascia in upper chest	Lower border of mandible	Facial (VII) nerve	Draws angle of mouth downward

CHAPTER 5.1

Table 5.1-2. Origin, insertion, nerve supply and actions of muscles of mastication

Muscle	Origin	Insertion	Nerve supply	Actions
1. Masseter	Lower border of zygomatic arch	Lateral surface of mandible	Mandibular division of trigeminal (V) nerve	Raises jaw
2. Temporalis	Temporal bone	Coronoid process and anterior ramus of mandible	Mandibular division of trigeminal (V) nerve	Raises jaw
3. Internal pterygoid	Sphenoid, palatine, and maxilla bones	Medial surface of mandible	Mandibular division of trigeminal (V) nerve	Closes jaw, pulls jaw sideways
4. External pterygoid	Sphenoid bone	Anterior surface of mandibular condyle	Mandibular division of trigeminal (V) nerve	Pulls jaw forward

Origin, insertion and actions of muscles of mastication are depicted in Table 5.1-2.

Muscles that move the head

The muscles in the neck and upper back which attach the head to the trunk are responsible for movements of the head (flexion, extension, tilt and rotation). These muscles include (Fig. 5.1-1) :
- Sternocleidomastoid,
- Splenius capitis,
- Semispinalis capitis,
- Longissimus capitis.

Origin, insertion and actions of these muscles are summarized in Table 5.1-3.

- Trapezius,
- Rhomboideus major,
- Levator scapulae,
- Serratus anterior
- Pectoralis minor.

Origin, insertion, nerve supply and actions of these muscles are summarized in Table 5.1-4.

Muscles that move the upper arm

Shoulder joint being multiaxis (ball and socket type) joint makes the upper arm move freely movable part of the body. The muscles which attach the humerus with various regions of pectoral girdle, ribs and vertebral column are

Table 5.1-3. Origin, insertion, nerve supply and actions of muscles that move the head

Muscle	Origin	Insertion	Nerve supply	Actions
1. Sternocleidomastoid	Anterior surface of sternum and upper surface of clavicle	Mastoid process of temporal bone	Accessory (XI) nerve	Pulls head to one side, pulls head toward chest, or raises sternum
2. Splenius capitis	Spinous processes of lower cervical and upper thoracic vertebrae	Mastoid process of temporal bone	Cervical spinal nerves	Rotates head, bends head to one side, or brings head into upright position.
3. Semispinalis capitis	Processes of lower cervical and upper thoracic vertebrae	Occipital bone	Cervical spinal nerves	Extends head, bends head to one side, or rotates head.
4. Longissimus capitis	Processes of lower cervical and upper thoracic vertebrae	Mastoid process of temporal bone	Cervical spinal nerves	Extends head, bends head to one side, or rotates head

MUSCLE OF SHOULDER GIRDLE AND UPPER LIMB

These can be divided into following subgroups :
- Muscles that move the pectoral girdle
- Muscles that move the upper arm
- Muscles that move the forearm
- Muscles that move the wrist, hand and fingers.

Muscles that move the pectoral girdle

Muscles that move the pectoral girdle are those which attach the scapulae to the trunk, humerus to the scapula and humerus to the chest wall. These muscles are responsible for upward, downward, forward and backward movements of the scapula. These include the following (Fig. 5.1-2) :

involved in the movements of upper arm. Depending upon their primary action, these muscles can be grouped as below (Fig. 5.1-3):
- *Flexors* of upper arm, e.g., pectoralis major and coracobrachialis,
- *Extensors* of upper arm, e.g., teres major, latissimus dorsi.
- *Abductors* of upper arm, e.g., supraspinatus and deltoid.
- *Rotators* of upper arm, e.g., subscapularis, infraspinatus, and teres major.

Origin, insertion, nerve supply and actions of these muscles are summarized in Table 5-1-5.

Table 5.1-4. Origin, insertion, nerve supply and actions of muscles that move the pectoral girdle

Muscle	Origin	Insertion	Nerve supply	Actions
1. Trapezius	Occipital bone and spines of cervical and thoracic vertebrae	Clavicle and spine and acromion process of scapula	Accessory (XI) nerve and cervical spinal nerves (C_3 - C_5)	Raises scapula, pulls scapula medially, or pulls scapula and shoulder downward
2. Rhomboideus major	Spines of upper thoracic vertebrae	Medial border of scapula	Dorsal scapular nerve	Raises and adducts scapula.
3. Levator scapulae	Transverse processes of cervical vertebrae	Medial margin of scapula	Dorsal scapular nerve and cervical spinal nerves C_3 - C_5	Elevates scapula
4. Serratus anterior	Outer surfaces of upper ribs	Medial border of scapula	Long thoracic nerve	Pulls scapula anteriorly and downward
5. Pectoralis minor	Sternal ends of upper ribs	Coracoid process of scapula	Medial pectoral nerve	Pulls scapula forward and downward or raises ribs

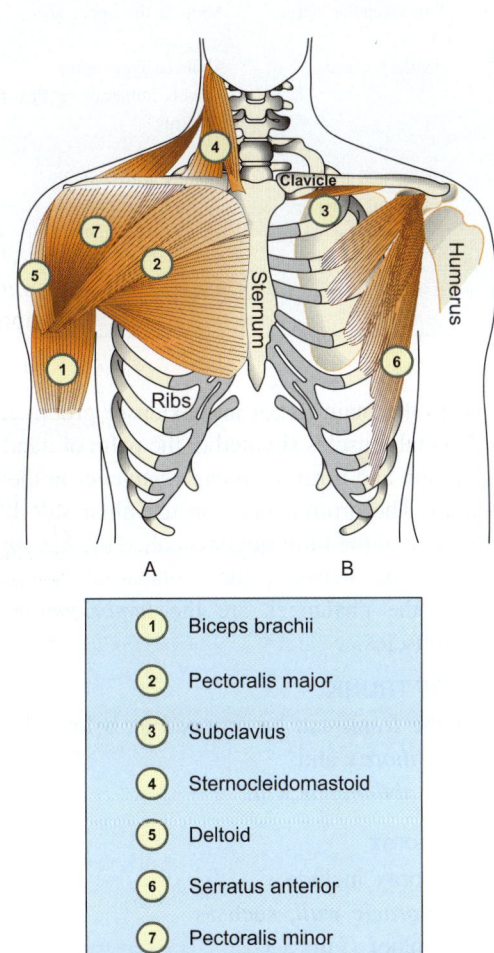

1. Biceps brachii
2. Pectoralis major
3. Subclavius
4. Sternocleidomastoid
5. Deltoid
6. Serratus anterior
7. Pectoralis minor

Fig. 5.1-2. Muscles that move the pectoral girdle (shoulder): A, anterior superficial view; and B, anterior deep view.

Muscles that move the forearm

Movers of the forearm are those muscles which attach the radius and ulna to the humerus or pectoral girdle. Depending upon their primary action these muscles can be grouped as below (Fig. 5.1-3):

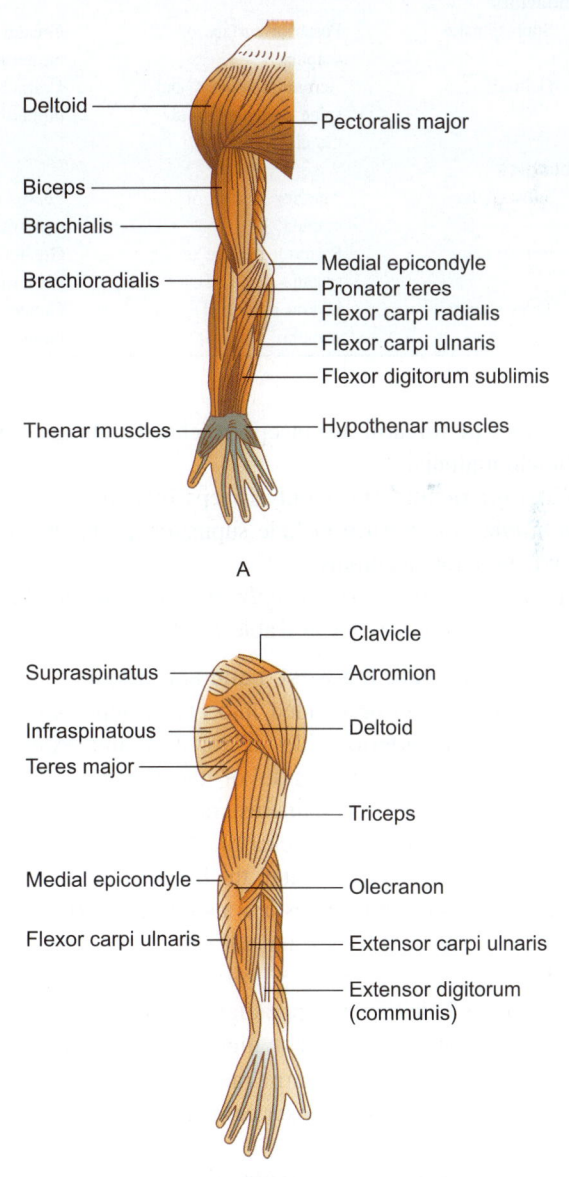

Fig. 5.1-3. Muscles of the right upper limb: A, anterior aspect; and B, posterior aspect.

Table 5.1-5. Origin, insertion, nerve supply and actions of muscles that move the upper arm

Muscle	Origin	Insertion	Nerve supply	Actions
Flexors				
1. Coracobrachialis	Coracoid process of scapula	Shaft of humerus	Musculocutaneous nerve	Flexes and adducts the upper arm.
2. Pectoralis major	Clavicle, sternum, and costal cartilages of upper ribs	Intertubercular groove of humerus	Medial and lateral pectoral nerves	Pulls arm forward and across chest, rotates humerus, or adducts arm.
Extensors				
1. Teres major	Lateral border of scapula	Intertubercular groove of humerus	Lower subscapular nerve	Extends humerus, or adducts and rotates arm medially
2. Latissimus dorsi	Spines of sacral, lumbar and lower thoracic vertebrae, iliac crest, and lower ribs	Intertubercular groove of humerus	Thoracodorsal nerve	Extends, adducts, and rotates humerus medially, or pulls the shoulder downward and back.
Abductors				
1. Supraspinatus	Posterior surface of scapula	Greater tubercle of humerus	Suprascapular nerve	Abducts the upper arm
2. Deltoid	Acromion process and spine of scapula and the clavicle	Deltoid tuberosity of humerus	Axillary nerve	Abducts upper arm, extends humerus, or flexes humerus.
Rotators				
1. Subscapularis	Anterior surface of scapula	Lesser tubercle of humerus	Upper and lower subscapular nerves	Rotates arm medially
2. Infraspinatus	Posterior surface of scapula	Greater tubercle of humerus	Suprascapular nerve	Rotates arm laterally.
3. Teres minor	Lateral border of scapula	Greater tubercle of humerus	Axillary nerve	Rotates arm laterally.

- *Flexors* of forearm are biceps brachii, brachialis, and brachioradialis.
- *Extensor* of forearm is only triceps brachii.
- *Rotators* of forearm include supinator, pronator teres and pronator quadratus.

Origin, insertion, nerve supply and action of these muscles are summarized in Table 5.1-6.

Muscles that move the wrist, hand and fingers

These muscles can be divided into two groups—flexors present on the arterior side of forearm and extensor present on the posterior side of the forearm. These muscles *arise* from the humerus, radius and ulna. The tendons of the flexor muscles in front and extensor muscles behind are inserted into the bases of the terminal phalanges of the digits. Slips are also given to the other phalanges. These muscles include the following (Fig. 5.1-3) :

- *Flexors* include flexor carpi radialis, flexor carpi ulnaris, palmaris longus, and flexor digitorum profundus.
- *Extensors* are extensor carpi radialis longus, extensor carpi radialis brevis, extensor carpi ulnaris and extensor digitorum.

Origin, insertion, nerve supply and actions of these muscles are summarized in Table 5.1-7.

Note : The thumb has separate muscles which, however, correspond to the main flexor and extensor groups in the forearm. Special muscles situated in the palm of hand also move the thumb and form the *thenar eminence* at the base of the thumb. The prominence on the ulnar side of the hand at the base of the little finger is called the *hypothenar eminence.* Arising between the metacarpal bones and inserted into the phalanges are the *lumbrical* and *interosseous* muscles.

MUSCLES OF TRUNK

Muscles of the trunk can be grouped as below :

- *Muscles of thorax* and
- *Muscles of abdominal wall*

Muscles of thorax

Muscles of thorax include :

Muscles of thoracic wall, such as

- Pectoralis major (Fig. 5.1-2),
- Pectoralis minor (Fig. 5.1-2),
- Serratus anterior (Fig. 5.1-2), and
- Intercostal muscles

Diaphragm

It is a large dome-shaped muscle separating the cavity of thorax from that of abdomen. It consists partly of muscle (around the circumference) and partly of membrane or flat tendon (in the centre) (Fig. 5.1-4).

Table 5.1-6. Origin, insertion, nerve supply and actions of muscles that move the forearm

Muscle	Origin	Insertion	Nerve supply	Actions
Flexors				
1. Biceps brachii	Coracoid process and tubercle above glenoid cavity of scapula	Radial tuberosity of radius	Musculocutaneous nerve	Flexes arm at elbow and rotates the hand laterally.
2. Brachialis	Anterior shaft of humerus	Coronoid process of ulna	Musculocutaneous and radial nerves	Flexes arm at elbow
3. Brachioradialis	Distal lateral end of humerus	Lateral surface of radius above styloid process	Radial nerve	Flexes arm at elbow.
Extensors				
1. Triceps brachii	Tubercle below glenoid cavity and lateral and medial surfaces of humerus	Olecranon process of ulna	Radial nerve	Extends arm at elbow
2. Anconeus	Lateral epicondyle of humerus	Olecranon and superior portion of shaft of ulna	Radial nerve	Extends forearm at elbow joint
Rotators				
1. Supinator	Lateral epicondyle of humerus and crest of ulna	Lateral surface of radius	Deep radial nerve	Rotates forearm laterally.
2. Pronator teres	Medial epicondyle of humerus	Lateral surface of radius	Median nerve	Rotates arm medially.
3. Pronator quadratus	Anterior distal end of ulna	Anterior distal end of radius	Median nerve	Rotates arm medially.

Table 5.1-7. Origin, insertion, nerve supply and actions of muscles that move the wrist, hand and fingers

Muscle	Origin	Insertion	Nerve supply	Actions
Flexors				
1. Flexor carpi radialis	Medial epicondyle of humerus	Base of second and third metacarpals	Median nerve	Flexes and abducts wrist.
2. Flexor carpi ulnaris	Medial epicondyle of humerus and olecranon process	Carpal and metacarpal bones	Ulnar nerve	Flexes and adducts wrist.
3. Palmaris longus	Medial epicondyle of humerus	Fascia of palm	Median nerve	Flexes wrist
4. Flexor digitorum	Anterior surface of ulna	Bases of distal phalanges in fingers (except thumb)	Median and ulnar nerves	Flexes distal joints of fingers
Extensors				
1. Extensor carpi radialis longus	Distal end of humerus	Base of second metacarpal	Radial nerve	Extends wrist and abducts hand
2. Extensor carpi radialis brevis	Lateral epicondyle of humerus	Base of second and third metacarpals	Radial nerve	Extends wrist and abducts hand
3. Extensor carpi ulnaris	Lateral epicondyle of humerus	Base of fifth metacarpal	Deep radial nerve	Extends and adducts wrist.
4. Extensor digitorum	Lateral epicondyle of humerus	Posterior surface of phalanges in fingers two through five	Deep radial nerve	Extends fingers
5. Extensor digitii minimi	Lateral epicondyle of humerus	Tendon of extensor digitorum on fifth phalanx	Deep radial nerve	Extends proximal phalanx of little finger and hand at wrist joint

C H A P T E R   5 . 1

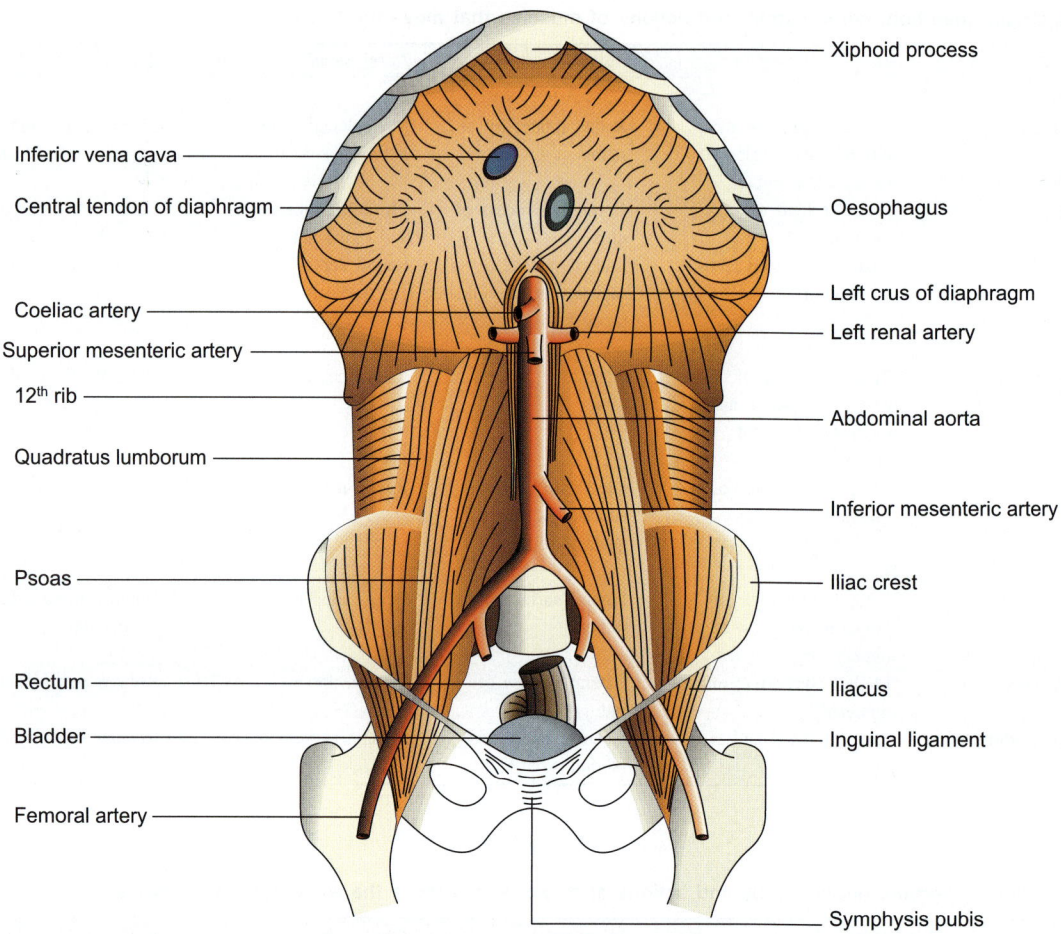

Inferior vena cava

Central tendon of diaphragm

Coeliac artery

Superior mesenteric artery

12th rib

Quadratus lumborum

Psoas

Rectum

Bladder

Femoral artery

Xiphoid process

Oesophagus

Left crus of diaphragm

Left renal artery

Abdominal aorta

Inferior mesenteric artery

Iliac crest

Iliacus

Inguinal ligament

Symphysis pubis

Fig. 5.1-4. *Diagram showing under surface of diaphragm and muscles of posterior abdominal wall.*

Parts and attachments of diaphragm :
- *Sternal part* is attached in front to the lower end of sternum.
- *Costal part* is attached to the lower six ribs on either side.
- *Lumbar part* is attached to the first two lumbar vertebrae by two slips called the crurae (legs) of the diaphragm .

Surfaces. Diaphragm has two surfaces :
- *Upper surface* is related to the heart and pericardium in the centre and to the pleura and base of lung on either side.
- *Under surface* (Fig. 5.1-4), largely covered by peritoneum, is related on the right side and centrally to the upper surface of liver; and on the left side to the fundus of stomach and the spleen.

Openings in diaphragm (Fig. 5.1-4) are :
- For aorta in the midline.
- For oesophagus slightly to the left,
- For inferior vena cava, slightly to the right.

Nerve supply and actions. The diaphragm is a very important muscle of respiration. It is supplied by *phrenic nerve* from the cervical plexus.

- *During inspiration,* the muscle part of diaphragm contracts and it becomes flattened towards the abdomen; and thereby helping to enlarge the size of thoracic cavity.
- *During expiration,* the diaphragm relaxes and resumes its dome-shaped appearance.

Muscles of abdominal wall
Anterior abdominal wall

These include following muscles (Fig. 5.1-5) :
- Rectus abdominis,
- External oblique,
- Internal oblique, and
- Transverse abdominis

Salient features. Muscels of the anterior abdominal wall are :
- They connect the rib cage and vertebral column to the pelvic girdle.
- Linea alba, a tough connective tissue which extends from the xiphoid process of the sternum to symphysis pubis, serves as an attachment for some of the abdominal wall muscles.

- Contraction of these muscles help in forceful expiration, defecation, urination, vomiting and childbirth.

Origin, insertion, nerve supply and actions of these muscles are summarized in Table 5.1-8.

Posterior abdominal wall

Muscles of posterior abdominal wall include :

- Psoas muscle,
- Iliacus muscle, and
- Quadratus lumborum (Fig. 5.1-5).

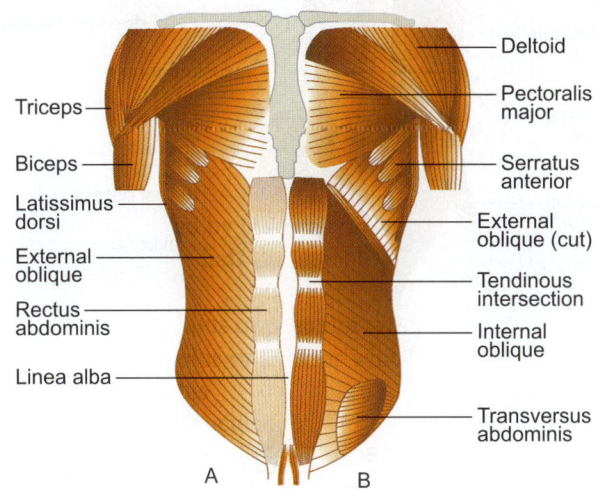

Fig. 5.1-5. Muscles of anterior abdominal wall : A, superficial view; and B, deep view.

Origin, insertion, nerve supply and actions of these muscles are summarized in Table 5.1-8.

MUSCLES OF THE BACK

Muscles of the back include several group of muscles which are placed on either side of the spine and extend the varying distances between the occiput above and the sacrum below (Fig. 5.1-6).

Muscles of upper back extend the neck. These include:

- Splenius capitis,
- Semispinalis capitis, and
- Longismus capitis

Muscles of lower back which straighten the spine, consist of three groups of muscles :

- *Iliocostalis group* is laterally placed,
- *Longissimus group* is intermediately placed, and
- *Spinalis group* is medially placed.
- Combined these muscles constitute the *erector spina*.

MUSCLES OF PELVIS AND PERINEUM

Muscles of pelvis form the floor of the abdominal cavity, just as the diaphragm forms it roof. These include levator ani and coccygeus. The muscles of pelvic floor, together with the fasciae covering their internal and external surfaces are collectively referred to as the *pelvic diaphragm*.

Muscles of perineum. The perineum is the entire outlet of pelvis. The muscles of pelvis include superficial transversus perinei, bulbospongiosus and ischio-cavernosus.

C H A P T E R   5 . 1

Table 5.1-8. Origin, insertion, nerve supply and actions of muscles of the abdominal wall

Muscle	Origin	Insertion	Nerve supply	Actions
Of anterior abdominal wall				
1. External oblique	Outer surfaces of lower ribs	Outer lip of iliac crest and linea alba	Thoracic spinal nerve T_7-T_{12} and ilio-hypogastric nerve	Tenses abdominal wall and compresses abdominal contents
2. Internal oblique	Crest of ilium	Cartilages of lower inguinal ligament, ribs, linea alba, and crest of pubis	Thoracic spinal nerves T_8-T_{12}, ilio-hypogastric nerve and ilioinguinal nerve	Same as above
3. Transversus abdominis	Costal cartilages of lower ribs, processes of lumbar vertebrae, lip of iliac crest, and inguinal ligament	Linea alba and crest of pubis	Thoracic spinal nerves T_8-T_{12}, ilio-hypogastric nerve and ilioinguinal nerve	Same as above
4. Rectus abdominis	Crest of pubis and symphysis pubis	Xiphoid process of sternum and costal cartilages	Thoracic spinal nerve T_7-T_{12}	Same as above, also flexes vertebral column
Of posterior abdominal wall				
1. Psoas major	Transverse processes and bodies of lumbar vertebrae	With iliacus into lesser trochanter of femur	Lumbar spinal nerves L_2-L_3	Flexes thigh at hip joint
2. Iliacus	Iliac fossa of ilium	Lesser trochanter of femur	Femoral nerve	Flexes thigh
3. Quadratus femoris	Ischial tuberosity	Quadrate tubercle on posterior femur	Nerve to quadratus femoris	Laterally rotates and stabilizes hip joint

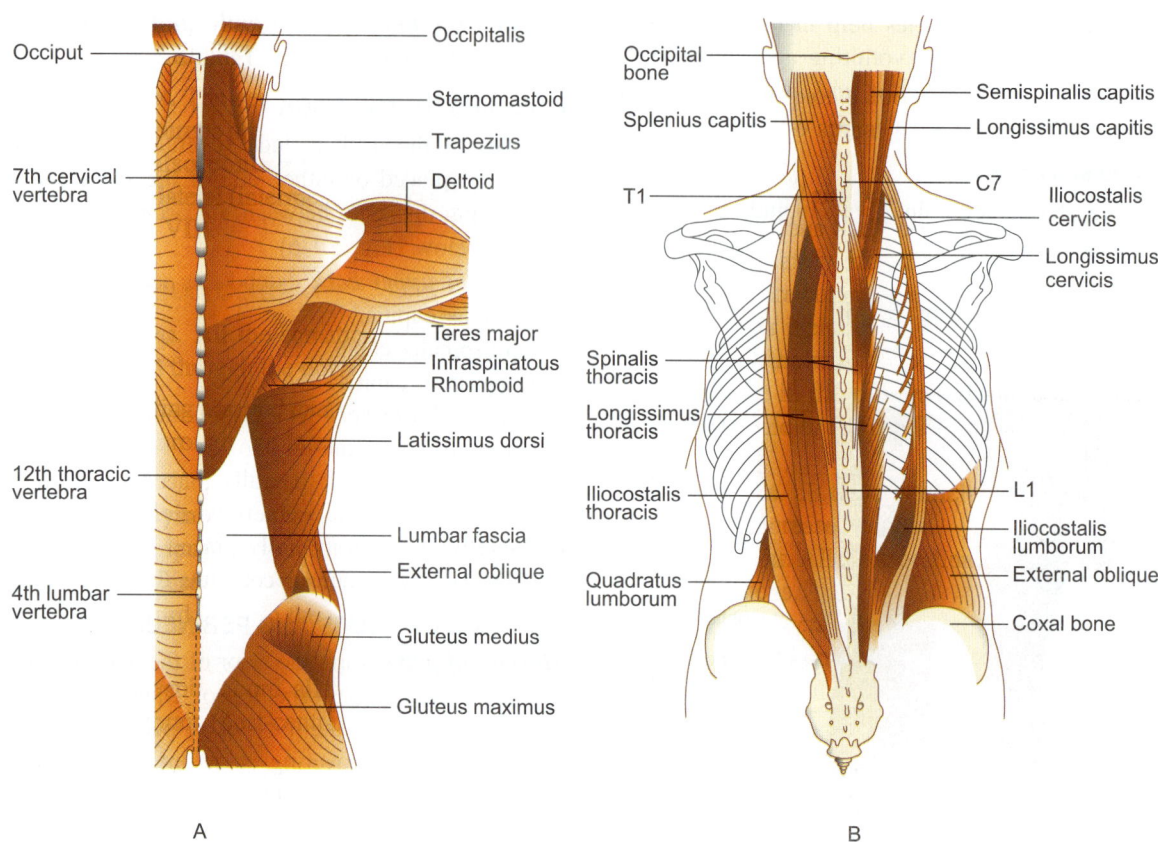

Fig. 5.1-6. Muscles of the back : A, superficial view; and B, deep view.

These muscles along with their fascia constitute the *urogenital diaphragm.*

Muscles of male and female pelvis and perineum are shown in Figs. 5.1-7 and 5.1-8 and their salient features are summarized in Table 5.1-9.

MUSCLES OF PELVIC GIRDLE AND LOWER LIMB

These can be divided into following subgroups :
* Muscles that move the thigh,
* Muscles that move the leg, and
* Muscles that move the ankle, foot and toes.

Muscles that move the thigh

Muscles that move the thigh are attached to the femur and to some part of the pelvic girdle. These can be divided into three groups :

Flexors of thigh or muscles of anterior group include psoas major and iliacus (Fig. 5.1-9A). They primarily flex the thigh.

Abductors of thigh or muscles of posterior group also known as *muscles of the buttock* make up the rounded eminence of buttock. They include gluteus maximus, gluteus medius and gluteus minimus (Fig. 5.1-9B). These abductors rotate the thigh.

Adductors of thigh include adductor longus, adductor magnus and gracilis.

Origin, insertion, nerve supply and actions of the muscles that move the thigh are summarized in Table 5.1-10.

Muscles that move the leg

The muscles that move the leg connect the tibia and fibula to the femur or pelvic girdle. These are the muscles of thigh region which can be arranged in two groups :

Anterior group muscle of thigh or extensors of leg lie in front of the femur. These include rectus femoris, vastus lateralis, vastus medialis and vastus intermedius (Fig. 5.1-10A). These combined constitute the *quadriceps femoris.*

2. Posterior group muscles of thigh or flexors of leg lie behind the femur. These include biceps femoris semitendinosus, and semimembranosus (Fig. 5.1-10B). These combined constitute the *hamstring* muscles.

Origin, insertion, nerve supply and actions of muscles that move the lower leg are summarized in Table 5.1-11.
Muscles that move the ankle, foot and toes or the muscles located in lower leg region, attach the femur, tibia, and fibula to various bones of foot. These include (Table 5.1-12 and Fig. 5.1-11) :
* *Dorsiflexors of foot.* Tibialis anterior, peroneus tertius, and extensor digitorum longus.

Fig. 5.1-7. *Muscles of male perineum.*

Fig. 5.1-8. *Muscles of female pelvic floor.*

- *Plantar flexors of foot.* Gastrocnemius, soleus and flexor digitorum longus.
- *Invertor of foot.* Tibialis posterior.
- *Evertor of foot.* Proneus longus.

Small muscles of foot. There are a number of small muscles in foot similar to those in the hands, viz, short muscles in the sole which are attached to the big toe, *interosseous* and *lumbrical* muscles for the toes.

Table 5.1-9. Origin, insertion, nerve supply and actions of muscles of the pelvic outlet

Muscle	Origin	Insertion	Nerve supply	Actions
Muscles of pelvic floor				
1. Levator ani	Pubic bone and ischial spine	Coccyx	Sacral spinal nerves S_1-S_4	Supports pelvic viscera, and provides sphincter-like action in anal canal and vagina
2. Coccygeus	Ischial spine	Sacrum and coccyx	Sacral spinal nerves S_1 S_4	Same as above
Superficial muscles of perineum				
1. Superficial transversus perinei	Ischial tuberosity	Central tendon	Perineal branch of pudendal nerve of the sacral plexus	Supports pelvic viscera
2. Bulbospongiosus	Central tendon	Males: Urogenital diaphragm and fascia of penis	Perineal branch of pudendal nerve of the sacral plexus	Males : assists emptying of urethra
		Females: pubic arch and root of clitoris		Females : constricts vagina
3. Ischiocavernosus	Ischial tuberosity	Pubic arch	Perineal branch of pudendal nerve of the sacral plexus	Same as above
Deep muscles of perineum				
1. Deep transversus perinei	Ischial rami	Perineal body of perineum	Perineal branch of pudendal nerve of the sacral plexus	Helps to expel last drop of urine.
2. External urethral sphincter	Ischial and pubic rami	Median raphe in male and vaginal wall in female	Sacral spinal nerves S_4 and inferior rectal branch of pudendal nerve	Helps to expel last drop of urine.
3. External anal sphincter	Anococcygeal ligament	Perineal body of perineum	Sacral spinal nerve S_4 and inferior rectal branch of pudendal nerve	Keep anal canal and anus close

Fig. 5.1-9. *Muscles that move the thigh : A, anterior view; and B, posterior view.*

Fig. 5.1-10. *Muscles of thigh region that move the lower leg : A, anterior view; and B, posterior view.*

Table 5.1-10. Origin, insertion, nerve supply and actions of muscles that move the thigh.

Muscle	Origin	Insertion	Nerve supply	Actions
Flexors				
1. Psoas major	Lumbar intervertebral	Lesser trochanter of femur, disks, bodies and transverse processes of lumbar vertebrae	Lumbar spinal nerves L_2-L_3	Flexes thigh
2. Iliacus	Iliac fossa of ileum	Lesser trochanter of femur	Femoral nerve	Flexes thigh
3. Gluteus maximus	Posterior surface of ileum	Posterior surface of sacrum & coccyx	Inferior gluteal femur and iliotibial tract	Extends leg at hip nerve
Abductors				
1. Gluteus medius	Lateral surface of ileum	Greater trochanter of femur	Superior gluteal nerve	Abducts and rotates thigh medially
2. Gluteus minimus	Lateral surface of ileum	Greater trochanter of femur	Superior gluteal nerve	Same as above
3. Tensor fasciae latae	Anterior iliac crest	Lateral condyle of tibia by fascia	Superior gluteal nerve	Abducts, flexes, and rotates thigh medially
Adductors				
1. Adductor longus	Pubic bone near symphysis pubis	Posterior surface of femur	Obturator nerve	Adducts, flexes, and rotates thigh laterally
2. Adductor brevis	Inferior ramus of pubis	Linea aspera of femur	Obturator nerve	Adducts, flexes and rotates thigh medially.
3. Adductor magnus	Ischial tuberosity	Posterior surface of femur	Obturator and sciatic nerve	Adducts, extends, and rotates thigh medially
4. Gracilis	Lower edge of symphysis pubis	Medial surface of tibia	Obturator nerve	Adducts thigh, flexes and rotates leg at knee

Table 5.1-11. Origin, insertion, nerve supply and actions of muscles that move the lower leg

Muscle	Origin	Insertion	Nerve Supply	Actions
Flexors (Hamstring group)				
1. Biceps femoris	Ischial tuberosity and posterior surface of femur	Head of fibula and lateral condyle of tibia	Tibial and common paroneal nerves from sciatic nerve	Flexes and rotates leg laterally and extends thigh
Semitendinosus	Ischial tuberosity	Medial surface of tibia	Tibial nerve	Flexes and rotates leg medially and extends thigh
Semimembranosus	Ischial tuberosity	Medial condyle of tibia	Tibial nerve	Flexes and rotates leg medially and extends thigh
2. *Sartorius*	Spine of ileum	Medial surface of tibia	Femoral nerve	Flexes leg and thigh, abducts thigh, rotates thigh laterally, and rotates leg medially
Extensors (Quadriceps femoris group)				
1. Rectus femoris	Spine of ileum and margin of acetabulum	Patella by common tendon which continues as patellar ligament to tibial tuberosity	Femoral nerve	Extends leg at knee
2. Vastus lateralis	Greater trochanter and posterior surface of femur	Lateral border of patella		
3. Vastus medialis	Medial surface of femur	Medial border of patella		
4. Vastus intermedius	Anterior and lateral surfaces of femur	Upper border of patella		

Vastus medialis

Biceps tendon

Patella

Ligamentum patellae

Peroneus longus

Subcutaneous surface of tibia

Extensor digitorum longus

Gastrocnemius (medial head)

Tibialis anterior

Soleus

Extensor hallucis longus

Lateral malleolus

A

Semi-tendinosus

Biceps

Semi-membranosus

Gracilis

Popliteal artery

Gastrocnemius (medial head)

Gastrocnemius (lateral head)

Soleus

Soleus

Peronus longus

Flexor digitorum longus

Medial malleolus

Achilles tendon

Lateral malleolus

B

Gastrocnemius (cut)

Gastrocnemius (cut)

Soleus (cut)

Soleus (cut)

Tibialis posterior

Flexor digitorum longus

Peroneus longus

Flexor hallucis longus

Peroneus brevis

C

Fig. 5.1-11. *Muscles of the leg region which move the ankle, foot and toes : A, anterior view; B, superficial posterior view; and C, deep posterior view.*

Table 5.1-12. Origin, insertion, nerve supply and actions of muscles that move the ankle, foot and toes

Muscle	Origin	Insertion	Nerve supply	Actions
Dorsiflexors				
1. Tibialis anterior	Lateral condyle and lateral surface of tibia	Tarsal bone (cuneiform) and first metatarsal	Deep fibular (peroneal) nerve	Dorsal flexion and inversion of foot
2. Fibularis (peroneus) tertius	Anterior surface of fibula	Dorsal surface of fifth metatarsal	Deep fibular (peroneal) nerve	Dorsal flexion and eversion of foot.
3. Extensor digitorum longus	Lateral condyle of tibia and anterior surface of fibula	Dorsal surfaces of second and third phalanges of four lateral toes	Deep fibular (peroneal) nerve of toes.	Dorsal flexion and eversion of foot and extension of toes.
Plantar flexors				
1. Gastrocnemius	Lateral and medial condyles of femur	Posterior surface of calcaneus	Tibial nerve	Plantar flexion of foot and flexion of leg at knee
2. Soleus	Head and shaft of fibula and posterior surface of tibia	Posterior surface of calcaneus	Tibial nerve	Plantar flexion of foot
3. Flexor digitorum longus	Posterior surface of tibia	Distal phalanges of four lateral toes	Tibial nerve	Plantar flexion and inversion of foot and flexion of four lateral toes
Invertor of foot				
1. Tibialis Posterior	Lateral condyle and posterior surface of tibia and posterior surface of fibula	Tarsal and meta-tarsal bones	Tibial nerve	Plantar flexion and inversion of foot.
Evertors of foot				
1. Fibularis (peroneus) longus	Lateral condyle of tibia and head and shaft of fibula	Tarsal and metatarsal bones	Superficial fibular (peroneal) nerve	Plantar flexion and eversion of foot; also supports arch
2. Fibularis (peroneus) brevis	Body of fibula	Base of fifth metatarsal	Superficial fibular (peroneal) nerve	

Neuromuscular Junction and Muscle Physiology

5.2

NEUROMUSCULAR JUNCTION

STRUCTURE

Neuromuscular junction refers to intimate contact of nerve endings with the muscle fibres to which they innervate. It is constituted by following structures (Fig. 5.2-1) :

Terminal button. The axon of a neuron supplying a skeletal muscle loses its myelin sheath and divides into a number of fine branches which end in small swellings (knobs) called *terminal buttons* or end feet which form a neuromuscular junction, at the centre of muscle fibre. The terminal knob contains large number of vesicles containing acetylcholine and mitochondria. The acetylcholine is synthesized by the mitochondria.

Presynaptic membrane. This refers to the axonal membrane lining the *terminal buttons* of the nerve endings.

Synaptic cleft. It is a 50 to 100 nm wide space between the presynaptic membrane and the postsynaptic membrane. It is filled by extracellular fluid with reticular fibres forming the matrix. It contains the enzyme cholinesterase which can degrade acetylcholine.

Postsynaptic membrane. This is the name given to the muscle fibre membrane (sarcolemma) in the region of neuromuscular junction. The muscle membrane in this

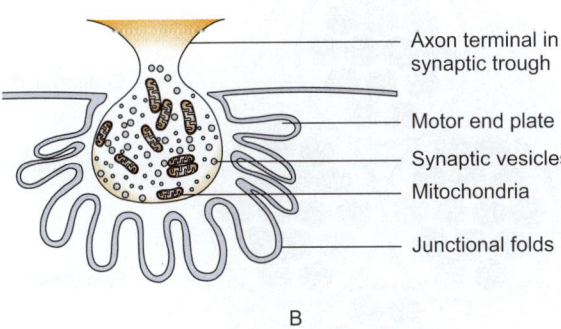

Fig. 5.2-1. *Structure of neuromuscular junction: A, the axon of the neuron loses its myelin sheath and divides into fine branches; and B, structure of terminal button and motor end plate.*

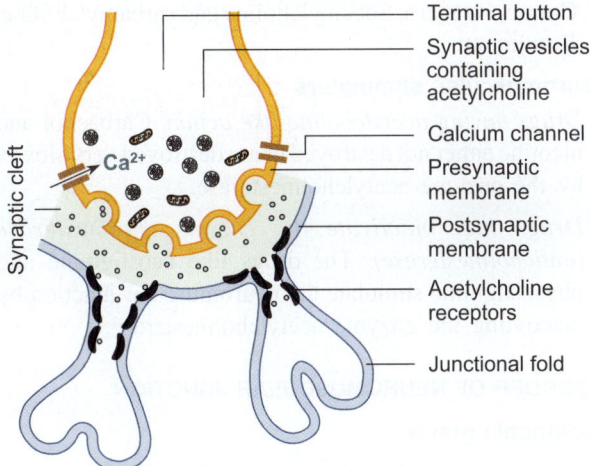

Fig. 5.2-2. *Detailed structure of neuromuscular junction showing Ca^{2+} channels on presynaptic membrane and ACh receptors on postsynaptic membrane.*

region is thickened and depressed to form the *synaptic trough* in which the terminal button fits. This thickened portion of the muscle membrane is also called *motor end plate*. The postsynaptic membrane contains *receptor sites* for acetylcholine called the *nicotinic receptors*.

NEUROMUSCULAR TRANSMISSION

The skeletal muscle is stimulated only through its nerve. The neuromuscular junction transmits the impulses from the nerve to muscle. The *sequence of events* which causes transmission of impulse through neuromuscular junction are:

Release of acetylcholine by the nerve terminals. When the nerve impulse (action potential) travelling in the nerve fibre (axon) reaches the terminal buttons, the voltage-gated Ca^{2+} channels present on the presynaptic membrane open up. Consequently the Ca^{2+} ions present in the ECF of synaptic cleft enter the terminal buttons.

The elevated Ca^{2+} levels in the cytosol of terminal buttons trigger a marked increase in exocytosis of vesicles releasing acetylcholine in the synaptic cleft (Fig.5.2-2).

Effect of acetylcholine on the postsynaptic membrane. The acetylcholine so released diffuses in the synaptic cleft

and binds to the nicotinic-acetylcholine receptors located mainly on the junctional folds of the motor end plate (postsynaptic membrane) leading to opening up of the tubular channels.

Development of end plate potential. Due to opening of the acetylcholine-gated channels in the end plate membrane, a large number of Na^+ ions from the ECF enter inside the muscle fibre following the electrochemical gradient.

When sodium ions enter inside, carrying with them large numbers of positive charges, there occurs depolarization causing a local positive potential change inside the muscle fibre membrane called the *end plate potential.*

The end plate potential is non-propagative but when a critical level of –60mV is reached, it triggers the development of action potential in the muscle fibre and is conducted away from the end plate in both the directions along the muscle fibres thus causing muscle contraction.

Removal of acetylcholine. The actylcholine released in the synaptic cleft stays for short period and is removed within one millisecond by the enzyme acetylcholinesterase which is present in the matrix of synaptic cleft.

It is important to note that the rapid removal of acetylcholine prevents the repeated excitation of muscle fibre.

DRUGS AFFECTING NEUROMUSCULAR JUNCTION

Neuromuscular blockers

Neuromuscular blockers are the drugs that block transmission at the neuromuscular junction. Some of the common neuromuscular blockers, which are commonly used in clinical practice and research, are:

- Curare, Bungaro, Succinylcholine and carbamylcholine, Botulinum

Neuromuscular stimulators

1. *Drugs having acetylcholine-like action.* Carbachol and nicotine either not destroyed or are destroyed very slowly by the enzyme acetylcholinesterase.

2. *Drugs that inactivate the enzyme cholinesterase (anticholinesterase).* The drugs like neostigmine and physostigmine stimulate the neuromuscular junction by inactivting the enzyme acetylcholinesterase.

DISORDER OF NEUROMUSCULAR JUNCTION

Myasthenia gravis

Myasthenia gravis is a disorder in which the myoneural junction is unable to transmit signals from the nerve fibre to muscle fibres, thereby causing paralysis of the involved muscles. Myasthenia is probably an autoimmune disease. In this disease the antibodies are produced against the acetylcholine-gated channels (receptors) present on the motor end plate which destroy these channels. Thus, the acetylcholine released at the nerve terminal is not able to produce adequate end plate potential to excite the muscle fibre. If the disease is intense enough, the patient dies of paralysis, in particular, the paralysis of respiratory muscles.

MUSCLE PHYSIOLOGY

GENERAL CONSIDERATIONS

The muscle cell, like the neuron, is an excitable tissue, i.e. an action potential is generated when it is stimulated.

There are three different types of muscles in the body: skeletal muscles, cardiac muscles and smooth muscles. Based on certain distinctive features the muscles can be grouped as:

Striated versus non-striated muscles

Striated muscle cells show large number of cross striations at regular intervals when seen under light microscope. Skeletal and cardiac muscles are striated.

Non-striated muscle cells do not show any striations. Smooth muscles or the so-called plain muscles are non-striated.

Voluntary versus involuntary muscles

Voluntary muscle's can be made to contract under our will to perform the movements we desire. All skeletal muscles are voluntary muscles. These are supplied by somatic motor nerves.

Involuntary muscle's activities cannot be controlled at will. Cardiac and all smooth muscles are involuntary muscles. These are innervated by autonomic nerves.

Skeletal muscles

The skeletal muscles, as the name indicates, are attached with the bones of the body skeleton and their contraction results in the body movements. The skeletal muscles constitute about 40 per cent of the total body mass.

STRUCTURAL ORGANIZATION OF SKELETAL MUSCLE

Structurally, the skeletal muscle consists of a large number of muscle fibres and a connective tissue framework organized as (Figs. 5.2-3 and 5.2-4):

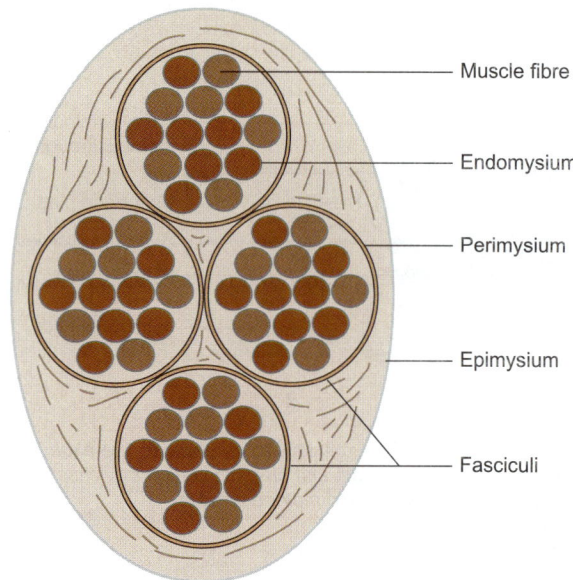

Fig. 5.2-3. Transverse section of skeletal muscle seen under light microscope.

- Each *muscle fibre* is surrounded by delicate connective tissue called *endomysium.*
- The muscle fibres are grouped into a number of bundles called *fasciculi.* Each fasciculus is surrounded by a sheath called *perimysium.*
- All the fasciculi collectively form the *muscle belly.* The connective tissue that surrounds the entire muscle belly is called *epimysium.*
- At the junction of the muscle with its tendon the fibres of endomysium, perimysium and epimysium become continuous with the fibres of the tendon.
- *Tendons* are fibrous terminal ends of the muscles made up of collagen fibres.

STRUCTURE OF A MUSCLE FIBRE

Each muscle fibre is basically a long (1 to 4 cm), cylindrical (10-100 μm in diameter) multinucleated cell. Its cell membrane is called *sarcolemma* and the cytoplasm is called *sarcoplasm.* The sarcoplasm contains number of *myofibrils* which form the main structure of a muscle

Fig. 5.2-4. *Schematic diagram showing structural organization of skeletal muscle: A, muscle belly; B, muscle fibres grouped into fasciculi; C, muscle fibre; D, myofibril; and E, arrangement of thick and thin filaments.*

fibre. The sarcolemma along with the sarcoplasmic reticulum form the so-called *sarcotubular system.*

Myofibril

Each muscle fibre consists of a large number of myofibrils which are arranged parallel to each other and running along the entire length of the muscle fibre.

Each myofibril consists of many thick and thin filaments (myofilaments) made up of contractile proteins. Thick filaments are made up of myosin, while thin filaments are made of actin.

Striations of muscle fibres

The dark and light bands result from a difference in the refractive index of its different parts. The arrangement is as below (Fig. 5.2-4).

- The dark band is called *A band.* In the area of A band the thick (myosin) filaments line up the thin filaments.
- In the centre of each A band there is a lighter H zone where thin filaments do not overlap the thick filaments.
- In the centre of each H zone is seen M line which is more pronounced during muscle contraction.
- The light band is called *I band.* This area contains only thin (actin) filaments.
- Each I band is bisected by a narrow dark Z *line.* The portion of myofibril between two successive Z lines is called a *sarcomere.* Thus a sarcomere includes ½ I band + A band + ½ I band and is about 2.5 µm in length at rest. The sarcomere is the structural and functional unit of the muscle fibre. During muscle contraction the sarcomere reduces in length to 1.5 µm and during stretching of the muscle it increases in length to 3.5 µm.

Thick and thin filaments

The thick and thin filaments (Fig. 5.2-4E) form the *contractile apparatus* of a striated muscle. These are made up of three types of proteins:

- *Contractile proteins* are *myosin* and *actin* which interact to generate the contractile force in a muscle.
- *Regulatory proteins* also called relaxation proteins include *tropomyosin* and *troponin.* These regulate the interaction between the myosin and actin.
- *Anchoring proteins,* as the name indicates, anchor the different proteins to each other as well as to sarcolemma.

Thick filament

A thick filament is made up of hundreds of molecules *myosin.*

Structure of myosin molecule. The myosin molecule is made up of 6 polypeptide chains, 2 heavy chains and 4 light chains. The two heavy chains form a double helix which constitutes the *tail* and *body* of the myosin molecule. The light chains form the globular *head* of myosin molecule. The myosin molecule present in the skeletal muscle has two heads and is called *myosin-II.*

Arrangement of myosin molecules in a thick filament. In a thick filament, half of the myosin molecules are oriented with their heads in one direction and the remaining half in opposite direction (Fig. 5.2-5 A & B).

Thin filament

Each thin filament is made up of contractile protein molecules (actin) and two types of regulatory protein molecules (tropomyosin and troponin) (Fig. 5.2-6).

A

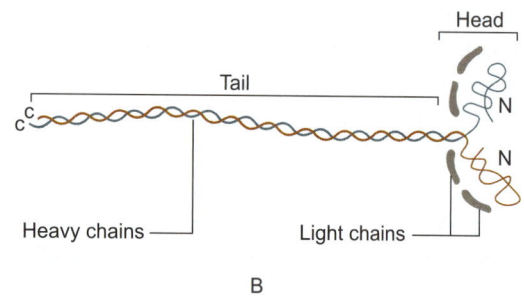

B

Fig. 5.2-5. *Arrangement of myosin molecules in thick filament (A) and structure of myosin molecule (B).*

Fig. 5.2-6. *Structure of a thin filament.*

Actin. About 300 to 400 actin molecules are present in each thin filament. The actin molecules form a long double helix consisting of two chains of globular units.

Tropomyosin. About 40-60 tropomyosin molecules are present in each thin filament. The tropomyosins are long filaments which lie in the groove between the two chains of actin molecules. It covers the binding site of actin where myosin head comes in contact with actin which prevents the interaction between actin and myosin filaments.

Troponin. Troponin molecules are small globular units located at intervals along the tropomyosin molecule. The troponin molecule has three subunits:

- *Troponin-T* binds the other troponin components to tropomyosin.
- *Troponin-I* prevents the interaction of myosin heads with active sites on actin.
- *Troponin-C* contains binding site for Ca^{2+} that initiates muscle contraction.

SARCOTUBULAR SYSTEM

The sarcolemma (cell membrane of muscle cell) along with the sarcoplasmic reticulum (the endoplasmic reticulum of muscle cell) forms a highly specialized system called sarcotubular system. This plays an important role in the internal conduction of depolarization within the muscle fibre. The sarcotubular system is primarily formed by a transverse tubular system (T-system) and a longitudinal sarcoplasmic reticulum (Fig. 5.2-7).

Fig. 5.2-7. *Sarcotubular system showing transverse tubules and longitudinal sarcoplasmic reticulum.*

PROCESS OF EXCITATION-CONTRACTION COUPLING

The process by which depolarization of a muscle fibre initiates contraction is called excitation-contraction coupling. The sequence of events during this process are:

- Action potential initiated in the plasma membrane of a muscle fibre spreads rapidly on the surface as well as into the interior of the muscle fibre through the T-tubules.
- When the action potential reaches the tip of T-tubule, calcium ions diffuse into the cytoplasm. The concentration of Ca^{2+} in the ICF is increased by some 2000 times.
- The Ca^{2+} ions get attached to troponin-C and start a chain of events which produce contraction. Thus the calcium ions act as linking or coupling material between the excitation and the contraction of the muscle.

PROCESS OF MUSCLE CONTRACTION

Molecular basis of muscle contraction

AF Huxley and HE Huxley in 1954 put forward the *sliding theory* or *ratchet theory.* This theory explains that the sliding of filaments is brought about by a repeated cycle of formation of the *cross-bridges* between the head of myosin and actin molecules.

Initiation of cross-bridge cycling. During resting stage, troponin-I is lightly bound to actin and the tropomyosin molecules are located in the groove between the strands of actin filaments in such a way that they block the myosin-binding sites on actin (Fig. 5.2-8A). When activation takes place, the Ca^{2+} ions get attached to *troponin-C* subunit of the protein troponin. This causes the tropomyosin molecule to move laterally, uncovering the binding sites on the actin molecules for head of the myosin molecules. Thus the cross-bridge cycle is switched on (initiated) by the lateral movement of tropomyosin (Fig. 5.2-8B and Fig. 5.2-9).

A

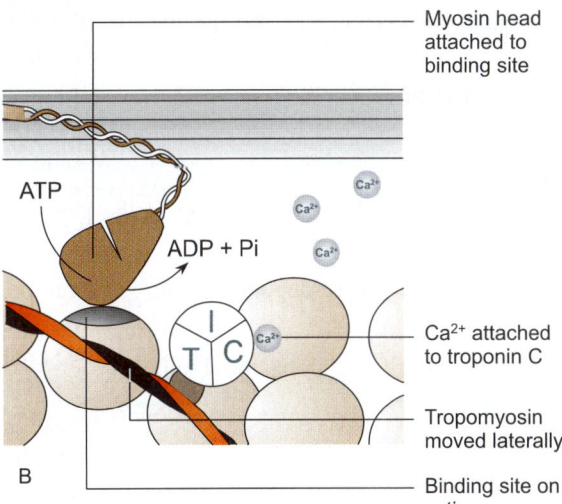

B

Fig. 5.2-8. *Initiation of cross-bridge cycling : A, resting state (myosin binding site on actin is covered by troponin -tropomyosin complex); and B, on activation Ca^{2+} binds to troponin-C subunits resulting in conformational change and lateral displacement of tropomyosin (causing uncovering of binding site for myosin—head of myosin) on actin (initiation of cross-bridge cycle).*

Stage i

Stage ii

Stage iii

Stage iv

Stage v

Fig. 5.2-9. *Stages of cross-bridge cycling.*

Muscle Relaxation within a few milliseconds of the action potential, the calcium pump transports Ca^{2+} ions present in sarcoplasm during contraction back into the longitudinal portion of the sarcoplasmic reticulum.

SEQUENCE OF EVENTS DURING MUSCLE CONTRACTION AND RELAXATION WHEN STIMULATED BY A NERVE

The events which occur during contraction and relaxation in a skeletal muscle, when excited by a nerve, are summarized sequence-wise:

Nerve excitation

Stimulation of motor neuron

↓

Initiation of action potential in motor neuron's axon

↓

Nerve conduction

Propagation of action potential in the motor nerve

↓

Impulse reaching nerve ending (at synaptic button)

↓

Neuromuscular transmission

Increased permeability of presynaptic membrane to Ca^{2+} ions

↓

Inflow of Ca^{2+} ions from ECF into the nerve terminals

↓

Release of ACh from microvesicles present at nerve terminal

↓

Diffusion of ACh into synaptic cleft

↓

Binding of ACh to receptors on the motor end plate (postsynaptic membrane)

↓

Opening of ACh-gated channels in the motor end plate membrane

↓

Entry of mainly Na^+ ions and to a lesser extent Ca^{2+} ions through these channels into the muscle fibre

↓

Development of end plate potential (EPP)

↓

Muscle excitation

Local EPP when reaches a threshold magnitude, voltage-gated Na^+ channels are opened up at the site.

↓

Generation of action potential (AP) in the muscle fibre by end plate depolarization.

↓

Propagation of AP in muscle fibre along the surface and into the fibre along the T-tubules

↓

Excitation contraction coupling

Release of Ca^{2+} ions from terminal cistern

↓

Diffusion of Ca^{2+} ions into the sarcoplasm

↓

Binding of Ca^{2+} ions to troponin-C

Muscle contraction (molecular theory)

Uncovering of binding sites for myosin on actin
↓
Cross-bridge formation between myosin head and actin
↓
Angular movement of cross-bridges (Power stroke)
↓
Sliding of thin filaments over thick filaments.
↓
Initiation of muscle contraction
↓
Muscle relaxation

Active transport of Ca^{2+} into sacrcoplasmic reticulum
↓
Decreased concentration of Ca^{2+} in sarcoplasm
↓
Removal of Ca^{2+} ions from troponin-C
↓
Cessation of cross-bridge cycling
↓
Relaxation of muscle fibre

C H A P T E R   5 . 2

Removal of calcium from troponin restores blocking action of troponin-tropomyosin complex. Myosin cross-bridge cycle closes and muscle relaxes.

CONTRACTILE RESPONSE

A typical contractile response consists of a brief contraction followed by relaxation, and is referred to as *single muscle twitch*.

Isometric contraction

As the name indicates (iso = same, metric = measure, i.e. length), in this type of contraction, the length of muscle remains same but tension is developed in the muscle. Thus there is no movement of the object. Since work done is the product of *force* and *distance*, therefore, in isometric contraction *no external work is done*.

Examples of isometric contraction of muscles

- Contraction of muscles which help in maintaining posture against gravity, and
- Contraction of arm muscles when trying to push a wall.

Isotonic contraction

As the name indicates (iso = same, and tonic = tone or tension), in this type of contraction, the tension in the muscle remains same whereas its length decreases. Since the muscle length is shortened, so the *external work is done* in isotonic contraction.

Examples of isotonic muscle contraction

- Contraction of leg muscles during walking and running,
- Contractions of muscles while lifting a weight, and
- Contraction of muscles during flexion of arm.

SOME CHARACTERISTICS OF THE SKELETAL MUSCLES IN THE INTACT BODY

Muscle tone

Muscle tone is the state of slight contraction with certain degree of vigour and tension. All the skeletal muscles exhibit muscle tone. However, it is more marked in the antigravity muscles, viz. extensors of the lower limbs, trunk muscles, and muscles of the neck.

Maintenance of muscle tone. Muscle tone is maintained by asynchronous discharge of impulses from gamma motor neurons in the anterior grey horn of the spinal cord concerned with the motor nerve supply of the muscles. The gamma motor neurons in turn are controlled by some higher centres in brain.

Abnormalities of the muscle tone include:

- *Hypertonic state* or the spastic paralysis of the skeletal muscles occurs in upper motor neuron lesions. Spasticity results due to exaggerated activity of lower motor neurons following or loss of inhibitional activity of upper motor neurons.

- *Hypotonic state* or the flaccid paralysis of the muscles occurs in lower motor neuron lesions. The tone of the affected muscles is decreased or totally lost and ultimately the muscles undergo wasting.

Gradation of force of muscle contraction in the intact body

For performing different kinds of work, e.g. picking up a pen from the table, or lifting 10 kg weight, same muscles are involved but on these different situations, muscles can generate different degree of power. This property of skeletal muscles is known as gradation of force of contraction. Gradation of muscle power in muscles is made possible by certain factors which affect the force of contraction. These are:

1. *Recruitment of motor units.* The force of contraction produced in a muscle depends upon the number of motor units recruited. When minimal activity is required, only a few motor units are recruited. With increasing effort, more and more motor units from the *motor neuron pool* of a muscle are recruited into activity. This phenomenon is called multiple motor unit summation.

2. *Frequency of nerve impulses.* The motor control system in the brain can vary the force of contraction by varying the frequency of nerve impulses stimultaing the muscle. As the impulse frequency increases, its effects are summated (*wave summation)* and the muscle tension increases.

3. *Synchronization of impulses.* At any one time, the motor units are in different phases of activity, i.e. some are contracting and others are relaxing. Due to algebraic summation the muscle gives a steady but weak pull. With increasing synchronization of the motor units, the force of contraction increases.

4. *Effect of initial length of muscle fibre.* According to Starling's law, upto an optimal limit, the greater the initial length of the muscle fibres, greater is the force of contraction. This, however, is not the usual method of varying the force of contraction in the intact body.

5. *Warming up.* Warming up is the term used in the parlour of sports persons for the exercises performed before actually participating in any game event. These pregame 'warm up' due to beneficial effects of the exercise increase the muscle performance when the person takes part in the actual event.

Muscle fatigue

Failure of a muscle to maintain tension as a result of previous contractile activity is known as muscle fatigue. If the muscle is allowed to rest after the onset of fatigue it recovers its ability to contract.

It refers to the fatigue of the most of muscles that develops after prolonged general exercise such as marathon running, and competitive football match playing.

Onset and recovery of fatigue depends on:
- Intensity and duration of exercise, and
- Type of muscle fibres. Fast glycolytic fibres fatigue early and also recover rapidly from fatigue. Slow oxidative fibres do not fatigue early but they also require longer time of rest (upto 24 hours) for complete recovery.

COMMON DISORDERS OF MUSCLES AND ELECTROMYOGRAPHY

DISORDERS OF SKELETAL MUSCLES

1. *Muscular dystrophy.* Muscular dystrophy is a syndrome which occurs due to genetic mutation and is characterized by progressive muscle weakness.

2. *Myotonia.* Myotonia is a disorder which occurs due to abnormalities of the sodium and chloride channels caused by abnormal genes on chromosomes 7, 17 or 19. It is characterized by an abnormally prolonged muscle relaxation after voluntary contraction.

3. *Myasthenia gravis.* It is a disorder of neuromuscular junction, characterized by a grave weakness of the muscles (see page 138).

4. *Fibrillation and denervation hypersensitivity.* The denervation of skeletal muscles in lower motor neuron lesions causes flaccid paralysis of the muscle, fibrillation and denervation hypersensitivity.
- *Fibrillation* is characterized by fine, irregular contractions of individual muscle fibres.
- *Denervation hypersensitivity* refers to when the muscle becomes highly sensitive to acetylcholine.

ELECTROMYOGRAPHY

Electromyography refers to the technique of recording the total electrical activity of the motor nerve and the muscle under study. The machine used to record the said electrical activity is called *electromyograph* and the record obtained is called the *electromyogram.*

Cardiovascular System

Anatomy of Cardiovascular System: The Heart and Blood Vessels

6.1

ORGANIZATION AND FUNCTIONS OF CARDIOVASCULAR SYSTEM

ORGANIZATION OF CARDIOVASCULAR SYSTEM

The cardiovascular system (CVS) consists of the heart and the blood vessels. The *heart* acts as a system of two pumps working in series and forms the driving force for blood flow. The blood vessels that take blood from the heart to various tissues are called *arteries*. The smallest arteries are called *arterioles*. Arterioles open into a network of *capillaries* which constitute the microcirculation. The most important function of blood vessels, i.e. the rapid exchange of materials between the blood and extracellular fluid bathing the tissue cells is served by the capillaries. In other words, capillaries serve as the *exchange region*. In some situations capillaries are replaced by slightly different vessels called *sinusoids*. Blood from capillaries (or from sinusoids) is collected by small *venules* which join to form *veins*. Veins serve as the blood reservoir and return the collected blood to the heart. Functionally the cardiovascular system consists of two main divisions (Fig. 6.1-1):

- *Systemic circulation*
- *Pulmonary circulation*

FUNCTIONS OF CARDIOVASCULAR SYSTEM

Primary functions of the cardiovascular system are:
1. Distribution of nutrients and oxygen (O_2) to all body cells, and

147

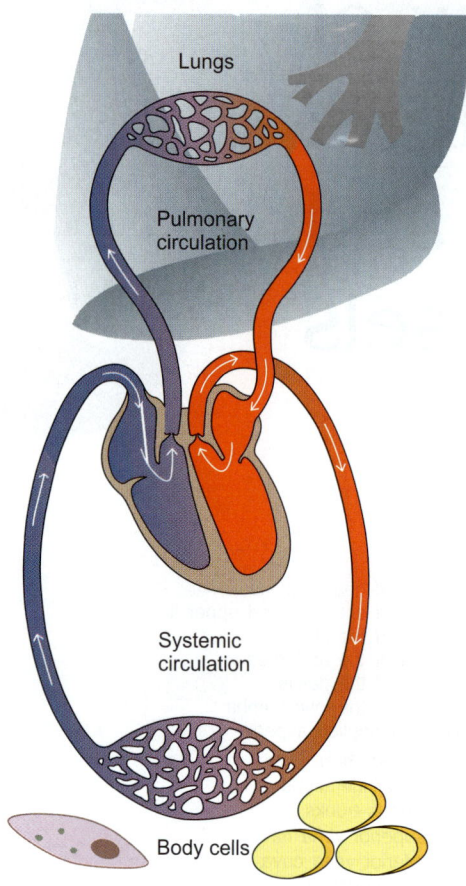

Fig. 6.1-1. *General pattern of cardiovascular system comprising systemic and pulmonary circulation.*

2. Collection of waste products and CO_2 from different body cells and to carry them to excretory organs for excretion.
Secondary functions that are subserved by the cardiovascular system are :
1. Thermoregulation
2. Distribution of hormones to the target tissues, and
3. Delivery of antibodies, platelets and leucocytes to aid body defence mechanism.

THE HEART

GROSS APPEARANCE, SIZE AND LOCATION

The heart is a cone-shaped, hollow muscular pump designed to ensure the circulation of blood through the tissues of the body.

Size. In an adult, the heart is as large as a clenched fist, being approximately 14 cm (5.5 inches) long and 9 cm (3.5 inches) wide. It weights about 300 gm.

Location. The heart lies in the mediastinal area of thoracic cavity between the lungs. It is situated obliquely behind the sternum, a little more to the left than the right (Fig. 6.1-2).

Fig. 6.1-2. *Location of heart in the thorax.*

Gross appearance and immediate relations. Being conical in shape, it is described as having base, apex, sternocostal surface and diaphragmatic surface (Fig. 6.1-3).
- *Sternocostal surface* of the heart is facing anteriorly and is related to the body of sternum and costal cartilages.
- *Diaphragmatic surface* is facing inferiorly and is in contact with the diaphragm.
- *Apex* refers to the bluntly pointed terminal part of the heart which is directed downwards and to the left. The apex is about 9 cm to the left of the midline at the level of the 5th intercostal space, i.e. a little below and medial to the left nipple. Apex of the heart is formed by the left ventricle.
- *Base* i.e. posterior aspect of the heart is related to the structures in posterior mediastinum, i.e., descending aorta, inferior vena cava, oesophagus and trachea. Base is directed upwards and to the right (e.g. apex which is directed downwards and to the left).
  Laterally the heart is enclosed by lungs.
  Superiorly the heart is associated with aorta, superior vena cava, pulmonary artery and pulmonary veins.

CHAMBERS OF HEART

Each half of heart consists of an inflow chamber called the *atrium* and an outflow chamber called the *ventricle* (Fig. 6.1-4). Thus, there are four chambers in the heart.

Atria

Interatrial septum separates the right and left atria which are thin-walled chambers.

Right atrium receives deoxygenated blood from tissues of the entire body through the *superior* and *inferior vena cavae*. This blood passes into the right ventricle through the right *atrioventricular orifice* which is guarded by *tricuspid valve*. The right atrium has got the pacemaker

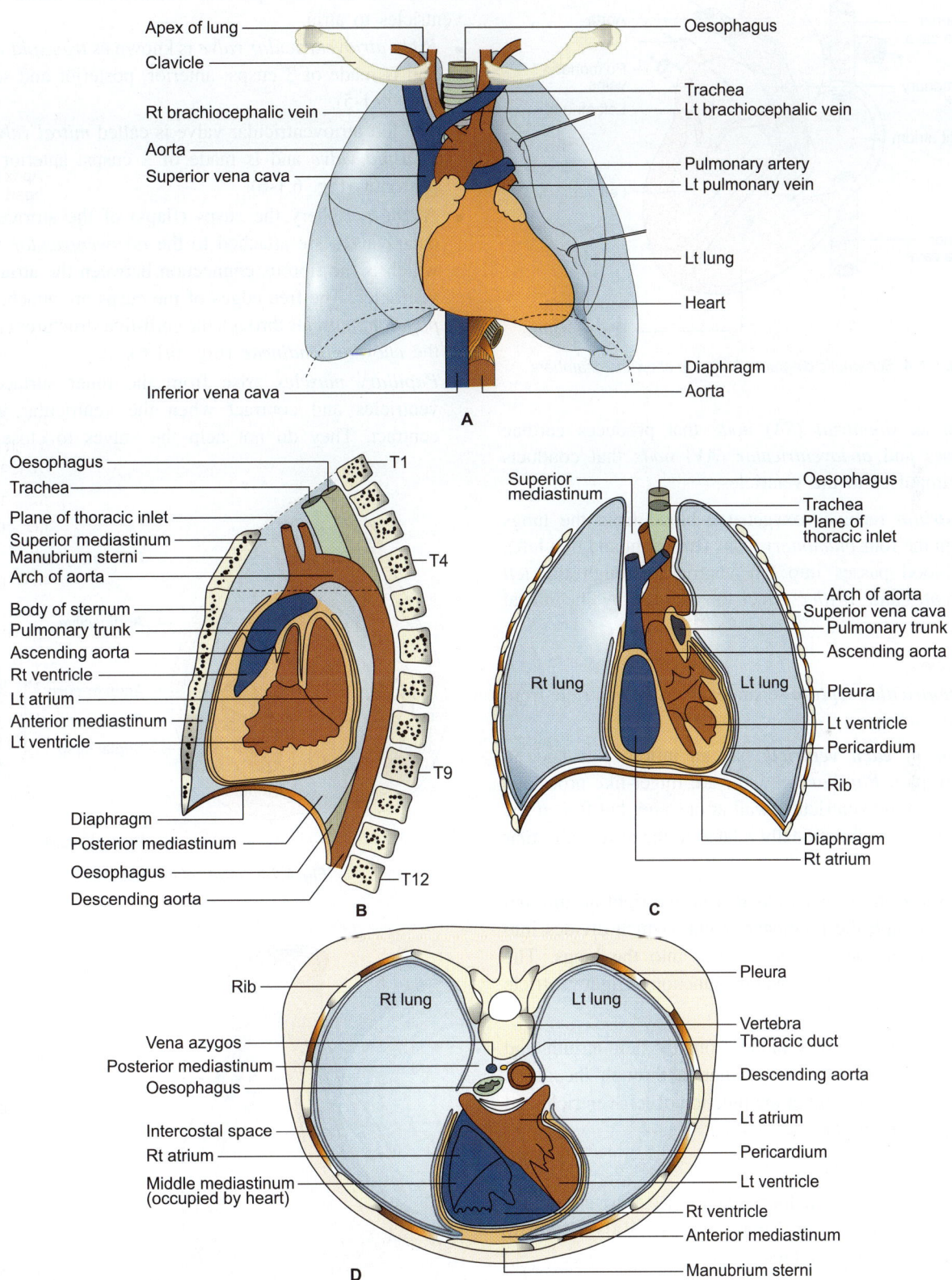

Fig. 6.1-3. *Gross appearance and structures related to heart : A; front view; B, coronal section through heart and lungs; C, sagittal section of thorax in the area of heart; and D, transverse section of thorax through heart.*

C
H
A
P
T
E
R

6
.
1

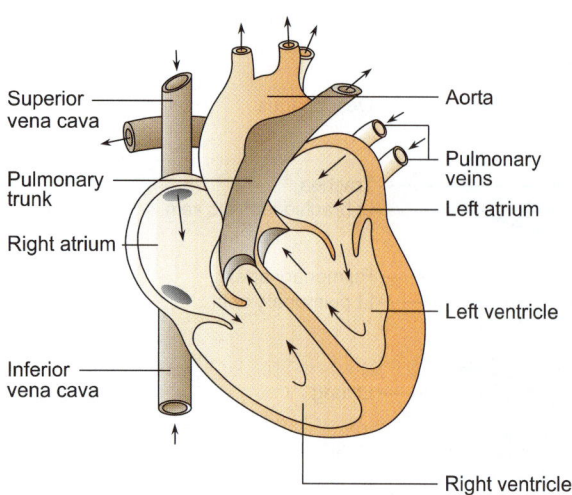

Fig. 6.1-4. Schematic diagram of heart to show the chambers.

known as *sinoatrial (SA) node* that produces cardiac impulses and *atrioventricular (AV) node* that conducts these impulses to the ventricles.

Left atrium receives oxygenated blood from the lungs through the four *pulmonary veins* (two right and two left). This blood passes into left ventricle through the *left atrioventricular orifice* which is guarded by the mitral valve.

Ventricles

Interventricular septum separates the right ventricle from left ventricle.

Interior of each ventricle has an inflow part and an outflow part. *Papillary muscles* are finger-like processes attached to the ventricular wall at one end, but free at the other. They are functionally related to the atrioventricular valves.

Right ventricle receives blood from the right atrium and pumps through the pulmonary trunk (which divides into right and left pulmonary arteries) into the lungs. The *pulmonary valve* is present at the junction of right ventricle and pulmonary trunk.

Left ventricle receives blood from the left atrium and pumps out into systemic circulation through the aorta. *Aortic* valve is present at the junction of left ventricle and the *ascending aorta.*

VALVES OF HEART

There are four valves in human heart, two atrioventri-cular valves and two semilunar valves. Valves allow unidirectional flow of blood.

Atrioventricular valves

The atrioventricular valves open towards the ventricles and close towards the atria. They allow blood to flow

from atria to ventricles. But when ventricles contract, they are closed and thus prevent backflow of blood from ventricles to atria.

- *Right atrioventricular valve* is known as *tricuspid valve* and is made of 3 cusps: anterior, posterior and septal (Fig. 6.1-5).
- The left atrioventricular valve is called *mitral valve* or *bicuspid valve* and is made of 2 cusps: anterior and posterior (Fig. 6.1-6).
- At the periphery the cusps (flaps) of the atrioventri-cular valves are attached to the *atrioventricular ring,* which is the fibrous connection between the atria and ventricles. The free edges of the cusps are attached to *papillary muscles* through the cord-like structures called the *chordae tendineae* (Fig. 6.1-6).
- *Papillary muscles* arise from the inner surface of ventricles and contract when the ventricular walls contract. They do not help the valves to close but

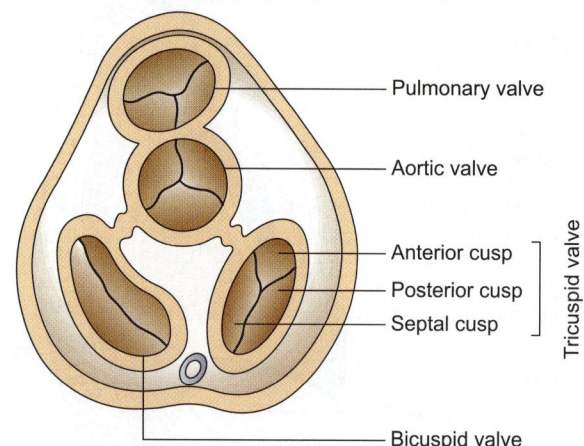

Fig. 6.1-5. Valves of the heart.

Fig. 6.1-6. Bicuspid valve attached with papillary muscle and chordae tendineae.

prevent the bulging of the valves into the atria when ventricles contract.

Semilunar valves

- *Aortic valve* is the semilunar valve present at the opening of aorta in left ventricle. It is made of three semilunar cusps: one anterior and two posterior (Fig. 6.1-5).
- *Pulmonary valve* is the semilunar valve present at the opening of pulmonary trunk into the right ventricle. It is also made of three semilunar cusps: one posterior and two anterior (Fig. 6.1-5).
- *Semilunar valves open* away from ventricles and close towards the ventricles. These valves open when ventricles contract allowing the blood to flow from left ventricle to aorta and from right ventricle to pulmonary trunk.
- *Semilunar valves close* when ventricles relax thus preventing backflow of blood from aorta or pulmonary trunk into the ventricles.

STRUCTURE OF THE WALLS OF HEART

Walls of the heart are composed of thick layer of cardiac muscle, the *myocardium*, covered externally by the epicardium, and lined internally by the *endocardium*.

- Walls of the atrial portion of the heart are thin.
- Walls of the ventricular portion of the heart are thick.

Skeleton of the heart consists of fibrous rings that surround the atrioventricular, pulmonary, and aortic orifices and are continuous with the membranous part of the ventricular septum.

Pericardium

The heart and roots of the great vessels are enclosed by a fibroserous sac called pericardium. Its function is to restrict excessive movements of the heart as a whole and to serve as a lubricated container in which different parts of the heart can contract. Pericardium consists of two layers: outer fibrous and inner serous (Fig. 6.1-7).

Fibrous pericardium surrounds the heart like a bag and is attached with the surrounding structures.

Serous pericardium has parietal and visceral layers. The *parietal layer* of serous pericardium lines the fibrous pericardium and is reflected around the roots of the great vessels to become continuous with the *visceral layer of serous pericardium* that closely cover the heart and is often called the *epicardium*. The slit-like space between the parietal and visceral layers of the serous pericardium is called *pericardial cavity* which contains small amount of *pericardial fluid* that acts as a lubricant to facilitate movement of the heart.

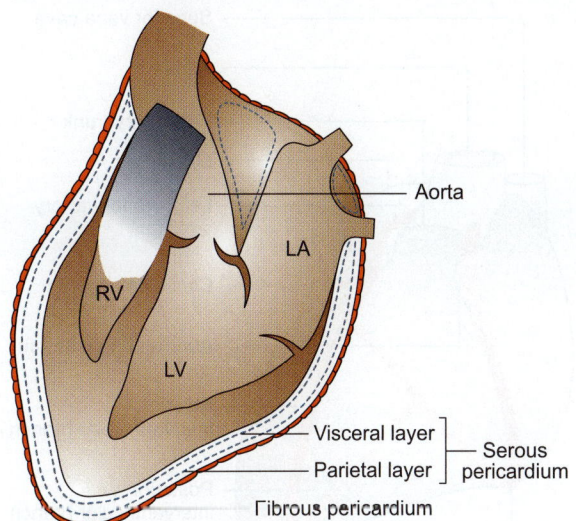

Fig. 6.1-7. *Schematic sagittal section of heart showing fibrous and serous pericardium.*

Myocardium

The myocardium (muscular tissue of the heart) is the main tissue constituting the walls of the heart. It consists of three types of muscle fibres:

- *Cardiac muscles* forming the walls of the atria and ventricles (see page 169),
- Muscle fibres forming the *pacemaker* which is the site of origin of cardiac impulse (see page 172), and
- Muscle fibres forming the *conducting system* which transmits the impulse to the various parts of the heart (see page 172).

Endocardium

Endocardium is thin smooth and glistening membrane lining the myocardium internally. It consists of a single layer of endothelial cells. The endocardium continues as the endothelium of great vessels opening in the heart.

BLOOD SUPPLY TO THE HEART

The blood is supplied to the heart by coronary arteries.

CORONARY BLOOD VESSELS

Coronary arteries

Two coronary arteries (right and left) arise from the root of ascending aorta and supply blood to the myocardium (Fig. 6.1-8).

Right coronary artery (RCA) supplies blood to the right ventricle, right atrium, the posterior part of left ventricle, posterior part of interventricular septum and major portion of the conducting system of heart including SA node.

Left coronary artery (LCA) thus supplies mainly to the anterior part of left ventricle, left atrium, anterior part of the interventricular septum and a part of the left branch of bundle of His.

C H A P T E R   6 . 1

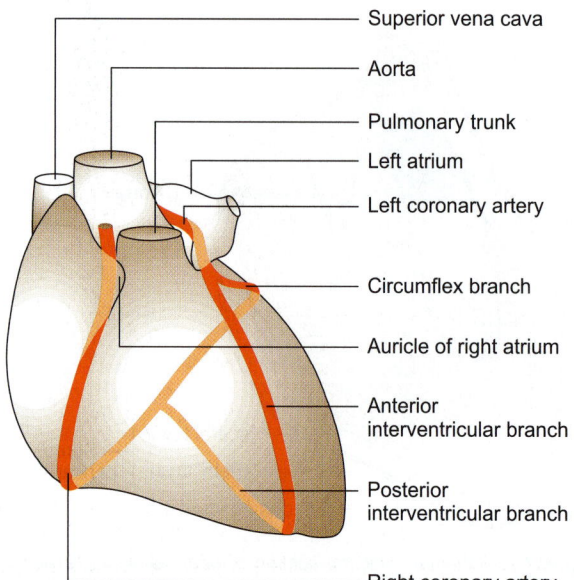

Fig. 6.1-8. Major coronary arteries and their branches.

Coronary veins

Coronary sinus is a wide vein about two centimetres long which drains most of the venous blood from the myocardium (mainly left ventricle) into the right atrium. Its tributaries are the *great cardiac vein,* the *small cardiac vein,* the *posterior vein of left ventricle,* and the *oblique vein of left ventricle* (Fig. 6.1-9).

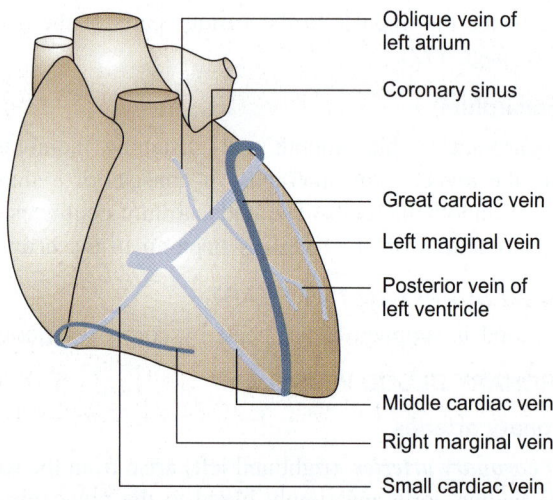

Fig. 6.1-9. Coronary sinus and its tributaries.

Anterior cardiac vein draining venous blood mainly from the right ventricle opens directly into the right atrium.

Thebesian veins and *coronary-luminal vessels* (connections between the coronary vessels and the lumen of heart) constitute the deep venous system. These vessels drain only less than 10 per cent of the venous blood from

myocardium directly into the various cardiac chambers, contributing to an *anatomic shunt effect.* The coronary luminal connections carry a larger proportion of the flow in the right ventricle than in the left ventricle.

CORONARY BLOOD FLOW: CHARACTERISTIC FEATURES

Normal coronary blood flow and oxygen demand

A continuous flow of blood to the heart is essential to maintain an adequate supply of O_2 and nutrients.

Normal coronary blood flow at rest is about 250 ml (70 ml/100 gm tissue/min), i.e. about 5% of the resting cardiac output (5 L). Three- to six-fold increase in the coronary blood flow may occur during exercise.

Phasic changes in coronary blood flow

The coronary blood flow shows changes during phases of cardiac cycle. The blood flow is determined by the balance between *pressure head* (i.e. aortic pressure) and the resistance (i.e. extravascular pressure exerted by the myocardium on the coronary vessels) offered to blood flow during various phases of cardiac cycle as shown in Fig. 6.1-10 and described below:

Blood flow to left ventricle

During systole the tension developed in the left ventricle is so high that it has throttling effect on the branches of coronary arteries. As a result, the average blood flow through the capillaries of left ventricles falls.

During diastole the cardiac muscles relax and blood flow increases. Thus, most of the coronary blood flow (over 70%) occurs during diastole.

Blood flow to right ventricle and atria

Blood passing through coronary capillaries of right ventricle also shows phasic changes similar to left ventricle. However, the changes in right ventricular flow are far less because force of contraction of the right ventricle is much less. Thus, the blood flow to the right ventricle and atria occurs both during systole and diastole.

INNERVATION OF THE HEART

Heart is innervated by both divisions (sympathetic and parasympathetic) of the autonomic nervous system. For details (see page 173 and 197).

THE BLOOD VESSELS

The blood vessels that comprise the vascular system can be grouped into two systems :
• The arterial system, and
• The venous system

The arterial and venous trees of the body functionally constitute two different systems of circulation—the pul-

Phases

1 Atrial systole
2 Isovolumic contraction phase ⎤
3 Rapid ejection   ⎬ **Ventricular systole**
4 Slow ejection   ⎦
5 Protodiastole   ⎤
6 Rapid filling   ⎥
7 Diastasis   ⎬ **Ventricular diastole**
1 Late rapid filling ⎦

Fig. 6.1-10. *Blood flow in right and left coronary arteries and coronary sinus during different phases of cardiac cycle.*

monary circulation and systemic circulation. The blood vessels described in this section belong to systemic circulation.

THE ARTERIAL SYSTEM

The arterial tree of systemic circulation includes the aorta and its branches that lead to all body tissues.

AORTA

Aorta is the largest artery of the body. It arises from the left ventricle, arches over the heart to the left, and descends just in front of the vertebral column through the thorax and abdomen upto 4th lumbar vertebra, where it ends by dividing into the left and right common iliac arteries (Figs. 6.1-11 and 6.1-12).

PARTS AND MAIN BRANCHES OF AORTA

The aorta is divided into three main parts :
• The ascending aorta,
• The arch of aorta, and
• The descending aorta.

The ascending aorta

Course. The ascending aorta, about 5 cm (2.1 inches) long, after leaving the left ventricle, passes upwards and to the right. It then becomes continuous with arch of aorta (Fig. 6.1-13).

Branches. The only branches that arise from the ascending aorta are :
• Right coronary artery, and
• Left coronary artery.

Coronary arteries. The coronary arteries arise from the aorta just above the level of the aortic valve and supply blood to the heart. The right and left coronary arteries and their main branches travel in the epicardium of heart and subdivide sending penetrating branches through the myocardium.

Clinically applied aspect

The coronary arteries supply the myocardium with oxygen and nourishment. They are, therefore, of great practical importance because disease of their walls may result either in narrowing of the artery or complete blockage of one of the branches. Both conditions cause cardiac pain (angina). If the block is complete, as in coronary artery thrombosis (myocardial infarction), and if the patient survives, the part of the myocardium, supplied by the affected branch, will become deprived of its blood supply and the muscle will be replaced by a fibrous tissue scar. If this is extensive it will weaken the pumping power of the heart.

The arch of aorta

Course. The ascending aorta turns backwards and to the left to form the arch of aorta which is convex upwards. The arch of aorta lies behind the manubrium sterni and becomes continuous with descending thoracic aorta (Fig. 6.1-13).

Branches. Three large branches arise from the arch of aorta (Fig. 6.1-13).

1. Brachiocephalic artery. The brachiocephalic (innominate) artery after arising from the arch of aorta runs

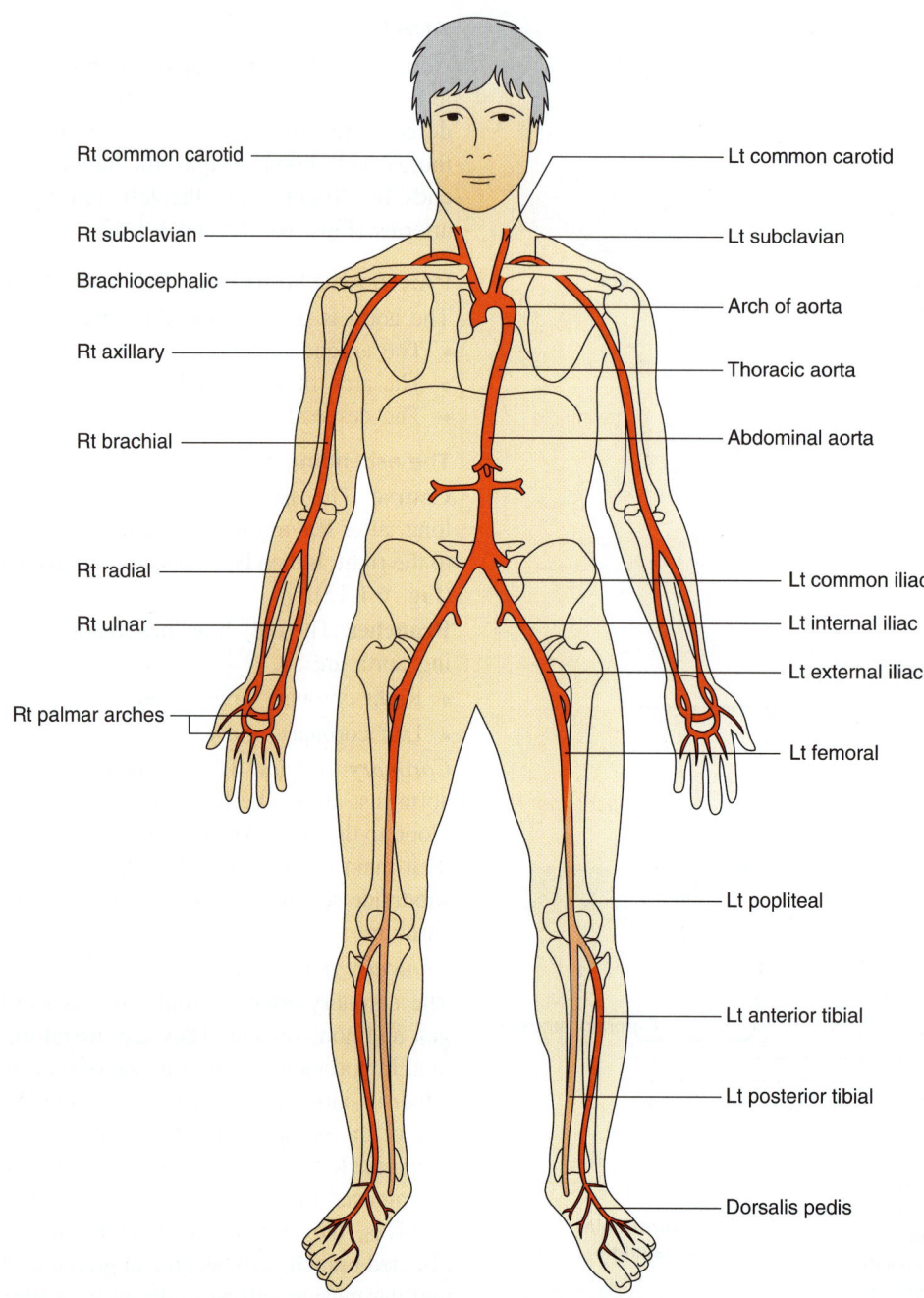

Fig. 6.1-11. The aorta and its main branches.

upwards and to the right for about 5 cm. At the level of sternoclavicular joint it ends by dividing into two branches:

- *The right common carotid artery,* which supplies blood to the right half of the head and neck (see page 158).
- *The right subclavian artery.* It carries blood to the right upper arm (see page 159).

2. *Left common carotid artery,* the second branch from arch of aorta, supplies blood to the left side of neck and head (see page 158).

3. *Left subclavian artery,* the third branch from the arch of aorta, supplies blood to the left upper limb.

The descending aorta

The descending aorta can be divided into two parts:
- Descending thoracic aorta, and
- Descending abdominal aorta.

Thoracic aorta

Course. The arch of aorta becomes continuous with descending aorta at the level of 4th thoracic vertebra. The

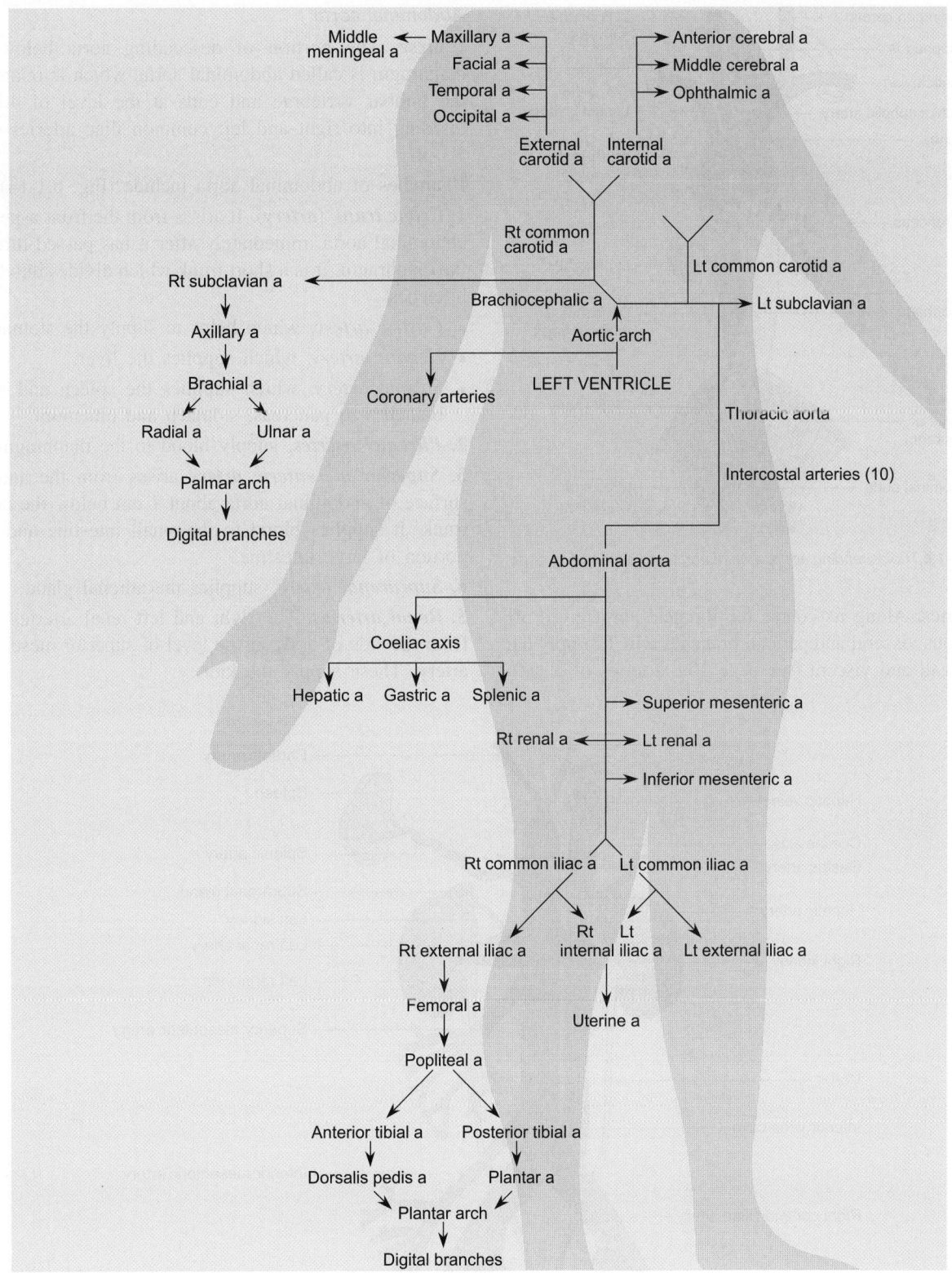

Fig. 6.1-12. Plan of the arterial system

portion of the descending aorta above the diaphragm is called thoracic aorta. The thoracic aorta continues downwards in the thorax in front of the remaining thoracic vertebrae and passes through an opening in the diaphragm at the level of 12th thoracic vertebra to become the abdominal aorta (Fig. 6.1-13).

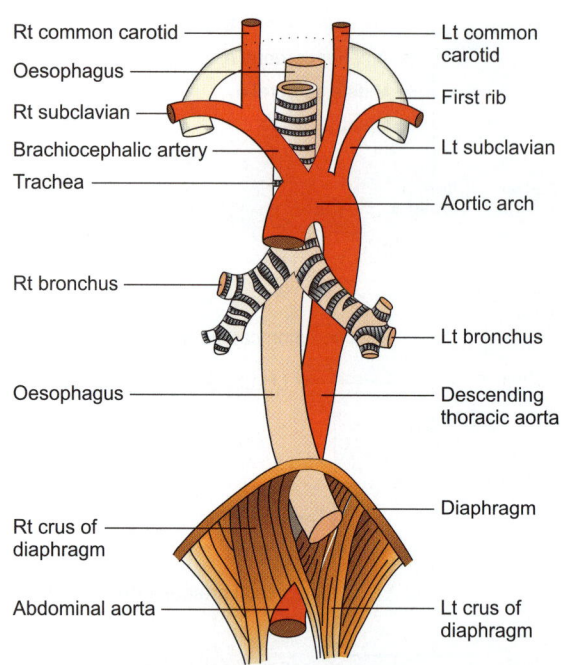

Fig. 6.1-13. *The ascending aorta, arch of aorta and descending aorta.*

Branches. Along its course the thoracic aorta gives off numerous visceral and parietal branches which supply the chest wall and viscera (see page 159, arteries of chest).

Abdominal aorta

Course. The portion of descending aorta below the diaphragm is called abdominal aorta, which is related to the lumbar vertebrae and ends at the level of 4th by dividing into right and left common iliac arteries (Fig. 6.1-14).

Branches of abdominal aorta include (Fig. 6.1-14):

1. *Celiac trunk (artery).* It arises from the front aspect of abdominal aorta immediately after it has passed through the diaphragm. It is a short trunk which divides into three branches :

- *Gastric artery,* which helps to supply the stomach.
- *Hepatic artery,* which supplies the liver.
- *Splenic artery,* which supplies the spleen and gives branches to pancreas, stomach and omentum.

2. *Phrenic arteries,* supply blood to the diaphragm.

3. *Superior mesenteric artery* arises from the anterior surface of abdominal aorta about 1 cm below the celiac trunk. It supplies blood to the small intestine and first portion of large intestine.

4. *Suprarenal artery,* supplies the adrenal gland.

5. *Renal arteries.* The right and left renal arteries arise from the side of aorta at the level of superior mesenteric artery. These supply the kidney.

Fig. 6.1-14. *Abdominal aorta and its branches.*

6. *Inferior mesenteric artery.* It arises lower down from the anterior surface of aorta and sends branches to the lower parts of the colon and to the rectum.

7. *Gonadal arteries.* Ovarian arteries in females and spermatic arteries in males supply the ovaries or testis.

8. *Lumbar arteries* (3-4 pairs). These arise from the posterior surface of aorta in the region of lumbar vertebrae. These arteries supply the posterior abdominal wall.

9. *Middle sacral artery.* This small, single vessel supplies the sacrum and coccyx.

10. *Common iliac arteries.* These are terminal branches of abdominal aorta. These vessels supply blood to the lower regions of the abdominal wall, the pelvic organs and the lower extremities (see page 159).

REGIONAL ARTERIAL SUPPLY

After studying the different parts and branches of aorta, it will be useful to study the regional arterial supply as below :

- Arteries of head and neck,
- Arteries of shoulders and upper limbs,
- Arteries of the chest,
- Arteries of the abdomen,
- Arteries of the pelvis, and
- Arteries of the lower limbs.

ARTERIES OF HEAD AND NECK

Arteries supplying the head and neck area are branches of (Fig. 6.1-15) :

- Subclavian arteries, and
- Common carotid arteries.

Branches of subclavian artery to head and neck area

Branches of subclavian artery supplying the head and neck area are :

- Vertebral arteries,
- Thyrocervical arteries,
- Costocervical arteries.

Vertebral arteries

The vertebral arteries (one each, right and left), after arising from the subclavian arteries, pass upwards through the special foramina in the transverse processes of upper six cervical vertebrae. Then, they wind behind the atlas, enter the skull through the foramen magnum, and unite to form a single basilar artery (Fig. 6.1-15 and 6.1-16).

Basilar artery. The basilar artery runs along the ventral brain stem and gives branches that supply pons and cerebellum. It terminates by dividing into two posterior cerebral arteries which take part in formation of circle of Willis along with the anterior cerebral arteries (branches of internal carotid arteries) (Fig. 6.1-16).

C H A P T E R 6.1

Fig. 6.1-15. *Main arteries of head and neck.*

Superficial temporal

Posterior auricular

Occipital

Internal carotid

External carotid

Carotid sinus

Vertebral

Thyrocervical axis

Subclavian

Ophthalmic

Maxillary

Facial

Lingual

Superior thyroid

Common carotid

Brachiocephalic

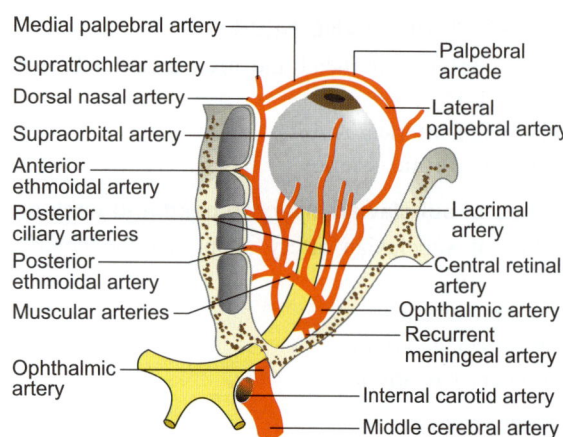

Fig. 6.1-16. Ophthalmic artery and its branches.

Thyrocervical arteries

Thyrocervical arteries (Fig. 6.1-15) are short branches of subclavian artery which gives off branches to the thyroid gland, parathyroid gland, larynx, trachea, oesophagus, and pharynx, as well as to various muscles in the neck, shoulder and back.

Costocervical arteries

Costocervical arteries are the third vessels to branch from the subclavian. These give off branches which supply to muscles in the neck, back and thoracic wall.

Common carotid arteries

The right common carotid artery is a branch of brachio-cephalic artery, while left common carotid artery arises directly from the arch of aorta. Thereafter, the right and left common carotid arteries ascend deeply within the neck ensheathed in the *carotid sheath* along with the internal jugular vein and vagus nerve. At the level of thyroid cartilage of larynx, they divide to form the external and internal carotid arteries (Fig. 6.1-15).

External carotid artery

External carotid artery, as its name suggests, supplies the structure of outer surface of the head and neck through following branches (Fig. 6.1-15) :

1. *Superior thyroid artery,* supplies to the hyoid bone, larynx and thyroid gland.

2. *Lingual artery,* supplies to the tongue, and salivary glands beneath the tongue.

3. *Facial artery :* It passes up over the outer surface of the lower jaw just in front of the angle and supplies the lower part of face i.e. chin, lips, nose, pharynx and palate.

4. *Occipital artery.* It passes behind the ear and supplies the occipital part of scalp, mastoid process, and various muscles in the neck.

5. *Superficial temporal artery,* the terminal branch of external carotid artery, passes in front of the ear to supply

the parotid salivary gland and frontal, temporal and parietal portions of the scalp.

6. *Maxillary artery,* the other terminal branch of the external carotid artery, supplies the structures around the jaws (teeth, gums, cheeks, nasal cavities), and gives off the important *middle meningeal artery* to the interior of the skull.

Note. It is clinically applied aspect that the pulse can be felt both in the facial artery as it crosses the lower jaw and in the temporal artery where it is placed immediately in front of the external auditory meatus.

Internal carotid artery

Internal carotid artery, a terminal branch of common carotid artery, lies deep in the muscles in the neck. It extends upwards to enter the interior of the skull through the carotid foramen in the petrous portion of the temporal bone. In the middle cranial fossa of the skull it ends by dividing into anterior and middle cerebral arteries. It provides major blood supply to the brain. Its branches include:

1. *Ophthalmic artery.* Ophthalmic artery arises from the internal carotid artery at the level of anterior clenoid process. It enters the orbit through the optic canal and constitutes the main source of blood supply to eyeball and other orbital structures (Fig. 6.1-16).

2. *Posterior communicating artery.* It is a small branch which joins the posterior cerebral artery to form circle of Willis (Fig. 6.1-17).

3. *Choroidal artery.* It is also a small branch which gives off branches to chiasma, optic tract and lateral geniculate body.

4. *Anterior cerebral artery.* It is the smaller terminal branch of internal carotid artery.

5. *Middle cerebral artery* is the largest branch of internal carotid artery.

Fig. 6.1-17. Circle of Willis.

The anterior and middle cerebral arteries communicate with each other and also with basilar artery to form *circle of Willis* (Fig. 6.1-17) which ensures the even distribution of blood to the brain.

ARTERIES OF SHOULDER AND UPPER LIMB

Arteries of axilla and upper arm

The axillary artery. The *subclavian artery,* after giving off branches to the neck, continues as axillary artery into the upper arm (Fig. 6.1-18). The axillary artery supplies branches to structures in the axilla, chest wall and shoulder. At the lower boundary of axilla it continues as brachial artery.

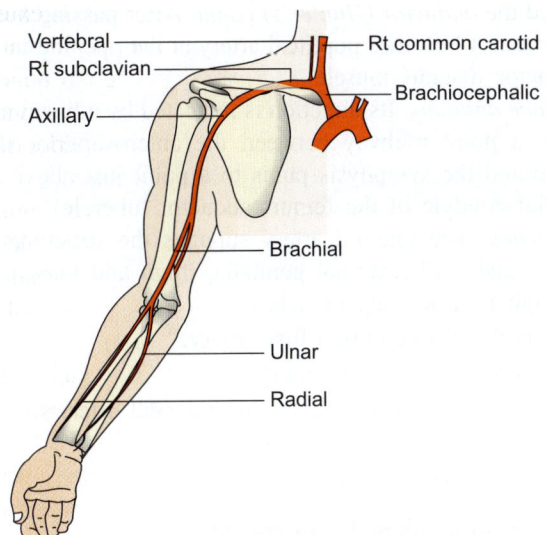

Fig. 6.1-18. *Main arteries of shoulder and upper limb.*

Brachial artery. Brachial artery extends along the humerus from the lower border of axilla to the bend of elbow. It supplies to the upper arm structures through its branch *(deep brachial artery)* and shorter branches.

In the cubital fossa (bend of elbow) it ends by dividing into radial and ulnar arteries.

Arteries of forearm

Radial artery. It extends from the elbow to wrist along the radial (lateral) side of the forearm. Near the wrist it becomes superficial and can be felt lying in front of the bone and thus provides a convenient site for taking pulse (*radial pulse*).

Ulnar artery. It runs from the elbow to the wrist along the ulnar (medial) side of the forearm.

Arteries of hands

Palmar arches. Just in front of the wrist, in the palm, the ends of radial and ulnar arteries anastomose to form two transverse arches :
- Superficial palmar arch, and
- Deep palmar arch.

Branches from the palmar arches supply the structures in hands and fingers.

ARTERIES OF CHEST

The walls and viscera of thorax are supplied by branches of subclavian artery and thoracic aorta (Figs. 6.1-19 and 6.1-13).

Fig. 6.1-19. *Schematic drawing to show arteries supplying to chest wall. (2 and 3) Second and third ribs, (AIA) Anterior intercostal artery, (GR) grey ramus, (IA) Intercostal artery, (RIT) Right internal throacic, (S) Sternum, (SG) Sympathic ganglion, (VSB) ventral somatic branch of spinal nerve*

Branches of subclavian artery for chest

Internal thoracic artery, a branch of subclavian artery, supplies the chest wall through its branches:
- *Anterior intercostal branches* are six paired arteries (right and left), which supply to the muscles and other structures of six upper intercostal spaces. They also supply the mammary glands.

Branches of descending thoracic aorta to chest

Visceral branches
- *Pericardial arteries* (2-3 in number) supply the pericardium.
- *Bronchial arteries* (3 in number) supply the bronchial tree.
- *Esophageal arteries* (4-5 in number) supply the eosophagus.
- *Mediastinal arteries* (numerous) supply structures in mediastinum.

Parietal branches of thoracic aorta include :
- *Posterior intercostal arteries,* supply thoracic wall.
- *Subcostal arteries,* supply thoracic wall.
- *Superior phrenic arteries*, supply the superior and posterior surface of diaphragm.

ARTERIES OF ABDOMEN

Arteries to abdominal wall

Anterior abdominal wall is primarily supplied by branches of :

- Internal thoracic artery, and
- External iliac arteries.

Posterior abdominal wall is supplied by following paired branches from abdominal aorta (see page 156, Fig. 6.1-14):

- Inferior pherenic arteries,
- Lumbar arteries, and
- Middle sacral arteries.

Arteries to abdominal viscera

The abdominal viscera is supplied by following branches of abdominal aorta (see page 156, Fig. 6.1 -14):

- Celiac artery (trunk),
- Superior mesenteric artery,
- Suprarenal arteries,
- Renal arteries,
- Inferior mesenteric artery.

ARTERIES OF PELVIS

Internal iliac artery, a branch of common iliac artery (see page 157, Fig. 6.1-14), supplies the various structures of pelvis and gluteal region through its following branches (Fig. 6.1-20) :

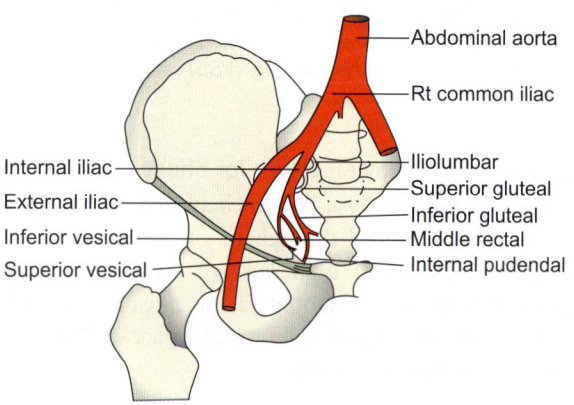

Fig. 6.1-20. *Main branches of internal iliac artery.*

- *Iliolumbar artery,* supplies to the ilium and muscles of the back.
- *Superior and inferior gluteal arteries,* supply to the gluteal muscles, pelvic muscles and skin of the buttocks.
- *Internal pudendal artery,* supplies to distal portion of alimentary canal, the external genitalia and the hip joint.
- *Superior and inferior vesical arteries,* supply to the bladder. In the males these vessels also supply to seminal vesicles and the prostate gland.
- *Middle rectal artery,* supplies to the rectum.
- *Uterine artery,* supplies to uterus and vagina in females.

ARTERIES OF LOWER LIMB

External iliac artery, the direct continuation of the ab-

dominal aorta, mainly supplies the structures of lower limb. It extends downward from the pelvis in the lower limb and is named, in successive part of its course, the femoral, the popliteal and the posterior tibial artery (Fig. 6.1-21) :

Arteries in the thigh

Femoral artery. The external iliac artery after passing below the inguinal (Poupart's) ligament becomes the femoral artery.

Course. In the upper half of thigh the femoral artery is comparatively superficial and lies in the space known as *femoral triangle* where pulsations can be felt. The lower part lies more deeply among muscles in a special tunnel called the *adductor (Hunter's) canal.* After passing out of the canal it becomes popliteal artery at the opening in the adductor magnus muscle.

Surface anatomy. Its direction is indicated by a line drawn from a point midway between the anterosuperior iliac spine and the symphysis pubis to a point just above the medial condyle of the femur (adductor tubercle).

Branches. The femoral artery supplies the structures of abdominal wall, external genitalia, thigh and knee joint through its following branches :

- Superficial circumflex iliac artery,
- Superficial epigastric artery,
- Superficial and deep external pudendal arteries,
- Profunda femoris artery, and
- Deep genicular artery.

Arteries in popliteal fossa and leg

Popliteal artery. The femoral artery becomes popliteal artery at the proximal border of popliteal fossa (space behind the knee). Branches of this artery supply blood to the knee joint and to certain muscles in the thigh and calf. Its branches also participate in an anastomosis around the knee joint. At the lower border of popliteal fossa, the popliteal artery ends by dividing into anterior and posterior tibial arteries (Fig. 6.1-21).

Anterior tibial artery. It passes downwards between the tibia and fibula to supply the front of the leg and is continued downwards on the dorsum of foot as the *dorsalis pedis artery.*

Posterior tibial artery, the larger branch of popliteal artery, is in fact the direct continuation of the popliteal artery in the back of leg where it lies deep in the calf muscle and gives off following branches:

- *Small branches* to skin, muscles and other tissues of the lower leg along the way.
- *Peroneal artery* is a large branch of the posterior tibial artery which supplies structures of the medial side of fibula and contribute to the anastomosis of the ankle.
- *Terminal branches.* The posterior tibial artery divides into medial and lateral plantar arteries.

Abdominal aorta
Rt common iliac
Deep circumflex iliac
Superficial circumflex iliac
External iliac
Profunda femoris
Deep femoral
Lateral femoral
Internal iliac
Superficial pudendal
Deep external pudendal
Femoral
Deep genicular
Anterior tibial
Dorsalis pedis

Femoral
Popliteal
Anterior tibial
Peroneal
Posterior tibial
Medial plantar
Lateral plantar

Anterior view

Posterior view

Fig. 6.1-21. *Main arteries of lower limb.*

Arteries to the ankle and foot

The dorsalis pedis artery (continuation of anterior tibial artery) anastomoses with the medial and lateral plantar arteries to form the *plantar arch,* similar to the palmar arch of hand. Digital branches from the plantar arch supply blood to the toes.

CLINICALLY APPLIED ASPECTS

Pressure points are the areas where the arteries are near the surface and can be felt and/or compressed against some firm underlying structure. By compressing the arteries at pressure points, it is sometimes possible to arrest severe haemorrhage. Some examples of pressure points in the body are mentioned below :

Pressure points in head and neck area

- *Facial artery* : Against the lower jaw.
- *Temporal artery* : In fornt of the external auditory meatus.
- *Occipital artery* : Against the occipital bone 6.5 cm behind the ear.
- *Common carotid* : Against the cervical vertebrae to the side of larynx.

Pressure points in upper limb area

- *Subclavian artery.* Against the first rib in the hollow above the clavicle.
- *Brachial artery.* Against the medial aspect of humerus in the middle of arm.
- *Radial artery.* At the lower end of radius just above the wrist on its anterior surface
- *Ulnar artery.* Against the anterior surface of ulna.

Pressure points in lower limb area

- *Femoral artery.* Against the pubic bone under the inguinal (Poupart's) ligament.
- *Posterior tibial artery.* Against the posterior surface of medial malleolus.
- *Dorsalis pedis artery.* Against the upper surface of the navicular bone.

THE VENOUS SYSTEM

GENERAL CONSIDERATIONS

The venous system is concerned with collection of deoxygenated blood from the various tissues of the body and returning it to heart. We have seen that the arteries begin as large vessels which gradually become smaller and they end in arterioles which merge into capillaries. In contrast to it, the veins begin as very small vessels, the *venules,* which unite to form progressive large veins.

Divisions of venous system

The venous system can be considered to consist of three sets of veins : the pulmonary, the coronary, and the systemic.

Pulmonary veins carry oxygenated blood from the lungs to the left atrium. These form part of pulmonary circulation which is discussed separately (see page 150).

Coronary veins collect the deoxygenated blood from the myocardium. These veins unite to form the *coronary sinus* which opens into the right atrium directly.

Systemic veins. The systemic veins can be divided into two main groups :

- *Superficial veins.* These are situated on the surface of the body, just under the skin. These are commonly interconnected in irregular networks, so that many unnamed tributaries may join to form a relatively large vein. Some superficial veins can be easily seen through the skin.

- *Deep veins.* These are situated deep in the tissue.
  Mainly large veins typically follow the course of main arteries, and often have the same names as their companion in the arterial system. For example, renal veins follow the renal arteries.

MAJOR VENOUS TRUNKS

The veins of systemic circulation unite to form larger and larger vessels until two major venous trunks are formed which drain the blood into the right atrium of the heart. These venous trunks are:

- Superior vena cava, and
- Inferior vena cava.
  Fig. 6.1-22 shows the main veins constituting the venous systems.

SUPERIOR VENA CAVA

The superior vena cava is formed at the level of lower border of first right costal cartilage by the union of right and left brachiocephalic veins (Fig. 6.1-23). It is about 7 cm long and ends by opening in the right atrium at the level of third right costal cartilage.

Tributaries of superior vena cava

The superior vena cava drains blood from the head, neck, chest and upper limb through following tributaries (Fig. 6.1-23) :

1. *Right brachiocephalic vein.* It is only 2.5 cm long. It is formed by the union of right internal jugular and subclavian veins. The various tributaries which drain into right brachiocephalic vein are (Fig. 6.1-23) :

- *Right subclavian veins* bringing deoxygenated blood from the right upper limb.
- *Right internal jugular vein* bringing blood from the right half of head and neck area.
- *Right vertibral vein* draining blood from the structures supplied by vertebral artery.
- *Right internal thoracic vein* draining blood from the area supplied of internal thoracic artery.
- *Right inferior thyroid vein* draining the area supplied by the artery of same name.
- *Right first intercostal vein* draining blood from the structures of first intercostal space.

Note : In addition to the above veins the right brachiocephalic vein, the thoracic or right lymphatic duct also drains into it.

2. *Left brachiocephalic vein.* It is formed by the left internal jugular and subclavian veins. Its *tributaries* are similar to right brachiocephalic vein, except that it also receives blood from the left superior intercostal vein (Fig. 6.1-23).

3. *Azygos vein* opens into the superior vena cava on the right side about its middle (Fig. 6.1-23). It is a large vein which drains blood from the thorax and abdominal wall. The *azygos system* of veins may also serve as a bypass for the inferior vena cava in case of obstruction (for details see veins of thorax page 167).

INFERIOR VENA CAVA

This is the largest vein in the body. It is formed by the union of the right and left common iliac veins at the body of the 5th lumbar vertebra (Fig. 6.1-22). It ascends upwards along the posterior abdominal wall lying to the right of the abdominal aorta. It ends by piercing the diaphragm to open into the right atrium of heart.

Tributaries. It drains the blood from the following structures through various tributaries from :

- *From the lower limbs* the blood is drained into inferior vena cava (for detail see page 165).
- *From the abdomen* the blood is brought into the inferior vena cava through the tributaries which have the names of the parietal and visceral branches of abdominal aorta. These veins are the lumbar, renal, suprarenal, inferior phrenic, hepatic, and right spermatic or ovarian (For details see page 166 and Fig. 6.1-22).

REGIONAL VENOUS DRAINAGE

Till now we have studied the plan of venous system and two major venous trunks which ultimately pour the deoxygenated blood collected from various parts of the body into the right atrium. At this juncture, it will be useful to study the venous drainage from the different regions of the body as below :

Rt subclavian

Rt brachiocephalic

Rt axillary

Rt cephalic

Rt brachial

Rt basilic

Rt median cubital

Rt radial

Rt median

Rt ulnar

Rt cephalic

Rt femoral

Rt popliteal

Rt anterior tibial

Rt posterior tibial

Lt internal jugular

Lt external jugular

Lt brachiocephalic

Superior vena cava

Hepatic

Inferior vena cava

Renal

Gonadal

Lt common iliac

Lt internal iliac

Lt external iliac

Lt great saphenous

Lt small saphenous

Superficial veins

Deep veins

Fig. 6.1-22. Main veins constituting venous system of the body.

- Venous drainage from head and neck.
- Venous drainage from the upper limbs.
- Venous drainage from the thorax and abdominal wall.
- Venous drainage from the abdominal viscera.
- Venous drainage from the pelvis.
- Venous drainage from the lower limbs.

VENOUS DRAINAGE FROM THE HEAD AND NECK

Venous blood drained from the head and neck area reaches the superior vena cava through two main veins:

- External jugular vein, and
- Internal jugular vein

External jugular vein

External jugular vein is formed in the neck at the level of angle of jaw by the union of *superficial veins* of the scalp. This vein passes downwards in front of the sternomastoid muscle and ends by entering the subclavian vein (Fig. 6.1-24).

Tributaries of external jugular vein which return venous blood from the superficial structures of face scalp are the superficial veins of the same name as the branches of external carotid artery.

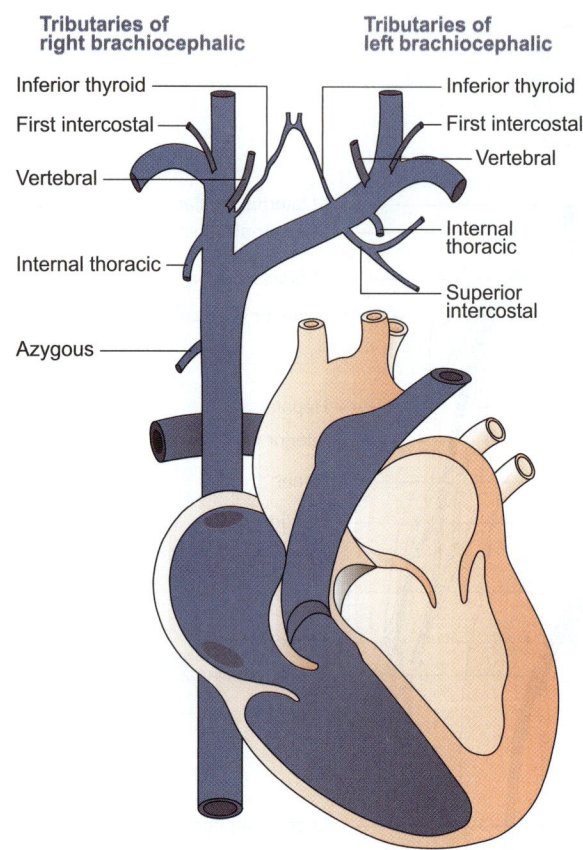

Tributaries of right brachiocephalic

Inferior thyroid
First intercostal
Vertebral
Internal thoracic
Azygous

Tributaries of left brachiocephalic

Inferior thyroid
First intercostal
Vertebral
Internal thoracic
Superior intercostal

Fig. 6.1-23. Superior vena cava and brachiocephalic veins with their tributaries.

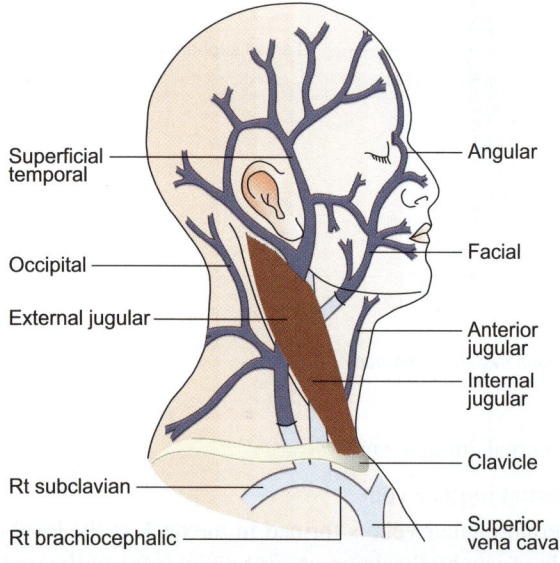

Superficial temporal
Occipital
External jugular
Rt subclavian
Rt brachiocephalic

Angular
Facial
Anterior jugular
Internal jugular
Clavicle
Superior vena cava

Fig. 6.1-24. Veins of head and neck.

Internal jugular veins

Internal jugular veins begin at the jugular foramen in the base of skull as direct continuation of the sigmoid portion of the transverse (lateral) sinus. They run downwards in the neck, deep to the sternomastoid muscle, in close association with the carotid artery with which it is included in the carotid sheath. Finally the internal jugular veins join with the subclavian veins, carrying blood from the upper limbs, to form the *brachiocephalic veins* which open in the superior vena cava.

Tributaries of internal jugular vein are :

1. *Facial veins.* Facial vein is downward continuation of the angular vein which collects blood from the upper part of face through various small veins (Fig. 6.1-24). There is also a communication between the angular vein and the veins inside the skull which pass through the orbit. It is for this reason that boils and carbuncles on the face may be particularly dangerous, for infection may spread through this connection and cause cavernous sinus thrombosis.

2. *Intracranial venous sinuses.* The venous blood from the deep area of brain is collected into channels called the dural venous sinuses. These sinuses, lined by endothelium, are formed by layer of dura mater. The main venous sinuses are as below (Fig. 6.1-25) :

Superior sagittal sinus
Straight sinus
Left transverse sinus
Inferior sagittal sinus
Left internal jugular vein

Fig. 6.1-25. Venous system of brain viewed from the right.

- *Superior sagittal sinus.* It begins in the frontal region of the skull, carries the blood from the superior part of brain, and runs directly backwards in the midline to the occipital region in a fold of dura mater called the *falx cerebri.* Then it turns to the right side and continues as *right transverse sinus.*

- *Inferior sagittal sinus* collects blood from the deeper parts of brain and passes backward to continue as *straight sinus.*

- *Straight sinus* runs backwards and downwards and continues as *left transverse sinus.*

- *Transversus sinuses* run forward and medially from the occipital region on each side to continue with the sigmoid sinus.

- *Sigmoid sinuses* continue inferiorly as internal jugular veins.

VENOUS DRAINAGE FROM THE UPPER LIMB

The veins draining blood from different structures of upper limb are arranged in two groups : superficial and deep veins (Fig. 6.1-26).

Fig. 6.1-26. Superficial veins of right upper limb.

Superficial veins of upper limb

These lie below the skin and are interconnected in complex networks. The superficial veins begin mainly on the back of hand, and some of them converge in cubital space in fornt of elbow joint. The main superficial veins are :

- *Cephalic vein* runs upwards from the hand to shoulder on the lateral side of the arm. In the shoulder it pierces the tissues and opens into the *axillary veins.*
- *Basilic vein* runs upwards from the back of hand on ulnar side for a distance and then curves forwards to the anterior surface. It continues ascending in the medial side until it reaches the middle of upper arm. There it penetrates deep and joins the axillary vein.
- *Median vein* is a small vein that is not always present. It commences at the palmar surface of the hand, runs upwards on the front of forearm and ends in the basilic vein.
- *Median cubital vein* is a small but prominent vein which in the cubital fossa ascends from the cephalic vein on lateral side to join the basilic vein on the medial side. This vein is often used as a site for *venipuncture* for the collection of blood sample and for the injection of fluids or drugs into the blood stream.

Deep veins of upper limb

The deep veins generally parallel the arteries in each region of the upper limb and are given similar names as below :

In the hands blood is collected by *palmar metacarpal veins and deep palmar venous arches* and emptied in the ulnar and radial vein.

In the forearm
- *Ulnar veins* run upwards on the medial side, and
- *Radial vein* runs upwards on the lateral side.

In the upper arm
- *Brachial vein* in formed by the union of ulnar and radial veins just above the elbow. The brachial vein continues upward along with the brachial artery.
- *Axillary vein* is the continuation upward of brachial vein. As mentioned above, the superficial basilic and cephalic veins open into the axillary vein in the upper part of upper arm.
- *Subclavian vein* is a continuation of the axillary vein and unites with the internal jugular vein to form the brachiocephalic vein. At the junction with internal jugular vein and left subclavian vein it receives thoracic duct and the right subclavian vein receives the right lymphatic duct.
- *Brachiocephalic veins* of the two sides join to form the superior vena cava which opens in the right atrium of the heart.

VENOUS DRAINAGE FROM THORAX AND ABDOMINAL WALL

The veins draining blood from the thorax include (Fig. 6.1-27):

1. *Internal thoracic veins* receive blood from the tributaries corresponding to branches of internal thoracic artery. These veins open into *brachiocephalic veins.*

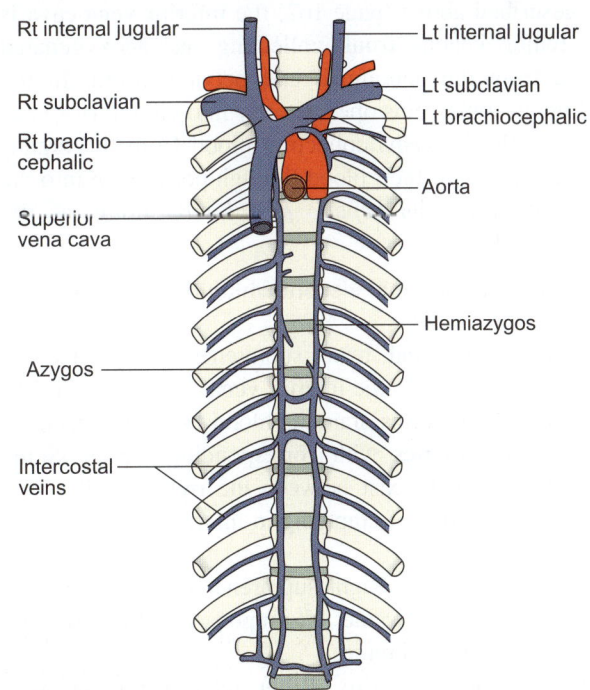

Fig. 6.1-27. Superior vena cava and main veins of the thorax.

C H A P T E R 6 . 1

2. Intercostal veins. Some of the intercostal veins directly open into the brachiocephalic veins. However, most of the intercostal veins open into the internal thoracic veins.

3. Lumbar veins drain blood from the thoracic and abdominal wall and open into the inferior vena cava.

4. Azygos vein. Most of the blood from right side of thoracic cavity and abdominal wall is drained by azygos vein, which ascends on the right side of vertebral column, from the level of 2nd lumbar to 4th thoracic vertebrae, where it empties in the superior vena cava. Tributaries of azygos vein include :

- *Posterior intercostal veins,* which drain the intercostal spaces on the right side.
- *Ascending lumbar veins,* both right and left, open in azygos vein. These drain blood from the thoracic wall and abdominal wall.

5. Hemiazygos vein. Most of the blood from the left side of thoracic cavity and abdominal wall is drained by hemiazygos vein, which ascends on the left side of vertebral column from the left side of lumbar region to the level of left brachiocephalic vein in which it empties. The hemiazygos vein also sends tributaries to the right azygos vein.

The azygos system. The azygos vein (on right side) and hemiazygos vein (or left side) communicate with each other and also with many veins which drain into inferior vena cava. Thus, the azygos system bypasses the blood from inferior vena cava to superior vena cava in case the former is blocked.

VENOUS DRAINAGE FROM ABDOMINAL VISCERA

As described above (page 162) the inferior vena cava is the major venous trunk collecting the deoxygenated blood from the abdominal and pelvic viscera. In the abdomen, some veins open directly into the inferior vena cava, while the veins collecting blood from the organs of digestion pour their blood through portal vein into the liver and form the *hepatic portal circulation,* as described below :

Veins from abdominal viscera which directly open into inferior vena cava

The lumbar, gonadal, renal, suprarenal, phrenic and hepatic veins open into the inferior vena cava (Fig. 6.1-22). Generally, these veins drain the blood from the structures supplied by arteries with corresponding names. Some differences which exist between the right and left side veins, in the mode of emptying in inferior vena cava, are as below :

- *Suprarenal veins.* Right suprarenal vein empties into inferior vena cava; the left empties into the left renal or left inferior phrenic.
- *Inferior phrenic veins.* Right inferior phrenic vein empties into the inferior vena cava, one of which

empties into the left renal, suprarenal vein and other into the inferior vena cava.

- *Gonadal veins.* The right gonadal (spermatic or ovarian) empties into the inferior vena cava, but the left empties into the left renal vein.

Hepatic portal circulation

The veins collecting blood from the spleen and abdominal organs of digestion are unique and differ from rest of the veins. These veins originate from the capillary net-work of the organs of digestion and carry blood from these organs through the *portal vein* to the liver. In the liver, this blood passes through a second capillary bed, the *hepatic sinusoids.* This unique venous pathway constitutes the *hepatic portal circulation.* The importance of this is that the digested foodstuffs absorbed from the alimentary canal go to the liver first. Passage of the blood containing absorbed foodstuffs from the hepatic sinusoids allows the liver cells to absorbs, modify and store them.

Portal vein

Portal vein itself is quite small (about 8 cm long), and is formed behind the pancreas by the union of splenic vein and superior mesenteric vein and opens into the liver (Fig. 6.1-28).

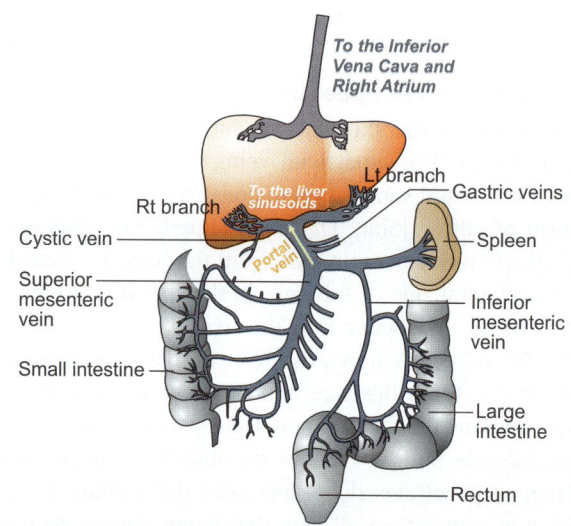

Fig. 6.1-28. Portal vein, its tributaries and termination.

Tributaries of portal vein include the following veins, each of which drains blood from the area supplied by the corresponding artery :

- *Superior mesenteric vein* drains blood from the small intestine, ascending colon, and transverse colon. It unites with the splenic vein to form the portal vein.
- *Splenic vein.* It drains the blood from the spleen, the pancreas and part of stomach. It unites with superior mesenteric vein to form the portal vein.
- *Inferior mesenteric vein.* It drains blood from the

descending colon, sigmoid colon and rectum. It opens into the splenic vein.

- *Gastric veins* (right and left) drain blood from the stomach and distal end of oesophagus. They drain into the portal vein.
- *Cystic vein* drains blood from the gall bladder, and joins the portal vein.

Note: It is important to note that :

- *Blood supplied by hepatic artery* to the liver does not take part in portal circulation. This blood supplies oxygen and nutrients to the liver cells.
- *Obstruction of the portal vein* or its branches causes a rise in blood pressure in the portal venous system, a condition known as *portal hypertension*. This results in enlargement of the spleen, oesophageal varices and haemorrhoids.

VENOUS DRAINAGE FROM PELVIS

Internal iliac veins

Most of the blood from the pelvis is drained by internal iliac veins through their tributaries. The internal iliac veins begin deep within the pelvis and ascend to the pelvis brim where they unite with external iliac veins to form the *common iliac veins*. The right and left common iliac veins unite to form the inferior vena cava (Fig. 6.1-22).

Tributaries that drain blood from the organs of reproductive, urinary and digestive systems in the pelvic region are the veins corresponding to the branches of internal iliac artery such as the gluteal, pudendal, vesical, rectal, uterine and vaginal. Typically these veins have many interconnections and form plexuses in the region of rectum, urinary bladder, and prostate gland (in the male) or uterus and vagina (in the female).

VENOUS DRAINAGE FROM LOWER LIMBS

The veins draining blood from different structures of the lower limbs (as in the case of upper limbs) are arranged in two groups: superficial and deep (Fig. 6.1-22).

Superficial veins of lower limb

The superficial veins of the foot and leg lie below the skin and are interconnected to form complex network. These vessels drain into two major trunks: the small and great saphenous veins.

1. *Small saphenous vein* (Fig. 6.1-29). It begins on the lateral side of the foot, receives many small tributaries and passes upwards along the centre of the back of calf and pierces the deep fascia of the limb over the popliteal space at the back of knee joint to empty into the popliteal vein.

2. *Great saphenous vein* (Fig. 6.1-29). It begins in the marginal vein of the dorsum of foot, extends along the medial side of leg and thigh, receiving many tributaries on the way. Just below the medial end of the inguinal ligament it passes deeper to enter the *femoral vein.*

Fig. 6.1-29. *Superficial veins of lower limb.*

The point where it pierces the deep fascia of the limb is called the *saphenous opening.*

Deep veins of the lower limb

The deep veins generally parallel the arteries in each region of the lower limb and are given similar names as below (Fig. 6.1-22) :

Anterior and posterior tibial veins begin at the lower end of the leg and ascend upwards upto the popliteal fossa accompanied by the corresponding arteries.

Popliteal vein is formed by the union of anterior and posterior tibial veins at the level of knees and pass upwards in company with the popliteal artery.

Femoral vein. The popliteal vein enters the Hunter's canal and continues upward through the thigh as the femoral vein. In the femoral triangle, the femoral vein lies along with femoral artery in a sheath of fibrous tissue, called the *femoral sheath.* Here it receives the long saphenous vein and passes under the inguinal ligament to become the *external iliac vein.*

Note. It is important to note that :

- Both superficial and deep veins of the lower limb are provided with valves which are more numerous in the deep veins.

- The saphenous veins communicate extensively with the deep veins of the legs. As a result, there are many pathways by which blood can be returned to the heart from the lower extremities.

- Saphenous veins are subjected to increased blood pressure in standing posture because of gravitational force. Therefore, in persons with prolonged period of standing (e.g. traffic police), these veins are prone to develop abnormal dilatations or varicosities (varicose veins).

Physiological Activities of the Heart

6.2

PHYSIOLOGY OF CARDIAC MUSCLE

STRUCTURAL ORGANIZATION OF CARDIAC MUSCLE

- The cardiac muscle fibres are *striated*. However, unlike the skeletal muscles, the cardiac muscles are *involuntary* (like smooth muscles). Thus cardiac muscles share some characteristics with skeletal muscles and others with smooth muscles.

- The cardiac muscle fibres are *ribbon-like, branched* and interdigitate freely with each other. The branches from the neighbouring fibres join together. At the point of contact of two muscle fibres, the membranes of both the muscle fibres are fused together and thrown into extensive infolding forming the so-called *intercalated disc* (Fig. 6.2.1).

- Along the sides near the outer border of intercalated disc the two adjacent muscle fibres are connected with each other through the *gap junctions*. The action

169

Fig. 6.2-1. *Structure of cardiac muscle.*

potential passes from one cardiac muscle cell to the other through gap junctions which provide *low resistance bridges* and thus the cardiac muscle acts as a *functional syncytium* of many cardiac cells. In this way the cardiac impulse spreads throughout the muscle mass quickly resulting in a coordinated contraction of the whole tissue.

Structure of a cardiac muscle fibre

Each muscle fibre is about 80 μm long and about 15 μm broad. Its cell membrane is called *sarcolemma* and the cytoplasm is called *sarcoplasm*. Each muscle fibre is made up of number of *myofibrils* which lie parallel to each other. Each myofibril is 2 μm is diameter, and consists of thick and thin filaments. Essentially the structure and striations are similar to that of a skeletal muscle (see page 138).

Sarcotubular system

The sarcotubular system in cardiac muscles is well developed like that of skeletal muscle (see page 140). However, the tubules of the T-system penetrate the sarcomere at Z-line. Therefore, in cardiac muscles, there is only one triad per sarcomere as compared to two in skeletal muscle.

PROCESS OF EXCITABILITY AND CONTRACTILITY: AN ELECTRO-MECHANICAL PHENOMENON

The cardiac muscle being an excitable tissue produces an action potential (*electrical phenomenon*) when stimulated and responds by contracting (*mechanical phenomenon*). The events which link the electrical phenomenon with mechanical phenomenon constitute the *excitation-contraction coupling phenomenon*.

ELECTRICAL POTENTIALS IN CARDIAC MUSCLE

Resting membrane potential

The resting membrane potential (RMP) of a normal cardiac muscle fibre is –85 to –95 mV (negative interior with reference to exterior).

Action potential

When stimulated, each cardiac muscle fibre shows an electrical activity known as propagated action potential. The action potential recorded from a single cardiac muscle fibre is unusually long and can be divided into five distinct phases (Fig. 6.2-2).

Fig. 6.2-2. *Various phases of action potential and ion conductance: Phase 0 = depolarization; Phase 1 = rapid repolarization; Phase 2 = plateau phase; Phase 3 = late rapid repolarization; and Phase 4 = resting potential.*

Phase 0: Rapid depolarization. The phase 0 (upstroke) is characterized by the depolarization which proceeds rapidly, as in skeletal muscle and nerve. The rapid depolarization and the overshoot are due to rapid influx of Na^+ ions similar to that occurring in nerve and skeletal muscle.

Phase 1: Initial rapid repolarization. Rapid depolarization is followed by a very short-lived slight rapid repolarization. The membrane potential reaches from +30 mV to –10 mV during this phase. The initial rapid repolarization is due to closure of Na^+ channels and opening of K^+ channels resulting in transient outward current.

Phase 2: Plateau. During plateau phase the cardiac muscle fibre remains in the depolarized state. The membrane potential falls very slowly. The plateau phase lasts for about 100-200 msec. This phase occurs due to slow influx of Ca^{2+}.

Phase 3: Repolarization. During this phase complete repolarization occurs and the membrane potential falls to the approximate resting value.

Ionic basis. The slow repolarization results from closing of Ca^{2+} channels and opening of K^+ channels.

Phase 4: Resting potential. In this phase of resting membrane potential (also called as polarised state) the potential is maintained at –90 mV.

Duration of action potential

The duration of action potential is about 250 msec at a heart rate 75 beats/minute. The duration of action potential decreases with increased heart rate (150 msec at a heart rate of 200 beats/min).

Spread of action potential through cardiac muscle

The cardiac muscle acts as physiological syncytium due to presence of gap junctions amongst the cardiac muscle fibres. Because of this the action potential spreads through the cardiac muscles very rapidly. Further, as there are two syncytia (the atrial and the ventricular) in the heart, so the action potential is transmitted from atria to ventricles only through the fibres of specialized conductive system.

EXCITATION-CONTRACTION COUPLING PHENOMENON IN CARDIAC MUSCLES

The sequence of events during excitation-contraction coupling in the cardiac muscle are similar to those observed in a skeletal muscle (see page 140), with the following exception:

In cardiac muscle (as against that in skeletal muscle) extra calcium ions diffuse into the sarcoplasm from T-tubules without which the contraction strength would be considerably reduced, whereas skeletal muscle contraction is hardly affected by calcium concentration in ECF.

PROCESS OF CARDIAC MUSCLE CONTRACTION

The molecular mechanism of cardiac muscle contraction by cross-bridge cycling and sliding of filaments is primarily similar to that of skeletal muscles (see page 140) and smooth muscles. However, in cardiac muscle:

- Troponin-tropomyosin complex controls the onset and offset of cross-bridge cycling, similar to that in skeletal muscles, and
- Like smooth muscles, the contractility of cardiac muscle is sensitive to *phosphorylation.*

RELAXATION OF CARDIAC MUSCLE

Relaxation of cardiac muscle (diastole) occurs when levels of Ca^{2+} ions fall in the cardiac muscle fibres. During diastole the Ca^{2+} ions are extruded out of the cardiac muscle fibre by a carrier system operating at the sarcolemma in which two Na^+ ions are exchanged for each Ca^{2+} ion extruded. Thus, the rate of Ca^{2+} ion extrusion depends on the gradient of Na^+ created by Na^+-K^+ ATPase.

Inhibition of this secondary active transport of Ca^{2+} ions, e.g. by digitalis or other cardiac glycosides raises the intracellular Ca^{2+} concentration and thereby increases myocardial contractility. This effect is utilized in patients with congestive heart failure.

PROPERTIES OF CARDIAC MUSCLE

The basic properties of cardiac muscle include:
- Excitability (bathmotropism),
- Contractility (inotropism),
- Autorythmicity (see page 173), and
- Conductivity (see page 173).

EXCITABILITY

Excitability (bathmotropism) is the property by which tissues respond to stimuli. The cardiac muscle responds by development of action potential.

The characteristics of cardiac muscle excitability which needs a special emphasis is its refractory period.

Refractory period

Refractory period refers to the period following action potential during which the cardiac muscle does not respond to a stimulus. Cardiac muscle has a long refractory period (250-300 msec in ventricles and about 150 msec in atria). It is of two types:

1. *Absolute refractory period (ARP).* During this period the cardiac muscle does not show any response at all. It extends from phase 0 to half of phase 3 of action potential, i.e. until the membrane potential reaches approximately –50 mV during repolarization (Fig. 6.2-3). Normal duration of absolute refractory period (ARP) in ventricles is about 180-200 msec.

2. *Relative refractory period.* During this period the muscle shows response if the strength of stimulus is increased to maximum. It extends from second half of the phase 3 to phase 4 of the action potential. Normal

Fig. 6.2-3. *Record of action potential (A) and mechanical response (B) from the cardiac muscle fibre shown on same time scale depicting the significance of long refractory period. ARP: Absolute refractory period; and RRP: relative refractory period.*

duration of relative refractory period in ventricles is about 50 msec.

Significance of long refractory period in cardiac muscle

As shown in Fig. 6.2-3, the cardiac muscle is refractory to any stimulus during the contraction phase (systole), therefore, the complete summation of contractions and thus tetanus cannot be produced in cardiac muscle. This property is very useful. Since the heart has to function as a pump, it must relax, get filled up with blood and then contract to pump out the blood. A tetanized heart would be useless as a pump.

CONTRACTILITY

Contractility is the ability of the cardiac muscle to actively generate force to shorten and thicken to do work when sufficient stimulus is applied. Process of myocardial contractility is discussed on page 171.

Characteristic features of myocardial contractility and factors affecting are:

- All or none law, and
- Starling law of heart.

1. All or none law. The response of cardiac muscle to a stimulus is all or none in character, i.e. when a stimulus of subthreshold intensity is applied, the heart does not contract at all (none response), when stimulus of threshold or suprathreshold intensity is applied, it contracts to its maximum ability (all response). This is because of the syncytial arrangement of the cardiac muscle fibres. Therefore, the 'all or none' law in heart is applicable to whole of functional syncytial unit, i.e. the entire atria or entire ventricle, while in skeletal muscle it is applicable only to a single muscle fibre.

2. Starling's law of heart. According to Starling's law the force of contraction is the function of the initial length of the muscle fibres; and upto physiological limits the greater the initial length, greater is the force of contraction. In the case of heart muscle the end diastolic volume forms the preload. The effect of changing end diastolic volume on force of cardiac contraction has been studied by Frank and Starling in 1910. *The Frank-Starling law of heart* states that within physiological limits the force of cardiac contraction is proportional to its end diastolic volume (venous return).

Clinical significance of Frank-Starling law of heart is in control of cardiac output as discussed (see page 181).

ORIGIN AND SPREAD OF CARDIAC IMPULSE

CONDUCTING SYSTEM OF THE HEART

Autorhythmicity refers to the property of cardiac muscle

which enables the heart to initiate its own impulse at constant rhythmical intervals. Because of this property the heart continues to beat even after all nerves to it are sectioned. This is because of the presence of specialized *pacemaker tissue* in the heart that can initiate repetitive action potentials. The pacemaker tissue makes a *conduction system* that normally spreads impulses through the heart.

The conducting system of the heart consists of specialized fibres of the heart muscle. These include (Fig. 6.2-4):

Fig. 6.2-4. *Specialized conducting tissues of the heart.*

1. Sinoatrial node. Sinoatrial (SA) node is located in the wall of right atrium just to the right of opening of superior vena cava. Spontaneous rhythmical electrical impulses arise from the SA node and spread in all directions.

2. Interatrial tract (Bachman's bundle). It is a band of specialized muscle fibres that run from SA node to left atrium. It causes simultaneous depolarization of the left atrium.

3. Internodal conduction pathway. Three internodal conduction paths which connect SA node to atrioventricular (AV) node include (Fig. 6.2-4):

- Anterior internodal pathway of Bachman,
- Middle internodal pathway of Wenckebach, and
- Posterior internodal pathway of Thorel.

4. Atrioventricular node. The atrioventricular (AV) node is located just beneath the endocardium on the right side of lower part of atrial septum, near the tricuspid valve. It is stimulated by the excitation wave that travels through internodal tracts and atrial myocardium.

5. Atrioventricular bundle of His. The atrioventricular bundle arises from the AV node, descends through the fibrous skeleton of the heart and divides into right bundle branch (RBB) for right ventricle and left bundle branch (LBB) for the left ventricle. The branches break up and become continuous with the plexus of Purkinje fibres.

6. Purkinje fibres. These are spread out deep to the endocardium and reach all parts of the ventricles, including the bases of papillary muscles.

INNERVATIONAL CHARACTERISTICS OF HEART

- Both SA node and AV node are richly supplied by the sympathetic as well as parasympathetic nerves. Parasympathetic fibres come from the vagus nerve and most sympathetic fibres come from the stellate ganglion.
- SA node is supplied by right vagus nerve and right-sided sympathetics.
- AV node is supplied by left vagus and left-sided sympathetic nerves.

MECHANISM OF ORIGIN OF RHYTHMIC CARDIAC IMPULSE

PACEMAKER

The part of the heart from which rhythmic impulses for heart beat are produced is called *pacemaker*. In mammalian heart, *SA node acts as a pacemaker* because the rate of impulse generation by SA node is highest. However, when there occurs blockage of transmission of impulse from SA node to AV node, the pacemaker activity may shift from SA node to other sites, e.g. AV node. When pacemaker is other than SA node it is called as *ectopic pacemaker*. Ectopic pacemaker causes abnormal sequence of contraction of different parts of the heart.

Rate of production of rhythmic impulses by different parts of the heart is:

- SA node: 70 to 80 per minute,
- AV node: 40 to 60 per minute,
- Atrial muscle: 40 to 60 per minute, and
- Ventricular muscles: 20 to 40 per minute.

ELECTRICAL POTENTIAL IN PACEMAKER TISSUE

In pacemaker (SA node) fibres, the resting membrane potential is only of –55 to –60 mV; and that this is not steady, due to slow depolarization which is due to slow diffusion of Na^+ followed by Ca^{2+} influx because of leakage channels (Fig. 6.2-5). Due to this slow depolarization the threshold level – 40 mV is reached very slowly. Once the threshold level of – 40 mV is reached there occurs a rapid depolarization upto +5 mV followed by rapid repolarization, i.e. there occurs action potential and generation of an impulse. After rapid repolarization (phase 3 of action potential), once again the resting membrane potential (phase 4 of action potential) is reached which is not stable and starts rising slowly to again reach at threshold level to produce the second impulse. This slow rising resting membrane potential in between the action potentials is called *prepotential* or *pacemaker potential* (Fig. 6.2-5). Presence of this unique feature in the cells of pacemaker tissue is the underlying mechanism

Fig. 6.2-5. *Phases of action potential in cardiac muscle fibre (0, 1, 2, 3, 4) and sinoatrial node showing pacemaker potential. AP = action potential.*

responsible for self-generation of rhythmic impulses (autorhythmicity).

SPREAD OF CARDIAC IMPULSE

The cardiac impulse which originates in the SA node in the form of action potential spreads throughout the heart through the conduction system (property of conductivity).

SA node and atria. The impulse travels over the muscle fibres of atria from SA nodal fibres, and through the interatrial tract to the left atrium. Conduction through these fibres causes simultaneous depolarization of both the atria. Atrial depolarization is completed in about 0.1 sec. The impulse reaches to AV node from SA node within 0.03 sec after its origin.

AV node. Conduction through AV node is slow, there is a delay of about 0.1 sec. This AV nodal delay is useful, for it provides time for completion of atrial contraction and their emptying (i.e. ventricular filling) before the ventricles contract.

Ventricular conduction. The impulses conducted through the AV node are distributed to ventricles through bundle of His, its branches, and Purkinje fibres in 0.08 to 0.15 sec. In humans, depolarization of the ventricular muscle proceeds as follows (Fig. 6.2-6):

- Starts at the left side of interventricular septum.
- Moves first to the right across the mid portion of the septum.
- The wave of depolarization then spreads down the septum to apex of heart.
- It, then, returns along the ventricular walls to the AV groove, proceeding from the endocardial to the epicardial surface.

CHAPTER 6.2

SA Node

AV Node

Atrial activation

Septal activation
from left to right

Right   **Left**

Activation of anteroseptal
region of the ventricular
myocardium

Activation of major
portion of ventricular
myocardium from
endocardial surfaces

Late activation of
posterobasal portion
of the left ventricle,
the pulmonary conus
and uppermost portion
of septum

Fig. 6.2-6. Spread of cardiac impulse.

- The last parts of the heart to be depolarized are the posterobasal portion of the left ventricle, the pulmonary conus, and the uppermost portion of the septum.

Thus, total time required for conduction from SA node to endocardial surface is 0.22 sec.

ELECTROCARDIOGRAPHY

William Einthoven, a Dutch physiologist, originally developed the technique of electrocardiography. He was awarded Nobel Prize in 1924 for his contribution and is called the father of modern electrocardiography.

Electrocardiography refers to extracellular recording of the summed-up electrical events of all the cardiac muscle fibres generated with each heart beat. Electrically heart behaves as a *dipole,* i.e. two-terminal battery in which the excited part (depolarized segment) forms a negative pole and the non-excited part forms the positive pole. Thus, ECG is nothing but the surface recording of the potential difference between the two poles of the heart dipole at a given time. The record of the potential fluctuations during the cardiac cycle is called the *electrocardiography* (ECG). The machine used to record these potential fluctuations is called *electrocardiograph.*

ELECTROCARDIOGRAPH

The electrocardiograph (ECG machine) is essentially a sophisticated string galvanometer. A modern electro-cardiograph amplifies and records the potential fluctuations on a moving strip of paper. Special paper is used which turns black on exposure to heat. The stylus (recording pen) is made hot by electrical current flowing through its tip.

NORMAL ELECTROCARDIOGRAM

Electrocardiogram (ECG) refers to the record of the potential fluctuations during the cardiac cycle. As a result of sequential spread of the excitation in the atria, the interventricular septum and the ventricular walls (Fig. 6.2-7) and finally repolarization of the myocardium, a series of positive and negative waves designated as P, Q, R, S and T are recorded during each cardiac cycle.

Waves of ECG

P wave. P wave is the positive (upright rounded) deflection. It is produced by the depolarization of atrial musculature so also called atrial complex.

Fig. 6.2-7. Normal electrocardiogram showing various waves.

QRS complex. QRS complex consists of three consecutive waves. Q wave is a small negative wave which may be absent normally quite often. It is continued as a tall positive R wave which is followed by a small negative S wave. The QRS complex is caused by ventricular depolarization.

T wave. T wave is the last, positive, dome-shaped deflection. T wave represents ventricular repolarization.

U wave. It is a small round positive wave. It occurs due to slow repolarization of papillary muscle. It is rarely seen normally. It becomes prominent in hypokalaemia.

Note: Since atrial repolarization coincides with ventricular depolarization, so it is merged with QRS complex and thus not recorded as a separate wave.

Intervals and segments of ECG

P-R interval. It is measured from the onset of P wave to the onset of the QRS complex. It measures the *AV conduction time,* including the AV nodal delay. Its *duration* varies from 0.12 to 0.21 sec depending on the heart rate.

Clinical significance. Prolonged PR interval indicates AV conduction block.

QT interval. It is the time from the start of the QRS complex to the end of T wave. It indicates total *systolic time of ventricles,* i.e. ventricular depolarization and repolarization.

ST segment. It is an isoelectric period between the end of QRS complex and beginning of T wave.
- Its *duration* is about 0.32 sec.
- It corresponds with *ventricular repolarization.*

Clinical significance. ST segment is elevated in patients with myocardial infarction.

CLINICAL APPLICATIONS OF ELECTROCARDIOGRAPHY

Electrocardiography is an indispensable tool in the diagnosis, prognosis and planning treatment of the cardiac disorders such as :
- Cardiac arrhythmias,
- Myocardial infarction,
- Hypertrophy of various cardiac chambers, and
- Effects on ECG of changes in the ionic composition of blood.

HEART AS A PUMP

The heart as a pump can be considered actually comprising two separate pumps in the series: a *right heart* that pumps the blood through the lungs and a *left heart* that pumps the blood through the peripheral organs. Further, each sided pump consists of an atrium and a ventricle. The atria act as *primary pumps* for the ventricles. The ventricles in turn provide the major force that propels the blood through pulmonary and systemic circulations. To act as a pump, the heart contracts and relaxes rhythmically. The terms *systole* (contractile phase) and *diastole* (relaxation phase) are used for different phases. The electrocardiogram records the *electrical events* that precede and initiate the corresponding *mechanical events* as:
- *P wave* is followed by *atrial contraction.*
- *QRS waves* are caused by depolarization of the ventricles which initiates *contraction of the ventricles.*
- *T wave* occurs slightly before the end of ventricular contraction.

CARDIAC CYCLE

The cardiac cycle thus includes both electrical and mechanical events that occur from the beginning of one heart beat to the beginning of the next.

PHASES OF CARDIAC CYCLE

Duration of each cardiac cycle at a normal heart rate of 75 beats/min is 60/75 = 0.8 sec.

During each cardiac cycle both atria contract (*atrial systole*) and relax (*atrial diastole),* and both ventricles contract (*ventricular systole*) and relax (*ventricular diastole*).

Therefore, each cardiac cycle can be considered to consist of simultaneously occurring atrial and ventricular cycles with following phases (Figs. 6.2-8 and 6.2-9):

Atrial cycle
1. Atrial systole or atrial contraction phase (0.1 sec)
2. Atrial diastole (0.7 sec).

Ventricular cycle
Ventricular systole (0.3 sec) consists of:
1. Isovolumic (isometric) contraction phase (0.05 sec), and
2. Phase of ventricular ejection which can be further divided into rapid ejection phase (0.1 sec), and slow ejection phase (0.15 sec).

Ventricular diastole (0.5 sec) consists of:
1. Protodiastole (0.04 sec),
2. Isovolumic (isometric) relaxation phase (0.06 sec),
3. Rapid passive filling phase (0.11 sec),
4. Reduced filling phase or diastasis (0.19 sec), and
5. Last rapid filling phase which coincides with the atrial systole (0.1 sec).

ATRIAL CYCLE

Atrial systole
- Atrial systole or the atrial contraction phase lasts for 0.1 sec and coincides with the last rapid filling phase of ventricular diastole (Figs. 6.2-8 and 6.2-9).

C H A P T E R 6.2

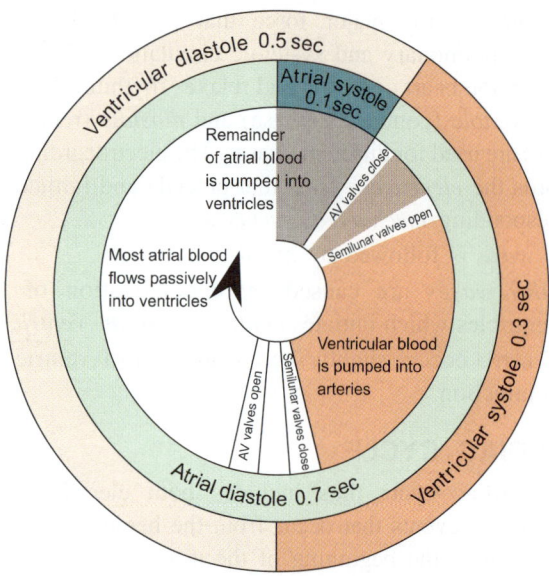

Fig. 6.2-8. Duration of phases of cardiac cycle.

- Before the beginning of atrial systole, the ventricles are relaxing, AV valves are open and blood is flowing from the great veins into the atria and from the atria into the ventricles. Thus the atria and ventricles are forming a continuous cavity.

The contraction of atria causes:
- *Increase in intra-atrial pressure* by 4 to 6 mm of Hg pressure rise in right atrium is reflected into the veins and is recorded as *a-wave* from the jugular vein.
- *Increase in the ventricular pressure* occurs slightly due to pumping of blood in the ventricles.
- *Narrowing of origin of great veins* and decreasing venous return to the heart.

Atrial diastole
After the atrial systole, there occurs atrial diastole (0.7 sec). This period coincides with the ventricular systole and most of the ventricular diastole (Fig. 6.2-8).

- During atrial diastole, atrial muscles relax and there occurs gradual filling of the atria due to continuous venous return and the pressure gradually increases in the atria (Fig. 6.2-10).

VENTRICULAR CYCLE
Ventricular systole
After the atrial contraction phase is over, the ventricles start contracting. The ventricular systole lasts for 0.3 sec, and has following phases:

1. *Phase of isovolumic (isometric) contraction*
- With the beginning of ventricular contraction, the ventricular pressure exceeds atrial pressure very rapidly causing closure of AV valves (this event is responsible for production of first heart sound).
- Since the AV valves have closed and semilunar valves have not opened, pressure inside the ventricles rises rapidly to a high level, but the volume of blood in the ventricles does not change, so this phase is called *isovolumic contraction phase.*
- During this phase, due to sharp rise in ventricular pressure, there occurs bulging of AV valves into the atria producing a small but sharp rise in intra-atrial pressure called *c-wave.*
- This phase lasts for 0.05 sec, until the pressure in the left and right ventricles exceeds the pressure in the aorta (80 mm of Hg) and pulmonary artery (10 mm of Hg) and the aortic and pulmonary valves open.

2. *Phase of ventricular ejection*
The ventricular ejection phase begins with the opening of semilunar valves and lasts for about 0.25 sec. It can be further divided into two phases:
- *Rapid ejection phase.*
- *Slow ejection phase.*

Ventricular diastole
1. *Protodiastole.* When the ventricular systole ends, the ventricles start relaxing and intraventricular pressure falls

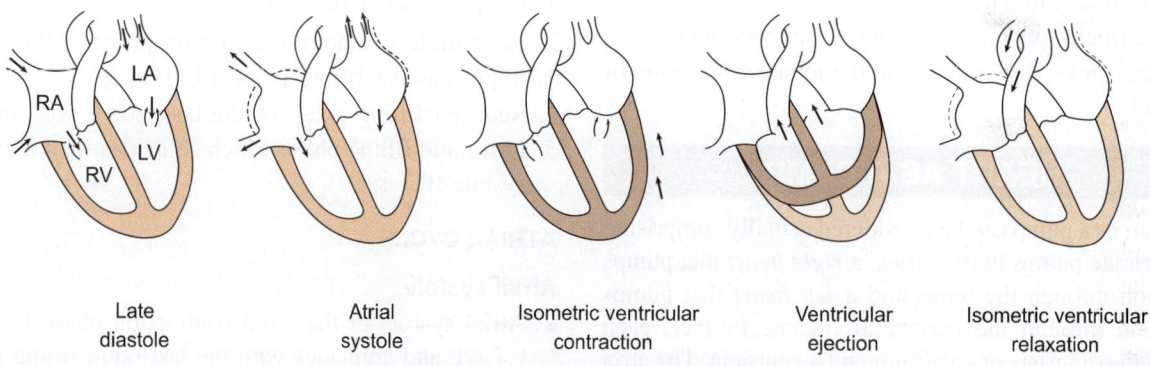

| Late diastole | Atrial systole | Isometric ventricular contraction | Ventricular ejection | Isometric ventricular relaxation |

Fig. 6.2-9. Phases of cardiac cycle.

Fig. 6.2-10. *Phases and events during cardiac cycle.*

rapidly. This phase lasts for 0.04 sec. During this phase the elevated pressure in the distended arteries (aorta and pulmonary artery) immediately pushes the blood back towards ventricles which snaps the semilunar valves to close. Closure of semilunar (i.e. aortic and pulmonary) valves prevents the movement of blood back into the ventricles and produces the *second heart sound* (S₂). It also causes *dicrotic notch* in the down slope of aortic pressure called the *incisura*.

2. Isovolumic or isometric relaxation phase

- This phase begins with the closure of semilunar valves and lasts for about 0.06 sec.
- Since semilunar valves have closed and the AV valves have not yet opened, so the ventricles continue to relax as closed chambers in this phase.

- But the ventricular volume remains constant, so this phase is called isvolumic or isometric relaxation phase.
- This phase ends when the AV valves open, as indicated by the peak of *v-wave* on the atrial pressure tracing (Figs. 6.2-9 and 6.2-10).

3. Rapid passive filling phase (0.11 sec)

- During ventricular systole, the atria are in diastole and venous return continues so that the atrial pressure is high. When the AV valves open, the high atrial pressure causes a rapid, initial flow of blood into the ventricles. The rapid passive filling phase produces the *third heart sound (S₃)*.
- Once the AV valves open, the atria and ventricles are a common chamber and pressure in both cavities falls as ventricular relaxation continues.

4. Reduced filling and diastasis (0.19 sec). In this phase, pressure in atria and ventricles reduces slowly and remains little above zero. This decreases the rate of blood flow from atria to ventricle causing a very slow filling called *diastasis.*

5. Last rapid filling phase (0.1 sec). The last rapid filling phase of ventricular diastole coincides with the atrial systole. During this phase additional 25 per cent of the blood enters the ventricles. With this phase the ventricular cycle is completed.

EVENTS DURING CARDIAC CYCLE

The events associated with contraction and relaxation of the heart during a cardiac cycle include pressure changes in the ventricles, atria and aorta; volume changes in the ventricles and valvular events. Most of these have been described during various phases of cardiac cycle.

Pressure changes in the aorta

Pressure in the aorta varies between 80 to 120 mm of Hg during the cardiac cycle. Aortic pressure changes during various phases of cardiac cycle (Fig. 6.2-10) are:

During atrial systole. During atrial systole the pressure in the aorta is about 80 mm of Hg.

During ventricular systole. During ventricular systole the aortic pressure starts rising along with the intraventricular pressure and during rapid ejection phase and reaches maximum (120 mm of Hg) at the end of rapid ejection phase.

During ventricular diastole. Due to sudden closure of semilunar valve the backflowing blood collides against the closed aortic valve. This collision causes a small but sharp rise in aortic pressure. This small rise produces a notch called *incisura.* This sharp pressure rise is recordable even from peripheral arteries and is called *dicrotic notch.*

During rest of the diastole the aortic pressure smoothly declines to about 80 mm of Hg.

Pressure changes in pulmonary artery

Pressure curve in the pulmonary artery is similar to that of aorta but pressures are low. Pulmonary artery systolic pressure averages 15-18 mm of Hg and its pressure during diastole is 8-10 mm of Hg.

Volume changes in the ventricles during cardiac cycle

During atrial systole. Atrial systole coincides with the last rapid filling phase of ventricular diastole. When the atrial contraction begins about 105 ml (75%) of the blood has already flown into the ventricles. The atrial contraction causes additional 25 ml (25%) filling of the ventricles. Thus at the end of atrial systole, i.e. at the end of ventricular diastole the ventricular volume is about 130 ml. This is called *end-diastolic volume.*

During ventricular systole

During isovolumic contraction phase, as the name suggests, there occurs no change in the ventricular volume.

During ventricular ejection phase about 80 ml of the blood is ejected out by each ventricle. This is called *stroke volume.* The percentage of the end-diastolic volume that is ejected out with each stroke during systole (about 65%) is called *ejection fraction.* Thus, about 50 ml of the blood in each ventricle at the end of ventricular systole is called *end-systolic volume.*

Valvular events (Heart sounds)

A total four heart sounds (1st, 2nd, 3rd and 4th) are produced by certain mechanical activities during each cardiac cycle. The heart sounds can be heard with stethoscope (auscultation) and can be recorded (phonocardiography).

First heart sound (HS$_1$). First heart sound is produced by vibrations set up by the sudden closure of AV valves at the start of ventricular systole (Fig. 6.2-10). It sounds like the spoken word 'LUBB'.

Second heart sound (HS$_2$). It is caused by vibrations associated with closure of the semilunar valves just at the onset of ventricular diastole. It sounds like the spoken word 'DUBB'.

Third heart sound (HS$_3$). Third heart sound is caused by vibrations set up in the cardiac wall by inrush of blood during *rapid filling phase* of ventricular diastole. It cannot be heard by auscultation with stethoscope.

Fourth heart sound (HS$_4$) It is caused by vibrations set up during atrial systole. It is normally not audible.

ARTERIAL PULSE

Arterial pulse is also an event related to cardiac cycle. The blood forced into the aorta during systole not only moves the blood in the vessels forward but also sets up a pressure wave that is transmitted along the *arteries to the periphery.* The pressure wave expands the arterial walls as it travels, and expansion is palpable as the *pulse.*

Examination of arterial pulse

Examination of the arterial pulse is an essential feature of clinical examination. Arterial pulse can be palpated from any superficial artery, e.g. radial, femoral, dorsalis pedis and carotid, etc. Most frequently, pulse is examined from the radial artery because it is conveniently approached without exposing the body, and can be easily palpated as it is placed superficially against the bone.

Examination of the pulse should include following aspects:

1. *Pulse rate* refers to number of pulses per minute.

- *Normal pulse rate* varies with age being 150-180/min in fetus, 130-140/min at birth, about 90/min at the age of 10 years and about 72/min in adults.

- *Increased pulse rate* represents tachycardia and occurs during exercise, in anxiety, in fever, in hyperthyroidism and in atrial and ventricular tachycardias.

- *Decreased pulse rate* represents bradycardia and is seen in hypothyroidism and incomplete heart blocks.

2. *Volume of pulse* also known as strength of arterial pulse or amplitude or impact that can be felt. It represents stroke volume or the pulse pressure (i.e. systolic-diastolic pressure).

- *Rapid and thready pulse* occurs in hypovolaemia as in severe haemorrhage.

- *Increased volume pulse* is seen during exercise and in ventricular hypertrophy.

3. *Rhythm of pulse* is noted as regular or irregular. Under normal conditions and during sinus bradycardia or sinus tachycardia pulse appears at regular intervals.

- *Irregular pulse rhythm* is a feature of extra systole, atrial fibrillation and other cardiac arrhythmias.

4. *Character of pulse* is felt on palpation. It denotes the tension and waves in the pulse.

CARDIAC OUTPUT AND VENOUS RETURN

DEFINITION OF CARDIAC OUTPUT AND RELATED TERMS

The main function of the heart is to pump blood to meet the metabolic needs of the body. The measure of the heart's ability to pump blood is cardiac output. The *cardiac output* refers to the amount of blood ejected by each ventricle per minute. The *stroke volume* is the amount of blood pumped out by each ventricle per beat or per contraction. Therefore, cardiac output (CO) can be calculated by multiplying the stroke volume (SV) by the heart rate (HR):

CO = SV × HR

Under normal conditions the average heart rate is about 70 beats/min and stroke volume is about 80 ml and thus cardiac output is 80 × 70 = 5.6 L.

The cardiac output is expressed in litres per minute and normally varies from 5 to 6 L per min. In health, the right and left ventricular outputs are nearly equal. Thus, each ventricle pumps about 5-6 L of blood into the circulation per minute. This is made possible because of the fact that the right and left side pumps act in series.

Cardiac index is the cardiac output expressed in relation to the body surface area. The normal cardiac index is about 3.2 L/min/m².

Distribution of the cardiac output

Of the total cardiac output, about 75% is distributed to the vital organs of the body and rest of 25% to the skeletal muscles, other organs of the body and skin. The distribution of the cardiac output to various organs of the body is shown in Table 6.2-1.

Table 6.2-1. Distribution of cardiac output to various organs

Body organ	Amount of blood flow (ml/min)		Percentage of total cardiac output	
Liver	1500		25	
Kidney	1300		about 25	75
Brain	750			
Heart	250	1500	25	
Lungs	500			
Skeletal muscles and other body organs	1000	1500	25	
Skin	500			

REGULATION OF CARDIAC OUTPUT

The cardiac output increases or decreases in various physiological and pathological conditions as described above. The variations in the cardiac output are brought about by certain factors operating through certain mechanisms by an integrated role.

The cardiac output (CO), as we know, is the product of stroke volume (SV) and heart rate (HR), i.e. CO = SV × HR. Therefore, variations in the cardiac output can be produced by the factors which change stroke volume or heart rate, or both. (Fig. 6.2-11).

Cardiac output control mechanisms

The stroke output is regulated by two mechanisms: intrinsic and extrinsic.

1. Intrinsic autoregulation (Frank-Starling mechanism).

According to *Frank-Starling law* of heart, 'within physiological limits' the force of contraction of *cardiac muscle* is proportionate to the initial length of muscle fibres. In the heart, end-diastolic volume forms the preload. Therefore, precisely the Frank-Starling law of heart can be stated as, within physiological limits, the force of cardiac contraction is proportional to its end-diastolic volume (EDV). Since, in this intrinsic regulation mechanism, cardiac muscle fibres are stretched to increase their initial length, it is also termed as *heterometric mechanism*.

Factors affecting end-diastolic volume (venous return)

The end-diastolic volume refers to the *venous return* to the heart during diastole. For individual at rest, the cardiac

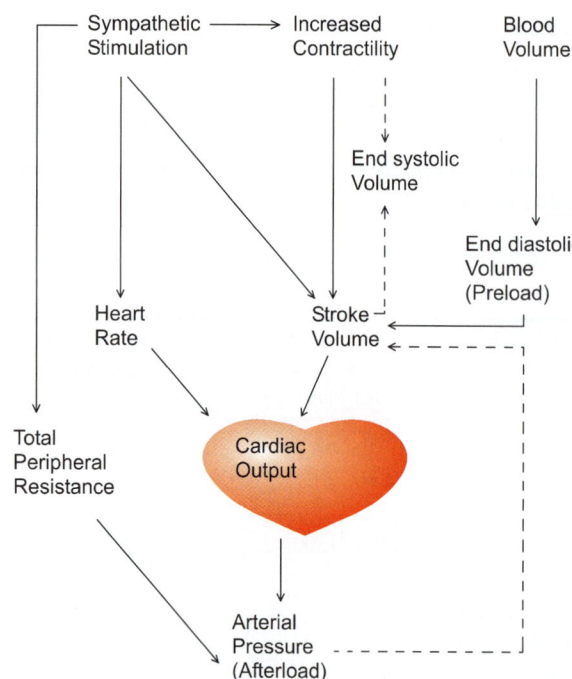

Fig. 6.2-11. *Interaction between the factors that regulate cardiac output and arterial pressure. Solid lines indicate increase and dotted lines indicate a decrease.*

output and venous return are approximately 5 L/min. Factors affecting venous return (Fig. 6.2-12) are:

1. *Respiratory pump.* During inspiration the intrathoracic pressure becomes more negative and there occurs descent of diaphragm which increases the intra-abdominal pressure. The decreased pressure inside the inferior vena cava coupled with increased intra-abdominal pressure during inspiration results in increased flow of blood into the right atrium. This mechanism of increased blood flow during inspiration is called *respiratory pump*. This respiratory pump operates strongly in forced respiration and in severe muscular exercise increasing the venous return.

2. *Cardiac pump.* The cardiac pump influences the venous return by two kinds of forces the 'vis-a-tergo' and 'vis-a-fronte'.

- *Vis-a-tergo* refers to the forward push from behind, i.e. the propelling force. Vis-a-tergo results from the myocardial contraction during systole and is supplemented by the elastic recoil of the arterial wall (Windkessel effect).
- *Vis-a-fronte* refers to the suction force acting from the front which basically pulls the blood from the great veins into the right atrium. This suction force is created by ventricular contraction.

3. *Muscle pump.* The muscle pump mechanism is responsible for flow of blood from the veins of the limbs to the heart.

Working of muscle pump. Two types of veins are present in the limbs: superficial and deep veins. Blood flows from the superficial veins into deep veins through communicating veins. Due to the presence of valves in the limb veins the blood flows in one direction, i.e. from periphery towards heart and not in reverse direction.

- *When the skeletal muscles contract*, the deep veins present in between the muscles are compressed and due to increased pressure the valve present proximal to the contracting muscle is opened up while the valve present on distal end is tightly closed and in this way the blood is propelled up towards the heart (Fig. 6.2-13A).
- *When the skeletal muscle relaxes* a negative pressure is created in the segment of veins. So due to back flow the proximal valve is closed and the distal valve is opened and blood is sucked up (Fig. 6.2-13B).
- *With rhythmic contractions of skeletal muscles* in this way, the blood is squeezed out of the limbs towards the heart.

Applied aspect. In certain professions (e.g. nurses, traffic police, etc.) the individuals have to keep standing for a long time of a day. In such persons, veins of lower limbs

Fig. 6.2-12. *Frank-Starling curve (A) and factors affecting end-diastolic volume (B). Blue arrows indicate increase and green arrows indicate decrease.*

Fig. 6.2-13. *Mechanism of muscle pump: A, during contraction of muscles; and B, during relaxation of muscles.*

become large, tortuous and bulbous. This condition is called *varicose veins.*

4. *Blood volume.* The increased blood volume increases the venous return and a decreased blood volume decreases the venous return.

5. *Sympathetic discharge.* On sympathetic stimulation there occurs increase in the venous tone which decreases the capacity of the venous system (veins are capacitance vessels).

6. *Standing body position* is associated with a decreased venous return due to peripheral pooling of the blood.

Clinical significance of Frank-Starling mechanism

- *For small, momentary adjustments necessary for keeping the outputs of two ventricles equal* and adjusting them to match the venous return the intrinsic regulation works continuously.
- *Maintenance of constant stroke volume when the peripheral resistance is increased is carried out by intrinsic mechanism.* When the peripheral resistance (blood pressure) is increased, initially the heart is unable to pump all the blood it normally does. The accumulated blood in the ventricle stretches the muscle fibres leading to great force of contraction and thus the stroke volume is restored to normal in spite of greater resistance to the outflow.
- *Intrinsic control mechanism serves as a life-saving device in cardiac failure.* Left ventricular failure causes accumulation of blood within left ventricle, thereby

decreases blood supply to vital organs. Soon, accumulation of blood in the left ventricle increases the initial length of muscle fibres leading to greater cardiac output according to Frank-Starling mechanism in initial stage.

2. Extrinsic regulation (autonomic neural mechanism)

In this mechanism stroke volume increases due to *increased myocardial contractility* without any increase in the initial muscle length. Therefore, it is also called *homometric mechanism.* The homometric regulation is governed by autonomic neural mechanism as described below:

Sympathetic activity

Stimulation of the sympathetic nerves to the heart results in increased myocardial contractility and is known as *positive inotropic effect.* The positive inotropic effect of the norepinephrine liberated at the sympathetic nerve endings is augmented by circulating norepinephrine.

Inhibition of sympathetic system has opposite effects.

Characteristics of increased myocardial contractility

- The ventricles contract more forcefully and more rapidly. As a result the ventricles are able to do more work per stroke, i.e. ejection fraction increases at the same end-diastolic volume (without increase in venous return).
- Due to more complete emptying of ventricles during each systole the *end-systolic volume is decreased.*
- Due to increased stroke output, *arterial pressure is increased.*

Parasympathetic activity

There is a negative inotropic effect of parasympathetic (vagal) stimulation. This effect, however, is not much because vagal fibres are mainly distributed to the atria and not much to the ventricles.

Role of heart rate in control of cardiac output

Since, cardiac output is the product of stroke volume and heart rate, it is tempting to attribute the increase in cardiac output to increase in the heart rate. However, in fact it is not so. It has been seen that when heart rate alone is increased, the cardiac output does not increase at all. The progressive increase in the heart rate is associated with a proportionate decrease in stroke volume because of reduced diastole time and thus reduced end-diastolic volume. Conversely, when the heart rate is reduced the ventricular diastole is prolonged leading to more ventricular filling and thus an increased stroke volume.

During exercise the sympathetic stimulation produces a marked increase in the heart rate (200-300%) due to positive chronotropism and moderate increase (50-60%) in the stroke volume due to positive inotropism leading to manifold increase in cardiac output.

Physiology of Circulation

6.3

INTRODUCTION

Physiology of circulation is concerned with flow of blood and the pressure in the various segments of the vascular system of the body. It can be discussed under following headings:
- Functional organization and structure of vascular system,
- Haemodynamics,
- Blood flow and pressure in different segments of circulatory system, and
- Blood pressure.

FUNCTIONAL ORGANIZATION AND STRUCTURE OF VASCULAR SYSTEM

ORGANIZATION OF VASCULAR SYSTEM

The vascular system is organized into two separate circulations (systemic and pulmonary), arranged in series.

Systemic circulation

Systemic circulation supplies blood to various systemic organs through parallel distribution channels (Fig. 6.3-1). This parallel arrangement of vessels ensures the supply of

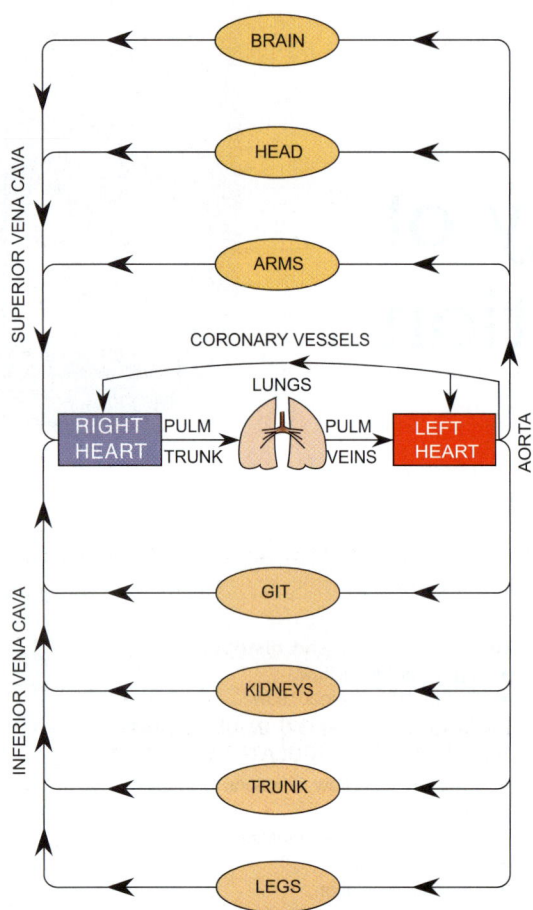

Fig. 6.3-1. *A schematic illustration of the organization of cardiovascular system depicting in series arrangement of pulmonary and systemic circulation and parallel arrangement of vessels supplying blood to organs.*

blood of the same arterial composition (i.e. same O_2 and CO_2 tension, pH, glucose level and essentially the same arterial pressure) to various body organs. In systemic circulation, from the left ventricle, blood is pumped through the arteries and arterioles to the capillaries, where it equilibrates with the interstitial fluid. The capillaries drain through the venules into the veins and ultimately to the right atrium.

Pulmonary circulation

Pulmonary circulation is meant for oxygenation of blood. Since pulmonary circulation is arranged in series with systemic circulation, so it receives the same amount of blood over any significant time period. In pulmonary circulation, from the right ventricle, blood is pumped through the pulmonary arteries to the pulmonary capillaries. In the pulmonary capillaries, the blood equilibrates with the O_2 and CO_2 of alveolar air. The capillaries then drain the oxygenated blood through venules and then through pulmonary veins into the left atrium.

Systemic vascular tree

From functional point of view the systemic vascular tree can be divided into following types of blood vessels:

- *Large elastic arteries* (Windkessel vessels) include aorta and its main branches such as carotid, iliac and axillary arteries,
- *Large muscular arteries* (distribution vessels) which include most of the arteries of the body, e.g. arteries like radial, ulnar, popliteal.
- *Arterioles* and precapillary sphincters (resistance vessels).
- *Meta-arterioles* and capillaries (exchange vessels),
- *Venules* (postcapillary resistance vessels),
- *Veins* (capacitance vessels), and
- *Arteriovenous anastomoses* (shunt or thoroughfare vessels).

STRUCTURE OF BLOOD VESSELS

General structural characteristics

Histologically, walls of most of the blood vessels except the capillaries consist of three coats (Fig. 6.3-2):

Fig. 6.3-2. *Histological structure of an artery.*

1. *Tunica intima.* It is the innermost coat of the vessel wall. In large arteries, from inside-out, it consists of:

- *Endothelial lining,* which is very smooth and silky, and consists of single layer of cells. It lies in contact with blood.
- *Basal lamina* is a thin layer of glycoprotein which lines the external aspect of the endothelium.
- *Subendothelial connective tissue* is a delicate layer of connective tissue which lies outside the basal lamina.
- *Internal elastic lamina* is a thin membrane formed by elastic fibres.

2. *Tunica media.* It is the middle, thickest coat of the vessel wall. It consists of smooth muscles and elastic tissue. The ratio of these two tissues varies from vessel to vessel. On the outside, tunica media is limited by a membrane formed by elastic fibres called the *external elastic lamina.*

3. Tunica adventitia. It is the outermost coat of the vessel wall. It is made of connective tissue in which collagen fibres are prominent. This layer prevents undue stretching or distension of the blood vessel.

Essential characteristics

Essential characteristics of blood vessels like lumen diameter, wall thickness, approximate total cross-sectional area and percentage of blood volume contained are shown in Table 6.3-1.

Table 6.3-1. Essential characteristics of various types of blood vessels

Vessel	Lumen diameter	Wall thickness	Approximate cross-sectional area (cm²)	Percentage of total blood volume contained in all vessels of each type
Aorta	2.5 cm	2 mm	45	2
Artery	0.4 cm	1 mm	20	8
Arteriole	30 µm	20 µm	400	1
Capillary	5 µm	1 µm	4500	5
Venule	20 µm	2 µm	4000	54
Vein	0.5 cm	0.5 mm	40	
Vena cava	3 cm	1.5 mm	18	
Heart				12
Pulmonary circulation				18

HAEMODYNAMICS

Haemodynamics, which refers to study of blood flow in various segments of the vascular system, can be discussed under following headings:

- General principles governing (factors affecting) blood flow,
- Types of blood flow, and
- Regulation of blood flow in different situations.

GENERAL PRINCIPLES GOVERNING (FACTORS AFFECTING) BLOOD FLOW

FLOW-PRESSURE-RESISTANCE RELATIONSHIP

Relationship between flow of a fluid with the pressure and resistance offered to it through a rigid tube was studied by a French physiologist Poiseuille in 1842 and Hagen, and is known as Poiseuille's law or Poiseuille-Hagen law.

Poiseuille's law

Poiseuille's law expressing the relation between the flow (Q) and pressure gradient (ΔP) in a long narrow tube of length (L), the viscosity of fluid (η), and the radius (r) of the tube is as:

$$Q = \frac{\Delta P\, \pi r^4}{8\, \eta L}$$

Thus, according to Poiseuille's law the flow (Q) of a Newtonian fluid through a rigid tube is determined by:

1. Pressure gradient (ΔP), i.e. difference in the pressure between the two ends of the tube. In other words, fluid always flows from an area of high pressure (P_1) to one of lower pressure (P_2), i.e. Q α ΔP or (P_1–P_2).

2. Radius of tube (r). The flow of fluid varies directly as the fourth power of radius (r^4). Thus if the radius is halved the flow will decrease by 16 times and vice versa. Thus this factor is very important for flow of blood through the blood vessels.

3. Viscosity of fluid (η). The flow of fluid varies inversely with the viscosity of fluid, i.e. greater the viscosity, lesser the flow and vice versa.

4. Length of the tube (L). The flow is inversely proportional to the length of the tube. Longer the length greater will be the total resistance offered.

Resistance (R). According to mathematical calculation in principles of physics, resistance (R) is represented by 8 Lη/πr⁴. By replacing 8 Lη/πr⁴ with R in Poiseuille's law, it becomes:

$$Q = \frac{\Delta P}{R}$$

Thus, Poiseuille's law can be considered analogous to Ohm's law of current.

The Poiseuille's law is valid for straight rigid tubes with Newtonian fluid flowing through them. Since, blood vessels are not rigid and the blood is not a Newtonian fluid, therefore, strictly speaking the Poiseuille's law does not apply to flow of blood through the vascular system. Nevertheless, the important principles relating flow, pressure gradient and resistance remain applicable, so they are discussed in relation to blood flow as:

BLOOD FLOW AND PRESSURE GRADIENT RELATIONSHIP

The relationship between flow of blood and pressure in the blood vessels is not linear because blood vessels are distensible (e.g. aorta) (Fig. 6.3-3B) and show active myogenic contractile response to stretch (e.g. arterioles) (Fig. 6.3-3C). Such arterioles serve to stabilize the blood flow over a wide range of pressure (80 mm of Hg to 200 mm of Hg). This phenomenon is called *autoregulation.*

BLOOD FLOW AND RESISTANCE RELATIONSHIP

From Poiseuille's law it can be derived that flow is inversely proportional to the resistance, i.e. Q α 1/R. In vascular system resistance is represented by peripheral resistance unit (PRU).

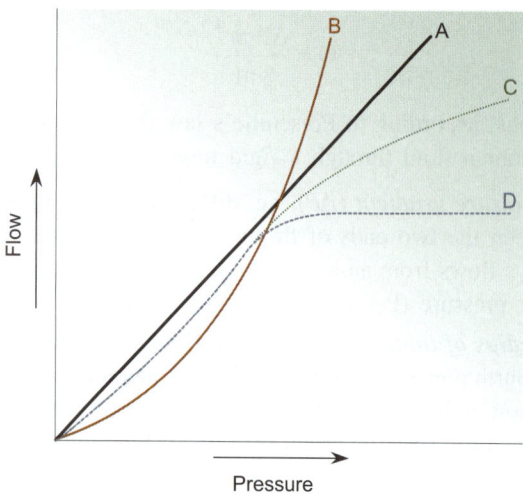

Fig. 6.3-3. *Relationship of pressure to flow: A, in a rigid tube; B, in a distensible blood vessel (aorta); and C, distensible blood vessel containing active myogenic contractile element.*

Factors that affect resistance to blood flow

The major factors that determine the resistance to flood flow are:

I. The viscosity of blood, and

II. The radius of vessels.

I. Blood viscosity and resistance

Definition and unit of viscosity

Viscosity was described by Isaac Newton in 1713 as internal friction to flow in a fluid or lack of slipperiness. The resistance met by the fluid moving through a tube in a streamlined flow is due to the friction between adjacent laminae and not due to the friction between vessel wall and fluid. Thus, greater the internal friction, greater is difference in velocity (shear rate) between two laminae and greater the coefficient of viscosity.

Unit of viscosity is *Poise* (after Poiseuille), but *Relative viscosity* is a more often used term; and refers to the viscosity of a fluid relative to the viscosity of water at body temperature (37°C).

- Plasma, has a relative viscosity of 1.7, and
- Blood (plasma plus cells) has a relative viscosity of about 4-5.

Pathological conditions associated with high blood viscosity are:

- Severe polycythaemia
- Abnormal shaped RBCs (congenital spherocytosis)
- Abnormally high immunoglobulin level
- Lowered body temperature (in frost bite).

II. Radius of blood vessels and resistance

As mentioned earlier, the rate of flow is proportional to the fourth power of the radius (r^4) of the blood vessels.

Thus, even a small change in the calibre of the blood vessels will produce a marked change in blood flow. For example, at a pressure head of 100 mm of Hg, the change in flow rate with change in the radius is:

Radius	Flow rate
1 mm	1 ml/min
2 mm	16 ml/min
4 mm	256 ml/min

Among the blood vessels, in aorta and large arteries there is little resistance. Arterioles are the major seat of vascular resistance.

VELOCITY OF BLOOD FLOW

The velocity of blood flow refers to displacement of blood per unit time, i.e. cm/sec.

Velocity and cross sectional area relationship

- The relationship between velocity (V), quantity of blood flow (Q) and cross sectional area (A) of the blood vessel is:

$$V = \frac{Q}{A}$$

Thus if quantity of blood flow (Q) remains constant and cross sectional area (A) increases then velocity of blood flow will decrease.

- Since, cross-sectional area of capillaries is 1000 times as that of aorta, so the velocity of blood flow in capillaries is approximately 1 mm/sec as compared to 40 cm/sec in aorta (Fig. 6.3-4 and Table 6.3-1).

BLOOD FLOW : TYPES AND DISTRIBUTION

TYPES OF BLOOD FLOW

Blood flow in the vascular system is of two types:

Laminar blood flow. Blood flow in the blood vessels is normally streamline, like the flow of liquids in narrow rigid tubes. Such a blood flow is called laminar blood flow and is considered to consist of a series of thin laminae slipping over one another (Fig. 6.3-5A). The laminar blood flow being streamlined is noiseless.

Turbulent blood flow. In turbulent blood flow, the blood moves in irregular varying paths continuously mixing within the vessel and colliding with the vessel wall. This causes a greater energy loss as compared to laminar flow. The turbulent blood flow is noisy.

Conditions associated with turbulent blood flow are:

- Constriction of the artery by an atherosclerotic plaque (Fig. 6.3-5B) or by any other cause, e.g. application of external pressure while measuring the blood pressure with sphygmomanometer. The turbulent flow generates vibrations (sounds) which can be heard over the artery

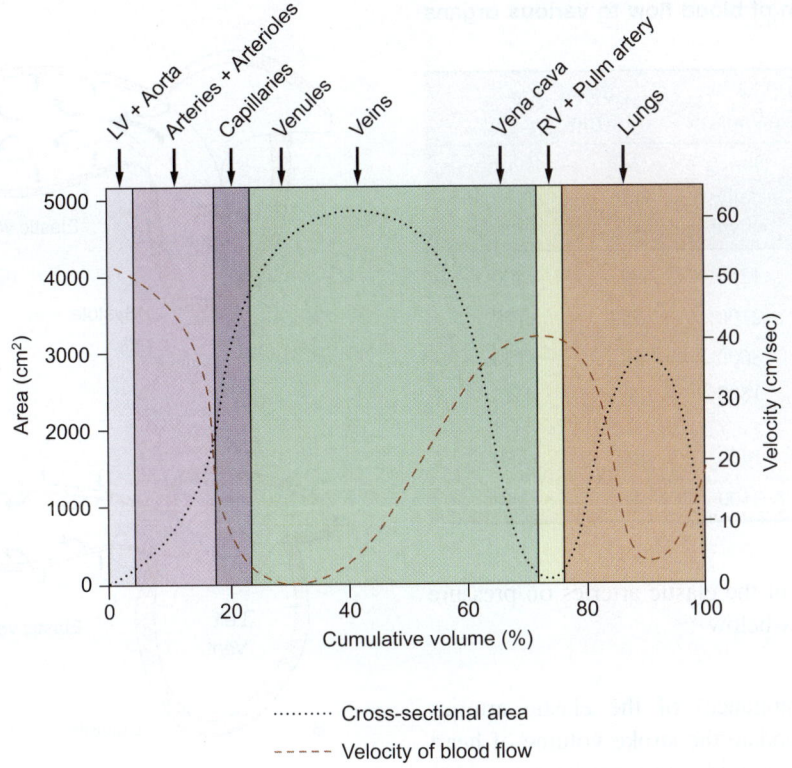

Fig. 6.3-4. *Relationship between cross-sectional area, velocity of blood flow and pressure as a function of cumulative blood volume.*

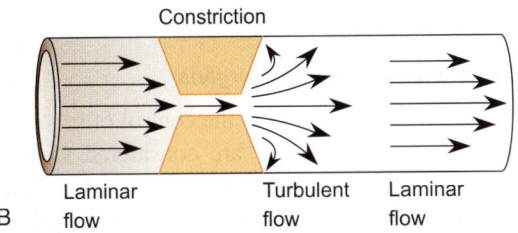

Fig. 6.3-5. *Laminar blood flow (A) and turbulent blood flow caused by constriction of the lumen of blood vessel.*

by a stethoscope, e.g. *Korotkoff sounds* heard while recording the blood pressure or the *murmur* heard over a constricted artery.

- Anaemia

DISTRIBUTION OF BLOOD FLOW TO VARIOUS REGIONS OF THE BODY

At rest about 5 litres of blood enters aorta per minute. In terms of tissue weight, blood flow to liver, brain and heart is very high. Kidney has high blood flow because it is related to excretory function rather than metabolic requirement. The distribution of blood flow to various organs and regions of the body during resting conditions and during maximum activity conditions is shown in Table 6.3-2.

PRESSURE AND FLOW IN DIFFERENT SEGMENTS OF CIRCULATORY SYSTEM

PRESSURE AND FLOW FUNCTIONS OF ELASTIC ARTERIES

The large elastic arteries (Windkessel vessels) include aorta and its main branches such as carotid, iliac and axillary arteries. These vessels contain elastic tissue in their walls in abundance which provides them two properties of distensibility and elastic recoil. The effect

C H A P T E R   6.3

Table 6.3-2. Distribution of blood flow to various organs of the body

Organs	Blood flow per organ (ml/min)		Blood flow (ml/100 gm/min)	
	At rest	During maximum activity	At rest	During maximum activity
Heart	250	1200	80	400
Brain	750	2100	55	150
Liver	1500	3000	58	120
Skeletal muscles	150	1800	4	70
Kidney	1200	1400	400	450
Skin	200	3500	8	150

of these two properties of the elastic arteries on pressure and flow of blood is as below :

Distensibility

The distensibility (compliance) of the elastic arteries allows them to accommodate the stroke volume of heart during systole with only a moderate increase in pressure (from 80 mm Hg to 120 mm Hg) (Fig. 6.3-6A). Due to distension of these vessels a part of energy released from the heart is stored as potential energy in the wall of aorta.

Elastic recoil

During diastole the stretched elastic wall of the aorta recoils and the potential energy stored in the wall is released onto the blood. This causes the blood to flow during diastole also; in this way the pressure in the aorta does not fall below 80 mm Hg (Fig. 6.3-6B).

Functions of elastic vessels

1. They reduce velocity of blood flow to some extent during ventricular contraction (systole) due to property of distensibility.

2. They cause increase in velocity of blood flow to some extent during ventricular diastole by elastic recoil. Thus, the Windkessel effect reduces the energy expenditure of heart.

3. Pumping action of the heart along with elastic recoil of aorta together constitutes a driving force for blood to move forward (towards periphery). This force is called *vis-a-tergo force,* and is an important determinant for venous return.

4. Conversion of pulsatile blood flow from heart to a steady continuous flow. The elastic vessels act together with arterioles (resistance vessels) to convert this pulsatile flow into a steady continuous flow in the tissue capillaries, which allows maximum exchange between the blood and tissues.

Fig. 6.3-6. *Distensibility (A) and elastic recoil (B) seen in aorta and its main branches maintain arterial pressure and flow during diastole.*

Clinically applied aspects

Due to age-related degenerative changes the elasticity of large vessels is decreased and so is the Windkessel effect. Therefore, in old age systolic blood pressure increases. and diastolic blood pressure decreases. Thus, in normal healthy individual aged about 70 years, typical blood pressure is 160/70 mm of Hg. That is, there occurs *systolic hypertension* with *increased pulse pressure* (SBP–DBP).

PRESSURE AND FLOW FUNCTIONS OF ARTERIOLES

Structural characteristics

Each arteriole is only a few millimetre long and branches many a time to supply about 10-100 capillaries.

Functions of arterioles

1. Control of blood flow to the organs

The arterioles play major role in the control of blood flow to organs or tissues. So, they are considered *stopcocks (valves) of circulation.* The constriction of arterioles increases the resistance and decreases the blood flow while dilation of arterioles decreases the resistance and increases the blood flow. The arterioles control blood flow to organs by autoregulation.

Autoregulation. It is the ability of an organ or tissue to adjust its vascular resistance and maintain a relatively constant blood flow over a wide range of arterial pressure (Fig. 6.3-7). Autoregulation is well developed in the kidney, brain, heart, skeletal muscle, and mesentery.

Fig. 6.3-7. *Autoregulation of blood flow. Note the blood flow remains relatively constant over a wide range of arterial pressure. This is accomplished by change in resistance proportionate to change in arterial pressure.*

2. Conversion of pulsatile flow from heart to a steady continuous flow

As described in functions of the elastic vessels, the arterioles along with the elastic vessels convert the pulsatile flow in the arteries to a steady flow in capillaries.

MICROCIRCULATION

ARCHITECTURE OF MICROCIRCULATION

The microcirculation involves a meshwork of vessels less than 100 μm in diameter. These include small arterioles, meta-arterioles, capillaries, postcapillary venules and arteriovenous shunts (Fig. 6.3-8):

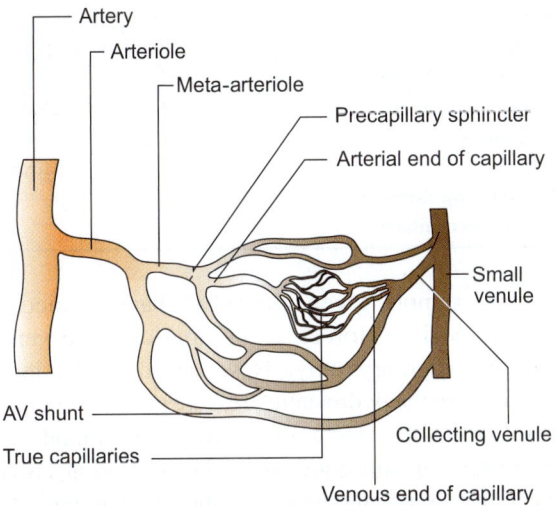

Fig. 6.3-8. *Architecture of microcirculation.*

Meta-arterioles. The arterioles divide into smaller muscle-walled vessels, sometimes called meta-arterioles and these in turn feed into capillaries.

Precapillary sphincters refer to a cuff of smooth muscle cells that surround the origin of capillaries. These determine the size of capillary exchange area at one particular moment in the tissue. For example, increase in the sphincter patency increases number of open capillaries. Precapillary sphincters respond to local or circulating vasoconstrictor substances.

Capillaries arise directly from arterioles or meta-arterioles. These vessels allow easy exchange of gases and nutritive substances across them and so are also called as *exchange vessels*. Capillaries constitute the most important segment of the circulatory system. Their structure and functions will be discussed in detail.

Postcapillary venules, which measure 20-60 μm in diameter, are the *most permeable part* of the micro-circulation.

Arteriovenous anastomosis (shunt or thoroughfare vessels). These are short, low-resistance connections between the arterioles and veins, bypassing the capillaries. These are abundantly innervated by vasomotor sympathetic fibres. These vessels are especially found in the skin of fingers, toes and earlobes where they are involved in the regulation of body temperature.

STRUCTURAL CHARACTERISTICS OF CAPILLARIES

Each capillary has an average diameter of 5 μm, length of 50 μm, wall thickness of 1 μm and cross-sectional area of 40 μm^2.

The capillary wall essentially consists of a single layer of endothelial cells which are lined on the outside by a basal lamina (glycoprotein), overlying the basal lamina there may be isolated branching perivascular cells called *pericytes.*

The endothelial structure of capillaries varies in different organs depending on the function of the particular tissue. Under electron microscope, three types of capillaries have been identified :

1. *Continuous capillaries* are characterized by a single layer of endothelial cells which are almost continuous, except for small clefts of 6-7 nm in size in between the cells (Fig. 6.3.9A). These are the most common type of capillaries and are found in most of the body tissues viz. skeletal muscle, adipose tissue, connective tissue, pulmonary circulation and so on.

2. *Fenestrated capillaries* consist of thin endothelial cells with large fenestrations (20-100 nm in diameter) (Fig. 6.3-9B) which make the capillaries porous. Fenestrated capillaries are found in renal glomeruli, intestinal villi, most endocrinal glands.

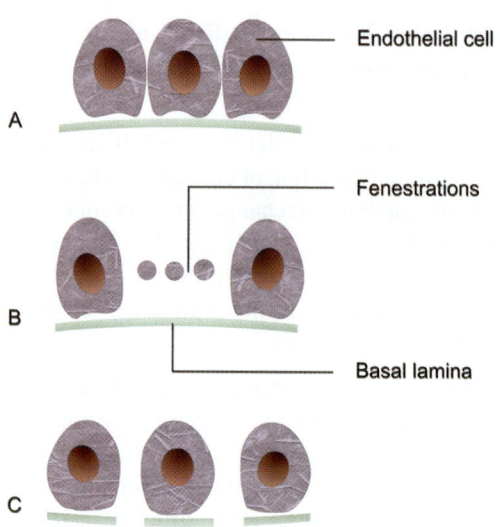

Fig. 6.3-9. Structure of different types of capillaries: A, continuous; B, fenestrated; and C, discontinuous.

3. Discontinuous capillaries are characterised by large gaps (600-3000 nm in diameter) between endothelial cells (Fig. 6.3-9C). Through these gaps even-formed elements of blood can pass freely. Such capillaries are also called sinusoids and are found in bone marrow, liver and spleen.

TRANSCAPILLARY EXCHANGE

The capillary blood brings oxygen, electrolytes and nutrients to the tissues and removes the waste products of cellular metabolism. The exchange of these substances occurs across the thin membrane formed by the endothelial cells.

Filtration and reabsorption across microvascular endothelium

The rate of filtration and absorption at any point along the capillary wall depends on the balance of forces known as *Starling forces*. According to Starling hypothesis the filtration absorption is expressed as:

$$K (P_c + \pi_i) - (P_i + \pi_c)$$

K = the permeability-surface area coefficient

P_c = the hydrostatic capillary pressure,

P_i = the hydrostatic interstitial pressure,

π_c = oncotic pressure of blood, and

π_i = oncotic pressure of the interstitium.

Thus, P_c–P_i, represents the hydrostatic pressure gradient, and

π_c – π_i, represents the oncotic pressure gradient.

1. Hydrostatic capillary pressure (P_c) tends to force the fluid out through the capillary membrane. The values of hydrostatic capillary pressure in most of the tissues are:

- At the arterial end = 30-40 mm Hg,
- At the venous end = 10-15 mm Hg, and
- In the middle = 25 mm Hg.

2. Hydrostatic interstitial pressure (P_i) tends to force fluid inward through the capillary membrane. It is about –2 mm Hg in subcutaneous tissue.

3. Oncotic pressure of blood or plasma colloid osmotic pressure (π_c) results from the osmotic pressure of plasma proteins. It tends to pull fluid inward through the capillary membrane. It is about 25-27 mm of Hg.

4. Oncotic pressure of the interstitium (π_i) is due to the presence of proteins in the interstitial space. It tends to pull fluid out of the capillary membrane. The effective oncotic pressure in the interstitium is estimated to range between 5-10 mm Hg (average 8 mm Hg).

Calculation of net filtration at the capillaries

From the above description, the net forces acting on the fluid at the arteriolar and venous end of a typical muscle *capillary* can be calculated (Table 6.3-3):

- Thus at arteriolar end the filtering force of 15 mm Hg moves the fluid out of capillary (filtration) into the interstitium while at venous end the filtering force of –10 mm Hg moves the fluid into the capillary (reabsorption) from the interstitium.
- The net filtering force for the whole capillary is 5 mm Hg.

Table 6.3-3. Calculation of net filtration force at the capillaries

	At the arteriolar end (mm Hg)	At the venous end (mm Hg)
• **Forces tending to move fluid outward**		
– Capillary hydrostatic pressure (P_c)	35	10
– Interstitial oncotic pressure (π_i)	3	3
Total outward force ($P_c + \pi_i$)	**38**	**13**
• **Forces tending to move fluid inward**		
– Oncotic pressure of blood (π_c)	25	25
– Interstitial hydrostatic pressure (P_i)	–2	–2
Total inward force ($\pi_c + P_i$)	**23**	**23**
• **Filtering force**	38 – 23	13 – 23
	15	– 10
• **Net filtering force of the whole capillary**	(15 – 10)	
	= 5	

In the example given above we have studied the balance of Starling forces at the arteriolar and venous end of the capillary only. However, over the length of the capillary the hydrostatic pressure gradually declines to zero near the middle of capillary. From here the inward forces become dominant and reabsorption process starts to reach its maximum at the venular end (Fig. 6.3-10).

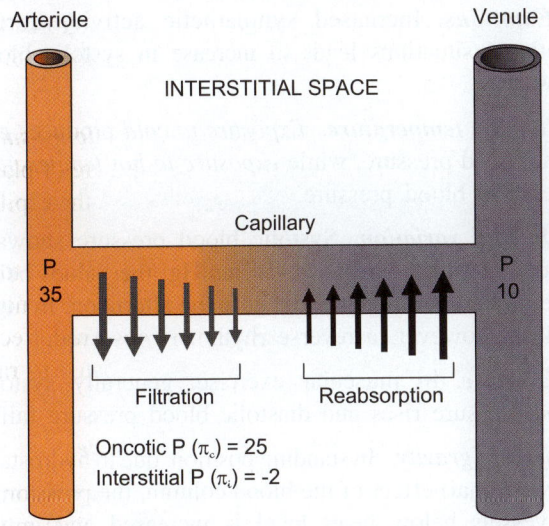

Arteriole   Venule

INTERSTITIAL SPACE

Capillary

P 35

P 10

Filtration   Reabsorption

Oncotic P (π_c) = 25
Interstitial P (π_i) = -2

Fig. 6.3-10. *Filtration and reabsorption in a capillary due to balance of Starling forces.*

VENOUS CIRCULATION

STRUCTURAL CHARACTERISTICS OF VEINS

Walls of veins, as compared to arteries, at equivalent levels in the vascular tree are thin-walled and contain small amount of elastic tissue and smooth muscle, and have larger lumen. Because of their structural characteristics they are more distensible and collapsible.

Lumen of the veins is larger than the equivalent arteries.

Valves are present in the veins of the dependent parts of the body (Fig. 6.2-13) that prevent the backflow of venous blood.

FUNCTIONS OF THE VEINS

1. Blood reservoirs

Because of their feature of *distensibility and collapsibility* the veins serve as blood reservoirs. About 60 to 70 per cent of the circulating blood is present in the venous system. Due to this property veins are also called the *capacitance vessels.*

2. Conduits

The systemic veins carry blood from the tissues to the right atrium, and the pulmonary veins collect blood from the lungs and return it to the left atrium.

3. Maintenance of cardiac output

Veins help to maintain the cardiac output whenever there is loss of blood. After blood loss from an external or internal injury reflex increase in sympathetic discharge produces contraction of the smooth muscles in the walls of the veins. As a result of venular contraction, there occurs a decrease in their capacity leading to increased venous return to heart. In this way veins help to maintain

cardiac output by maintaining normal venous return in spite of blood loss.

Venous return has been discussed in detail on page 179.

BLOOD PRESSURE

DEFINITIONS (TERMINOLOGY)

Blood pressure is the lateral pressure exerted by the flowing blood on the walls of the vessels. It is usually measured in mmHg. Without any further qualification the term blood pressure denotes the *arterial pressure*. While describing the pressure exerted by the blood column in other types of blood vessels, the type of vessel is also mentioned, e.g. *capillary pressure* and *venous pressure.*

Systolic blood pressure

- The maximum arterial pressure during systole is called *systolic blood pressure,* and occurs during ventricular ejection.
- Normal systolic blood pressure in a young adult is 120 mmHg (range: 105-135 mmHg).
- Systolic blood pressure undergoes considerable fluctuations, e.g. it is increased during excitement, exercise and meals, and is decreased during sleep and rest.

Diastolic blood pressure

- Diastolic blood pressure refers to the minimum arterial pressure during diastole and occurs just before the onset of ventricular ejection.
- Normal diastolic blood pressure in a young adult is 80 mmHg (range 60-90 mmHg).

Conventional expression of blood pressure

Conventionally, systolic and diastolic blood pressures are denoted as numerator and denominator, respectively. For example, blood pressure of a normal person is written as 120/80 mmHg.

Pulse pressure

- Pulse pressure is the arithmetic difference between systolic and diastolic blood pressures.
- Normally, average pulse pressure is 40 mmHg.

Mean arterial pressure

- Mean arterial pressure (MAP) is the average of all pressures measured millisecond by millisecond throughout the cardiac cycle.
- Practically, MAP is roughly equal to diastolic pressure (DP) plus one third of pulse pressure (PP), i.e.

$$DP + \frac{1}{3} PP$$

- Normal value of MAP is 93 mmHg (range: 90-100 mmHg).

C H A P T E R   6.3

DETERMINANTS OF (FACTORS AFFECTING) ARTERIAL BLOOD PRESSURE

- The arterial blood pressure (BP) is a function of the product of cardiac output (CO) and total peripheral resistance (PR), i.e.

  Arterial BP = cardiac output (CO) × peripheral resistance (PR)

- Therefore, arterial blood pressure is affected by conditions that affect either cardiac output or peripheral resistance.

- Changes in cardiac output affect the systolic pressure more than diastolic pressure while changes in peripheral resistance affect diastolic pressure more than the systolic pressure.

- As discussed in the section on cardiac output (see page 179), the cardiac output is a function of *heart rate* and *stroke volume,* so these two are important determinants of the blood pressure.

- The peripheral resistance (see page 186) depends upon the viscosity of blood, elasticity of the vessel wall, and velocity of the blood flow. Thus, these factors are also important determinants of the blood pressure.

Effect of some of the important determinants of the blood pressure is shown in Fig. 6.2-11 and described here briefly:

VARIATIONS IN BLOOD PRESSURE

Physiological factors affecting blood pressure

1. *Age.* In healthy humans, both systolic and diastolic pressures rise with age.

- *At birth* systolic blood pressure is 40 mmHg (range: 20-60 mmHg). It then rises rapidly upto one month of age.

- *At one month* of age the systolic blood pressure becomes about 80 mmHg and then rises slowly.

- *At about 17 years* of age normal adult level of blood pressure is 120/80 mmHg.

- *At about 70 years of age* the normal value of blood pressure is 160/90 mmHg. The increase in blood pressure associated with advancing age is due to increase in rigidity of vessel wall.

2. *Sex.* *Before menopause,* females have little lower (4-6 mmHg) systolic blood pressure than males of corresponding age. *After menopause,* systolic blood pressure in females is little higher (4-6 mmHg) than males of same age group.

3. *Effect of meals.* *Systolic blood pressure* increases by 4-6 mmHg after meals and this effect lasts for about one hour.

Diastolic blood pressure either remains unchanged or decreases slightly due to vasodilatation in splanchnic vessels.

4. *Emotions.* Increased sympathetic activity during emotional situations leads to increase in systolic blood pressure.

5. *Climatic temperature.* *Exposure to cold* produces rise in the blood pressure, while *exposure to hot temperature* lowers the blood pressure.

6. *Diurnal variation.* Systolic blood pressure shows a diurnal variation of about 6-10 mmHg; the values being lower in the morning and higher in the afternoon. In night workers, however, a reverse rhythm is observed.

7. *Exercise.* In muscular exercise, generally systolic blood pressure rises and diastolic blood pressure falls.

8. *Effect of gravity.* In standing position, due to hydrostatic (gravitational) effect of the blood column, the pressure in the vessels below heart level is increased and in the vessels above heart level it is decreased.

9. *Effect of change in posture.* Immediately on standing there occurs peripheral pooling of blood in dependant parts leading to decreased venous return and decreased cardiac output and momentary fall in systolic blood pressure.

10. *Sleep.* In complete relaxed state during early hours of sleep there occurs fall in blood pressure up to 15 to 20 mmHg. However, in disturbed sleep blood pressure increases due to increased sympathetic discharge.

11. *Body built.* Systolic blood pressure is slightly higher in obese individuals as compared to thin-built individuals.

Pathological variations in blood pressure

1. Hypertension

Definition. Hypertension (HT) refers to a condition in which value of systolic blood pressure is persistently more than 140 mmHg and/or that of diastolic blood pressure is above 90 mmHg. If there is increase only in systolic blood pressure, it is called *systolic hypertension* in which pulse pressure is raised.

Types of hypertension. It is of two types : primary and secondary hypertension.

1. *Primary hypertension* also known as *essential hypertension* is characterized by a raised blood pressure without any underlying disease. Risk factors for primary HT include: heredity, obesity, mental tension and smoking.

2. *Secondary hypertension* refers to a condition in which blood pressure is raised due to some other underlying disease. Common causes of secondary hypertension are:

- *Cardiovascular diseases* e.g. atherosclerosis.
- *Renal diseases* e.g. glomerulonephritis and tumour of juxtaglomerular cells leading to formation of excess of angiotensin II.

- *Endocrinal disorders* like hyperaldosteronism (excessive secretion of aldosterone from adrenal cortex), phaeochromocytoma (tumour of adrenal medulla) and Cushing's syndrome (excessive secretion of glucocorticoids from adrenal cortex).
- *Neurologic disorders* which may produce hypertension include raised intracranial pressure.
- *Pregnancy-induced hypertension (PIH)* is noticed in some of the pregnant women. Its exact cause is not known.

2. Hypotension

Hypotension refers to a condition in which values of blood pressure are below the normal range. Clinically when the systolic blood pressure is less than 90 mmHg, it is considered hypotension. It is of following types :

Primary hypotension also known as essential hypotension is a disorder of unknown aetiology.

Secondary hypotension, occurs secondary to some other underlying diseases such as myocardial infarction, neurogenic shock, haemorrhagic shock, hypoactivity of pituitary gland and hypoactivity of adrenal glands.

Postural hypotension refers to sudden fall in blood pressure when patients stand up from lying down posture. It occurs due to some dysfunction of autonomic nervous system.

REGULATION OF BLOOD PRESSURE

Arterial blood pressure is controlled by several mechanisms which under physiological conditions maintain the normal mean arterial pressure (MAP) within a narrow range of 95 to 100 mmHg. Various mechanisms controlling arterial pressure can be grouped as:

A. Rapid blood pressure control mechanisms,
B. Intermediate blood pressure control mechanisms, and
C. Long-term blood pressure control mechanisms.

Rapid blood pressure control mechanism (Nervous regulating mechanism)

Rapid blood pressure control mechanism or the so-called short-term control mechanism primarily includes the following three nervous reflexes:

1. Baroreceptor reflexes (see page 199),
2. Central nervous system ischaemic response (see page 201), and
3. Chemoreceptor reflexes (see page 201).

Salient features of rapid control mechanisms are:

- These *act very rapidly,* i.e. within seconds to few minutes of alterations in the blood pressure.
- These are *short-term mechanisms,* i.e. these act for few hours to few days and are thus insignificant in long-term regulation of blood pressure.
- These are useful in preventing *acute decreases in blood pressure* (e.g. during severe haemorrhage) as

well as in preventing *excessive increases in blood pressure* (e.g. as might occur in response to excessive blood transfusion).

Intermediate blood pressure control mechanisms

The intermediate blood pressure control mechanisms that are important in blood pressure control after several minutes of acute pressure changes are:

1. Renin-angiotensin vasoconstrictor mechanism (for details see page 202),
2. Stress relaxation and reverse stress relaxation mechanism, and
3. Capillary fluid shift mechanism.

Salient features of intermediate blood pressure control mechanisms are:

- These mechanisms come into play after several minutes of acute pressure changes and reach full function within a few hours.
- These mechanisms play their role from few days to few weeks.
- All these mechanisms basically try to control the alterations in blood pressure by altering the blood volume.

Stress relaxation and reverse stress relaxation mechanisms

Stress relaxation mechanism refers to vasodilatation occurring due to stress on the vascular smooth muscles. When pressure in the vessels becomes too high (e.g. following massive slow intravenous transfusion), the vessels become stretched and continue to stretch for minutes or hours. This causes relaxation of blood vessels simply by vascular tone adjustment. This leads to an increase in the capacity of the arterial system with a concomitant fall in blood pressure.

Reverse stress relaxation mechanism operates when the blood pressure is low due to less stress on the vessel walls and tries to restore it back to normal. For example when blood pressure falls due to prolonged slow bleeding, there occurs tightening of blood vessel walls by vascular tone adjustment secondary to less stress on the vessel wall (reverse stress relaxation mechanism). This mechanism tries to restore the blood pressure back to normal. This mechanism can correct upto 15% change in blood volume below normal.

Capillary fluid shift mechanism

Capillary fluid shift mechanism helps in restoring both low and high blood pressure back to normal:

When blood pressure is raised, the mean capillary pressure is also high resulting in shift of fluid from circulation to the interstitial fluid compartments. This reduces the blood volume to restore the arterial pressure.

When blood pressure is lowered, the mean capillary pressure is also low, resulting in absorption of fluid from the interstitial compartments to circulation. Thus the blood volume is increased which helps to return the blood pressure back to normal.

The capillary fluid shift mechanism is about two times more effective than baroreceptor reflex mechanism in controlling the blood pressure, but it acts much more slowly (intermediate acting mechanism) than baroreceptor mechanism (rapid acting mechanism).

Long-term blood pressure control mechanisms

Kidneys play main role in the long-term control of blood pressure by following mechanisms:

1. *Direct mechanism,* i.e. 'Renal-body fluid feedback mechanism'.
2. *Indirect mechanisms* control kidney functions indirectly via following hormonal mechanisms:
   i. Aldosterone system, and
   ii. Renin-angiotensin system (see page 364).

Renal-body fluid system for arterial pressure control

The most important mechanism for the long-term control of blood pressure is linked to control of circulatory volume by the kidney. In fact, it is similar to the capillary fluid shift mechanism except that only the renal glomerular capillaries are involved in the process. The renal-body fluid system corrects blood pressure by causing appropriate changes in blood volume through *diuresis* and *natriuresis:*

The salient features of the renal-body fluid feedback mechanism can be summarized as:

- The renal-body fluid feedback mechanism takes several hours to show any significant response.
- These mechanisms operate very powerfully to control arterial pressure over days, weeks, and months.
- The effectiveness of these mechanisms becomes steadily greater with time.
- These mechanisms, if given sufficient time, control arterial pressure at the level that provides normal output of salt and water by the kidneys.

Cardiovascular Regulation and Adjustments During Health and Disease

6.4

CARDIOVASCULAR REGULATION
- Circulatory adjustments
- Cardiovascular control mechanisms

Neural control mechanisms
- Medullary cardiovascular control centres
- Autonomic nerve supply to heart and blood vessels.
- Afferent impulses to medullary cardiovascular control centres
- Role of skeletal nerves and muscles in control of blood pressure

Humoral control mechanisms
- Circulating vasodilators
- Circulating vasoconstrictors
- Ions and other chemical factors

Local control mechanisms
- Mechanisms involved in acute control of blood flow
- Mechanisms involved in long-term blood flow regulation

- Angiogenesis
- Development of collateral blood vessels

CARDIOVASCULAR HOMEOSTASIS IN HEALTH

Cardiovascular adjustments during gravitational changes
- Posture change from lying to standing
- Prolonged quiet standing
- Postural hypotension

Cardiovascular adjustments during muscular exercise
- Changes in muscle blood flow
- Other cardiovascular changes

CARDIOVASCULAR HOMEOSTASIS IN DISEASES

Circulatory shock
- Types and causes
- Stages and clinical features
  - Non-progressive shock
  - Progressive shock
  - Refractory shock
- Physiology in treatment of shock

CARDIOVASCULAR REGULATION

CIRCULATORY ADJUSTMENTS

Cardiovascular control makes *circulatory adjustments* which are essential to cope up with the timely needs of each and every organ of the body and is thus of fundamental importance for survival.

Circulatory adjustments which ensure that all of the organs receive sufficient blood flow are: (1) control of blood volume, and (2) control of arterial pressure. These circulatory adjustments are made by the cardio-vascular control mechanisms primarily by regulating following parameters.

A. *Regulation of cardiac performance,* i.e. alterations in the activities of heart which include:

1. *Chronotropic action,* i.e. effect on heart rate which may be in the form of:
- Increased heart rate (tachycardia) or positive chronotropic effect.
- Decreased heart rate (bradycardia) or negative chronotropic effect.

2. *Inotropic action,* i.e. effect on force of contraction which may be in the form of:
- Increase in the force of contraction (positive inotropic effect), or
- Decrease in the force of contraction (negative inotropic effect).

3. *Dromotropic action,* i.e. effect on conduction of impulse through the heart, which may be in the form of:
- Increase in the velocity of impulse conduction (positive dromotropic effect), or
- Decrease in the velocity of impulse conduction (negative dromotropic effect).

4. *Bathmotropic action,* i.e. effect on the excitability of the cardiac muscle, which may be in the form of:
- Increased excitability of cardiac muscle (positive bathmotropic effect), or
- Decreased excitability of cardiac muscle (negative bathmotropic effect).

B. *Regulation of performance of blood vessels* which primarily includes:

1. *Alterations in diameter of arterioles* which change the peripheral resistance and also the hydrostatic pressure in the capillaries, and

2. *Alteration in diameter of veins* which changes the venous pressure and thus venous return and the cardiac output.

CARDIOVASCULAR CONTROL MECHANISMS

The cardiovascular control mechanisms which play their role in making circulatory adjustments during the routine and emergency cardiovascular stresses can be grouped as:
- Neural control mechanism,
- Humoral control mechanisms, and
- Local control mechanisms.

NEURAL CONTROL MECHANISM

Neural regulation of circulation is of fundamental importance since it responds within seconds.

Components of neural control mechanism

The neural cardiovascular regulating mechanism consist of:
- A. Medullary cardiovascular control centres.
- B. Autonomic nervous system supplying the heart and blood vessels.
- C. Afferent impulses to medullary centres.
- D. Role of skeletal nerves and muscles in controlling blood pressure.

MEDULLARY CARDIOVASCULAR CONTROL CENTRES

1. Vasomotor centre

It is the primary cardiovascular regulatory centre located in the medulla oblongata of brain stem. It consists of groups of neurons situated bilaterally in the reticular substance of medulla at the floor of fourth ventricle. The medullary cardiovascular centre is constituted by following different areas (Fig. 6.4-1):

Fig. 6.4-1. *Medullary cardiovascular control centres.*

Pressor area. Stimulation of pressor area produces:
- *Arteriolar constriction* which increases the systemic blood pressure,
- *Venoconstriction* which decreases blood stored in the venous reservoir and increases venous return,
- *Increase in heart rate* or positive chronotropic effect, and
- *Increase in force of contraction* or positive inotropic effect.

Depressor area. Stimulation of neurons forming depressor area produces decrease in the sympathetic activity due to inhibition of the tonically discharging impulses of the pressor area causing:
- *Arteriolar dilation* which decreases systemic blood pressure,
- *Venodilatation* which increases storage of blood in venous reservoir and decreases venous return and cardiac output,
- *Decrease in heart rate* or negative chronotropic effect, and
- *Decrease in force of contraction* or negative inotropic effect.

2. Medullary parasympathetic centre

Medullary parasympathetic centre or *cardiac vagal centre* earlier also called cardioinhibitory centre (CIC) is now called by its specific name, i.e. the *nucleus ambiguus* (NAm). Nucleus ambiguus receives afferents via nucleus tractus solitarius (NTS) and in turn sends inhibitory pathway in the form of vagal fibres to *heart* to decrease heart rate and force of cardiac contraction.

3. Medullary relay station for cardiorespiratory afferents

Nucleus tractus solitarius (NTS) of the vagus nerve forms

the so-called medullary relay station. It receives afferents from most of the baroreceptors and chemoreceptors. Cells of the NTS, in turn, relay the information to vasomotor centre and cardiac vagal centre (nucleus ambiguus) that control sympathetic and parasympathetic outputs, respectively.

AUTONOMIC NERVE SUPPLY TO HEART AND BLOOD VESSELS

AUTONOMIC NERVE SUPPLY TO HEART

Sympathetic supply

Spinal sympathetic centre is formed by neurons located in the intermediolateral horns of the spinal cord extending from T_1 to L_2 spinal segments. (Fig. 6.4-2).

Parasympathetic supply

Parasympathetic fibres to the heart are carried through two vagii (Fig. 6.4-3).

Fig. 6.4-3. Parasympathetic innervation of the heart.

Vagal tone. There is a good deal of tonic vagal discharge, called the *vagal tone*, in humans and other large animals. In adult humans the resting heart rate which is about 72 beats/min rises to 150-180 beats/min after the

Fig. 6.4-2. Sympathetic innervation to heart and blood vessels.

administration of vagolytic drugs such as atropine, because of the unopposed sympathetic tone.

AUTONOMIC NERVE SUPPLY TO BLOOD VESSELS

The autonomic efferents supplying the blood vessels produce two types of effects.

Vasoconstriction effect

Sympathetic vasoconstrictor fibres show tonic (i.e. continuous) discharge at the rate of about 1 impulse/sec. Therefore, when the sympathetic nerves are cut (*sympathectomy*), there occurs:

- *Vasodilatation*
- *Venodilatation* (increased venous capacity)

Stimulation of sympathetic fibres produces:

- *Constriction of arterioles*
- *Venoconstriction* (decreased venous capacity)

Vasodilatation effect. Neural vasodilatation effect on blood vessels is produced by following mechanisms:

1. *Decrease in discharge of noradrenergic vasoconstrictor nerves.*

2. *Sympathetic cholinergic vasodilator nerves.* Some of the organs of the body such as skeletal muscles, heart, lungs, liver, kidney and uterus in addition to adrenergic vasoconstrictor sympathetic fibres also receive innervation by *cholinergic vasodilator sympathetic* fibres having acetylcholine and vasoinhibitory peptide (VIP) as neurotransmitter.

3. *Parasympathetic vasodilator nerves.* Blood vessels, in general, do not have parasympathetic innervation with following exceptions:

- *Sacral outflow parasympathetic fibres* represented by *nervi erigentes* which supplies sexual erectile tissue, and
- *Cranial outflow of parasympathetic fibres* along chorda tympani branch of facial nerve to salivary glands.

4. *Vasodilation by axon reflex.* Conduction of normal sensory afferent impulses from the skin to spinal cord is called *orthodromic conduction.* However, in certain situations the antidromic conduction of impulses cause release of substance P from the nerve endings which produces vasodilation.

AFFERENT IMPULSES TO MEDULLARY CARDIOVASCULAR CONTROL CENTRES

The medullary control centres are influenced by afferent control impulses from the higher centres and a large number of other areas (Fig. 6.4-4). These include:

- Afferent impulses from higher centres controlling vasomotor centre,
- Afferent impulses from respiratory centres,

- Cardiovascular reflex mechanisms operating through medullary control centres are :
  - Baroreceptor reflex,
  - Chemoreceptor reflexes,
- Direct effects on vasomotor area
  - Central nervous system ischaemic response,
  - Cushing reflex,
- Afferents from nociceptive stimuli.

AFFERENT IMPULSES FROM HIGHER CENTRES CONTROLLING VASOMOTOR CENTRE AND CARDIAC VAGAL CENTRE

Cerebral cortex. There are descending tracts to the vasomotor area from cerebral cortex (particularly the limbic cortex) that relay in the hypothalamus. Some examples of the influence of limbic system on the VMC are:

- *Tachycardia and hypertension* produced by emotions,
- *Bradycardia and fainting* occurring during sudden emotional shock,
- *Fight or flight response* is a complex set of responses which increases cardiac output and raises blood pressure in anticipation of flight or physical defence.

Hypothalamus. The hypothalamus serves to integrate many somatic and autonomic responses. Examples are:

- *Temperature regulation.*
- *Emotional stresses.*

Reticular formation of pons, mesencephalon and diencephalon also influences the vasomotor area, for example:

- *Pain* usually causes rise in blood pressure via afferent impulses in the reticular formation converging on the vasomotor area. However, prolonged severe pain may cause vasodilation and fainting.

AFFERENT IMPULSES FROM RESPIRATORY CENTRES

Impulses arising from the respiratory centres affect the heart rate by changing the vagal tone and the alterations produced are known as *sinus arrhythmia* which occurs during forced breathing.

- *During inspiration,* the impulses arising from the respiratory centres inhibit the cardiac vagal centre causing reduced vagal tone and *sinus tachycardia.*
- *During expiration,* the respiratory centres stop sending inhibitory impulses to the cardiac vagal centre causing increased vagal tone and sinus bradycardia.

CARDIOVASCULAR REFLEX MECHANISMS AFFECTING MEDULLARY CONTROL CENTRES

Cardiovascular reflex mechanisms are multiple subconscious special nervous control mechanisms that operate

Fig. 6.4-4. *Scheme to show afferent impulses affecting medullary cardiovascular control centres.*

through medullary control centres all the time to maintain the arterial pressure within normal range. These include:

- Baroreceptor reflex mechanisms, and
- Chemoreceptor reflex mechanism.

Baroreceptor reflex mechanisms

Baroreceptors also known as mechanoreceptors or pressure receptors are the stretch receptors located in the walls of heart and large blood vessels. These are spray type nerve endings, i.e. they are extensively branched, knobby, coiled, and intertwined ends of myelinated nerve fibres.

Location of carotid and aortic arch baroreceptors

Carotid baroreceptors are located in carotid sinus which is a small dilatation of the internal carotid artery just above the bifurcation of the common carotid artery into external and internal carotid branches (Fig. 6.4-5).

Aortic arch baroreceptors are located in the wall of arch of aorta (Fig. 6.4-5).

Other systemic arterial baroreceptors (similar to carotid and aortic baroreceptors) are also found at the root of right subclavian artery and junction of thyroid artery and in the common carotid artery.

Innervation of baroreceptors *(Fig. 6.4-6)*

Carotid sinus baroreceptors are innervated by carotid sinus nerve (Hering's nerve) which is a branch of glossopharyngeal nerve, and

All other baroreceptors are supplied by the vagus nerve.

C H A P T E R   6 . 4

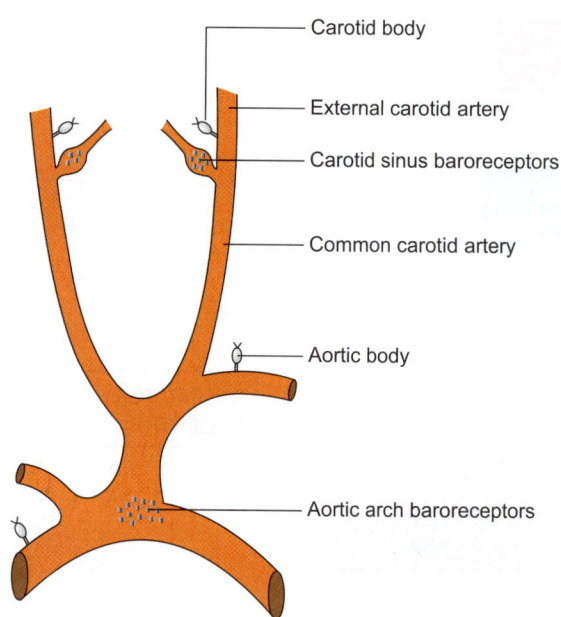

Fig. 6.4-5. *Location of baroreceptors (carotid sinus and aortic arch) and chemoreceptors (carotid bodies and aortic bodies).*

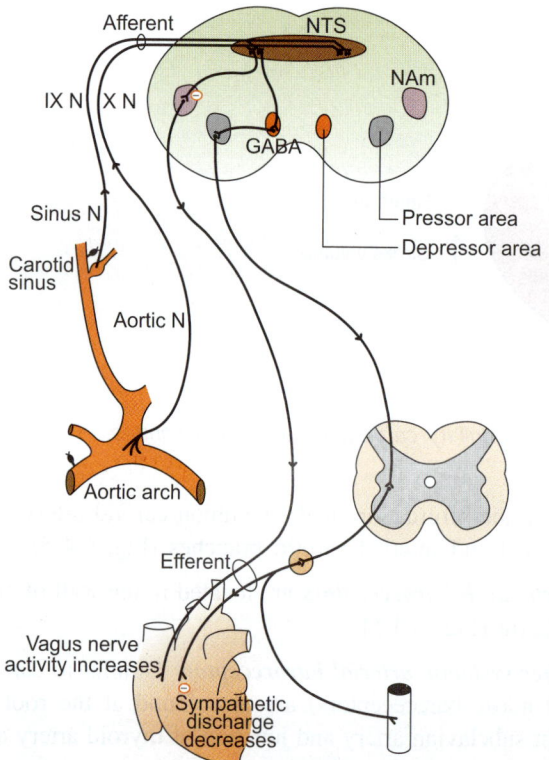

Fig. 6.4-6. *Neural pathway of baroreceptor reflex.*

Afferent fibres from the baroreceptors pass via the glossopharyngeal and vagus nerves to the medulla. Most of them end in the nucleus of the tractus solitarius (NTS),

where they secrete an excitatory transmitter, presumably glutamate.

Buffer nerves. The carotid sinus nerve and vagal fibres from the carotid sinus and aortic arch baroreceptors respectively are commonly called buffer nerves, as these are involved in buffering the blood pressure, i.e. preventing sudden rise and fall in blood pressure.

Projections from NTS terminate on to the:
- *Depressor area of VMC,*
- *Cardiac vagal centre* (nucleus ambiguus),

Response of carotid and aortic baroreceptors to pressure

Response from carotid baroreceptors have been studied in detail. Salient features of these receptor responses to pressure are:

Baroreceptor response. At normal blood pressure levels, the fibres of the buffer nerves discharge at a low rate which increases when the pressure in the carotid sinus and aortic arch rises, and declines when the pressure falls (Fig. 6.4-7).

Fig. 6.4-7. *Response of carotid sinus baroreceptors at different levels of arterial pressure.*

- The minimum pressure, about 60 mmHg, at which carotid baroreceptors are stimulated is called *threshold of baroreceptor reflex.*
- Above threshold level the baroreceptors respond progressively more rapidly till the discharge rate reaches a *plateau,* at 150–160 mmHg. Thus, the carotid baroreceptors exhibit a great sensitivity as they respond to pressure that varies approximately 50–160 mmHg.

Cardiac baroreceptors

Cardiac baroreceptors are located in the walls of heart subendocardially. All cardiac receptors are innervated by vagus nerve. These include:

Atrial stretch receptors

Atrial stretch receptors are present in the walls of atria. Atrial stretch receptors have been studied in detail by Prof. A.S. Paintal (an Indian scientist) in 1953. The atrial stretch receptors have been associated with following roles in the cardiovascular control:

1. As low-pressure receptors, the atrial stretch receptors along with pulmonary receptors play an important role to minimize arterial pressure changes in response to change in blood volume.

2. Atrial reflex control of heart rate (Bainbridge reflex). Bainbridge noted that sudden rise in atrial pressure after rapid infusion of saline or blood in anaesthetised animals produced tachycardia, if the initial heart rate was low. Thus, this reflex helps to prevent damming of blood in the veins, atria and pulmonary circulation.

3. Atrial reflex control of blood volume (volume reflex) when there is volume overload the atrial stretch receptors help to return the blood volume back towards normal by decreasing the secretion of antidiuretic hormone (ADH), which diminishes the reabsorption of water from tubules, and by release of a chemical *atrial natriuretic peptide* (ANP) which causes powerful diuresis and thus blood volume back to normal. This combined mechanism constitutes volume reflex.

Ventricular receptors

The ventricular baroreceptors are scattered throughout the left ventricle and interventricular septum. They discharge irregularly and no physiological significance can be attached to these receptors.

Pulmonary baroreceptors

Pulmonary baroreceptors are located in the walls of pulmonary trunk and its divisions—the right and left pulmonary artery play an important role to minimize arterial pressure changes in response to change in blood volume as discussed above.

Role of chemoreceptor reflexes in cardiovascular control

Chemoreceptors are chemosensitive cells that respond to following changes in blood:

- Oxygen lack (decreased PO_2),
- Carbon dioxide excess (increased pCO_2), and
- Hydrogen ion excess (decreased pH).

Location of chemoreceptors. The chemoreceptors are present in (Fig. 6.4.5):

1. *Carotid bodies.* These are 1 to 2 mm in size and are located in the bifurcation of each common carotid artery. These are innervated by carotid sinus nerve which is a branch of glossopharygeal nerve.

2. *Aortic bodies* are one to three in number located adjacent to arch of aorta. These are innervated by aortic nerve (branch of vagus nerve).

Functions of chemoreceptors

The chemoreceptors exert their role in cardiovascular regulation. In hypoxia there occurs increased chemoreceptor discharge, which not only produces hyperventilation but also excites the vasomotor centre (VMC) leading to peripheral vasoconstriction and increase in arterial blood pressure. Thus, unlike the inhibitory action of arterial baroreceptors, the chemoreceptors have an excitatory effect on the VMC.

NOTE. It is important to note that the chemoreceptors are not stimulated strongly until the arterial pressure falls below 60 mmHg. Therefore, it is at lower pressures that this reflex becomes important and help to prevent still further fall in pressure.

DIRECT EFFECTS ON VASOMOTOR AREA

The vasomotor centre is directly affected by locally produced hypoxia and hypercapnia. Examples of direct effects are central nervous system ischaemic response and Cushing reflex.

1. Central nervous system ischaemic response. When blood pressure falls below 60 mmHg, the blood flow to the vasomotor area is decreased enough to cause CNS ischaemia. As a result of CNS ischaemia, the CO_2/lactic acid are accumulated locally and excite the neurons of VMC which causes strong sympathetic stimulation leading to vasoconstriction. There occurs immediate increase in the blood pressure. This is called *CNS ischaemic response.* This acts as an emergency arterial pressure control system.

2. Cushing reflex. When intracranial pressure is increased it compresses the arteries in the brain and blood supply to the vasomotor area is compromised. The hypoxia and hypercapnia produced locally increase the discharge from VMC. The resultant rise in systemic pressure tends to restore the blood supply to medulla. This effect is called *Cushing reflex.* The resultant increase in blood pressure also causes reflex bradycardia via baroreceptor response. Thus, bradycardia is an important feature of raised intracranial pressure.

AFFERENTS FROM NOCICEPTIVE STIMULI

Afferents carrying pain sensations also affect VMC and evoke either pressor or depressor reflex effect as:

- Increase in the blood pressure and tachycardia is caused due to somatic pain afferents, and

- Hypotension and bradycardia are produced by *visceral pain afferents.*

ROLE OF SKELETAL NERVES AND MUSCLES IN CONTROLLING BLOOD PRESSURE

1. *Abdominal compression reflex.* Whenever VMC is stimulated, e.g. by baroreceptor reflex or chemoreceptor reflex, other areas of reticular formation of brain stem are also stimulated along with. They send simultaneous impulses through skeletal nerves to skeletal muscles of the body especially abdominal muscles. The contraction of abdominal muscles compresses the abdominal venous reservoirs increasing the venous return to heart and thereby the cardiac output. This response is called *abdominal compression reflex.*

2. *Role of skeletal muscles during exercise.* During exercise, the skeletal muscles especially that of limbs contract and compress the venous reservoirs. This causes translocation of large quantities of blood from the peripheral vessels into heart and lungs. This increases the cardiac output.

HUMORAL CONTROL MECHANISMS

Humoral regulation of circulation refers to the regulation by substances secreted into or absorbed into body fluids, e.g. hormones, ions, etc. Most important humoral factors affecting circulation are:

Circulating vasodilators

The circulating vasodilators include kinins and atrial natriuretic peptide (ANP).

- *Kinins* are peptides (bradykinin and lysyl-bradykinins) found in the plasma, and body tissues. They cause *vasodilation* by relaxing vascular smooth muscle (VSM) via NO and increase *capillary permeability.*
- *Atrial natriuretic peptide* (see page 374).

Circulating vasoconstrictor

The circulating vasoconstrictors include catecholamines, angiotensin II and vasopressin.

Catecholamines are released on sympathetic stimulation and include epinephrine and norepinephrine. Catecholamines stimulate both α and β adrenergic receptors. The catecholamines increase peripheral resistance and raise the diastolic blood pressure.

The renin-angiotensin system has important roles in the regulation of blood pressure and in the regulation of extracellular fluid volume. Renin, a protease enzyme, is secreted by *juxtaglomerular cells* of the kidney into the blood.

- *Renin* catalyzes the conversion of *angiotensinogen* (α_2-globulin substrate present in the plasma) to angiotensin I. Angiotensin I is converted into angiotensin II by the action of *angiotensin converting enzyme* (ACE) present in the endothelium of blood vessels throughout the body, especially in the lungs and kidneys.

$$\text{Angiotensionogen} \xrightarrow{\text{Renin}} \text{Angiotensin I} \xrightarrow{\text{ACE}} \text{Angiotensin II}$$

- *Angiotensin* II has three principal effects by which it can elevate the arterial pressure:
1. Vasoconstriction,
2. Decrease in salt and water excretion by kidney, and
3. Stimulation of thirst.

Vasopressin or antidiuretic hormone (ADH) is secreted in minute quantities and therefore mainly affects water reabsorption in renal tubules. However, after a severe haemorrhage its concentration rises to a high level and then it has vasoconstrictor effect.

Ions and other chemical factors

The increased concentration of many different ions and chemical factors can also alter local blood flow by causing vasodilation or vasoconstriction.

- Calcium ions cause vasoconstriction
- Potassium ions cause vasodilatation
- Hydrogen ions (decreased pH) cause vasodilation
- Carbon dioxide causes vasodilation in most tissues and marked vasodilation in the brain.
- Glucose or other vasoactive substances, when increased in quantities, raise the osmolarity of blood and cause vasodilation.

LOCAL CONTROL MECHANISMS

Local cardiovascular control mechanisms are primarily concerned with the control of blood flow to the tissues locally. These include :

A. Mechanisms involved in acute control of blood flow.
B. Mechanisms involved in long-term blood flow regulation.

MECHANISMS INVOLVED IN ACUTE CONTROL OF BLOOD FLOW

The mechanisms that are involved in most tissues of the body are:

1. Autoregulation, i.e. control of flow during changes in arterial pressure,
2. Role of local vasodilator metabolites and factors,
3. Role of local vasoconstrictors,
4. Role of substances secreted by endothelial cells.

1. Autoregulation (control of flow during changes in arterial pressure)

Autoregulation is the ability of an organ or tissue to adjust its vascular resistance and maintain a relatively constant blood flow over a wide range of arterial pressure. For details see page 189.

2. Role of local vasodilator metabolites

The accumulation of local vasodilator metabolites increase local blood flow. The greater the rate of metabolism in the tissue greater the rate of production of metabolites. These include :

- Decrease in O_2 tension and pH
- Increase in pCO_2 and osmolality
- Rise in temperature
- Potassium (K^+) and lactate ions
- Histamine
- Adenosine

Local vasodilator metabolites increase blood flow during following conditions :

Active hyperaemia It refers to the vasodilation which occurs when the tissue metabolic rate increases.

Reactive hyperaemia It is a phenomenon by which the local blood flow to the organ is controlled after a period of ischaemia

3. Role of local vasoconstrictors

Serotonin released from platelets in the injured tissue is responsible in part for the vasconstriction which occurs in haemostasis.

4. Role of substances secreted by endothelial cells

The vasoactive substances secreted by endothelial cells play important role in control of local blood flow. These include:

- Prostaglandins and thromboxane A_2,
- Endothelium-derived relaxing factor (EDRF), and
- Endothelins.

MECHANISMS INVOLVED IN LONG-TERM BLOOD FLOW REGULATION

The long-term blood flow regulation develops over a period of days to months to match the metabolic needs of the tissues. Long-term blood flow regulation is required by:

- Ischaemic tissues,
- Tissues that are growing rapidly, or
- Tissues that become chronically hyperactive.

The long-term blood flow regulation is brought about by an increase in the physiological size of the vessels in a tissue, and by an increase in the number of blood vessels. One of the major factors that stimulate the increased vascularity of the tissues is a low oxygen concentration.

Angiogenesis. The growth of the new vessels is called angiogenesis. *Angiogenic factors* such as vascular endothelial growth factor (VEGF), fibroblast growth factor (FGF), and angiogenin are the substances which are responsible for angiogenesis.

Development of collateral blood vessels. Collateral blood vessels refer to those new vessels which develop around a blocked artery or vein and allow the affected tissue to be at least partially resupplied with blood. An important example is the development of collateral blood vessels after thrombosis of one of the coronary arteries in old people.

CARDIOVASCULAR HOMEOSTASIS IN HEALTH

Cardiovascular homeostasis in health refers to the compensatory adjustments of the cardiovascular system to challenges faced by the circulation in everyday life. The common situations during which cardiovascular adjustments are required in day-to-day life include:

- Gravitational changes,
- Intrathoracic pressure changes, and
- Exercise.

CARDIOVASCULAR ADJUSTMENTS DURING GRAVITATIONAL CHANGES

Gravitational changes occur under following conditions in life:

- Posture change from lying to standing,
- Prolonged quiet standing,

ADJUSTMENTS DURING POSTURE CHANGE FROM LYING TO STANDING

When posture is changed from lying (recumbent) to standing (erect) the haemodynamic changes occur as a result of the effect of gravity on the blood column which tend to reduce the cardiac output and blood pressure. However, since in humans the compensatory mechanisms are so well developed that in normal persons no effect is felt on posture changes in day-to-day life. The sequence of events which occur during change in posture from lying to standing are (Fig. 6.4-8):

In standing position, due to *hydrostatic (gravitational) effect of blood column,* the blood pressure at the level of feet in both the arteries and veins is increased approximately by 80 mmHg.

Increased intraluminal pressure has no effect on thick-walled arteries, but the thin-walled veins distend and accommodate more blood (venous pooling).

Venous pooling (300-500 ml) results in decreased venous return and so the cardiac output and thence the blood pressure is also reduced.

A drop in the blood pressure in carotid sinus and aortic arch within seconds triggers the *baroreceptor- mediated compensatory mechanism* which causes following changes:

- *Heart rate* is increased by 5 to 10 beats/min.
- *Force of cardiac contraction* is increased leading to increase in stroke volume and cardiac output.
- *Peripheral resistance* is increased due to arteriolar constriction in the cutaneous, renal and splanchnic circulation. Increase in peripheral resistance increases the diastolic pressure.
- *Venoconstriction* in the body transfers blood from the capacitance vessels towards the heart increasing the venous return.
- *Increased secretion of renin and aldosterone* which also help in normalization of blood pressure.

In spite of the above mentioned compensatory changes the stroke volume and cardiac output in standing posture are about 25% less than in supine position.

However, due to a 25% increase in the total peripheral resistance the blood pressure becomes almost normal.

The above events are summarized in Fig. 6.4-8.

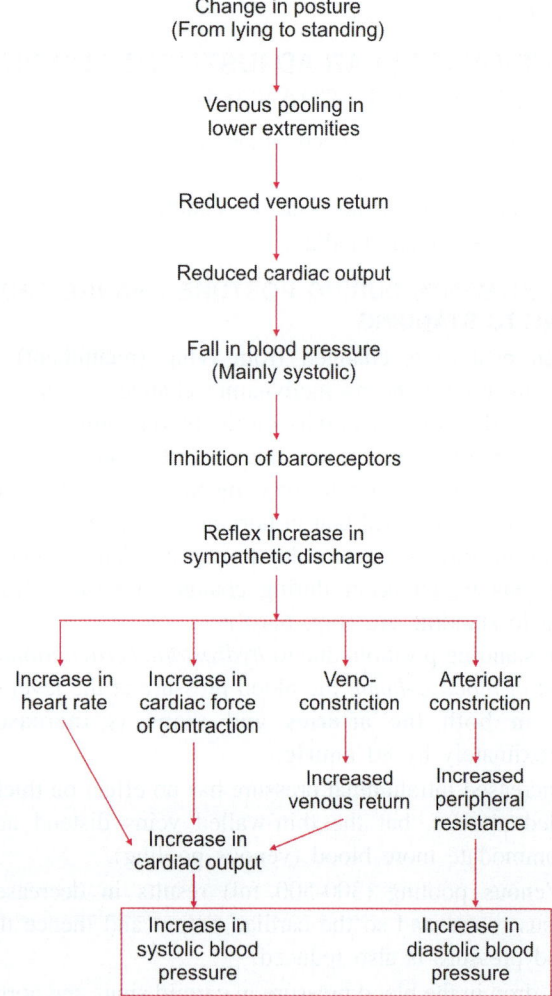

Fig. 6.4-8. *Summary of events maintaining normal blood pressure during change of posture from lying to standing.*

CHANGES DURING PROLONGED QUIET STANDING

During prolonged quiet standing (a situation particularly met with military or police personnel, i.e. standing in attention for long periods), along with the venous pooling the fluid begins to accumulate in the interstitial spaces because of increased hydrostatic pressure in the capillaries. The cardiac output is decreased due to decreased venous return. A stage may come when cerebral blood flow decreases to less than about 60% and symptoms of cerebral ischaemia develop. The individual may faint and fall down.

The fainting, in a sense, is also a homeostatic mechanism, because falling to horizontal position promptly restores venous return, cardiac output and cerebral blood flow to adequate levels.

Postural hypotension

Postural hypotension or orthostatic hypotension in which there occurs a sudden fall in blood pressue on changing posture from lying to erect, which causes symptoms of cerebral ischaemia. The individual experiences transient blurring of vision, dizziness or even fainting. It is diagnosed by recording blood pressure in lying and standing postures. A decrease in systolic blood pressure by 30 mmHg or more on standing from supine position is diagnostic. Postural hypotension develops in individuals in whom the cardiovascular compensatory mechanisms (described above) are very slow to develop.

CARDIOVASCULAR ADJUSTMENTS DURING MUSCULAR EXERCISE

Severe muscular exercise is the most stressful physiological condition that the cardiovascular homeostasis mechanisms face in everyday life, since, in addition to CVS adjustments, respiratory and other adjustments also occur in the body.

CARDIOVASCULAR RESPONSES TO EXERCISE

To meet the increased energy demand of muscles during exercise the primary cardiovascular response is in the form of:

- Increase in the skeletal muscle blood flow,
- Redistribution of blood flow in the body,
- Increase in the cardiac output,
- Blood pressure changes, and
- Changes in blood volume.

Skeletal muscle blood flow

At rest the blood flow to the skeletal muscle is about 2-4 ml/100 gm/min of muscle tissue. During strenuous exercise muscle blood flow can increase upto 20 times, i.e. about 50-80 ml/100 gm/min muscle tissue. This is called *exercise hyperaemia*. This tremendous increase in muscle blood flow during exercise is made possible by:

- Arteriolar dilatation, and
- Opening up of closed capillaries which greatly increase the surface area and the rate of blood flow.

Redistribution of blood flow

As mentioned earlier the tremendous increase in skeletal muscle blood flow is possible due to increased cardiac output and redistribution of cardiac output in the following manner (Table 6.4-1):

Table 6.4-1. Redistribution of cardiac output in standing posture during exercise

	At rest	During heavy exercise	Change
Cardiac output	5 L/min	24 L/min	Increased 5-6 times
Blood flow to:			
• Skeletal muscles	750-800 ml/min	20 L/min	25 times
• Heart	250 ml/min	1 L/min	4 times
• Brain	750 ml/min	750 ml/min	No change
• Viscera	2600 ml/min	500 ml/min	Decreased by 80%
• Skin	500 ml/min	400 ml/min	Initially decreased
		1000 ml/min	Later increased

Coronary blood flow. During exercise coronary blood flow is increased by 4 to 5 times with 100 per cent O_2 utilization. This occurs due to:

- *Increased coronary blood flow* due to sympathetic stimulation, and
- *Coronary vasodilatation*

Visceral blood flow is temporarily curtailed in coordination with increase in muscle blood flow. It is brought about by the increased sympathoadrenal discharge.

Splanchnic blood flow is decreased by 80% in severe exercise.

Renal blood flow is also decreased by 50-80% in severe exercise.

Cutaneous blood flow at rest is about 500 ml/min.

- *Decrease* in cutaneous blood flow occurs initially in the beginning of exercise due to reflex vasoconstric-tion.
- When body temperature rises, to dissipate the heat generated during exercise, the blood flow through the skin increases.

Cerebral blood flow remains unchanged.

Adipose tissue blood flow is increased by 4 times during exercise. This helps to deliver fatty acids mobilized from triglyceride stores to the working muscles.

INCREASE IN CARDIAC OUTPUT

Normal cardiac output is about 5-6 L/min. In maximum exercise it may increase by 5 to 6 times. Since, cardiac output is the product of heart rate and stroke volume, an increase in both contributes to the increase in cardiac output during exercise.

Factors contributing to tachycardia during exercise are:

- *Increased sympathetic discharge*
- *Peripheral reflexes* originating from the exercising muscles (muscle spindles, muscle-tendon receptors and organ of Corti) and joints.
- *Humoral factors,* such as release of adrenaline and noradrenaline and possibly thyroid hormones during exercise.
- *Increased temperature* in the myocardium due to increased activity of the heart during exercise may directly increase the rhythmicity of the pacemaker.

Mechanisms responsible for increase in stroke volume

It has been stated that increase in the stroke volume during exercise occurs due to gearing up of both the control mechanisms, i.e.

- Intrinsic autoregulation or Frank-Starling mecha-nism (for details see page 179).
- Extrinsic regulation or autonomic and neural mechanism (for details see page 181).

BLOOD PRESSURE CHANGES DURING EXERCISE

In systemic circulation

Systolic blood pressure is always raised by exercise since it depends upon the cardiac output which is increased in exercise.

Diastolic blood pressure which primarily depends upon the peripheral resistance may mildly increase or decrease or remain unchanged. Mostly the vaso-dilatation in the skeletal muscles balances the vasoconstriction in other tissues; so diastolic blood pressure is usually not changed much.

Mean blood pressure is usually increased.

In pulmonary circulation

- *Systolic blood pressure* in pulmonary artery may rise during heavy exercise to 25-30 mmHg from 15-20 mmHg at rest,
- *Diastolic blood pressure* may rise from 5-8 mmHg at rest to 8-10 mmHg, and
- *Mean blood pressure* may reach to 15 mmHg from 8-12 mmHg at rest.

CHANGES IN BLOOD VOLUME DURING EXERCISE

Blood volume during exercise is decreased by 15% resulting in haemoconcentration. Blood volume is decreased due to more plasma loss at the capillary level due to :

- Increased hydrostatic pressure in capillaries, and

● Increased tissue fluid osmotic pressure due to accumulation of osmotically active metabolites in tissue spaces.

SUMMARY OF CARDIOVASCULAR RESPONSES TO EXERCISE

The cardiovascular responses to exercise are summarized in Fig. 6.4-9.

Fig. 6.4-9. *Summary of cardiovascular responses to exercise.*

CARDIOVASCULAR HOMEOSTASIS IN DISEASES

Cardiovascular homeostasis mechanism operates in almost all cardiorespiratory and many other multiorgan diseases. The most important condition which needs special description is circulatory shock.

CIRCULATORY SHOCK

Circulatory shock or simply called as shock is a syndrome characterized by inadequate delivery of oxygen and nutrients to critical organs such as heart, brain, liver, kidneys and gastrointestinal tract.

TYPES AND CAUSES OF SHOCK

Depending upon the cause of inadequacy of cardiac output (relative or absolute) the circulatory shock may be of following types:

I.   Hypovolaemic shock,

II. Low-resistance or distributive or vasogenic shock,

III. Cardiogenic shock, and

IV. Obstructive shock.

I. Hypovolaemic shock

Hypovolaemic shock also known as cold shock is caused by a low blood volume resulting in decreased cardiac output.

Depending on the causes the hypovolaemic shock may be of following types:

1. *Haemorrhagic shock.* It occurs as a result of external or internal blood loss caused by ruptured vessels.

2. *Dehydration shock.* Fluid loss when insufficient amount can dehydrate the body and reduce the circulating blood volume. Fluid loss can occur from:
- *GIT* in diarrhoea or vomiting,
- *Kidney* in diabetes mellitus, diabetes insipidus, or excessive use of diuretics, and
- *Skin* in burns.

3. *Traumatic shock.* It is a special type of hypovolaemic shock in which there is associated neurogenic shock caused by severe pain which inhibits the vasomotor centre.

II. Low-resistance or distributive or vasogenic shock

Low-resistance or distributive or vasogenic shock occurs when neural reflexes or toxic substances cause excessive vasodilation within the vascular system. Low-resistance shock is also called *warm shock* because skin is warm and not cold and moist as it is in hypovolaemic shock. Depending upon the causes, the low-resistance shock is of following types:

1. *Neurogenic shock.* It occurs due to :
i. *Marked reduction in sympathetic vasomotor tone,* and
ii. *Pronounced increase in the vagal tone* as in vasovagal syncope or emotional fainting.

2. *Anaphylactic shock.* Anaphylaxis refers to an acute allergic reaction. Large quantities of histamine and histamine-like substances released in allergic reaction cause widespread and marked *vasodilation* reducing peripheral resistance. Also, there is marked *increase in capillary permeability* leading to fluid loss and adding hypovolaemic element to the low-resistance shock.

3. *Septicaemic shock.* Septicaemia is a condition in which bacteria circulate and multiply in the blood and form toxic products and cause high fever and marked vasodilatation due to peripheral arteriolar paralysis.

III. Cardiogenic shock

Cardiogenic shock occurs due to decreased pumping ability of the heart because of some cardiac abnormality.

Causes of cardiogenic shock are:
- Myocardial infarction,
- Cardiac arrhythmias,
- Congestive heart failure, and
- Severe valvular dysfunctions.

IV. Obstructive shock

Obstructive shock or, more precise, the extracardiac obstructive shock occurs due to impairment of ventricular filling during diastole due to some external pressure on the heart. Due to decreased ventricular filling the stroke volume and hence the cardiac output is decreased causing circulatory shock.

Causes of obstructive effusion shock are:
- Pericardial cardiac tamponade, i.e. bleeding into the pericardium with external pressure on the heart,
- Tension pneumothorax,
- Constrictive pericarditis, and
- Pulmonary embolism.

STAGES AND CLINICAL FEATURES OF SHOCK

Stages and clinical features of all types of shock are similar with minor differences. However, the haemorrhagic shock is more common. Depending upon the severity, the circulatory shock can be divided into three stages:
- First stage or non-progressive shock,
- Second stage or progressive shock, and
- Third stage or refractory shock.

I. First stage of shock or non-progressive shock

Non-progressive shock also known as *compensated shock* or initial stage of shock occurs when there is a moderate reduction in cardiac output.

Hypovolaemic shock due to acute blood loss, in other words, the *haemorrhagic shock,* occurs when at least 10 to 15% of total blood volume is lost. Thus, about 10% of the total blood volume may be lost without any significant effect.

Compensatory mechanisms of rapid onset (short-term mechanisms) are immediately set into motion following the acute loss of blood and try to maintain the blood flow to vital organs in spite of reduced cardiac output.

A. Rapid compensatory mechanisms (Neural mechanism)

Rapid or the so-called short-term control mechanisms primarily include the following three nervous reflexes:

1. Baroreceptor reflex. When the blood pressure is decreased there occurs decrease in the impulse discharge from the arterial baroreceptors (for detail see page 200).

2. Chemoreceptor reflex. Fall in blood pressure below 60 mmHg usually initiates chemoreceptor reflex.

3. CNS ischaemic response. When blood pressure falls below 50 mmHg this response is initiated (for details see page 201). It causes more powerful sympathetic stimulation.

The rapid compensatory mechanisms account for following symptoms and signs:

Symptoms and signs observed in patients with shock are:
- *Pale, cold and moist skin* occurs due to decreased blood flow to skin and increased sweating (due to increased sympathetic discharge).

- *Cyanotic tinge of skin* may sometimes occur because of increased O_2 extraction from the blood.
- *Tachycardia* and *fall in pulse pressure* produce *thin and thready pulse,* the characteristic feature of hypovolaemic shock.
- *Increased rate and force of respiration* is due to greater sino-aortic chemoreceptors' discharge.
- *Oliguria,* another important feature of hypovolaemic shock, is due to renal arteriolar constriction.
- *Restlessness and apprehension* may occur due to stimulation of brain stem reticular formation by circulating catecholamines, since haemorrhage is a potent stimulator of secretion of these hormones from the adrenal medulla.

B. Intermediate compensatory mechanisms

1. Renin-angiotensin vasoconstrictor mechanism (see page 202),
2. Reverse stress relaxation (see page 193), and
3. Capillary fluid shift mechanism (see page 193).

C. Long-term compensatory mechanisms

1. *Restoration of plasma volume and proteins.*
2. *Restoration of red cell mass.*

Note. Under normal circumstances the circulatory compensatory mechanisms described above eventually cause full recovery without help of outside therapy during the stage of non-progressive shock. However, a timely outside therapy may hasten the recovery.

II. Progressive shock

Second stage of the circulatory shock is progressive stage which occurs after a 15 to 25% loss of total blood volume. In this stage the compensatory mechanisms are not able to stop the progression of the shock. In progressive shock the structures of circulatory system begin to deteriorate and various types of *positive feedback mechanisms* develop. Therefore, timely therapeutic interventions are essential in this stage, otherwise the vicious cycle of positive feedback mechanisms will cause progressive decrease in the cardiac output and ultimately patient will go into stage of refractory shock.

Positive feedback cycles

Positive feedback cycles responsible for continuous progression of shock, if not interrupted by therapeutic intervention, leading to refractory stage are:

1. Cardiac failure.
2. Vasomotor failure.
3. Peripheral circulatory failure.
4. Septicaemia and toxaemia.

III. Refractory shock

As mentioned above, when the shock is in progressive stage and is not treated adequately, a vicious cycle of various positive feedback mechanisms set in and patient passes into the third stage of shock, the *refractory shock* (previously known as *irreversible shock*). In this stage all therapeutic interventions are usually ineffective and eventually the patient dies.

TREATMENT OF SHOCK WITH PHYSIOLOGICAL BASIS

The treatment of shock is aimed at correcting the cause and helping physiological compensatory mechanisms.

1. *General measures for shock treatment* are:
- *Room temperature.* Where the patients of shock are kept should be cold. If exposed to warmth there will be sweating which will cause further hypovolaemia and aggravate the shock.
- *Raising the foot end of the patient's bed* by 6 to 12″ (*Trendelenburg position*) helps in promoting the venous return and thereby increasing the cardiac output. It is especially useful in haemorrhagic and neurogenic shock when the blood pressure is too low.

2. *Replacement therapy* is very useful in hypovolaemic shock.

In haemorrhagic shock the best therapy is transfusion of whole *blood.* When whole blood is not available the *plasma* may be used. Plasma maintains the colloid osmotic pressure of the blood, but the haematocrit decreases with this therapy. If neither whole blood nor plasma is available a plasma substitute such as *dextran* may be used.

3. *Sympathomimetic drugs* are useful as:
- *Dopamine* should be the sympathomimetic drug of choice.
- Epinephrine or norepinephrine drug may also be used when dopamine is not available.

4. *Oxygen therapy.* Oxygen therapy may have some beneficial effects.

5. *Glucocorticoids.* Glucocorticoids are particularly useful in anaphylactic shock.

Lymphatic System

GENERAL CONSIDERATIONS
- Constituents of lymphatic system
- Functions of lymphatic system

THE LYMPH
- Formation and composition
- Lymph flow

LYMPH VESSELS
- Lymph capillaries
- Lymphatic vessels
- Lymphatic trunks and collecting ducts

LYMPHATIC ORGANS AND TISSUES
- Lymph nodes

GENERAL CONSIDERATIONS

The lymphatic system has been called the 'middle man' between blood and the body tissues. The whole of the tissues, however, are bathed in fluid called tissue fluid. All interchanges of nourishment and waste products between the blood and the body tissues take place through the medium of tissue fluid. Colloid material from the tissue fluid cannot re-enter the blood capillaries; hence lymph capillaries are ever present to receive colloids, as well as, electrolytes, water, and other substances and return them to the blood stream. The lymphatic system is, therefore, a subsidiary or second circulatory system, which drains the tissue fluids.

Constituents of lymphatic system

Lymph is, thus, the interstitial fluid that flows into the lymphatic capillaries. From the lymphatic capillaries, the lymph passes through vessels of successively increasing size and a large number of lymph nodes before entering the blood. The lymphatic system, thus, comprises of:
- The lymph,
- Lymphatic vessels,
- Lymph nodes, and other lymph organs.

Functions of lymphatic system

1. *Returns proteins from tissue spaces to blood.* The lymphatic system recovers approximately 200 gm of protein daily that has been lost from the microcirculation.

2. *Absorption of nutrients,* especially fats, from the gastrointestinal tract.

3. *Acts as transport mechanism* to remove red blood cells that have lost into the tissues as a result of haemorrhage.

4. *Supplies nutrients and oxygen* to those parts where blood cannot reach.

5. *Role in defence mechanism.* Lymph nodes associated with lymphatic system act as efficient filters. They have sinuses lined with phagocytic cells that engulf bacteria, red cells and other particulate material.

THE LYMPH

FORMATION AND COMPOSITION

Formation. Lymph is essentially the name given to the tissue fluid when it has entered the lymphatics. The formation of lymph is thus closely associated with the formation of tissue fluid.

As discussed in capillary exchange (see page 190), most (90%) of the fluid filtered at arterial end of the capillary is reabsorbed at its venous end; and the remaining 10% enters the circulation through lymphatics and is called lymph. Thus, the lymph is a transudate formed from blood in the tissue spaces, i.e. it is derived from the interstitial fluid.

Composition of lymph is similar to plasma except that:

- *Protein content* is usually lower than that of plasma (2-5 gm%). Protein content of the lymph usually varies with the region it drains.

- *Fat content.* Since, the lymphatic system also provides a route of absorption of long-chained fatty acids and cholesterol from the intestine (in the form of *chylomicrons)*, therefore, after a fatty meal these fat globules may be so numerous that lymph becomes milky and is then called *chyle*.

- *Cellular content.* Suspended in the lymph are cells that are chiefly lymphocytes. Most of these lymphocytes are added to the lymph as it passes through lymph nodes.

Lymph flow

Lymph enters the lymphatic capillaries under the influence of osmotic pressure of tissue fluid. The flow of lymph in the lymph vessels, like venous blood, is under low pressure and is controlled largely by the outside forces which include :

- Contraction of smooth muslces in the walls of large lymph vessels,
- Contraction of skeletal muscles,
- Movements of different body parts,
- Arterial pulsations,
- Compression of tissue by objects outside the body, and
- Negative intrathorcic pressure and action of respiratory muscles.

Normal lymph flow is 2-4 L/day (80 to 150 ml/hour) for the entire body.

Rate of lymph flow varies in different organs and is highest in the gastrointestinal tract and the liver.

In lymphatics rate of lymph flow is 100 ml/hour through thoracic duct and about 20 ml/hour through other lymphatic channels.

LYMPH VESSELS

The lymphatic system constitutes an accessory route for the removal of interstitial fluid. The small lymph vessels

are called lymph capillaries and the large lymph vessels are called lymphatic trunks and the largest lymph vessel is thoracic duct.

LYMPH CAPILLARIES

The lymph capillaries originate as closed endothelial tubes that are permeable to fluid and high-molecular weight compounds.

Structure of lymph capillaries (Fig. 6.5-1) is basically similar to that of blood capillaries with following differences:

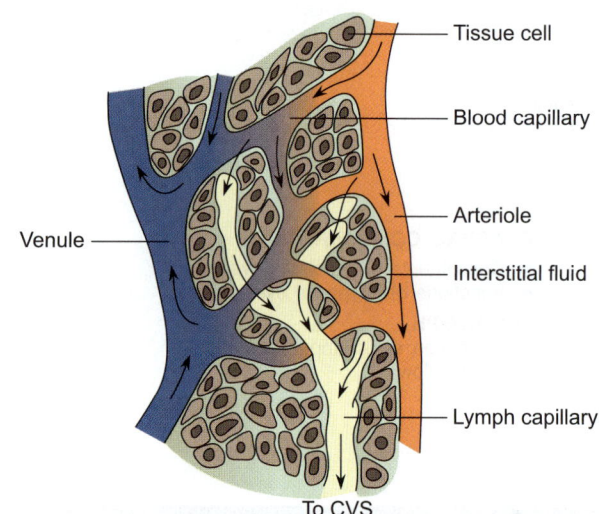

Fig. 6.5-1. Structure of lymph capillary.

- The basal lamina around the endothelial cells is absent or poorly developed,
- Pericytes or connective tissue are not present around the lymph capillaries,
- There are no visible fenestrations in the endothelium, and
- The junctions between endothelial cells are open. In fact, the edges of the endothelial cells overlap in such a way that they form minute flap valves.

LYMPHATIC VESSELS

The lymphatic capillaries are present in most tissues of the body except brain, cartilage, splenic pulp, bone marrow and avascular structures (e.g. cornea, crystalline lens, nail and hairs). The lymphatic capillaries join to form the lymphatic vessels. The lymphatic vessels are distributed throughout the body like the veins (Fig. 6.5-2). The lymphatics continue to unite and form larger and larger vessels until finally they converge to form the lymphatic trunks and collecting ducts.

LYMPHATIC TRUNKS AND COLLECTING DUCTS

Lymphatic trunks

The lymphatic trunks are larger lymph vessels which drain lymph from relatively large regions of the body, and they

Submaxillary nodes
Jugular trunk
Brachiocephalic vein
Axillary nodes
Cisterna chyli
Inguinal lymph nodes

Cervical nodes
Jugular vein
Subclavian trunk
Broncho-mediastinal trunk
Thoracic duct
Intercostal trunk
Intestinal trunk and nodes
Lumbar trunk and iliac nodes
Lymphatic vessels

Fig. 6.5-2. *Distribution of lymph vessels and lymph nodes in the human body.*

are named for the region with which they are associated. Examples of lymphatic trunks include (Fig. 6.5-2) :

- *Lumbar trunk.* It drains lymph from the lower limbs, lower abdominal wall, and the pelvic organs.
- *Intestinal trunk.* It drains lymph from the various viscera of abdomen.
- *Intercostal trunk.* It drains from portions of thorax.
- *Bronchomediastinal trunk.* It also receives lymph from the portion of thorax.
- *Subclavian trunk.* It drains lymph from the upper limb.
- *Jugular trunk.* It drains lymph from portions of the neck and head.

Collecting ducts

The lymphatic trunks then join to form two collecting ducts - the thoracic duct and right lymphatic duct (Figs. 6.5-2 and 6.5-3).

Thoracic duct is the largest lymph vessel in the body. It carries lymph from both sides of the body below the diaphragm and from the left side above the diaphragm. Near its termination it receives the *left subclavian lymphatic trunks* carrying lymph from left upper limb, the *left*

jugular lymphatic trunk carrying lymph from left half of head and neck, and sometimes the *left bronchomediastinal lymphatic trunk* carrying lymph from left half of thorax (usually this trunk enters the subclavian vein independently).

The thoracic duct ends by opening into the junction of the left subclavian vein and the internal jugular vein (Fig. 6.5-3).

Right lymphatic duct drains lymph from the right half of the body above the diaphragm. It is formed by the *right bronchomediastinal trunk* carrying lymph from the right half of thorax, *right jugular trunk* draining lymph from the right half of head and neck, and *right subclavian trunk* carrying lymph from the right upper limb. The right lymphatic duct ends by opening into the right subclavian vein (Fig. 6.5-3).

Structure of larger lymph vessels

Structure of larger lymph vessels is similar to that of veins:

- *Three coats,* i.e. tunica intima, tunica media and tunica adventitia can be distinguished.
- *Valves* similar to those in veins are present in abundance in small as well as large lymphatic vessels. The valves often give lymph vessels a beaded appearance.

LYMPHATIC ORGANS AND TISSUES

The lymphatic organs and tissues in the body include:
- Lymph nodes,
- Spleen,
- Thymus, and
- Mucosa - associated lymphoid tissue (MALT).

Note : Lymphatic organs have been described in the section on immunity (see page 54).

LYMPH NODES

The lymph nodes are small bean-shaped or oval structures which form part of lymphatic network distributed throughout the body.

Location of lymph nodes

There are many groups of lymph nodes in the body, arranged in superficial and deep sets (just as there are superficial and deep sets of lymphatics). Occasionally, a lymph node exists alone; mostly they are found in groups or chains. Superficial nodes are arranged along the veins and deep nodes along the arteries. Location of some of the important lymph node groups is as below:

Head and neck region

Superficial lymph nodes, draining the superficial tissues of the head and neck, are (Fig. 6.5-4) :
- Occipital lymph nodes
- Retroauricular lymph nodes

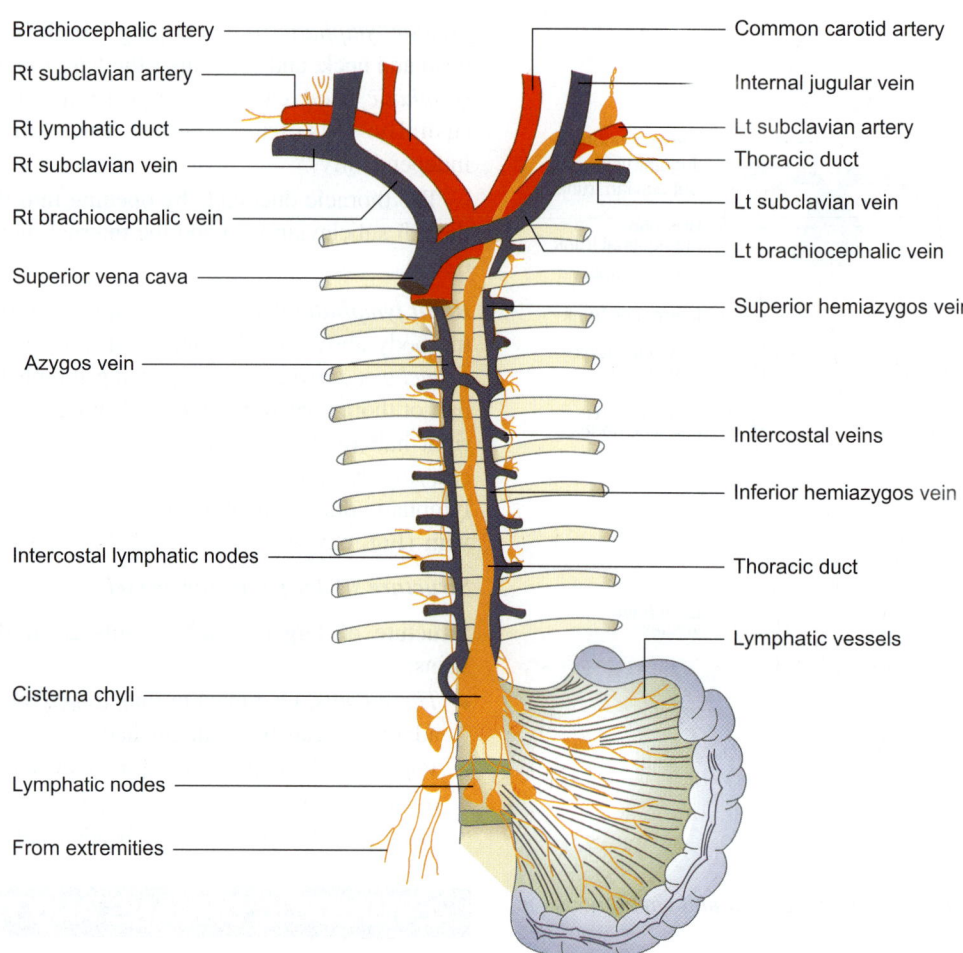

Fig. 6.5-3. *The thoracic duct and right lymphatic duct.*

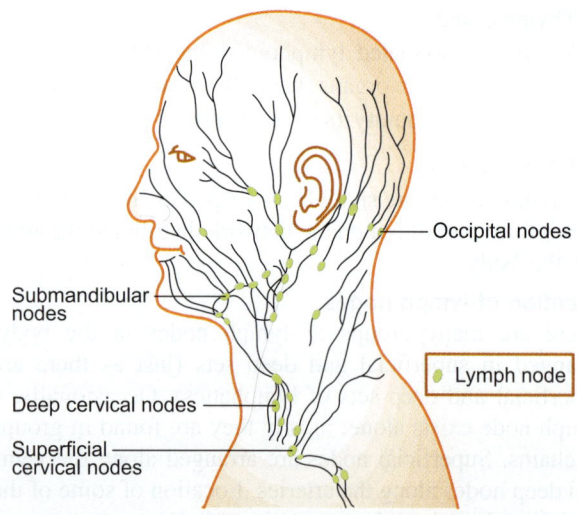

Fig. 6.5-4. *Lymph nodes of head and neck region.*

- Parotid lymph nodes
- Submandibular lymph nodes
- Submental lymph nodes
- Superficial cervical lymph nodes

Deep cervical lymph nodes. Lymph from all the superficial lymph nodes mentioned above drains into deep cervical lymph nodes which are located along the internal juguar vein (Fig. 6.5-2).

Shoulder girdle and upper limb region

Axillary lymph nodes, located in the axilla, are the chief lymph nodes draining the upper limbs, skin and muscle of chest, back and upper half of abdomen. Axillary lymph nodes are superficial nodes arranged in many groups (Fig. 6.5-2).

Other lymph nodes of upper limb not of much significance are :

- *Supratrochlear lymph nodes* (one or two nodes) lying just above the medial epicondyle of humerus.
- *Infraclavicular lymph nodes* (one or two nodes) lie just below the clavicle.

Thorax region

The lymph nodes of the thorax region are divided into:

- *Parietal nodes of thoracic region,* which drain the thoracic wall, include parasternal lymph nodes, intercostal lymph nodes and diaphragmatic lymph nodes.

- *Visceral sets of thoracic lymph nodes* include brachio-cephalic lymph nodes, posterior mediastinal lymph nodes and tracheobronchial lymph nodes which drain lymph from the thoracic viscera.

Abdominal and pelvic region

The lymph nodes draining the abdominal and pelvic viscera are arranged along the aorta and its major branches, and are named accordingly, e.g.:

- *Aortic lymph nodes (lateral, retro, and pre-aortic),*
- *Coeliac lymph nodes,*
- *Superior mesenteric lymph nodes,*
- *Inferior mesenteric lymph nodes,*
- *Common iliac lymph nodes,*
- *External iliac lymph nodes,*
- *Internal iliac lymph nodes.*

Lower limb region

Inguinal lymph nodes, located in the groin region, are the chief lymph nodes draining the lower limbs. They are arranged in following group (Fig. 6.5-2):

- *Superficial inguinal lymph nodes*
- Upper group lying along the inguinal ligament, and
- Lower group lying along the great saphenous vein.
- *Deep inguinal lymph nodes,* lying along the medial side of femoral vein.

Popliteal lymph nodes, one or two in number, of insignificant existence present in the popliteal fossa are the other lymph nodes of lower limb.

CHAPTER 6.5

Respiratory System

Anatomy, Organization and Functions of Respiratory System

RESPIRATORY PASSAGES

The chief organs of the respiratory system are right and left *lungs*. The oxygen contained in the atmospheric air reaches the lungs by passing through a series of *respiratory passages* which also serve for removal of CO_2 from the alveoli to the atmosphere. The respiratory system also includes a pump that ventilates the lung. This pump consists of the chest wall and respiratory muscles.

The respiratory passages include (Fig. 7.1-1) :
- Nose and nasal cavities,
- Pharynx,
- Larynx, and
- Tracheobronchial tree.

NOSE AND NASAL CAVITIES
EXTERNAL FEATURES OF NOSE

The nose is a special organ of the sense of smell, but it also serves as a passageway for air going to and from the lungs.

Shape and structure. The external nose is a projection of the face with a free tip. It is composed of a triangular framework of bone and cartilage, covered by skin and lined by mucous membrane.

Nostrils (anterior nares) are two oval openings on the undersurface of the nose. The anterior nares open into the right and left nasal cavities. These openings are guarded by numerous internal hairs that help to prevent the entrance of relatively coarse particles sometimes present in the air.

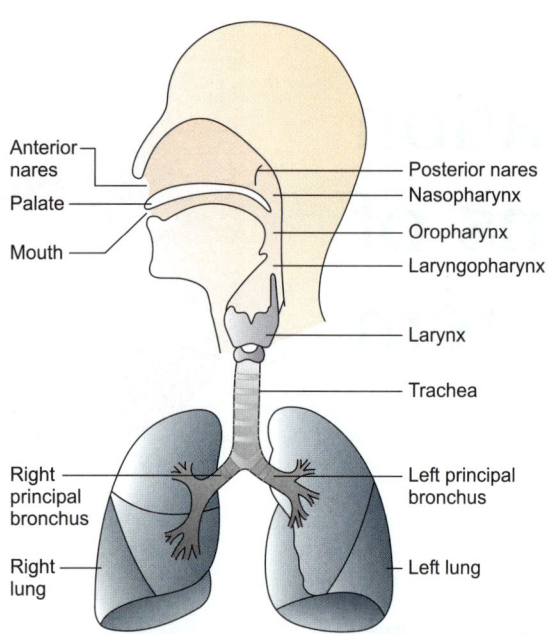

Fig. 7.1-1. *The air passages.*

THE NASAL CAVITY

The nasal cavity is divided into two parts (right and left) by the nasal septum. The nasal cavity extends from the anterior nares (nostrils) to the posterior nares (the choanae), through which it opens into the naso-pharynx.

Boundaries of nasal cavity

The bony and cartilagenous framework of each half of the nasal cavity forms its (Fig. 7.1-2):

- Roof,
- Floor,
- Medial wall, and
- Lateral wall.

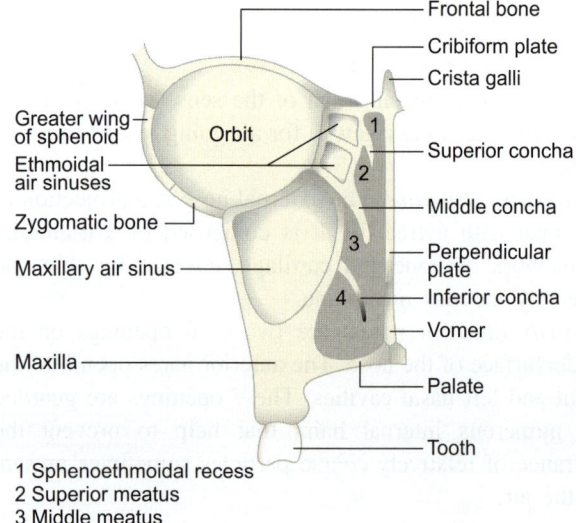

1 Sphenoethmoidal recess
2 Superior meatus
3 Middle meatus
4 Inferior meatus

Fig. 7.1-2. *Schematic coronal section through nasal cavity to show bone framework of its walls.*

Roof. Roof of the nose is very narrow about 1 cm in breadth posteriorly and about 6 cm long. It is formed anteriorly by the cartilage and posteriorly by nasal and ethmoid bones. The middle part of the roof is formed by cribriform plate of ethmoid bone which separates it from the cranial cavity.

Floor. Floor of nasal cavity is constituted by hard palate which separates it from the mouth. The hard palate is formed by palatine process of maxilla (anterior 2/3rd) and palatine bone (posterior 1/3rd).

Medial wall. Nasal septum (medial wall) divides the nasal cavity into right and left halves. It is made up of two parts:

- *Bony part,* is posterior and is formed by the vomer bone and perpendicular plate of ethmoid bone.
- *Cartilagenous part,* is anterior, and is formed by the septal cartilage.

Lateral wall. The bony framework of lateral wall is formed by the maxilla, the ethmoid bone and inferior conchae. On interior view of nasal cavity the lateral wall of nasal cavity presents following features :

Vestibule (Fig. 7.1-3). It is the lowest part of the lateral wall just above the anterior nares. It is lined by skin of the nose and is characterised by presence of long hair (vibrissae).

Conchae. These are three shelf-like projections called superior, middle and inferior conchae (Fig. 7.1-3). Each concha has a core of exceedingly light spongy bone covered by thick mucosa.

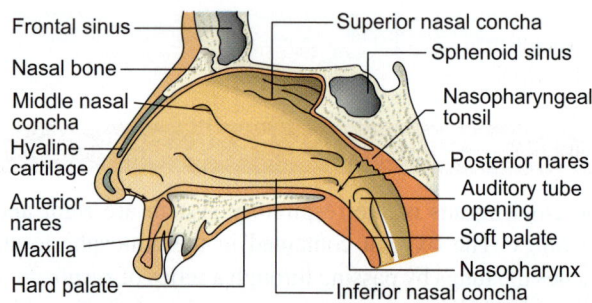

Fig. 7.1-3. *Features of lateral wall of nasal cavity.*

Meatuses. The conchae divide the nasal cavity into three spaces called the meatuses. These are :

- *Superior meatus.* It is the space below and in front of superior concha. The posterior ethmoidal air cells open into the superior meatus by one or more orifices (Fig. 7.1-4).
- *Middle meatus* is the space below and in front of middle concha. The frontal sinus, middle ethmoidal sinus and maxillary sinus open into this space (Fig. 7.1-4).

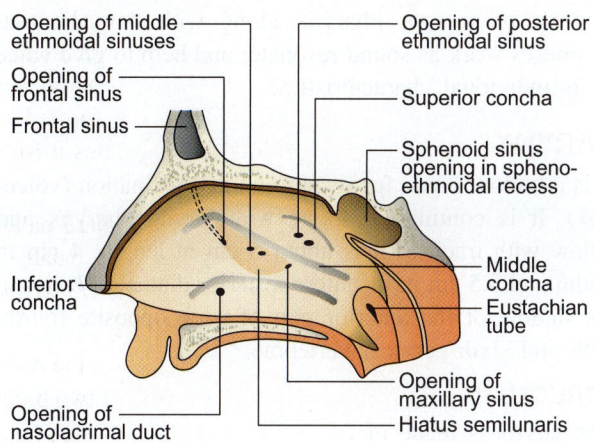

Fig. 7.1-4. *Lateral wall of nasal cavity with turbinate removed, showing the openings of various paranasal sinuses.*

- *Inferior meatus* is the space below the inferior concha. The nasolacrimal duct which drains the lacrimal sac opens in its anterior part (Fig. 7.1-4).

Lining of the nasal cavity

At the entrance the vestibule of the nasal cavity is lined with thick stratified squamous epithelium (skin) containing sebaceous glands and numerous coarse hairs.

Middle or respiratory portion of nasal cavity is lined by ciliated pseudostratified columnar epithelium which contains mucus-secreting goblet cells.

Upper or olfactory region, which includes the superior concha and adjacent part of nasal septum, is lined by neuroepithelium (olfactory epithelium) containing olfactory cells which are the receptors for smell.

The nasal mucosa, which is highly vascular, is continuous externally with the skin and internally with the mucous membrane lining the paranasal sinuses and nasopharynx.

Respiratory functions of nasal cavity

The nasal cavity is the first organ of respiration. It subserves following respiratory functions:

- *Warming the air.* Thick and highly vascular mucosa of nasal cavity warms the air to the body temperature.

- *Humidification* of the air to 100% saturation is caused when the air passes over the moist mucosa.

- *Filtration of air.* The hairs at the entrance to the nostrils and the cilia of the epithelium serve as filters to remove the particles which may be present in the air. The tortuous path between the turbinates also helps in filtering the air. The particles are deposited at the bends where they adhere to the mucous membrane of nasal cavity.

PHARYNX

The pharynx is a median passage that is common to gastrointestinal tract (GIT) and respiratory system. It is about 12-14 cm long and is continuous below with the oesophagus.

Parts of pharynx

It is divisible, from above downwards, into three parts (Fig. 7.1-5) :

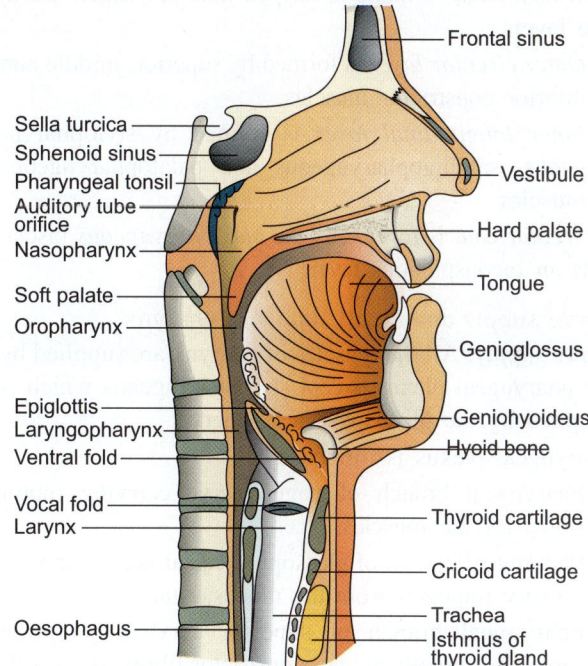

Fig. 7.1-5. *Sagittal section of nose, mouth and pharynx.*

1. *Nasopharynx* or nasal part of the pharynx into which nasal cavity opens through the posterior nares (choanae).
2. *Oropharynx* or oral part of the pharynx which is continuous with the posterior end of oral cavity. It lies below the nasopharynx separated from it incompletely by the soft palate. The communication between the nasopharynx and the oropharynx is called the *pharyngeal isthmus.*
3. *Laryngopharynx* or the laryngeal part of the pharynx is continuous in front with larynx, and below with oesophagus.

Structure of pharynx

The pharyngeal wall consists of four layers :

- Mucous coat,
- Fibrous coat,
- Muscular coat, and
- Areolar coat.

1. *Mucous coat* lining is as below :

- *Nasopharynx* is lined by ciliated columnar epithelium which is continuous with lining of nasal cavity.

- *Oropharynx and laryngopharynx* are lined by stratified squamous epithelium which is continuous with the lining of the mouth and oesophagus.

2. Fibrous coat is formed by the *pharyngobasilar fascia* which really is a dense thicknening of submucosa. It is thicker in the nasopharynx, where there is little muscle, and becomes thinner towards the lower end, where the muscle layer is thick.

3. Muscle coat is made of striped muscles which are in two layers :

- *Outer circular layer* is formed by superior, middle and inferior constrictor muscles.
- *Inner longitudinal layer* is formed by stylopharyngeous, salpingopharyngeous and palatopharyngeous muscles.

4. Areolar coat is formed by the *bucopharyngeous* fascia. It is an inconspicuous layer.

Nerve supply and blood supply of pharynx

Nerve supply. All the muscles of pharynx are supplied by the pharyngeal plexus except stylopharyngeous which is supplied by the glossopharyngeal nerve.

Pharyngeal plexus is formed by :

- Pharyngeal branch of vagus nerve carrying motor fibres for the muscles,
- Pharyngeal branch of glossopharyngeal nerve carrying sensory impulses from the mucosa, and
- Pharyngeal branch of superior cervical ganglion carrying sympathetic vasoconstrictor fibres for vessels of pharynx.

Blood supply. **Arterial supply** is from the branches of facial, lingual, maxillary and ascending pharyngeal arteries. *Venous blood* drains into facial veins and internal jugular veins.

Functions of pharynx

1. *Passageway for air.* Air from the nasal cavities enters the nasopharynx and passes down through the oropharynx and laryngopharynx to larynx. From the mouth the air can directly pass to oropharynx.
2. *Warming and humidification* of air occurs while passing through the pharynx, as like nasal cavities, its mucosa is also vascular and moist.
3. *Passage and taste of food.* The oropharynx serves as a passages for food, and some taste buds present here take part in taste sensation.
4. *Role in hearing.* The opening of eustachian tubes present in the nasopharynx equalizes the air pressure on tympanic membrane and thus plays important role in hearing (see page 494).
5. *Role in defence mechanism.* Lymphoid tissue present in the pharyngeal and laryngeal tonsils takes part in defense mechanism of the body (see page 55).

6. *Role of speech.* Pharynx along with the paranasal sinuses work as sound resonater and help to give voice its individual characteristics.

LARYNX

It is a hollow organ for respiration and phonation (voice-box). It is continuous above with laryngopharynx and below with trachea. It is about 5 cm in length, 4 cm in width and 3.5 cm in its anteroposterior diameter. It lies in the middle of the anterior part of neck opposite fourth, fifth and sixth cervical vertebrae.

STRUCTURE

The larynx is made of :
- Mucous membrane,
- Cartilages,
- Ligaments and membranes, and
- Muscles of larynx.

Mucous membrane

The larynx is made of rigid framework of cartilage, ligaments and muscles. These structures are covered on the inside by mucous membrane that is continuous above with that of the laryngeal part of pharynx and below with that of the trachea.

Cartilages of larynx

There are nine cartilages (3 single and 3 sets of paired cartilages) of larynx (Fig. 7.1-6).

Single cartilages are:

- *Thyroid cartilage.* It is the largest cartilage of larynx. It resembles a shield and rests on cricoid. It consists of two plates (laminae) joined at acute angle in midline forming laryngeal prominence (Adam's apple).
- *Cricoid cartilage.* It is shaped like a signet ring with a broad lamina posteriorly and a narrow arch anteriorly. The anterior part (arch) lies below the thyroid cartilage and its posterior part (broad lamina) extends upward into the interval between the laminae of thyroid cartilage.
- *Epiglottic cartilage.* It is tongue- or leaf-shaped, having a broad upper part, and a narrow lower end. Its lower narrow end is attached by thyroepiglottic ligament to the back of thyroid angle. Its upper broad end is free and rounded. In this way it guards the inlet of larynx.

Paired cartilages of larynx are :

- *Arytenoid cartilages.* These are pyramid-shaped cartilages which rest on the upper border of posterior lamina of cricoid cartilage (Fig. 7.1-6B).
- *Corniculate cartilages.* These are small conical nodules of elastic cartilage which are placed on either side above the apex of arytenoid cartilages.
- *Cuneiform cartilages.* These are small elongated pieces of elastic cartilages present within the aryepiglottic fold.

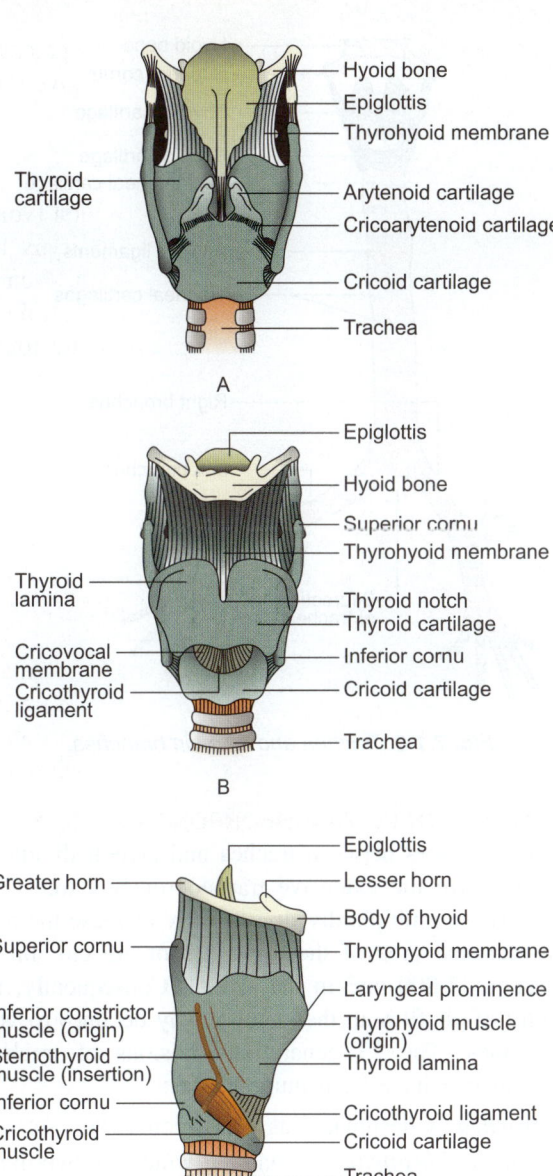

Fig. 7.1-6. *Cartilages of larynx : A, anterior view; B, posterior view; and C, lateral view.*

Ligaments and membranes of larynx

Various ligaments and membranes attach the cartilages of larynx to each other and to the hyoid bone above and to the tracheal ring below. Some important ligaments and membranes are (Fig. 7.1-6) :

- *Thyroid membrane.* It connects the upper border of thyroid cartilage with the body and greater corner of hyoid bone.
- *Anterior cricothyroid ligament.* It connects the lower border of thyroid cartilage to the arch of cricoid cartilage (Fig. 7.1-6A).
- *Cricotracheal ligament* connects the lower margin of cricoid cartilage to the trachea.

- *Thyroepiglottic ligament* connects thyroid cartilage to epiglottic cartilage.

Muscles of the larynx

The muscles of larynx are divided into extrinsic and intrinsic muscles :

Extrinsic muscles of larynx connect cartilages of larynx with the surrounding bones. These muscles raise or lower the larynx as a whole during deglutition. These include sternothyroid, thyrohyoid, sternohyoid, omohyoid and some pharyngeal muscles.

Intrinsic muscles. There are various intrinsic muscles which are confind to the larynx. Various actions of different intrinsic muscles of larynx are:

- Increase or decrease in the tension of vocal cords.
- Abducts or adducts the vocal cords.
- Opening or closing the glottis.
- Opening and closing of the inlet of larynx.

CAVITY (INTERIOR OF LARYNX)

The cavity (interior) of larynx is lined by mucous membrane and is divided into three parts by two pairs of upper vestibular and lower vocal folds lying approximately anteroposteriorly and projecting into the cavity of larynx. The three parts from above downward are (Fig. 7.1-7) :

- Vestibule,
- Ventricle or sinus, and
- Infraglottic cavity.

1. ***Vestibule*** is the upper part of laryngeal cavity which extends from its inlet to the vestibular folds.

Vestibular folds. The right and left vestibular folds are formed by the *vestibular ligaments* formed by bundle of fibres at lower free edge of a quadrangular membrane. These are directed downward and medially.

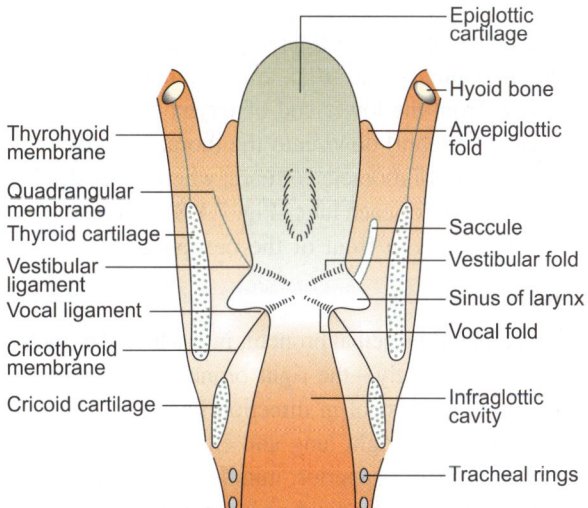

Fig. 7.1-7. *Coronal section of larynx viewed from behind showing three parts of the cavity of larynx.*

C H A P T E R 7.1

2. Ventricle or sinus. It is the middle part of laryngeal cavity which is limited above by the vestibular folds and below by vocal folds.

Vocal folds are formed by the vocal ligament lined by mucosa. These are directed upwards and medially. The space between the right and left vocal folds is called *rima glottidis.*

3. Infraglottic cavity. It is the lower part of laryngeal cavity which lies below the vocal folds. Inferiorly it widens and becomes continuous with the trachea.

FUNCTIONS OF LARYNX

1. Phonation i.e. production of vocal sounds is the main function of the larynx. Sound is characterized by pitch, volume and resonance.

- *Pitch* of voice depends upon the length and tightness of vocal cords.

- *Volume* of voice depends upon the force with which the vocal cords vibrate.

- *Resonance* and tone of the voice are determined by the shape of mouth, position of tongue and lips and air in the paranasal sinuses.

2. Protection of lower respiratory tract during deglutition is caused by closure of respiratory passages by the hinged epiglottis. This allows the food to pass into oesophagus and prevents it from entering the respiratory passages.

TRACHEOBRONCHIAL TREE

The tracheobronchial tree consists of :

- Trachea,

- Bronchi, and

- Branches of bronchi.

TRACHEA

Trachea, or windpipe, is a flexible, cylindrical tube about 2.5 cm in diameter and 12.5 cm in length. It extends downwards from the lower end of larynx (at the level of 6th cervical vertebra) down into the thoracic cavity up to the upper border of thoracic vertebra, where it divides into two bronchi, one for each lung (Fig. 7.1-8). In the thoracic cavity trachea lies in front of the oesophagus.

BRONCHI

The right and left principal bronchi, into which the trachea divides, differ slightly—the right bronchus being shorter wider, and more vertical in direction than left. The right bronchus enters the right lung and ends by dividing into three *lobar bronchi*—superior, middle and inferior, while the left bronchus ends by dividing into two lobar bronchi—superior and inferior, corresponding to two lobes of left lung (Fig. 7.1-8).

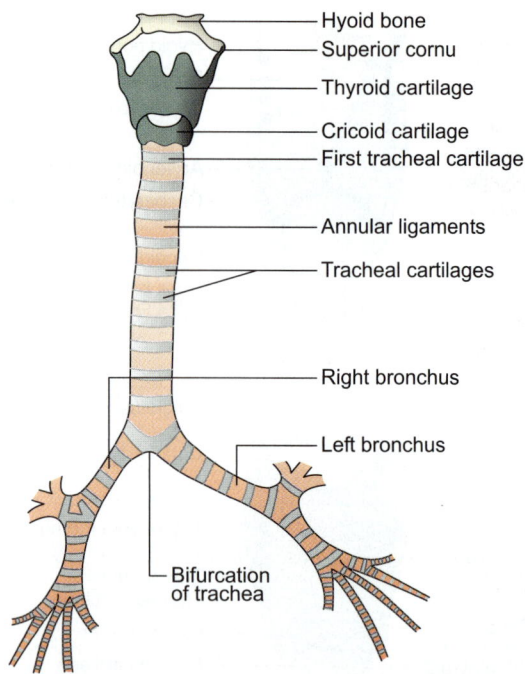

- Hyoid bone
- Superior cornu
- Thyroid cartilage
- Cricoid cartilage
- First tracheal cartilage
- Annular ligaments
- Tracheal cartilages
- Right bronchus
- Left bronchus
- Bifurcation of trachea

Fig. 7.1-8. *Trachea and its main branches.*

ORGANIZATION OF TRACHEOBRONCHIAL TREE

The air passages between trachea and alveoli divide 23 times to form the extensive tracheobronchial tree (Fig. 7.1-9). These multiple divisions greatly increase the total cross-sectional area of the airway from 2.5 cm^2 in the trachea to 11,800 cm^2 in the alveoli. Consequently, the velocity of air flow in the small airway declines to very low values. The 23 generation divisions of tracheobronchial tree have been numbered as:

The trachea is designated as generation zero.

The principal bronchi right and left which are two major divisions of trachea constitute the first generation.

- *Lobar bronchi,* which are divisions of the principal bronchus, form the 2nd generation.

- *Segmental bronchi*, which are further divisions of each lobar bronchus, forms the 3rd generation. Each segmental bronchus divides into several generations of branches that ultimately end in very small tubes called *bronchioles.*

- *Terminal bronchiole* is the name given to 16th generation of the divisions. Upto this generation of division no exchange of gases is possible.

- *Respiratory bronchiole* is the name given to 17th to 22nd generation of divisions. These are labelled as respiratory bronchioles because some exchange of gases is possible in these tubes.

- *Alveolar ducts* end in the alveoli or the alveolar sacs which form the 23rd generation division. It is here that most of the O$_2$ and CO$_2$ exchange occurs.

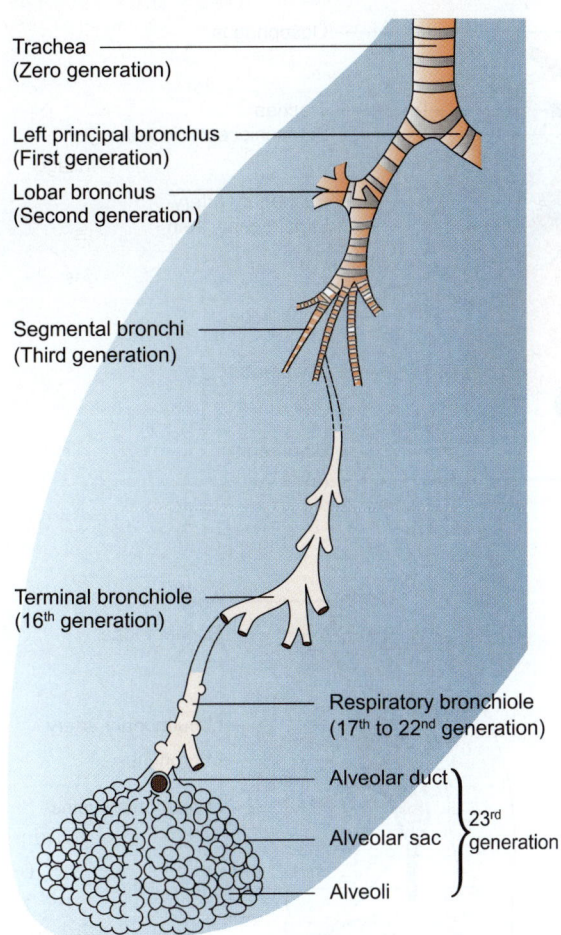

Trachea
(Zero generation)

Left principal bronchus
(First generation)

Lobar bronchus
(Second generation)

Segmental bronchi
(Third generation)

Terminal bronchiole
(16th generation)

Respiratory bronchiole
(17th to 22nd generation)

Alveolar duct

Alveolar sac — 23rd generation

Alveoli

Fig. 7.1-9. *The tracheobronchial tree.*

Zones of respiratory passages. Thus, from the functional point of view the tracheobronchial tree can be divided into two major zones:

i. *Conducting zone* of the air passages is formed by the first 16 generations of passages and it only transports gases from and to the exterior. Thus, conducting zone starts from trachea and extends upto terminal bronchioles. Since no exchange of gases is possible here, so starting from nose to the terminal brochioles forms the so-called *dead space* which has a total capacity of approximately 150 ml.

ii. *Respiratory zone.* The remaining 7 generations of tracheobronchial tree which includes the respiratory bronchioles, alveolar ducts and alveoli form the respiratory zone, where exchange of gases occurs. Its volume is approximately 4 L.

HISTOLOGICAL FEATURES OF TRACHEOBRONCHIAL TREE

1. *Cartilaginous rings* are present in trachea and initial bronchi of few generations. These are absent in terminal bronchioles and respiratory bronchioles. The cartilaginous rings of trachea are incomplete on their posterior aspect. This allows some contraction of trachea but tracheal lumen cannot be completely obliterated easily.

2. *Smooth muscles.* Ends of cartilaginous rings of trachea are approximated by transverse smooth muscle fibres. In terminal bronchioles they are present in large amount and form a sphincter. Smooth muscles are not present in alveoli.

3. *Epithelial lining* in trachea and large bronchi is columnar and becomes cuboidal in bronchioles and simple squamous in alveoli. The epithelial cells of tracheobronchial tree are ciliated. Cilia are absent in alveoli. Efficiency of ciliated cells of trachea and bronchi in propelling mucus and waste products is of higher order. Cilia are not influenced by nerve impulses. The mucus-secreting goblet cells and deep serous glands are present in trachea and bronchi but are absent in bronchioles and alveoli.

LUNGS AND PLEURA

THE LUNGS

GROSS ANATOMY

Shape, location, and associated structures
The right and left lungs (pulmones) are soft spongy, cone-shaped organs that lie in the corresponding halves of the thoracic cavity enclosed in a sac, the pleura. They are separated from each other by the mediastinal structures including the heart, the trachea, the oesopha-gus, great vessels, lymph nodes, lymph vessels and nerves.

External features
Each lung can be described to present the following external features : an apex, base, costal surface, medial surface and anterior, posterior and inferior borders (Fig. 7.1-10).

Apex refers to narrow upper end of the lung which is rounded and projects into the root of neck, about 2.5 cm above the level of middle third of clavicle.

Base refers to the broader inferior surface of the lung, which is concave to fit over the convex portion of diaphragm.

Costal surface, also called as lateral or outer surface of the lung, is convex and is closely associated with structures of thoracic wall which include the costal cartilages, the ribs and the intercostal muscles.

Medial surface is concave and associated with mediastinal structures. It presents following features :

• *Hilum* is a vertical triangular notch in the medial surface of each lung, which gives passage to the structures forming *root of the lung,* i.e. primary bronchus,

C H A P T E R 7 . 1

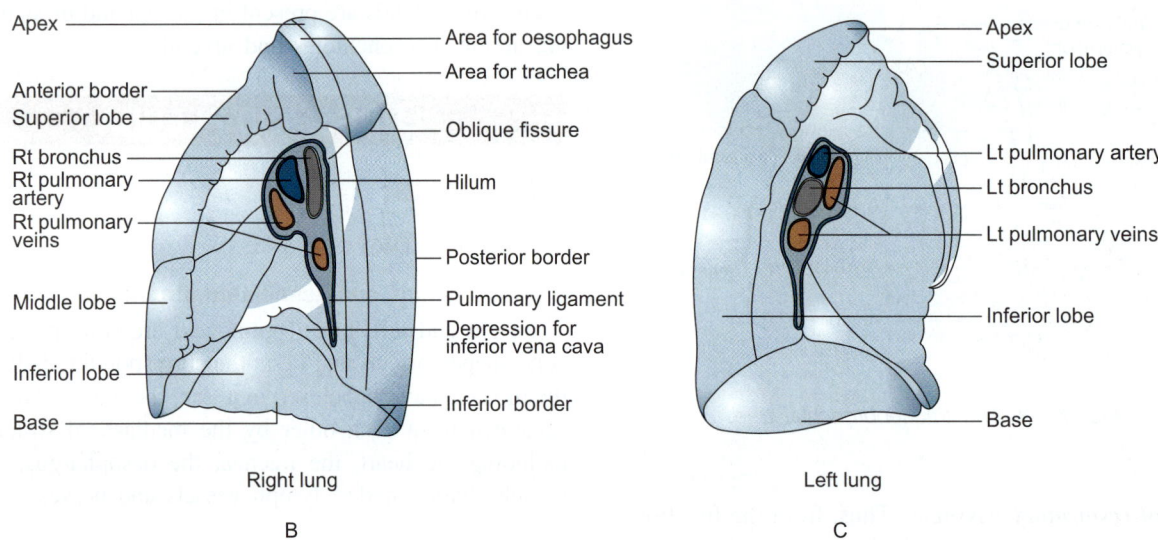

Fig. 7.1-10. *Gross features of the lungs : A, front view; B, medial view of right lung; and C, medial view of left lung.*

pulmonary artery and vein, bronchial arteries and veins, plexuses of nerves, lymphatics and lymph nodes. Structures forming root of the lung are covered by pleura and connect the lung to the trachea and heart.

- *Cardiac impression* is a deep concavity on the medial surface of lung just below and in front of the hilum where the heart lies. It is larger and deeper on the left than on the right lung, because the heart projects farther to the left side.

Borders of the lung. The costal surface meets the medial surface in front at the *anterior border* and behind at the *posterior border*. The costal and medial surfaces meet below with the base at the *inferior border*.

Fissures and lobes of the lungs

Right lung is divided into following three lobes by the oblique and horizontal fissures (Fig. 7.1-10) :

- Superior lobe,
- Middle lobe, and
- Inferior lobe.

Left lung is smaller than the right due to inclination of the heart to left side. It contains only the oblique fissure which divides it into two lobes (Fig. 7.1-10):

- Superior lobe, and
- Inferior lobe.

RESPIRATORY PARENCHYMA

Each respiratory unit consists of one respiratory bronchiole which opens into a number of alveolar ducts, and each alveolar duct in turn opens into number of alveoli. The two lungs contain about 300 million alveoli. Each alveolus has a diameter of about 0.2 μm. The alveoli are surrounded by pulmonary capillaries. The total area of the alveolar walls in contact with capillaries in both the lungs is about 70 m^2.

Microscopic structure of alveolus (Fig. 7.1-11)

Each alveolus is lined by two types of epithelial cells:

- *Type I cells* are flat cells with large cytoplasmic extensions and are the primary lining cells.
- *Type II cells* (granular pneumocytes) are thicker and contain numerous lamellar inclusion bodies. These cells secrete *surfactant*.

The alveolar wall also contains:

- Other *special type of epithelial cells,*
- *Pulmonary alveolar macrophages* (PAM) which are active phagocytic cells,
- *Lymphocytes,*
- *Plasma cells* which form and secrete immuno-globulins,
- *Amine precursor uptake and decarboxylation (APUD) cells* which store and secrete many biologically active peptidases, e.g. vasoactive intestinal peptide (VIP) and substance P, etc.,
- *Mast cells* which contain heparin, various lipids, histamine and various proteases that participate in allergic reactions.

Communication between the two alveoli occurs through small pores, called *pores of Kohn*.

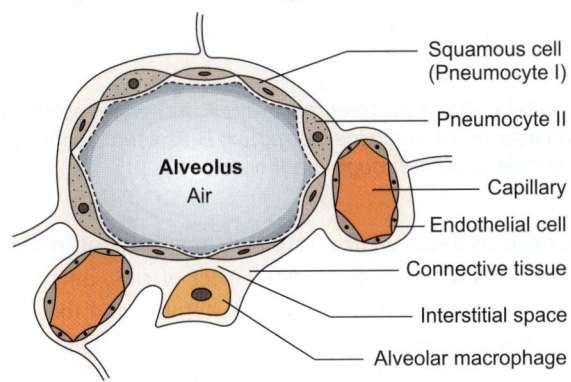

Fig. 7.1-11. Microscopic structure of alveolus.

BLOOD SUPPLY

Conducting airway is supplied by systemic blood, whereas respiratory zone of the lung is supplied by deoxygenated (venous) blood coming through pulmonary arteries to lungs. Blood is oxygenated in lungs and is returned to left atrium via pulmonary veins.

Bronchial circulatoin

The lungs receive oxygenated blood like other tissues in the body through *bronchial arteries* (two left and one right), which are branches of the descending thoracic aorta. Bronchial blood flow amounts to about 1 to 2 per cent of total cardiac output. The oxygenated blood in the bronchial arteries supplies the connective tissues, septa

and large and small bronchi of the lungs. Because the bronchial blood empties into the pulmonary veins and bypasses the right heart, the bronchial circulation, therefore, constitutes a *physiological shunt,* i.e. a channel that bypasses oxygenation in the lungs.

Pulmonary circulation

Pulmonary trunk arises from the right ventricle and divides into right and left pulmonary arteries which convey deoxygenated blood to the right and left lung, respectively. The blood circulates through a capillary plexus intimately related to the walls of alveoli and receives oxygen from the alveolar air. This blood which is now oxygenated is returned to the heart (left atrium) through four pulmonary veins.

Characteristic features of pulmonary circulation

- The pulmonary arteries and their branches are thin-walled and distensible, giving the pulmonary arterial tree a large compliance. The distensibility of pulmonary vessels makes the pulmonary circulation a *low- pressure, low-resistance and high-capacitance system.*
- The thickness of the right ventricle and pulmonary artery is approximately one third of the thickness of left ventricle and aorta, respectively.
- The pulmonary arterioles have very little smooth muscles in their walls. The pulmonary capillaries are larger in diameter than systemic capillaries and have multiple anastomoses.
- The pulmonary capillaries surround the alveoli and are sandwiched between their walls as a result each alveolus seems to be enclosed in a basket of capillaries (Fig. 7.1-12).
- *Pulmonary capillary pressure* is about 10 mmHg. Since this pressure is far below the colloid osmotic pressure (25 mmHg), so a net suction force of 15 mmHg tends

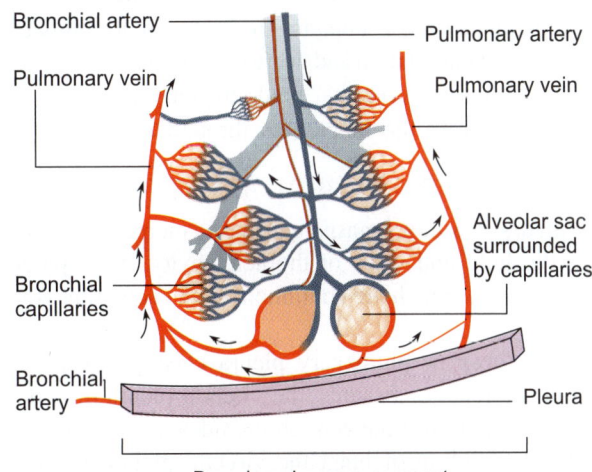

Fig. 7.1-12. Organization of pulmonary circulation.

to draw fluid from alveolar interstitial space into the pulmonary capillaries *which keeps the alveoli dry.* However, if the pulmonary capillary hydrostatic pressure rises above 25 mmHg fluid can escape into the interstitial space leading to *pulmonary oedema.* This can happen during exercise, particularly at high altitude, in left heart failure, mitral stenosis and pulmonary fibrosis which reduces the rate of gas exchange in the lungs. The resultant hypoxia may be fatal.

- *Pulmonary vessels contain* about 600 ml of blood at rest. Since the pulmonary vessels act as capacitance vessels their blood content can vary from 200 ml to 900 ml. Pulmonary blood volume *decreases* in conditions like standing and *increases* on changing posture from standing to lying.

LYMPHATIC CIRCULATION

Lungs are richly supplied by lymphatics. Lymphatics are present in the walls of the terminal bronchioles and in all the supportive tissues of the lungs. Particulate matter entering the alveoli during inspiration is removed by way of lymphatic channels. Lymphatics also remove the plasma proteins leaking from the lung capillaries and thus help to prevent the pulmonary oedema. The deep lymphatic vessels follow the bronchi and first drain into the *pulmonary nodes* (in the substance of the lungs) and then into *bronchopulmonary nodes.* The superficial lymph vessels lie near the surface of lungs and converge on to bronchopulmonary nodes. From bronchopul-monary node lymph drains into *tracheobronchial nodes* and from there into the *bronchomediastinal trunk.*

INNERVATION

- *Parasympathetic* fibres pass through vagus nerve. Their stimulation causes bronchoconstriction and increased bronchial secretion via muscarinic receptors.
- *Sympathetic nerves* supplying the lungs when stimulated cause bronchodilation and decreased bronchial secretion via adrenergic receptors, predominantly β_2.
- *Afferents* from the lungs pass through vagii.

PLEURA AND PLEURAL CAVITY

The pleura is a thin, transparent, moist membrane which lines the lung and walls of thoracic cavity. Thus pleura has two layers which are continuous with each other (Fig. 7.1-13):

Visceral layer or plumonary pleura closely covers the lung at the level of fissures, the visceral pleura dips into the fissure and lines the contiguous sides of the lobes. At the level of hilum of lung, the visceral pleura becomes continuous with the part of parietal pleura which covers the structures forming the root of lung (Fig. 7.1-10).

Parietal layer of pleura lines the walls of thoracic cavity and becomes continuous with the visceral pleura round the edges of hilum. Parietal pleura can be divided into following parts (Fig. 7.1-13):

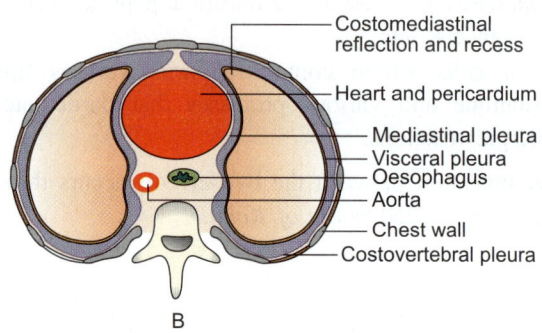

Fig. 7.1-13. *Pleura and pleural cavity : A, as seen in schematic coronal section through the thorax; and B, as seen in schematic transverse section through the thorax.*

- *Costovertebral pleura* refers to that part of parietal pleura which lines the inner aspect of ribs, intercostal spaces, part of inner surface of sternum and the sides of thoracic vertebrae.
- *Diaphragmatic pleura* refers to that part of parietal pleura that lines the convex part of diaphragm coming in contact with the base of lung.
- *Mediastinal pleura* lines the structures of mediastinum coming in contact with medial surface of the lung. The mediastinal pleura extends as a tube around the structures forming root of the lung and becomes continuous with visceral pleura round the edges of hilum.

Pleural cavity refers to the potential space between the visceral and parietal layer of pleura. The two layers of pleura are separated by only a very thin layer of serous fluid which helps these layers to move easily upon each other with respiratory movements of chest wall. Important *clinically applied aspects* are :

- *Pleurisy* i.e. when the surface of pleura becomes inflamed, friction results, and the sounds produced by this rubbing can be heard through the stethoscope.

- *Hydrothorax* refers to collection of fluid in the pleural cavity (e.g. as in pleurisy). It results in compression of the lung and possibly collapse of the portion of lung.
- *Pneumothorax* i.e. collection of air in the pleural cavity occurs following a puncture in the thoracic wall. It also results in collapse of lung. If the puncture in chest wall is closed, the air is gradually absorbed, and the lung resumes its normal position.

FUNCTIONS OF RESPIRATORY SYSTEM

A. Respiratory functions

The main function of the respiratory system in general and lung in particular is exchange of gases between atmosphere and blood.

B. Non-respiratory functions

I. Functions subserved by lung defence mechanisms

1. *Immunoglobulin-A (IgA)* secreted in the bronchial secretion protects against respiratory infections.

2. *Ciliary escalator action* is an important defence system against air-borne infections. The dust particles in the inhaled air are often laden with bacteria. While passing through the repeatedly branched bronchial tree the dust particles and the bacteria are caught in the mucous layer present at the mucosal surface of respiratory passages and are moved up towards pharynx by the rhythmic upward beating action of cilia (Fig. 7.1-14) and swallowed. Cigarette smoke disturbs the ciliary function.

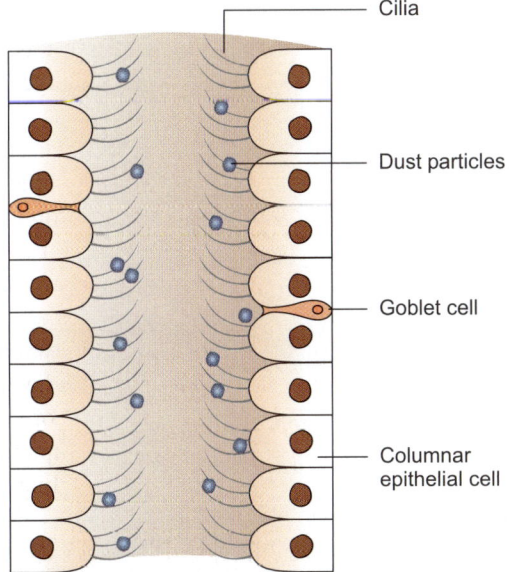

Fig. 7.1-14. Ciliary escalator action of the respiratory mucosa.

Cilia

Dust particles

Goblet cell

Columnar epithelial cell

3. *Pulmonary alveolar macrophages (PAM)* play important role in defence system by following mechanisms:
- Being actively phagocytic cells they ingest the inhaled bacteria and small particles.
- Help in processing inhaled antigens for immunologic attack.
- PAMs secrete substances that attract polymorphonuclear cells to the lungs.
- By some secretions they stimulate granulocyte and monocyte formation in the bone marrow.

4. *Cough reflex.* The laryngeal, tracheal, and bronchial mucous membranes contain vagal afferent terminals which act as *irritant receptors.* Stimulation of these receptors by chemical or mechanical stimuli (excessive mucus, inadvertently inhaled foodstuff etc.) produce a bout of coughing which helps in expulsion of foreign material.

II. Functions subserved by pulmonary circulation

1. *Reservoir for left ventricle.* When left ventricle output becomes transiently greater than systemic venous return, the blood stored in pulmonary circulation helps in maintaining the left ventricular output for few strokes.

2. *Pulmonary circulation acts as a filter* and filters out particles from the blood, which may include small fibrin or blood clots, detached cancer cells, fat cells, gas bubbles, agglutinated RBCs, masses of platelets and debris from stored blood.

3. *Removal of fluid from alveoli.* Because of low pulmonary hydrostatic pressure the fluid entering the alveoli is absorbed by the capillaries. This protects the gas exchange function of lungs and opposes transudation of fluid from capillaries to the alveoli.

4. *Role in absorption of drugs.* Certain drugs that rapidly pass through the alveolar capillary barrier by diffusion are administered by inhalation, e.g. anaesthetic gases, aerosol and other bronchodilators.

III. Metabolic functions of lungs

1. *Surfactant* produced in the lungs plays an important role in respiration (for details see page 236).

2. *Protein synthesis* for maintenance of structural framework.

3. *Conversion of angiotensin I to II* is performed by the enzyme angiotensin-converting enzyme (ACE) present in the pulmonary capillary endothelium.

4. *Inactivation partly or completely* of many vasoactive substances present in the blood is done by capillary endothelial cells as they pass through pulmonary circulation.

CHAPTER 7.1

5. *Fibrinolytic mechanism* present in the lung lyses clot in the pulmonary vessels.

6. *Storage of hormones and certain biologically active peptides* is done in the APUD cells and nerve fibres present in the alveoli. These substances include VIP, substance P, opioid peptides, cholecystokinin-pancreozymin (CCK-PZ) and somatostatin. These substances are later released into the systemic circulation.

IV. Functions subserved by respiratory muscles

Respiratory muscles are also used during laughing and singing.

Physiology of Respiration

INTRODUCTION

The word respiration has been derived from the Latin word 'respirare' which means to breathe.

The primary role of the respiratory system is to provide O_2 to the tissues for metabolic needs and remove the CO_2 formed by them. An adult body consumes about 250 ml of O_2 and produces about 200 ml of CO_2 per minute. Respiration entails two processes: the external respiration and internal respiration.

The *internal respiration* or tissue respiration refers to utilization of O_2 and production of CO_2 by the tissue.

The *external respiration* includes supply of O_2 to the tissues from the environment and excretion of CO_2 released by the tissues into the atmosphere. The process of external respiration involves three major events:

- *Pulmonary ventilation*, i.e. exchange of gases between the environment and lungs. It includes mechanics of respiration.
- *Pulmonary diffusion* refers to transfer of gases from alveoli to the blood by diffusion across the respiratory membrane.
- *Transport of gases* from the blood to the body cells and back.

PULMONARY VENTILATION

Pulmonary ventilation, as defined above, refers to the process of exchange of gases between the environment and lungs. Inflation and deflation of the lung occurring with each breath ensures this regular exchange of gases. The aspects and concepts related to pulmonary ventilation which need deliberation include :

- Mechanism of breathing,
- Pressure and volume changes during respiratory cycle,
- Lung volumes and capacities,
- Pulmonary elastance and compliance.

MECHANISM OF BREATHING

Pulmonary ventilation is accomplished by two processes:

- Inspiration, and
- Expiration.

Inspiration

Inspiration refers to inflow of atmospheric air into the lungs. This obviously occurs when the intrapulmonary pressure falls below the atmospheric air pressure.

It is an active process, normally produced by contraction of the *inspiratory muscles*. During tidal inspiration (quiet breathing) the diaphragm and external intercostal muscles contract and cause increase in all the three dimensions of thoracic cavity.

1. *Role of diaphragm.* In tidal inspiration (quiet breathing) 70-75% of expansion of chest is caused due to contraction of diaphragm. The diaphragm is a dome-shaped, musculotendinous partition between thorax and abdomen. The convexity of this dome is directed towards the thorax. When the diaphragm contracts following changes occur:

- The dome becomes flattened and the level of diaphragm is lowered *increasing the vertical diameter* of the thoracic cavity (Fig. 7.2.1A). During quiet breathing the descent of diaphragm is about 1.5 cm and during forced inspiration it increases to 7 cm.
- The descent of diaphragm causes rise in intra-abdominal pressure which is accommodated by the reciprocal relaxation of the abdominal wall musculature.
- Contraction of diaphragm also lifts the lower ribs causing thoracic expansion laterally and anteriorly (the bucket handle and pump handle effect, respectively) (Fig. 7.2-1B and C).

2. *Role of external intercostal muscles.* When the external intercostal muscles contract the ribs are elevated causing lateral and anteroposterior enlargement of thoracic cavity due to the so-called bucket handle and pump handle effects, respectively.

3. *Role of laryngeal muscles.* The abductor muscles of the larynx contract during inspiration pulling the vocal cords apart.

Forced inspiration is characterized by:

1. *Forceful contraction of diaphragm* leading to descent of diaphragm by 7 to 10 cm as compared to 1 to 1.5 cm during quiet inspiration.

2. *Forceful contraction of external intercostal muscles* causing more elevation of ribs leading to more increase in transverse and anteroposterior diameter of thoracic cavity.

3. *Contraction of accessory muscles of inspiration:* sternomastoid muscles, anterior serrati muscles, and scaleni muscles causes further expansion of thorax.

Expiration

Expiration refers to outflow of air from the lungs into the atmosphere. This obviously occurs when the intrapulmonary pressure rises above the atmospheric air pressure. Expiration in quiet breathing is largely a passive phenomenon and is brought about by the:

- Elastic recoil of the lungs,
- Decrease in size of the thoracic cavity due to relaxation of diaphragm and external intercostal muscles.

Forced expiration is required when respiration is increased during exercise or in the presence of severe respiratory disease. It is an active process caused by:

1. *Contraction of abdominal muscles, which causes:*

A. Vertical expansion   B. Transverse expansion   C. Anteroposterior expansion

Fig. 7.2-1. Mechanism of increase in diameter of thoracic cavity : A, increase in vertical diameter (descent of diaphargm); B, increase in transverse diameter (bucket handle effect); and C, increase in anteroposterior diameter (pump handle effect).

- Downward pull on the lower ribs and thus decrease the anteroposterior diameter of the thoracic cavity.
- Fixation of the lower ribs so that internal intercostal muscles act more effectively.

2. *Contraction of the internal intercostal muscles* tends to pull all the ribs downwards reducing anteroposterior diameter (because of falling of pump handle effect) as well as the transverse diameter (because of action of ribs like falling of bucket handle) of the thoracic cavity.

PRESSURE AND VOLUME CHANGES DURING RESPIRATORY CYCLE

Intrapulmonary pressure changes during respiratory cycle (Fig. 7.2-2)

The movement of air in and out of the lungs depends primarily on the pressure gradient between the alveoli and the atmosphere (i.e. *transairway pressure).* Intrapulmonary or alveolar pressure is the air pressure inside the lung alvceli. Intrapulmonary pressure changes during respiratory cycle are as below (Fig. 7.2-2) :

- *At end-expiration and end-inspiration,* i.e. when the glottis is open and there is no movement of air, the pressures in all parts of the respiratory tree are equal to atmospheric pressure, the intrapulmonary pressure is considered to be *zero* mm of Hg.

- *During inspiration* in quiet breathing, the pressure in the alveoli decreases to about –1 mm of Hg, which is sufficient to suck in about 500 ml of air into the lungs within 2 seconds period of inspiration. At the end-inspiration the intrapulmonary pressure again becomes zero.

- *During expiration* in quiet breathing, the elastic recoil of the lungs causes the intrapulmonary pressure to swing slightly to the positive side (+1 mm of Hg) which forces the 500 ml of inspired air out of the lungs during 2 to 3 seconds of expiration. At the end-expiration, once again the alveolar pressure regains the atmospheric pressure (zero mm of Hg).

Forceful expiration against closed glottis (Valsalva's manoeuvre) may produce intrapulmonary pressure of as much as 100 mmHg.

Intrapleural (pleural) pressure changes during respiratory cycle

Pleural pressure is the pressure of fluid in the space between the visceral pleura and parietal pleura. Intrapleural pressure changes during respiratory cycle are as below (Fig. 7.2-2) :

- *Normal pleural pressure* when the respiratory muscles are completely relaxed and the airways are open is about –2.5 mm of Hg. It is the result of balance of two opposite forces, the recoil tendency of the lungs and the recoil tendency of thoracic cage.

- *During inspiration* due to expansion of the chest wall the pleural pressure becomes still more negative (–6 mm of Hg) and pulls the surface of lungs with greater force creating negative intrapulmonary pressure.

- *During expiration.* At the end of inspiration, the inspiratory muscles relax and the recoiling force of lungs begins to pull the chest wall back to expiratory position. At end-expiratory position where the recoil force of the lungs and recoil force of thoracic cage

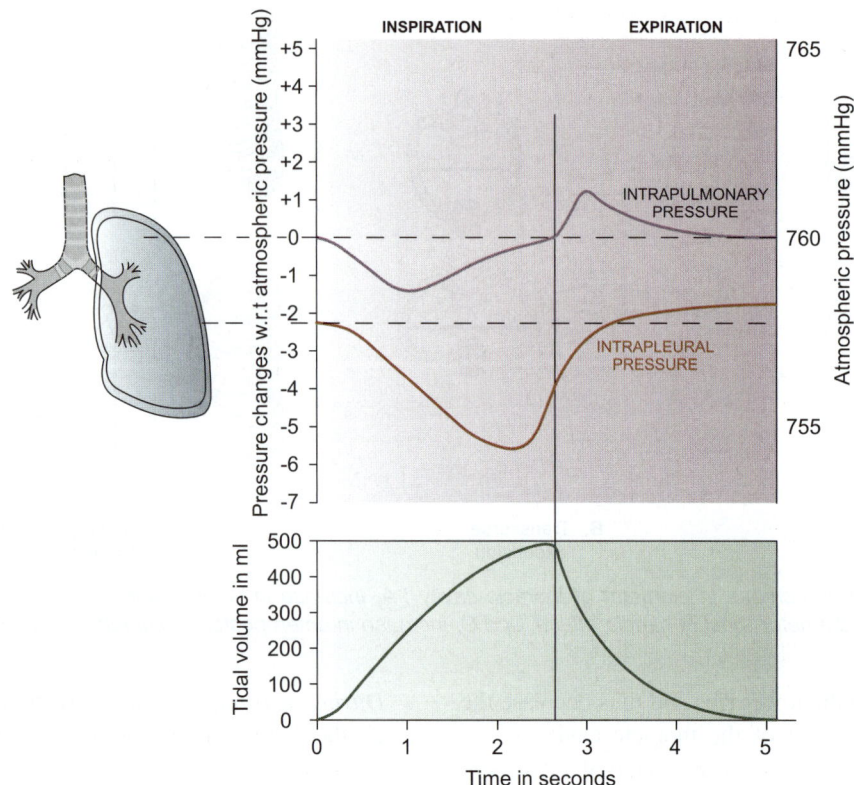

Fig. 7.2-2. *Pressure and volume changes during respiratory cycle.*

balance, the pleural pressure returns back to –2.5 mm of Hg.

Lung volume changes during respiratory cycle

- *During tidal inspiration* the volume of air in the lungs increases by 500 ml (tidal volume).
- *During tidal expiration*, the elastic forces compress the gas in the lungs which starts flowing out and at the end of expiration the volume of air in the lungs decreases by 500 ml (Fig. 7.2-2).

LUNG VOLUMES AND CAPACITIES

Lung volumes

The maximum volume to which a lung can be expanded has been divided into four non-overlapping volumes (Fig. 7.2-3).

1. Tidal volume (TV). It is the volume of air inspired or expired with each breath during normal quiet breathing. It is approximately 500 ml in normal adult male.

2. Inspiratory reserve volume (IRV). It is the extra volume of air that can be inhaled by a maximum inspiratory effort over and beyond the normal tidal volume. It is about 3000 ml in a normal adult male.

3. Expiratory reserve volume (ERV). It is the extra volume of air that can be exhaled by maximum forceful expiration over and beyond the normal tidal volume (i.e.

after the end of normal passive expiration). It is approximately 1100 ml in a normal adult male.

4. Residual volume (RV). It is the volume of the air that still remains in the lungs after the most forceful expiration. It is about 1200 ml in a normal adult male.

Lung capacities

Lung capacities are combination of two or more pulmonary volumes and include (Fig. 7.2-3):

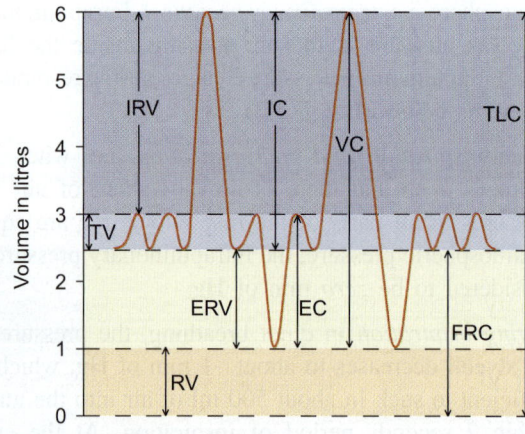

Fig. 7.2-3. *A spirogram showing various lung volumes and capacities.*

1. *Inspiratory capacity (IC).* This is the maximum volume of the air that can be inspired after normal tidal expiration. Therefore, it equals the tidal volume plus inspiratory reserve volume (TV + IRV) and is approximately 3500 ml in a normal adult male.

2. *Expiratory capacity (EC).* It is the maximum volume of air that can be expired after normal tidal inspiration. It equals tidal volume plus expiratory reserve volume (TV + ERV) and is approximately about 1600 ml in a normal adult male.

3. *Functional residual capacity (FRC).* It is the volume of air remaining in the lungs after normal tidal expiration. Therefore, it equals the expiratory reserve volume plus the residual volume (ERV + RV) and is about 2300 ml in a normal adult male.

Significance of functional residual capacity (FRC). The FRC (RV + ERV) of about 2300 ml represents the air that remains in the lungs most of the time. Even after the most forceful expiration about 1200 ml (residual volume) air is always present in the lungs. This has several advantages:

i. *Continuous exchange of gases* is possible due to presence of some air always in the lungs, and thereby concentration of O_2 and CO_2 in blood are maintained constant. Without FRC, pO_2 would have risen to 150 mmHg during inspiration, and reduced nearly to zero during expiration, which is maintained at about 100 mm of Hg due to the FRC.

ii. *Breath-holding* is made possible due to the FRC.

iii. *Dilution of toxic inhaled gases* occurs due to the reserve of 2300 ml of air in the lungs (FRC) most of the time.

iv. *Load on respiratory mechanism and left ventricle* would have been much more if there was no FRC.

4. *Vital capacity (VC).* This is the maximum amount of air a person can expel from the lungs after the deepest possible inspiration. Therefore it equals tidal volume plus inspiratory reserve volume plus expiratory reserve volume (TV + IRV + ERV) and is about 4600 ml in a normal adult male. Vital capacity depends on various factors. These include:

i. *Size of the thoracic cavity.* VC is more in males (2.6 L/m² body surface area) because of large chest size and more muscle power than females.

ii. *Age.* In old age VC is decreased due to decrease in elasticity of the lungs.

iii. *Strength of respiratory muscles.* In swimmers and divers VC is more because of the increased strength of the respiratory muscles.

iv. *Gravity.* In standing position VC is more than in sitting and lying position because of:

- Increased size of thoracic cavity in standing (diaphragm moves down), and
- Reduced pulmonary blood flow due to decreased venous return.

v. *In pregnancy* VC is reduced due to pushing up of diaphragm and reduced capacity of thoracic cavity.

vi. *In ascites* (accumulation of fluid in the abdominal cavity) VC is reduced due to same reason as in pregnancy.

vii. *Pulmonary diseases* like pulmonary fibrosis, emphysema, respiratory obstruction, pulmonary oedema, pleural effusion and pneumothorax are associated in decreased VC.

5. *Timed vital capacity (TVC) or forced vital capacities.* Forced vital capacity is the volume of the air that can be expired rapidly with a maximum force following a maximum inspiration. The volume of air expired can be timed by recording the vital capacity on a spirograph moving at the known speed. Components of TVC or FVC (Fig. 7.2-4) are:

Fig. 7.2-4. *Components of timed vital capacity.*

i. *Forced expiratory volume in 1 sec. (FEV_1).* It represents the volume expired in the first second of a FVC. FEV_1% is the per cent of FVC expired in one second (i.e. FEV_1% = FEV_1 / FVC × 100). Normally FEV_1% is about 80% of the FVC (Fig. 7.2-5A). Estimation of FEV_1 is the most commonly used screening test for airway diseases.

Clinical application. FEV_1 is useful in distinguishing between restrictive and obstructive lung diseases:

- Patients with *restrictive lung disease* (e.g. kyphoscoliosis and ankylosing spondylitis) have a reduced FVC but are able to achieve relatively high flow rates; therefore their FEV_1% exceeds 80% (Fig. 7.2-5B).
- Patients with *obstructive lung disease* (e.g. bronchial asthma) have low flow rates as a result of high airway

Fig. 7.2-5. *Forced expiratory volume in first sec (FEV$_1$) component of timed vital capacity: A, in normal subject; B, in a patient with restrictive lung disease; and C, in a patient with restrictive lung disease.*

resistance. Therefore their FEV$_1$% is abnormally low (Fig. 7.2-5C).

ii. *Forced expiratory volume in 2 sec. (FEV$_2$).* It represents the volume of air expired in first 2 sec. of FVC; FEV$_2$% is about 90% of FVC under normal condition.

iii. *Forced expiratory volume in 3 sec. (FEV$_3$).* It represents the volume of air expired in first 3 sec. Normally FEV$_3$% is 98-100% of FVC.

6. *Total lung capacity (TLC).* It is the volume of air present in the lungs after the maximal inspiration. It equals the vital capacity plus the residual volume (VC + RV) and is about 5800 ml in a normal adult male.

Minute ventilation (MV) or pulmonary ventilation (PV)

It is the volume of air inspired or expired per minute. It equals the tidal volume multiplied by respiratory rate (TV × RR). The TV at rest averages 500 ml (0.5 L), and the normal respiratory rate is 12-15 breaths/min; therefore normal minute volume is 6-7.5 L/min.

Maximum breathing capacity (MBC) or maximum voluntary ventilation or maximum ventilation volume (MVV). It is the maximum volume of air that can be ventilated on command during a given interval. Normal adult male can attain a maximum ventilation volume (MVV) of 80 to 170 L/min (average 100 L/min).

- MVV is profoundly reduced in patients with emphysema, airway obstruction and very poor respiratory muscle strength.

Measurement of static lung volumes and capacities

All volumes and capacities except residual volume, functional residual capacity and total lung capacity are recorded by *spirometer*. Functional residual capacity is determined by nitrogen washout method or helium dilution method and then residual volume and total lung capacity are calculated.

Recording of lung volumes and capacities are the important lung function tests.

PULMONARY ELASTANCE AND COMPLIANCE

Pulmonary elastance

Elastance refers to *recoil* (retractive) tendency of a structure. Both the thoracic cage and lungs have elastance.

Elastance or recoil tendency of the thoracic cage refers to constant tendency of the thoracic cage to expand (to pop outward). The elastance of the thoracic cage is because of the fact that the chest wall is an elastic structure which is normally kept partially pulled inward. The elastic property of the thoracic cage is because of the elastic nature of ribs, muscles and tendons.

Elastance of lungs. Elastance or recoil tendency of the lungs refer to the constant tendency of the lungs to collapse. The recoil forces in the lungs are generated by:

- *Tissue forces.* These are due to the presence of many elastic tissues such as smooth muscle, elastic and collagen in the lung parenchyma which are kept under constant stretch in the inflated lungs.

- *Surface forces.* These are generated at the alveolar surface lined by fluid (*alveolar surface tension*) due to which the alveoli tend to become progressively smaller and tend to collapse.

Alveolar surface tension

Alveolar surface tension is generated because of the unbalanced attraction of the liquid molecules at the surface of alveolar membrane.

Pulmonary surfactant. Pulmonary surfactant is a complex mixture of several phospholipids, proteins and ions. It is secreted by type II alveolar epithelial cells (granular pneumocytes). The presence of pulmonary surfactant in the fluid lining the alveoli reduces the surface tension markedly.

Respiratory distress syndrome (RDS) of newborn or the *hyaline membrane disease* occurs in the newborn babies (especially premature) due to inadequate formation of surfactant resulting in an elevated alveolar surface tension. In this condition it is extremely difficult to expand the lungs. Respiratory work is greatly increased and there is inadequate exchange of gases due to alveolar instability, pulmonary oedema, and collapse of alveoli (atelectasis) in many areas. This results in severe respiratory insufficiency and the infant may die.

Pulmonary compliance

- Compliance (C) refers to change in lung volume (ΔV) per unit change in transpulmonary pressure (ΔP), i.e

$$C = \frac{\Delta V}{\Delta P}$$

Transpulmonary pressure is the difference in the pressure between alveolar pressure and pleural pressure.

- Compliance expresses the distensibility (expansibility) of the lung and chest wall.
- Normal value of compliance for the lungs and chest wall combined is 0.13 L/cm of H_2O and for the lung alone it is 0.22 L/cm of H_2O.

PULMONARY DIFFUSION

INTRODUCTION

Pulmonary diffusion refers to transfer of gases from alveoli to capillary blood across the respiratory membrane.

To understand the intricacies of diffusion of gases across the respiratory membrane it is essential to have knowledge about the following related aspects and concepts:

- Pulmonary perfusion, i.e. pulmonary blood flow (see page 184).
- Physics of gas diffusion and gas partial pressures.
- Alveolar ventilation, i.e. the rate at which new air reaches the gas exchange area of the lungs.
- Alveolar ventilation-perfusion ratio.
- Diffusion of gases through the respiratory membrane.

PHYSICS OF GAS DIFFUSION AND GAS PARTIAL PRESSURES

Some of the important aspects concerning physics of gas diffusion and gas partial pressures are :

Gas pressure

The gas molecules have a kinetic energy so they are in a continuous random motion. These molecules bounce against each other and/or against the walls of container and exert a pressure. The gas pressure (P) exerted is denoted by the equation :

$$P = \frac{nRT}{V}, \text{ where}$$

P = Pressure of gas,
n = Number of molecules of gas,
T = Absolute temperature,
V = Volume of gas, and
R = Gas constant.

Partial pressure

According to *Dalton's law* of partial pressure, the total pressure exerted by a mixture of gases is equal to the sum of the partial pressure of all gases present in the mixture. Thus, the partial pressure (p) refers to the pressure exerted by any one gas present in a mixture of gases. Hence, the partial pressure (p) of a gas can be calculated by multiplying its fractional concentration by the total pressure. For example, environmental air which has atmospheric pressure (at sea level) of about 760 mmHg is a mixuture of 21% oxygen (O_2), and 79% nitrogen (N_2). Therefore, the partial pressure (p) of O_2 and N_2 respectively will be:

$$pO_2 = 760 \times \frac{21}{100} = 160 \text{ mmHg, and}$$

$$pN_2 = 760 \times \frac{79}{100} = 600 \text{ mmHg.}$$

Water vapour pressure

The atmospheric air entering the respiratory passages during inspiration is humidified by the water vapours from the conducting passages. By the time the atmospheric air reaches the alveoli it is saturated with water vapours. Thus, in the alveolar air, besides O_2 and N_2, water vapours also exert their partial pressure. Vapour pressure of water is dependant upon its temperature. At body temperature (37°C) the vapour pressure of water in alveolar air is 47 mmHg.

ALVEOLAR VENTILATION

Alveolar ventilation is the volume of the fresh air which reaches the gas exchange area of the lung each minute. During inspiration some of the air inhaled never reaches the gas exchange areas but instead fills the non-gas exchange areas (conducting zone) of the respiratory tract called the *dead space,* which is equal to about 150 ml.

During expiration out of 500 ml of tidal volume 150 ml of the alveolar expired air remains in the conducting passages. Therefore, of 500 ml air entering the lungs only

350 ml/breath is the fresh air which contributes to alveolar ventilation. Thus alveolar ventilation can be calculated as:

Alveolar ventilation (VA) = Respiratory rate × (Tidal volume – Dead space volume), with a normal tidal volume of 500 ml, a normal dead space of 150 ml, and a respiratory rate of 12 breaths per minute, alveolar ventilation equals 12 × (500 – 350), or 4200 ml/min.

ALVEOLAR VENTILATION-PERFUSION RATIO

Alveolar ventilation-perfusion ratio (VA/Q) is the ratio of alveolar ventilation per minute to quantity of blood flow to alveoli per minute. Normally, alveolar ventilation (VA) is 4.2 - 5.0 L/min, and the pulmonary blood flow (equal to cardiac output) is approximately 5 L/min. So, the normal VA/Q is about 0.84 to 0.9. At this ratio maximum oxygenation occurs.

ALVEOLAR AIR

Volume of air which is available for exchange of gases in the alveoli per breath is called alveolar air, which is equivalent to tidal volume minus dead space, i.e. (500 – 150) or 350 ml.

Composition of alveolar air

Alveolar air composition is considerably different than that of atmospheric air because of the following reasons:

- Water vapours dilute the other gases in the inspired air.
- Alveolar air is renewed very slowly by atmospheric air.
- Oxygen is constantly being absorbed from the alveolar air.
- Carbon dioxide is constantly diffusing from the pulmonary blood to alveoli.

Composition of expired air

As shown in Table 7.2-1, the composition of expired air is different than that of alveolar air. This is because of the fact that the expired air is a combination of dead space air and alveolar air.

DIFFUSION OF GASES THROUGH THE RESPIRATORY MEMBRANE

Respiratory unit and respiratory membrane

Each respiratory unit is composed of a respiratory bronchiole, alveolar ducts, atria and alveoli. There are about 300 million respiratory units in the two lungs. Gas exchange occurs through the membranes of all the structures forming a respiratory unit, not merely in the alveoli themselves.

Respiratory membrane or pulmonary membrane or the alveolocapillary membrane is the name given to the tissues which separate the capillary blood from the alveolar air. The exchange of gases between the capillary blood and alveolar air requires diffusion through this membrane.

Table 7.2-1. Composition and partial pressure of gases in atmospheric air, humidified air, alveolar air and expired air

Gas air	Partial pressure (mmHg) and concentration (percentage) of various gases			
	Atmospheric air	Humidified air	Alveolar air	Expired air
N₂	597.0 (78.62%)	563.4 (74.09%)	569.0 (74.9%)	566.0 (74.5%)
O₂	159.0 (20.84%)	149.3 (19.67%)	104.0 (13.6%)	120.0 (15.7%)
CO₂	0.3 (0.04%)	0.3 (0.04%)	40.0 (5.3%)	27.0 (3.6%)
H₂O	3.7 (0.5%)	47 (6.20%)	47.0 (6.2%)	47.0 (6.2%)
Total	760.0 (100%)	760 (100%)	760 (100%)	760 (100%)

Structure of respiratory membrane. It consists of following layers (Fig. 7.2-6):

- Layer of pulmonary surfactant and fluid lining the alveolus,
- Layer of alveolar epithelial cells,
- Basement membrane of the alveolar epithelial cells,

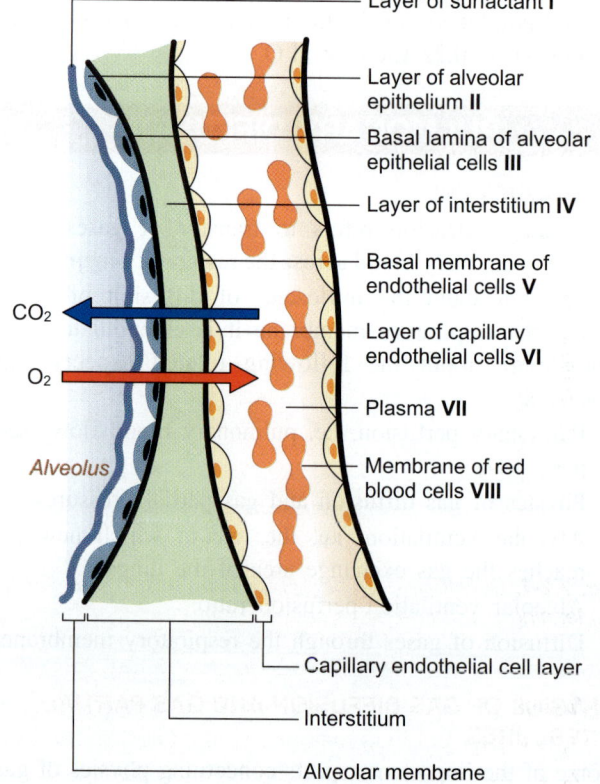

CO₂

O₂

Alveolus

Layer of surfactant **I**

Layer of alveolar epithelium **II**

Basal lamina of alveolar epithelial cells **III**

Layer of interstitium **IV**

Basal membrane of endothelial cells **V**

Layer of capillary endothelial cells **VI**

Plasma **VII**

Membrane of red blood cells **VIII**

Capillary endothelial cell layer

Interstitium

Alveolar membrane

Fig. 7.2-6. Layers of respiratory membrane.

- A very thin interstitial space between the epithelial and endothelial cells,
- Basement membrane of capillary endothelial cells, and
- Layer of capillary endothelial cells.

Surface area of the total respiratory membrane is about 70 square metres in the normal adult.

Diffusion and equilibration of gases across the respiratory membrane

Diffusion of O_2. The normal alveolar pO_2 is 104 mmHg, whereas the blood entering the pulmonary capillary normally has a pO_2 of 40 mmHg. Pressure gradient therefore is 64 mmHg in the beginning. After dissolving in the respiratory membrane, the O_2 molecules diffuse into the blood. As O_2 diffuses from alveoli to blood the pO_2 of blood becomes the same as in alveolar air (104 mmHg), the gradient becomes zero, and no diffusion occurs (Fig. 7.2-7). By the time blood passes to one-third of distance in capillary the pO_2 of blood equals that of alveoli.

Fig. 7.2-7. *Diffusion of oxygen across respiratory membrane (A) leading to progressive increase in capillary pO_2 (B).*

Diffusion of CO_2 occurs from blood to alveoli because pCO_2 is higher in blood than in alveolar air. The average pCO_2 in the pulmonary capillary blood is 46 mmHg as opposed to 40 mmHg in the alveoli. Therefore pressure gradient in the beginning is 6 mmHg and time integrated pressure gradient calculated for CO_2 (in a manner similar to O_2) across the respiratory membrane is only 1 mmHg. Although the pressure gradient for CO_2 is only one-tenth of the O_2 diffusion gradient, CO_2 diffuses almost 20 times more rapidly than O_2 because of higher diffusion coefficient.

Effect of alveolar ventilation-perfusion ratio on pulmonary gas exchange

- Optimum gas exchange across the respiratory membrane occurs when the alveolar ventilation-perfusion ratio (VA/Q) is normal, i.e. between 0.8 and 1.
- Both, a decrease as well as an increase, in VA/Q ratio reduces the gas exchange.

Diffusion capacity of lung

Diffusion capacity (DL) of the lung is quantitative expression of the ability of the respiratory membrane to exchange a gas between the alveoli and the pulmonary blood. It is defined as the volume of gas (V gas) that diffuses through the respiratory membrane of lung each minute for a pressure gradient of 1 mmHg.

TRANSPORT OF GASES

TRANSPORT OF OXYGEN

Transport of oxygen from the lungs to tissues occurs due to constant circulation of blood and diffusion of O_2 that occurs in the direction of concentration gradient which is represented by O_2 tension (pO_2) differences as given below:

- Alveolar air pO_2 : 104 mmHg
- Arterial blood pO_2 : 95 mmHg
- Venous blood pO_2 : 40 mmHg
- Tissue interstitial fluid pO_2 : 40 mmHg

UPTAKE OF OXYGEN BY PULMONARY BLOOD

As mentioned above, pO_2 of pulmonary arterial blood is about 40 mmHg and that of alveolar air is 104 mmHg. Therefore, due to this great concentration gradient oxygen readily diffuses from the alveoli into the blood.

TRANSPORT OF OXYGEN IN ARTERIAL BLOOD

Arterial blood contains about 20 ml of O_2 and venous blood about 15 ml of O_2 per 100 ml. Thus, about 5 ml of O_2 is transpoted per 100 ml of blood from lungs to the tissue cells. Oxygen is transported in the blood in two forms:

- As dissolved form, and
- In combination with haemoglobin.

Oxygen transport in dissolved form

The solubility of O_2 in water (plasma) is so little that at pO_2 value of 100 mmHg, out of the 20 ml of O_2 present in 100 ml of blood, only 0.3 ml is in dissolved form and rest is combined with haemoglobin (as oxyhaemoglobin).

Oxygen transport in combination with haemoglobin

Oxygenation of haemoglobin

After entering into the blood from the alveolar air, most of the oxygen combines with haemoglobin to form a *loose and reversible* combination. This process is called *oxygenation* (not oxidation) and converts deoxyhaemoglobin into oxyhaemoglobin. Each molecule of haemoglobin can combine with as many as *four O_2 molecules.*

Oxygen carrying capacity of haemoglobin

One gram of haemoglobin can bind with maximum of 1.34 ml of O_2. Thus 100 ml of blood with haemoglobin level of 15 gm% can carry 1.34×15, or 20.1 ml of oxygen. Practically 100 ml of the arterial blood carries about 19.8 ml of oxygen out of which about 19.5 ml as oxyhaemoglobin and 0.3 ml as dissolved form in plasma.

Oxygen-haemoglobin dissociation curve

Oxygen-haemoglobin dissociation curve refers to the curve obtained when the relation between the pO_2 and the percentage of haemoglobin saturation is plotted (Fig. 7.2-8). The O_2-Hb dissociation curve shows that percentage saturation of haemoglobin increases with the increase in pO_2 of arterial blood. However the relation is not linear but *sigmoid or S-shaped*

Shifts in O_2-Hb dissociation curve

Several factors affect the affinity for haemoglobin for O_2 and thus shift the O_2-Hb dissociation curve to either right or left.

Shift to right

Shift to right of O_2-Hb dissociation curve signifies decreased affinity of haemoglobin for O_2 (Fig. 7.2-8).

Thus at every level of pO_2, the oxygen saturation of haemoglobin is somewhat lower than the normal curve leading to more offloading of O_2.

Causes. The factors causing right shift are:

1. *An increase in pCO_2* shifts the curve to right, this phenomenon is known as *Bohr's effect* (Fig. 7.2-9A).
2. *A decrease in pH of blood,* as occurs in the tissues, also shifts the O_2-Hb dissociation curve to the right.
3. *Effect of temperature.* An increase in the temperature of blood shifts the curve to right.
4. *Effect of diphosphoglycerate.* The red blood cells are rich in 2,3-diphosphoglycerate (2,3-DPG) which is a highly charged anion that binds to β-chain of deoxygenated adult haemoglobin.

$$HbO_2 + 2,3\text{-DPG} \rightarrow Hb\ 2,3\text{-DPG} + O_2$$

Thus, an increase in the concentration of 2,3-DPG decreases the affinity of Hb for O_2 and shifts the normal O_2-Hb dissociation curve to the right. Causes of increased levels of 2,3-DPG are anaemia, exposure to chronic hypoxia at high altitude and certain pulmonary diseases.

Advantages versus disadvantages of right shift:

- Right shift is advantageous in the tissues where greater O_2 is released from haemoglobin (at the same pO_2).
- However, right shift is disadvantageous in the lungs because (at the same pO_2) blood takes up less oxygen.

Shift to left

Shift to left of O_2-Hb dissociation curve signifies increased affinity of haemoglobin for O_2 (Fig. 7.2-9B). Thus, at every pO_2 level the oxygen saturation of haemoglobin is somewhat greater than in normal curve.

Causes for left shift of the curve are:

- Decreased pCO_2 of blood,
- Increased pH of blood,
- Decreased temperature, and
- Fetal haemoglobin.

Advantages versus disadvantages of left shift. Left shift of the curve has limited advantage because though it allows greater uptake of O_2 at lungs (at same pO_2) but it decreases release of O_2 to the tissues (at same pO_2).

Effect of carbon monoxide on O_2 transport

- Carbon monoxide (CO) interferes with O_2 transport because it has about 200 times the affinity (of oxygen) for haemoglobin.
- CO combines with Hb at the same site on its molecule as O_2 and forms the *carboxyhaemoglobin*, and thus decreases the functional haemoglobin concentration.

RELEASE OF OXYGEN IN TISSUES AT REST

Oxygen delivery represents the amount of O_2 that is presented to body cells per minute. It is equal to the

Fig. 7.2-8 *Normal oxygen-haemoglobin dissociation curve.*

A

B

Fig. 7.2-9 *Right A and left B shift of oxygen-haemoglobin dissociation curve.*

arterial O_2 content multiplied by cardiac output. Since 100 ml of arterial blood at pO_2 of about 100 mmHg contains about 20 ml of oxygen, thus with a cardiac output of about 5 L/min the normal oxygen delivery to the entire body is about 1 L/min. The oxygen delivery to the tissues decreases with either decrease in arterial O_2 content or decrease in cardiac output.

Oxygen consumption. When the arterial blood with approximate pO_2 100 mmHg reaches the tissues with tissue fluid pO_2 40 mmHg, because of pressure gradient, about 5ml of O_2 diffuses from the tissue capillaries to the interstitial fluid out of 100 ml of blood (containing ~ 19 ml O_2) every minute. Thus, oxygen consumption of the whole body at rest with a cardiac output of 5 L/min is about $\dfrac{5 \times 5000}{100}$, or 250 ml of O_2 per minute.

Utilization coefficient. Utilization coefficient refers to the percentage of oxygen consumed out of oxygen delivered to the tissue, i.e.

$$\text{Coefficient of utilization} = \frac{\text{Oxygen consumed/min}}{\text{Oxygen delivered/min}} \times 100$$

So, at rest coefficient of utilization of whole body $= \dfrac{250 \text{ ml/min}}{1000 \text{ ml/min}} \times 100$

$$= 25\%$$

TRANSPORT OF CARBON DIOXIDE

Transport of carbon dioxide from tissue cells to the lungs occurs due to *constant circulation* of blood and diffusion of CO_2 that occurs at various sites in the direction of concentration gradient which is represented by CO_2 tension (pCO_2) differences as given below:

- Intracellular pCO_2 : 46 mmHg
- Interstitial fluid pCO_2 : 45 mmHg
- Arterial blood pCO_2 : 40 mmHg
  (in tissue capillaries)
- Venous blood pCO_2 : 45 mmHg
- Alveolar air pCO_2 : 40 mmHg

From the above pCO_2 levels, it is clear that:

Diffusion of CO_2 from the cells into the interstitial fluid occurs along a tension gradient of 1 mmHg.

Diffusion of CO_2 in blood. From the interstitial fluid the CO_2 diffuses into the capillaries at a tension gradient of 5 mmHg.

Transport of CO_2 in the blood occurs in three forms:

- In dissolved state (7%)
- In bicarbonate form (70%), and
- In carbamino compound form (23%).

Release of CO_2 in lungs. From the venous blood that is supplied to pulmonary capillaries the CO_2 diffuses across the respiratory membrane into the alveoli along a tension gradient of 5 mmHg.

Carbon dioxide dissociation curve

- Carbon dioxide dissociation curve is obtained by plotting the relationship between pCO_2 and total CO_2 content of the blood (Fig. 7.2-10).
- The graph shows that relationship between the two is nearly linear over wider range of pCO_2 (if compared with O_2-Hb dissociation curve, which is sigmoid-shaped).

Rate of total CO_2 transport

In resting conditions each 100 ml of blood transports about 4 ml of CO_2 from the tissues to the lungs. Thus, with an average cardiac output of 5 L/min, a total of (4×5000)/100 or 200 ml of CO_2 is transported/min.

During exercise the amount of CO_2 transported increases depending upon the severity of exercise. In severe exercise, as much as 4 L of CO_2 may be transported per minute.

Respiratory quotient

Definition. Respiratory quotient (RQ) refers to the ratio of the rate of CO_2 excretion and rate of O_2 consumption

Fig. 7.2-10. *Carbon dioxide dissociation curve for oxygenated (solid line) and for deoxygenated blood (dotted line) to demonstrate Haldane's effect.*

per minute. It is also called *respiratory exchange ratio.* **Normal value.** Normally, the rate of CO_2 excretion is 4 ml/100 ml/min, and rate of O_2 consumption is 5 ml/100 ml/min. So, respiratory quotient = 4/5, or 0.8.

REGULATION OF RESPIRATION

Respiration is regulated by a complex integration of neural control mechanisms which are modified by certain respiratory reflexes and chemical control mechanisms.

NEURAL REGULATION OF RESPIRATION

The involuntary neural control system regulates respiration by several groups of neurons situated bilaterally in medulla and pons which include medullary respiratory centres,

pontine respiratory centres, and reticular activating system (RAS).

I. Medullary respiratory centres

The medullary respiratory centres include two groups of neurons: the dorsal respiratory group (DRG), and ventral respiratory group (VRG) which generate the basic respiratory rhythm (Fig.7.2-11).

II. Pontine respiratory centres

The pontine centres include the apneustic centre (APN) and pneumotaxic centre (PNC), both of which modify the activity of medullary respiratory centres.

1. *Apneustic centre (APN).* Refers to a group of inhibitory neurons located bilaterally in the lower part of pons (Fig. 7.2-11). It sends signals to neurons of DRG. This increases the tidal volume and duration of inspiration, resulting in a deeper and more prolonged inspiratory effort termed as *apneusis.* However, normally the apneustic centre is inhibited by impulses carried by the vagus nerves and also by the activity of pneumotaxic centre.

2. *Pneumotaxic centre.* The pneumotaxic centres are located bilaterally in the upper pons. They inhibit the apneustic centre (APN). Therefore, stimulation of PNC shortens inspiration, leading to shallow and more rapid respiratory pattern.

Thus, though rhythm of respiration resides in DRG neurons in medulla, PNC and APN control these neurons to regulate the depth and rate of respiration.

III. Reticular activating system

The reticular activating system (RAS) stimulates the respiratory centres to increase respiratory drive. During sleep, RAS activity diminishes, decreasing respiratory

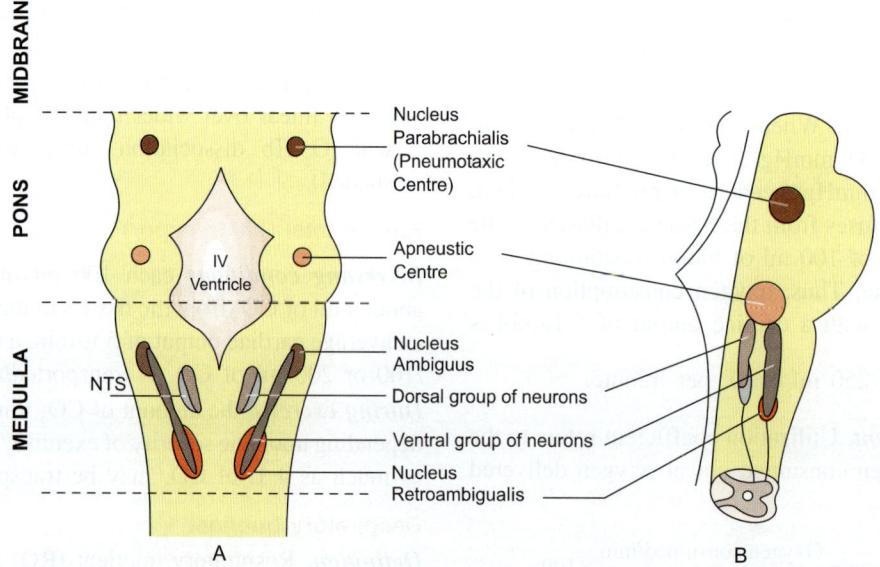

Fig. 7.2-11 *Medullary and pontine respiratory centres: A, front view; and B, lateral view.*

drive, which diminishes alveolar ventilation and results in a slight elevation of arterial CO_2 tension.

CHEMICAL REGULATION OF RESPIRATION

The chemical factors regulating respiration are pCO_2, pO_2 and pH of blood. These factors influence respiration in such a way that their own blood levels are maintained constant. The chemical mechanism of regulation operates through chemoreceptors.

Chemoreceptors

Chemoreceptors are the sensory nerve endings which are highly sensitive to changes in pCO_2, pO_2 and pH of blood. These are of two types:

- Peripheral chemoreceptors, and
- Central chemoreceptors.

Peripheral chemoreceptors

Location. Peripheral chemoreceptors include the carotid and aortic bodies (Fig. 7.2-12).

- *Carotid body* is located on either side near the bifurcation of common carotid artery.
- *Aortic bodies,* two or more in number, are located near the arch of aorta.

Functions. The peripheral chemoreceptors respond to lowered pO_2, increased pCO_2 and increased H^+ concentration in the arterial blood. The afferent impulses from the chemoreceptors stimulate the dorsal respiratory group (DRG) neurons, which lead to an increased rate and depth of respiration called *hyperventilation*. The peripheral chemoreceptors are the only sites that detect changes in pO_2.

Central chemoreceptors

Location. Central chemoreceptors are the cells (neurons) that lie just beneath the ventral surface of the medulla oblongata and are therefore also called medullary receptors (Fig. 7.2-13).

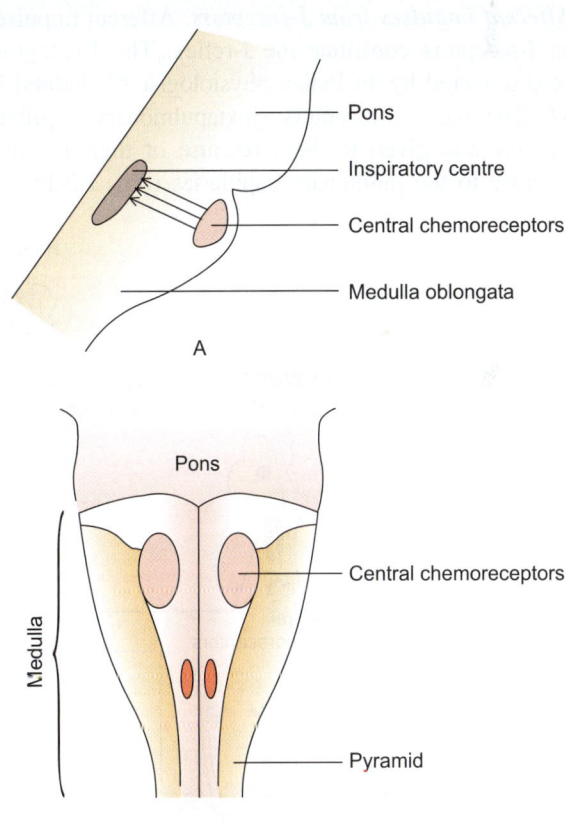

Fig. 7.2-13 *Location of central chemoreceptors in medulla: A, lateral view; and B, front view.*

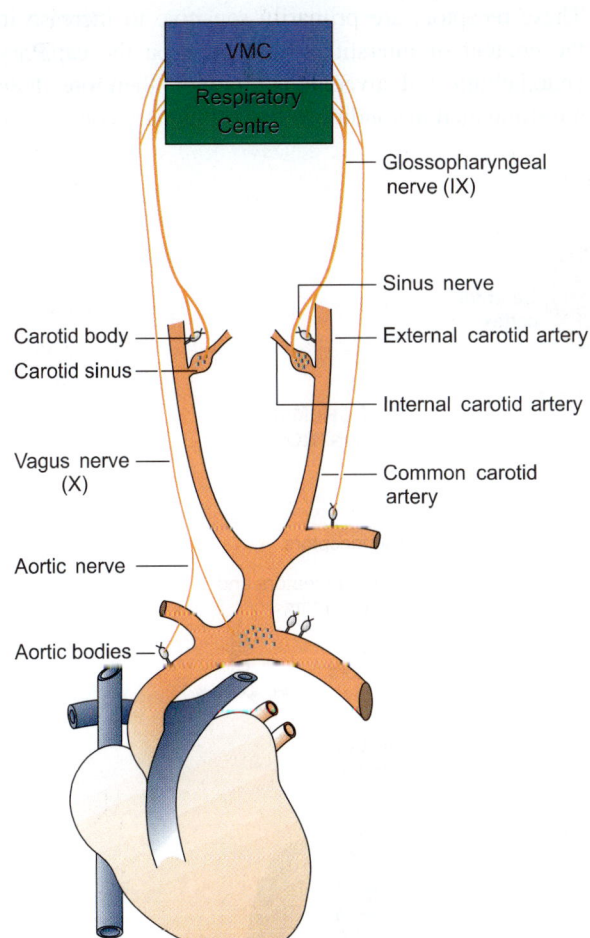

Fig. 7.2-12. *Location of carotid and aortic bodies (peripheral chemoreceptors).*

Stimulation characteristics of central chemoreceptors are:

- They respond to H^+ concentration in the surrounding interstitial fluid and CSF.

• The magnitude of stimulation is directly proportional to the local H^+ concentration, which in turn parallels arterial pCO_2.

OTHER FACTORS THAT INFLUENCE RESPIRATION

Afferent impulses from the receptors other than the chemoreceptors, i.e. from non-chemical receptors include the following (Fig. 7.2-14):

1. *Afferent impulses from pulmonary stretch receptors (Hering-Breuer reflex).* The Hering-Breuer inspiratory inhibitory reflex is initiated when the stretch receptors located in the smooth muscles of the bronchi and bronchioles are stimulated by inflation of the lungs. The impulses are then sent through *vagii nerves* to pontomedullary respiratory centres to inhibit respiration. This reflex is weakest in humans. It does not play any regulatory role in tidal respiration. This reflex is initiated only when the tidal volume is more than 1-1.5 L. Thus, the reflex tends to limit the tidal volume.

2. *Afferent impulses from J-receptors.* Afferent impulses from J-receptors constitute the J-reflex. The J-receptors were discovered by an Indian physiologist AS Paintal in 1954. The name J-receptors (juxtapulmonary capillary receptors) was given to them because of their location very close to the pulmonary capillaries (Fig. 7.2-15).

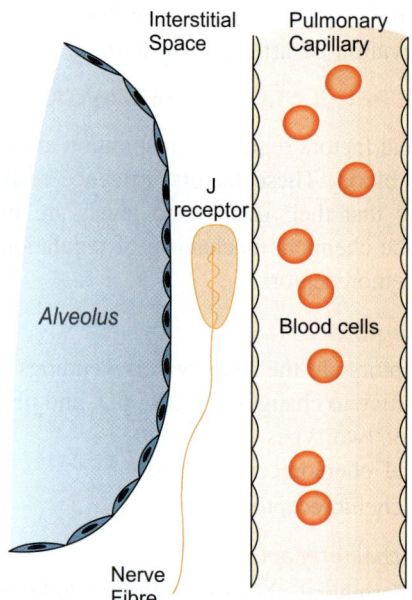

Fig. 7.2-15. *Location of J receptors.*

• These receptors are primarily sensitive to increase in the content of interstitial fluid between the capillary endothelium and alveolar epithelium, therefore, they are stimulated in conditions like pulmonary congestion,

Fig. 7.2-14. *Afferent impulses to respiratory centres.*

pulmonary oedema, pneumonia, hyperinflation of lungs and microembolism in pulmonary capillaries.

3. *Afferent impulses from proprioceptors.* Proprioceptors are the receptors present in the muscles, tendons and joints and are stimulated during change in the position of different parts of the body. This reflex helps in increasing ventilation during exercise. The paediatricians employ this reflex for initiating first breath in the newborn by slapping.

4. *Afferent impulses from thermoreceptors.* Thermoreceptors are those receptors which are stimulated by a change in the body temperature. When warm receptors are stimulated the impulses are conveyed to cerebral cortex via somatic afferent nerves. Cerebral cortex in turn stimulates the respiratory centres to produce hyperventilation.

Respiration helps to maintain body temperature, as some amount of heat is lost in the expired air. In dogs panting is one of the major mechanisms of thermoregulation.

Respiration: Clinically Applied Aspects

7.3

INTRODUCTION

RESPIRATORY ADJUSTMENTS TO STRESSES IN HEALTH
- Exercise
- High altitude
- High atmospheric pressure

DISTURBANCES OF RESPIRATION
Abnormal respiratory patterns
- Apnoea
- Hypoventilation
- Hyperventilation
- Dyspnoea
- Periodic breathing

Disturbances related to respiratory gases
- Hypoxia
- Hypercapnia
- Hypocapnia
- Asphyxia
- Carbon monoxide poisoning

ARTIFICIAL RESPIRATION AND CARDIOPULMONARY RESUSCITATION

Artificial respiration
Cardiopulmonary resuscitation

PULMONARY FUNCTION TESTS
- Ventilatory function tests
- Tests of diffusion
- Tests of ultimate purpose of respiration

INTRODUCTION

Applied respiratory physiology forms a link between the basics of respiration and clinical manifestations of respiratory diseases. This chapter is concerned with some of the important applied aspects of respiration which include:

- Respiratory adjustments to stresses in health,
- Disturbances of respiration,
- Artificial respiration,
- Pulmonary function tests.

RESPIRATORY ADJUSTMENTS TO STRESSES IN HEALTH

Respiratory adjustments to stresses in health illustrate the integrated operation of the respiratory regulatory mechanisms. The stresses faced by respiration requiring adjustments in day to day life include:

- Respiratory adjustments during excercise.
- Respiratory adjustments at high altitude.
- Respiratory adjustments to high atmospheric pressure.

RESPIRATORY ADJUSTMENTS DURING EXERCISE

Exercise is the most frequently faced stress in day-to- day life.

RESPIRATORY RESPONSES TO EXERCISE
I. Increase in pulmonary ventilation

The pulmonary ventilation increases linearly with the increases in intensity of exercise (O_2 consumption) until the anaerobic threshold is reached.

Mechanism of increased pulmonary ventilation

There are several factors which can account for the

marked increase in pulmonary ventilation occurring in severe exercise. The probable factors are :

1. *Neural control mechanisms* play main role in increasing pulmonary ventilation during exercise.

2. *Chemical mechanism* does not play the main role in exercise hyperpnoea, as the alveolar and arterial pO_2 and pCO_2 are well maintained during exercise. Following roles have been suggested, however :

- *Accentuations of the normal oscillations* in pO_2 and pCO_2 synchronous with respiration might stimulate the carotid body chemoreceptors and explains part of exercise hyperpnoea.

- *Acidosis produced due to accumulation of lactic acid* during severe exercise (above the aerobic threshold level) is responsible for increase in pulmonary ventilation.

II. Increase in oxygen uptake in the lungs

The oxygen uptake by blood in the lungs increases from 250 ml/min at rest to about 4 L/min during heavy exercise. This is made possible by :

- Increased pulmonary perfusion,
- Increased alveolar capillary pO_2 gradient, and
- Increased pulmonary diffusion capacity.

RESPIRATORY ADJUSTMENTS AT HIGH ALTITUDE

At high altitude barometric pressure is low and so the partial pressure of O_2 is also low, however, the amount of O_2 in the atmosphere is same as it is at the sea level. When a person is exposed to high altitude particularly by rapid ascent, the different systems of the body cannot cope with the lowered O_2 tension and the effects of hypoxia start. The changes in the body at high altitude are produced mainly by :

- Hypoxia produced by low pO_2, and
- Expansion of gases due to fall in atmospheric pressure.

HYPOXIA AT HIGH ALTITUDE

The effects of hypoxic hypoxia produced by decreasing pO_2 at high altitude depend upon:

- The level of altitude,
- Rate at which hypoxia develops, i.e. hypoxia occurs due to rapid ascent (acute hypoxia) or slow ascent (subacute hypoxia), and
- Duration of exposure to hypoxia, i.e. whether short-term stay or long-term stay (chronic hypoxia).

Clinical syndromes caused by high altitude

The three specific entities (clinical syndromes) which produce effects of low pO_2 at high altitude are:

- High altitude pulmonary oedema (HAPO),
- Acute mountain sickness, and
- Chronic mountain sickness.

High altitude pulmonary oedema

High altitude pulmonary oedema (HAPO) usually occurs as an effect of rapid ascent at high altitude (above 10,000 ft). It is usually seen in individuals who engage in heavy physical work during first 3 to 4 days after rapid ascent to high altitude due to sympathetic stimulation caused by hypoxia.

Acute mountain sickness

The characteristics of acute mountain sick-ness are headache, nausea, vomiting, irritability, insomnia, and breathlessness.

Chronic mountain sickness

Chronic mountain sickness (Monge's disease) occurs in some long-term residents of high altitude who develop extreme polycythaemia, cyanosis, malaise, fatigue and exercise intolerance.

Physiological compensatory responses to high altitude hypoxia

Two types of physiological compensatory responses known to occur in individuals exposed to high altitude hypoxia are accommodation and acclimatization.

Accommodation refers to immediate reflex adjustments of the respiratory and cardiovascular system to hypoxia. These are :

1. *Hyperventilation.* Hyperventilation occurs due to stimulation of peripheal chemoreceptors by low O_2 tension in the arterial blood. The hyperventilation improves arterial pO_2 and reduces pCO_2.

2. *Increase in 2,3-diphosphoglycerate (2,3-DPG)* concentration occurs in RBCs in response to hypoxia.

Acclimatization refers to changes in the body tissues in response to long-term exposure to hypoxia, with following changes occur in the tissues.

1. *Increase in red blood cell count (polycythaemia).* Occurs due to release of renal erythropoietin. This increase in RBC count leads to :
   – increase in haemoglobin concentration
   – increase in haematocrit value.

2. *Increase in pulmonary ventilation.* There is gradual increase in ventilation to an average of above five times as that of normal.

3. *Cardiovascular changes* in the form of tachycardia, and increased force of contraction of the heart.

4. *Pulmonary hypertension.* It occur in response to pulmonary vasoconstriction.

5. *Increase in total lung capacity and diffusion capcity* of lungs.

6. *Cellular and tissue acclimatization* occur by :
- Increase in oxidative enzymes concentration.
- Increase in mitochondrial density, and
- Increase in capillary density.

RESPIRATORY ADJUSTMENTS TO HIGH ATMOSPHERIC PRESSURE

Respiratory adjustments to high atmospheric pressure form a part of physiological problems faced by the body while going under the sea.

PHYSIOLOGICAL PROBLEMS UNDER DEPTH

If the appropriate preventive measures are not taken, then the individuals working at depth in sea will have to face following physiological problems:

Physiological problems due to effect of high pressure on respiratory gases

Air under high atmospheric pressure is breathed under the sea. At high atmospheric pressure of air the partial pressure of oxygen (pO_2), nitrogen (pN_2) and carbon dioxide (pCO_2) is also increased producing following physiological problems.

1. Effects of increased pO_2 (oxygen toxicity)

Oxygen toxicity may be acute or chronic.

Acute oxygen toxicity occurs on exposures to 4 atmosphere pressure of oxygen (pO_2 in lungs about 3000 mmHg).

- *Nervous complications of acute oxygen poisoning* include disorientation, dizziness, convulsions and even coma.
- *Irritation of airways* in the form of nasal congestion, sore throat, substernal discomfort, sneezing, coughing and bronchoconstriction,
- *Pulmonary oedema and atelectasis* begin to develop after 12 hours of exposure.
- *Bronchopneumonia* may be initiated when exposure is continued for more than 24 hours.

2. Effects of increased pN_2 (nitrogen narcosis)

Nitrogen narcosis is characterized by:

- *Euphoric symptoms.* The individual becomes jovial and carefree. These are followed by impairment of mental functions and intelligence, individual becomes drowsy and has poor muscular coordination.

PHYSIOLOGICAL PROBLEMS OF ASCENT

The two physiological problems which occur when an individual ascends back to sea level after sufficient exposure to high atmospheric presssure in the deep sea are:

- Decompression sickness, and
- Air embolism.

Decompression sickness

Decompression sickness is also known as Caisson's disease, dysbarism, compressed air sickness, the bends, and diver's palsy. When the individual ascends rapidly to sea level nitrogen is decompressed and escapes from the tissues at a faster rate. Being gas it forms bubbles while escaping rapidly from the tissues. The gas bubbles block the blood vessels producing tissue ischaemia and sometimes the tissue death. The symptoms produced by escaping gas bubbles constitute the *decompression sickness*. These are:

- *Pain in joints and muscles* of legs or arms.
- *Sensation of numbness,* tingling or pricking (paraesthesia) and itching.
- *The chokes*—shortness of breath.
- *Paralysis* of muscles.
- *Coronary ischaemia* or myocardial infarction.
- *Neurological symptoms* like dizziness and unconsciousness may occur.

Air embolism

Air embolism is another physiological problem which may occur during rapid ascent from a depth below the sea level.

Manifestations of air embolism include chest pain, tachypnoea, systemic hypotension and hypoxaemia. In severe cases, air emboli may travel to the systemic circulation, block the blood flow to some vital organs and may even result in death.

DISTURBANCES OF RESPIRATION

From the physiological viewpoint, disturbances of respiration can be discussed under following headings:

- Abnormal respiratory patterns, and
- Disturbances related to respiratory gases.

ABNORMAL RESPIRATORY PATTERNS

Eupnoea refers to normal respiratory pattern, which implies a normal rate, rhythm and depth of respiration. Various abnormal respiratory patterns (Fig. 7.3-1) can be produced by changes in the environment or diseases affecting the respiratory system, cardiovascular system, or brain. The common altered patterns of respiration are:

- *Tachypnoea* refers to increase in the rate of respiration.
- *Bradypnoea* means decrease in the rate of respiration.
- *Polypnoea* is used to denote the rapid but shallow breathing resembling panting in dogs. In this, the rate of respiration is increased but the force does not change significantly.
- *Apnoea* refers to temporary cessation of breathing.
- *Hypoventilation* term is used to describe a decrease in rate and force of respiration.

Fig. 7.3-1. *Various abnormal respiratory patterns.*

- *Hyperventilation* refers to increase in rate as well as force of respiration.
- *Hyperpnoea* signifies a marked increase in pulmonary ventilation due to increase in rate and/or force of respiration.
- *Dyspnoea.* When hyperpnoea involves 4-5 fold increase in pulmonary ventilation, an unpleasant sensation or discomfort is felt. This type of respiration is called dyspnoea.
- *Periodic breathing* refers to a respiratory pattern characterized by alternate periods of respiratory activity and apnoea. Some of the abnormal respiratory patterns are discussed in detail.

Apnoea

Apnoea refers to temporary cessation of breathing. Depending upon the cause apnoea may be of following types:

1. Voluntary apnoea refers to temporary arrest of breathing due to voluntary control of respiration. It is also called breath-holding.

2. Apnoea after hyperventilation occurs due to reduced stimulation of respiratory centre owing to CO_2 wash caused by hyperventilation.

3. Deglutition apnoea occurs reflexly during swallowing (about 0.5 sec). There is closure of glottis (the opening between vocal cords). This effect prevents aspiration of fluid or food into the lungs

4. Breath-holding attacks are attacks of brief period of apnoea which occur in infants and young children and are generally precipitated by emotional distress.

5. Adrenaline apnoea occurs after injection of high doses of adrenaline.

6. Sleep apnoea refers to cessation of breathing for a brief period (10 sec) during sleep in normal individual.

Hypoventilation

Hypoventilation refers to decrease in rate and force of respiration. Thus, in hypoventilation the amount of air moving in and out of lungs is reduced.

Hyperventilation

Hyperventilation refers to increase in rate as well as force of respiration. Thus, in hyperventilation the amount of air moving in and out of lungs is increased.

Causes of hyperventilation are:
- During exercise due to stimulation of respiratory centres by increased pCO_2
- Voluntary hyperventilation
- Secondary to hypoxia.

Dyspnoea

Dyspnoea literally means distressed breathing. Increased respiration without discomfort is called *hyperpnoea*. The word 'air-hunger' is used as synonym to dyspnoea in general language.

Dyspnoea point refers to the height of hyperpnoea at which dyspnoea appears.

Causes of dyspnoea are:
- *Respiratory disorders* such as bronchial asthma, emphysema, pneumonia, pulmonary oedema and penumothorax.
- *Cardiac failure* also causes dyspnoea.

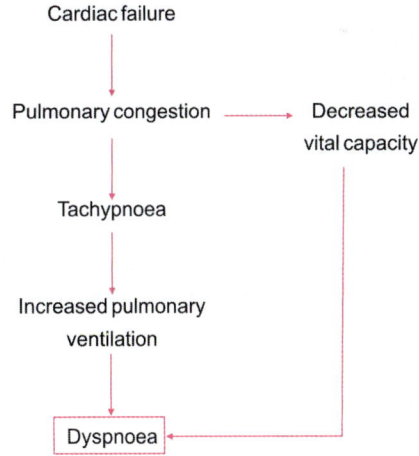

Periodic breathing

Periodic breathing is characterized by alternate periods of respiratory activity and apnoea.

Cheyne-Stokes respiration

Cheyne-Stokes respiration is periodic type of breathing in which the alternate periods of respiratory activity and apnoea occur at regular intervals; and during the period of respiratory activity there is waxing and waning of tidal volume (Fig. 7.3-2).

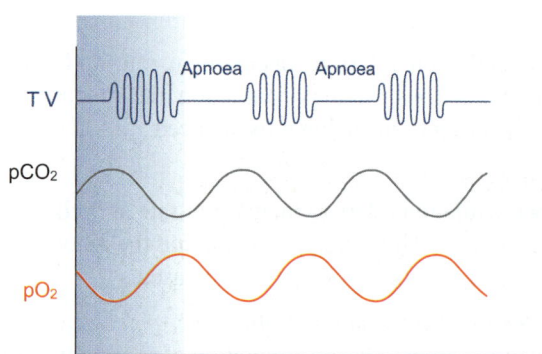

Fig. 7.3-2. *Periodic breathing (Cheyne-Stokes breathing).*

Causes of Cheyne-Stokes respiration are:

1. Physiological causes include:
- Voluntary hyperventilation,
- High altitude, and
- During sleep in some normal individuals especially infants.

2. Pathological causes are:
- Chronic heart failure,
- Brain damage,
- Uraemia, and
- Poisoning by narcotics.

DISTURBANCES RELATED TO RESPIRATORY GASES

Respiratory disturbances related to respiratory gases include:
- Hypoxia,
- Hypercapnia,
- Hypocapnia,
- Asphyxia, and
- Carbon monoxide poisoning.

Hypoxia

The term hypoxia is used to denote deficiency of oxygen supply at the tissue level. It has almost replaced the term anoxia (complete absence of oxygen), which rarely occurs practically.

Causes and types

Causes. Hypoxia can occur because of any one or more of the following defects:
- Decreased oxygen tension (pO_2) of the arterial blood,
- Decreased oxygen carrying capacity of the blood,
- Decreased rate of blood flow to the tissue, or
- Decreased utilization of oxygen by tissue cells.

Types. Depending upon the mechanism of occurrence there are four types of hypoxia:
- Hypoxic hypoxia,
- Anaemic hypoxia,
- Stagnant hypoxia, and
- Histotoxic hypoxia.

1. *Hypoxic hypoxia.* Hypoxic hypoxia occurs due to decreased oxygen tension (pO_2) of the arterial blood, hence also called *arterial hypoxia*. Therefore, in this condition O_2 carrying capacity of blood, rate of blood flow to tissue, and utilization of O_2 by tissues is normal.

Causes of hypoxic hypoxia are:

1. *Low oxygen tension (pO_2) in inspired air.* High altitude, where person is exposed to low atmospheric pO_2,

2. *Hypoventilation* due to any cause, e.g. obstruction in respiratory passages as in asthma,

3. *Reduced diffusion of oxygen across respiratory membrane* occurs due to :
   - Marked reduction in area of respiratory membrane as in emphysema,
   - Increased thickness of respiratory membrane as in pulmonary oedema, and
   - Non-functioning respiratory membrane as in fibrosis.

4. *Anatomical shunts,* i.e. when venous blood mixes with arterial blood lowering its pO_2, as occurs in congenital heart diseases such as Fallot's tetralogy.

2. *Anaemic hypoxia.* Anaemic hypoxia occurs due to the decreased O_2 carrying capacity of blood due to decreased haemoglobin content.

3. *Stagnant hypoxia.* Stagnant hypoxia occurs due to decreased blood flow to the tissues so that in spite of normal pO_2 and haemoglobin, adequate O_2 is not delivered to the tissues.

4. *Histotoxic hypoxia.* Histotoxic hypoxia occurs due to decreased ability of the tissues themselves to utilize the oxygen. So, strictly speaking, it is not a true hypoxia, because O_2 supply to the tissues is adequate e.g. as in cyanide poisoning.

Hypercapnia

Hypercapnia refers to increase in arterial pCO_2 (normal value 40 mmHg). When hypercapnia is the primary problem, it is associated with respiratory acidosis since an increase in CO_2 promptly generates excess H^+ through :

$$H_2O + CO_2 \xrightarrow{\text{Carbonic anhydrase}} H_2CO_3 \rightarrow H^+ + HCO_3^-$$

Hypercapnia occurs due to:

1. *Defective elimination of CO_2* as occurs in:
- Reduced pulmonary ventilation
- Reduced effective alveolar ventilation

2. *Accidental inhalation* of CO_2 in persons working in breweries and refrigeration plants.

Hypocapnia

Hypocapnia, i.e. reduced pCO_2 is usually associated with *respiratory alkalosis,* since decrease in CO_2 promptly drives the following reaction in backward direction, resulting in a decrease in H^+ concentration.

$$H_2O + CO_2 \xleftrightarrow{\text{Carbonic anhydrase}} H_2CO_3 \leftarrow H^+ + HCO_3^-$$

Causes. Hypocapnia occurs due to hyperventilation.

Asphyxia

Asphyxia refers to a condition in which hypoxia (decreased pO_2) is associated with hypercapnia (increased pCO_2).

Causes. Asphyxia can be general or local.

1. Local asphyxia occurs following complete obstruction or ligation of blood vessel.

2. General asphyxia can be chronic or acute.

- *Chronic asphyxia* may occur in patient with cor pulmonale i.e. right ventricular failure due to lung diseases.
- *Acute asphyxia* occurs due to sudden blockage in airways. Common causes are strangulation, drowning, acute tracheal obstruction (due to entry of food or due to choking), and paralysis of diaphragm, as in acute poliomyelitis.

Carbon monoxide poisoning

Carbon monoxide (CO) is a dangerous gas present in exhaust of gasoline engines, coal mines, gases from deep wells and underground drainage systems.

Toxic effects. Carbon monoxide produces anaemic hypoxia and derangement of cellular metabolic system.

ARTIFICIAL RESPIRATION AND CARDIOPULMONARY RESUSCITATION

ARTIFICIAL RESPIRATION

Artificial respiration (AR) alone is required as an emergency life-saving procedure:

I. *When there is sudden stoppage of breathing* as seen in:
- Drowning,
- Electrocution,
- Anaesthetic accidents,
- Carbon monoxide poisoning,
- Strangulation, and
- Accidents.

II. *Artificial respiration may also be needed when breathing is expected to stop gradually* as in paralysis of muscles in:
- Poliomyelitis,
- Diphtheria, and
- Ascending paralysis.

It is important to note that the tissues of brain, particularly cerebral cortex, develop irreversible damage if oxygen supply is stopped for 5 minutes. So, the resuscitation must be started quickly without any delay, before the development of cardiac failure.

Methods of artificial respiration

Mouth-to-mouth breathing method

Mouth-to-mouth breathing (exhaled air ventilation) is very useful because :
- It can be applied quickly without waiting for the availability of any aid.
- It is simple and effective measure of resuscitation.
- It can be applied in all age groups.
- It is the only technique capable of producing adequate ventilation.
- It also works by expanding the lungs.

Procedure

- To begin with patient's neck is extended by placing one hand under the neck and lifting it and pressing the forehead with the other hand (Fig. 7.3-3A). This prevents the flaccid tongue from falling back into the pharynx.
- Then the patient's nostrils are closed by the thumb and index finger of the hand (Fig. 7.3-3B).
- The resuscitator then takes a deep breath and exhales air into the patient's airway after tightly placing his mouth over patient's mouth, and noting the expansion of the chest at the same time. The volume of the air exhaled must be twice the normal tidal volume. This expands the patient's lungs.
- Then the resuscitator removes his mouth from that of the patient, allowing expiration to occur passively due to the elastic recoil of the lungs and chest (Fig. 7.3-3C).
- The above procedure is repeated 12 to 16 times per minute till spontaneous breathing returns, or till the patient is shifted to a hospital.

CARDIOPULMONARY RESUSCITATION

Cardiopulmonary resuscitation (CPR) is required in some patients when heart and respiration both stop. Breathing usually stops before the heart stops, so artificial respiration should be started immediately.

Emergency plan of cardiopulmonary resuscitation

The following plan called ABC of CPR has proved useful in reviving such patients:

A *Airway care*
B *Breathing* by artifical respiration (AR) method.
C *Cardiac massage* is required when carotid pulse cannot be felt (Fig. 7.3-4).

PULMONARY FUNCTION TESTS

Pulmonary function tests can be classified into following groups:
- Ventilatory function tests,

- Tests of diffusion,
- Tests of ultimate purpose of respiration, and
- Tests during exercise.

VENTILATORY FUNCTION TESTS

Ventilatory function tests are meant for assessment of the expansion of lungs and chest wall; and for assessment of restrictive and obstructive ventilatory defects. The assessment of ventilatory functions can be accomplished by measurement of various lung volumes and capacities by spirometry.

Spirometry

Spirometry refers to recording of volume changes during various clearly defined breathing manoeuvres. It can be performed using a simple spirometer, a modified spirometer called respirometer or computerized spirometer.

Simple spirometer (Fig. 7.3-5) is made of metal. It consists of following parts:

- *Outer chamber* or container which is filled with water.
- *Floating drum* or a gas bell, with 6 litre capacity, floats in the water in an inverted manner. It is attached to a chain which passes over a pulley bearing a balancing weight and a writing needle (pen). The needle (pen) moves with the movement of the floating drum. The

Fig. 7.3-3. Mouth-to-mouth breathing: A, the neck is extended by placing one hand under the neck and pressing the forehead with other hand; B, nostrils are closed with thumb and index finger and resuscitator exhales into the patient's airway by tightly placing his mouth over the patients mouth; and C, allows the patient to exhale passively by unsealing nose and mouth.

Fig. 7.3-4. Procedure showing external cardiac massage.

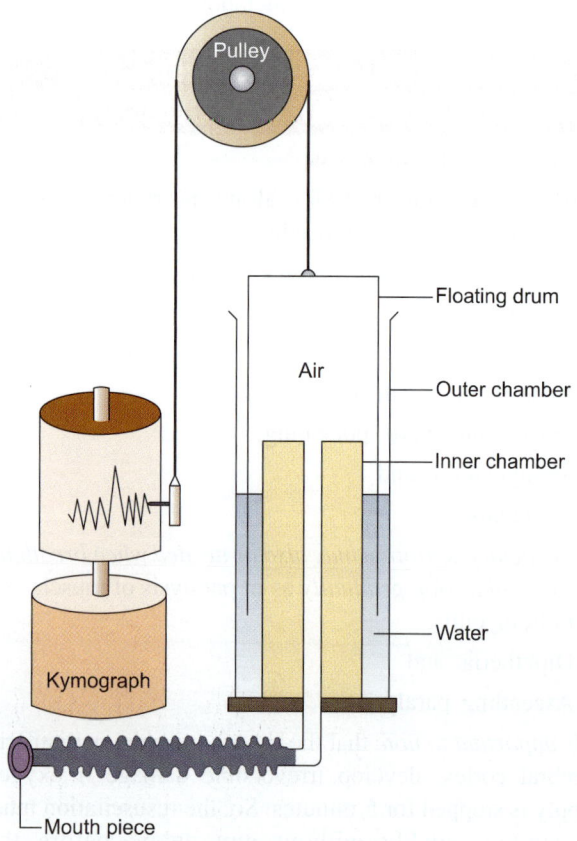

Fig. 7.3-5. Simple spirometer.

floating drum is thus counterpoised and has very little inertia and friction.

- *Inner chamber* is open at the top end which lies above the water level in outer chamber and is connected to a tube at the bottom end. At the end of tube, a mouthpiece is attached through which the subject is made to respire.

- *Kymograph* is a recording drum on which the movements of the needle are recorded.

For details of various lung volumes and capacities (see page 232).

TESTS OF DIFFUSION

Pulmonary diffusion refers to transfer of gases from alveoli to capillary blood across the respiratory membrane. The exchange of gases in the lungs was earlier believed to be dependent merely on the ability of the gases to diffuse across the respiratory membrane. This term led to the use of term *diffusion capacity*. Nowadays, the term *transfer factor,* rather than diffusion capacity, is used.

TESTS OF ULTIMATE PURPOSE OF RESPIRATION

Since the ultimate purpose of respiration is to supply O_2 from atmosphere to tissues and removal of CO_2 from the tissues into the atmosphere; so, the estimation of arterial blood pO_2, pCO_2 and pH (blood gas analysis) are most fundamental of all the pulmonary function tests.

Digestive System

Organization and General Characteristics of Digestive System

8.1

ORGANIZATION OF DIGESTIVE SYSTEM

To sustain life body needs a continual supply of water, electrolytes, and nutrients. This function is served by the gastrointestinal or the so-called digestive system. The digestive system comprises gastrointestinal tract (GIT) and accessory organs of digestion like teeth, tongue, salivary glands, liver and exocrine part of pancreas.

PARTS OF GASTROINTESTINAL TRACT

Gastrointestinal tract also known as alimentary canal is basically a muscular tube extending from the mouth to the anus (Fig. 8.1-1). At either end the lumen is continuous with external environment. It measures about 10 metres (30 feet) and comprises following parts:

Mouth. Mouth is loosely used term to denote the external opening and for the cavity it leads to. The cavity containing anterior two-thirds of tongue and teeth is the mouth cavity or oral cavity or buccal cavity.

Tongue, in the digestive system, plays two important roles:

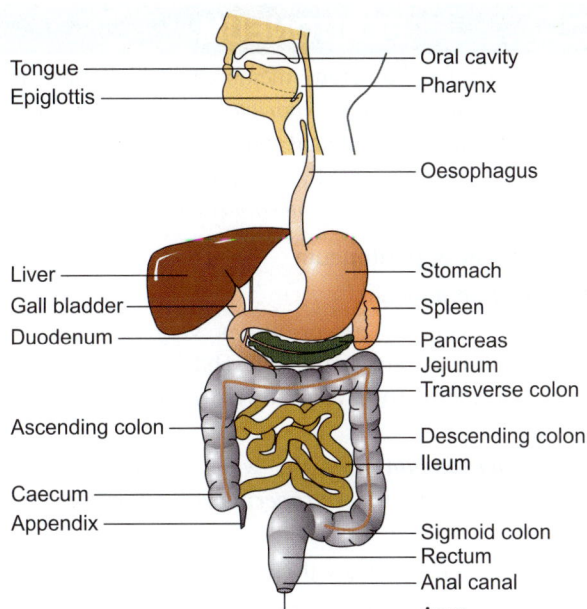

Fig. 8.1-1. The gastrointestinal system.

Tongue
Epiglottis

Oral cavity
Pharynx

Oesophagus

Liver
Gall bladder
Duodenum

Stomach
Spleen
Pancreas
Jejunum
Transverse colon

Ascending colon

Descending colon
Ileum

Caecum
Appendix

Sigmoid colon
Rectum
Anal canal
Anus

- Tells the taste of food, and
- Helps in chewing and swallowing of the food.

Teeth are accessory organ of digestion which help in chewing the food.

Pharynx. The pharynx is a median passage that is common to the gastrointestinal and respiratory systems.

Oesophagus. It is a fibromuscular tube about 25 cm long. At its junction to the pharynx upper oesophageal sphincter is present and at its junction with the stomach lower oesophageal sphincter is present.

Stomach. It is a hollow muscular bag connected to the oesophagus at its upper end and to the duodenum at the lower end.

Small intestine. It is a long tubular structure which can be divided into three parts:

- *Duodenum* is the first part of small intestine. It is C-shaped and measures about 25 cm in length,
- *Jejunum,* the middle part of the small intestine, is about 25 metres long, and
- *Ileum,* the last part of small intestine, is about 3.5 metres long.

Large intestine. It arches around and encloses the coils of the small intestine and tends to be more fixed than the small intestine. It is divided into following parts (Fig. 8.1-1):

- Caecum and appendix,
- Colon,
- Rectum, and
- Anal canal.

PERITONEUM

Peritoneum refers to serous membrane which lines the walls of abdominal cavity *(parietal layer)* and also the viscera contained in abdominal and pelvic cavities (visceral layer). The space between the parietal and visceral layers of peritoneum is called the *peritoneal cavity.*

Arrangement of peritoneum

Abdominal peritoneum

The arrangement of peritoneum is very complex. To simplify, for descriptive purpose the abdominal peritoneum can be considered to have following arrangements (Fig. 8.1-2) :

Parietal peritoneum lines the walls of the abdominal cavity and covers the *retroperitoneal structures,* e.g. kidneys.

Visceral peritoneum lines the abdominal viscera.

Folds and ligaments of peritoneum refer to those parts of the peritoneum which connect the viscera to the abdominal wall or to the other viscera. Some of the important folds and ligaments of peritoneum are (Fig. 8.1-2) :

1. *Lesser omentum.* It is fold of two layers of peritoneum which extends above from the liver to the lesser curvature of stomach below.

- *Superiorly* the two layers of peritoneum of lesser omentum are reflected to cover the liver.
- *Inferiorly* the two layers of peritoneum of lesser omentum separate to cover the anterior and superior surfaces of stomach and upper duodenum.
- *Right free margin* of the lesser omentum is formed by continuity of anterior and posterior layers. The bile duct, the hepatic artery, and the portal vein lie within this right free margin of lesser omentum (Fig. 8.1-2B).

2. *Greater omentum.* It is a fat-ladan apron-like fold of peritoneum which hangs from the stomach in front to the intestine. It consists of four layers of peritoneum. At the level of greater curvature of stomach the layers of peritoneum covering the anterior and posterior surfaces of the stomach meet and continue downwards as anterior two layers of the greater amentum. At the lower end of abdominal cavity these two layers of peritoneum get folded on themselves to form the posterior two layers of omentum. These extend upwards to reach the anterior border of pancreas where they gain attachment to the posterior abdominal wall.

3. *Mesentery* refers to the fold of peritoneum that connects the visceral peritoneum covering the small intestine to that covering the posterior abdominal wall. The attachment of mesentery along a short line of insertion on the posterior abdominal wall gives it the appearance of a ruffle or flounce. The mesentery supports the blood vessels and lymph vessels supplying the intestine.

4. *Transverse mesocolon* is the fold of peritoneum which attaches the transverse colon to the posterior abdominal wall. It lies posterior to the fourth layer of greater omentum (usually fused to it) in its upper part (Fig. 8.1-2).

5. *Sigmoid mesocolon* is the inverted V-shaped fold of peritoneum that connects sigmoid colon to the posterior abdominal and pelvic walls.

6. *Peritoneal folds connecting liver to the abdominal wall* include falciform ligament, coronary ligament and the right and left triangular ligaments.

7. *Gastrosplenic ligament.* The fold of peritoneum connecting stomach to spleen is called gastrosplenic ligament.

8. *Splinorenal ligments.* The fold of peritoneum that connects spleen to the left kidney is called splinorenal ligament (Fig. 8.1-2B).

9. *Gastrophrenic ligament* refers to the fold of peritoneum which connects the back of fundus of stomach to the diaphragm. It forms the superior boundary of lesser sac.

Fig. 8.1-2. Arrangement of peritoneum and peritoneal cavity as seen in : A, schematic sagittal section through abdominal and pelvic cavities; and B, transverse section across the abdomen at the level of foramen epiploicum.

The pelvic peritoneum

The peritoneum in the pelvis is continuous with that of the rest of the abdominal cavity. It covers the front aspect of the rectum. In the male it passes forwards over the posterior and upper surfaces of the bladder to become continuous with that on the anterior abdominal wall. In the female it passes from the rectum over the posterior and anterior surfaces of the uterus before reaching the bladder.

Peritoneal cavity

Peritoneal cavity refers to the space between the visceral and parietal layers of peritoneum. This space contains a thin film of fluid which allows free movement of the viscera against the abdominal wall and against each other. In the males the peritoneal cavity is a closed sac while in the females the uterine tubes open into the peritoneal cavity. The peritoneal cavity, for descriptive purposes, can be divided into following parts :

- The greater sac,
- The lesser sac, and
- Peritoneal pouches or recesses.

The greater sac refers to the main part of peritoneal cavity which extends from the roof of abdominal cavity to its floor.

The lesser sac is a fairly large isolated part of the peritoneal cavity which lies behind the stomach. The lesser sac opens on the right side into the greater sac through an opening called the *foramen epiploum* (Fig. 8.1-2A and B).

Peritoneal recesses are isolated areas of peritoneal cavity found in relation to the abdominal and pelvic viscera.

Functions of peritoneum

1. It is a serous membrane which enables the abdominal contents to glide over each other without friction.
2. It forms a partial or complete covering for the abdominal organs.
3. It forms ligaments and mesenteries which help to keep the organs in position.
4. The omentum and mesentery contain a considerable amount of fat and act as important fat stores for the body.
5. The omentum can move about inside the cavity and in the event of inflammation occurring tends to wrap itself round the affected part of the alimentary tract and prevent the infection from spreading to the rest of the peritoneum.
6. It has the power to absorb fluids in large quantities.

GENERAL CHARACTERISTICS OF GASTROINTESTINAL SYSTEM

STRUCTURAL CHARACTERISTICS OF GIT WALL

Different parts of the gastrointestinal tract are specialized for carrying out different functions particularly digestion and absorption, but the basic structural characteristics of the wall of whole gastrointestinal tract are similar. The intestinal wall from inside to outwards consists of following layers (Fig. 8.1-3):

1. *Mucosa* (mucous layer). It is innermost coat consisting of three layers:

- *Surface epithelium* lining the luminal surface consists of epithelial cells which vary in type from simple squamous to tall columnar depending upon the function of the part of GIT.

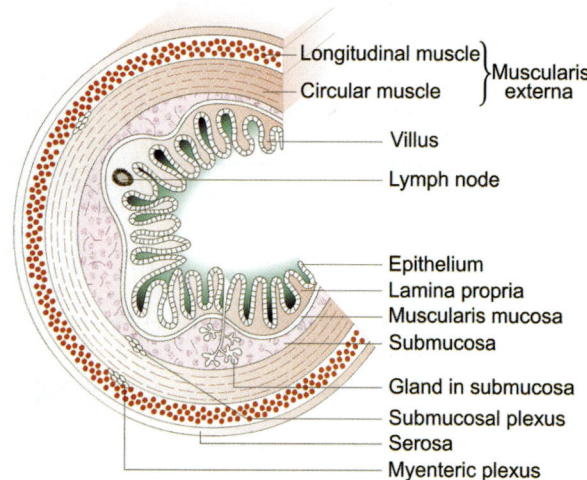

Fig. 8.1-3. *Cross-section of the alimentary canal depicting structural characteristics of its wall.*

- *Lamina propria* is composed of loose connective tissue which contains numerous glands, small blood vessels, lymphatics, and nerve fibres.
- *Muscularis mucosa* is composed of two thin layers of smooth muscle fibres which help in localised movements of the mucosa.

2. *Submucosa*. This refers to the layer of connective tissue present outside the mucosa. It contains blood vessels, lymphatics and a network of nerve fibres and nerve cells called submucosal nerve plexus (Meissner's plexus).

3. *Muscle coat*. It is formed by a thick layer of smooth muscle fibres surrounding the submucosa. The smooth muscle fibres are arranged in two layers:

- *Circular muscle fibres* form the inner layer, and
- *Longitudinal muscle fibres* form the outer layer.

In between the circular and longitudinal muscle fibres is present an extensive network of nerve cells and fibres named *Auerbach's plexus* (myenteric plexus).

4. *Serosa* (serous layer). This is the outermost layer consisting of a layer of connective tissue. This layer helps in the attachment of gut to the surrounding structures.

INNERVATION OF THE GIT

The innervation of the gastrointestinal tract includes intrinsic and extrinsic system (Fig. 8.1-4).

1. Intrinsic innervation

The intrinsic nervous system also called as *enteric nervous system* consists of nerve cells and fibres which originate and are located in the intestinal wall itself. This system supplies the smooth muscles of gastrointestinal tract (i.e. musculature of GIT except upper oesophagus and external anal sphincter which contain striated muscle). This system

Fig. 8.1-4. *Schematic illustration of the innervation of gut.*

controls most of the gastrointestinal functions like secretion and motility. The enteric nervous system is composed mainly of two plexuses:

Myenteric plexus or Auerbach's plexus is present in between the circular and longitudinal muscle fibres of muscular coat of the GIT. Stimulation of myenteric plexus causes increase in tone of the gut wall, intensity of rhythmical contractions of gut wall, rate of contraction, and velocity of contraction.

Meissner's plexus or submucosal plexus is present in the submucosal layer. It *controls the secretory activity* and blood flow to the gut.

The Auerbach's and Meissner's plexuses are interconnected with each other and are under the control of parasympathetic and sympathetic components of extrinsic nervous system. In both the plexuses, the axons branch profusely so that stimulation of one region produces a widespread response in the GIT.

2. Extrinisic innervation

The extrinsic system of nerves supplying the gut consists of the parasympathetic and sympathetic components of autonomic nervous system.

Parasympathetic innervation

The parasympathetic supply to the gut is made up of cranial and sacral divisions:

Chapter 8.1

1. *Cranial parasympathetic fibres* originate in medulla, come through vagus and supply the oesophagus, stomach, small intestine, pancreas and first half of the large intestine. They also make synaptic connections with intramural plexuses.

2. *Sacral parasympathetic fibres* originate in sacral spinal cord, pass through pelvic nerves to hypogastric (pelvic) ganglion as a postganglionic fibre, supply the distal half of large intestine and rectum. The sigmoid, rectal and anal regions have an especially rich supply of parasympathetic fibres that function in the defaecation reflex.

Functions of parasympathetics. Parasympathetic stimulation causes excitation of all the musculature of gut except the sphincters to which it inhibits. There occurs an increase in gastrointestinal motility and secretory activity.

Sympathetic innervation

The sympathetic fibres to gut arise from eighth thoracic (T_8) to second lumbar (L_2) spinal segments. The sympathetics innervate all portions of the gastrointestinal tract rather than being more extensively supplied to portions near the oral cavity and anus, as is true for parasympathetics.

Functions of sympathetic innervation. Sympathetic stimulation causes:

- Vasoconstriction,
- Excitation of ileocaecal and internal anal sphincters and smooth muscles of muscularis mucosa throughout (to increase number of folds); and
- Inhibition of motility in the gut.

Thus most of the effects of sympathetic stimulation are opposite to that of parasympathetic stimulation.

GASTROINTESTINAL BLOOD FLOW

The blood supply of the gastrointestinal tract forms part of splanchnic circulation. The main characteristic feature of the gastrointestinal blood flow is that it is *usually proportional to the level of local activity.*

GASTROINTESTINAL HORMONES

General characteristics

- Gastrointestinal hormones regulate the secretions and even to some extent the motility of gastrointestinal tract.
- The *glandular cells* secreting gastrointestinal hormones are individually scattered in the epithelium of the stomach and small intestine and not in the form of clusters of cells as in the endocrine glands.
- The luminal surface of glandular cells when stimulated by various chemicals present in the chyme release

hormone from the opposite surface into blood capillaries of portal circulation.

- Through portal circulation the released hormone reaches the target tissue situated in the nearby region of GIT and exhibits physiological actions on the target cells with specific receptors for the hormone. For example, the hormone gastrin released by G-cells present in mucosa of pyloric part of stomach in response to presence of peptides in chyme reaches the body of stomach via portal circulation and increases the acid secretion as well as motility of the stomach.
- The effects of gastrointestinal hormones persist even after nervous connections between the site of release and the site of action have been severed.

Classification of gastrointestinal hormones

The gastrointestinal hormones, based on their physio-anatomical similarities, can be broadly classified into three types:

1. *Gastrin family of hormones* includes:
   - Gastrin, and
   - Cholecystokinin PZ or CCK-PZ
2. *Secretin family of hormones* includes:
   - Secretin,
   - Gastric inhibitory polypeptide or GIP,
   - Vasoactive intestinal peptide or VIP,
   - Glucagon, and
   - Glucagon-like immune reactivity or GLI or glycentin.
3. *Other gastrointestinal hormones* includes:
   - Motilin,
   - Neurotensin,
   - Substance P,
   - Gastrin-releasing peptide or GRP, and
   - Somatostatin.

Actions of gastrointestinal hormones

The outlines of the action of each gastrointestinal hormone as well as the stimulus for secretion and site of secretion are depicted in Table 8.1-1.

FUNCTIONS OF DIGESTIVE SYSTEM

The functions of each part of the gastrointestinal tract (GIT) are described in the respective chapters. However, as introductory remarks to the digestive system, the various functions of GIT are summrized here.

I. Digestive functions

The major function of the gastrointestinal system is to transfer nutrients, minerals and water from external environment to the circulating body fluids for distribution to all the body tissues. This function is accomplished by following processes:

Table 8.1-1. Stimuli for secretion, site of action and actions of gastrointestinal hormones.

Hormone	Stimuli for secretion	Site of secretion	Actions						
			Gastric secretion	Gastric motility	Pancreatic secretion	Bile secretion	Gall bladder contraction	Small intestine secretion	Small intestine motility
• Gastrin	Small peptides, amino acids, gastric distention, vagal stimulation	G cells of gastric antrum	+	+	+	0	0	0	0
• Cholecysto-kinin (CCK)	Small peptides, amino acids, fatty acids	Type I cells of duodenum and jejunum	0	–	+	0	+	0	+
• Secretin	Acid in upper intestine Fatty acids	S cells of duodenum	–	0	+	+	0	0	0
• Gastric inhibitory polypeptide (GIP)	Fatty acids, amino acids, oral glucose	Duodenum and jejunum	–	–	0	0	0	+	–
• Vasoactive intestinal polypeptide (VIP)	Fatty acids	Jejunum	–	–	0	0	0	0	0
• Somatostatin	Acid in stomach	D cells of islets of Langerhans	–	–	–	0	–	0	0

0 (No action), + (stimulatory action) and – (inhibitory action)

1. *Ingestion of food.* It involves:

- Placing the food into the mouth. Most of the foodstuffs are taken into mouth as large particles mainly made of carbohydrates, proteins and fats.

- Chewing the food into smaller pieces is carried out with the help of teeth and jaw muscles. This process is called mastication.

- Lubrication and moistening of the food is done by the saliva.

- Swallowing the food (deglutition). It refers to pushing the bolus of food from mouth into the stomach. It is accomplished in three phases: oral phase, pharyngeal phase, and oesophageal phase.

2. *Digestion of food.* It refers to conversion of complex insoluble large organic molecules (food) into soluble, smaller and simpler molecules which can be easily absorbed. Digestion of food is accomplished with the help of hydrochloric acid and digestive juices containing various enzymes.

3. *Absorption of digested food.* Absorption of food refers to movement of digested molecules from the lumen of alimentary canal across its epithelial lining to the blood or lymph. The absorbed water, electrolytes and nutrients are carried away to the various tissues by the circulating blood.

4. *Egestion,* i.e. excretion of unwanted undigested food by the alimentary canal in the form of faeces is called defaecation.

II. Non-digestive functions

The main non-digestive function of the gastrointestinal system is its role as immune system. The lymphoid tissue in the tonsils, adenoids, and Peyer's patches constitute an important part of body's immune system. These provide both the humoral and cellular immunity which is specially effective against the microorganisms trying to enter the body from the alimentary canal.

CHAPTER 8.1

Anatomy and Physiology of Mouth, Pharynx and Oesophagus

8.2

ANATOMY OF MOUTH, PHARYNX AND OESOPHAGUS
Mouth
- The palate
- Tongue
- Gums and teeth
- Fauces

Pharynx
- Nasopharynx
- Oropharynx
- Laryngopharynx

Oesophagus

PHYSIOLOGICAL ACTIVITIES IN MOUTH, PHARYNX AND OESOPHAGUS

Mastication
- Chewing reflex
- Muscles of mastication
- Functions of mastication

Lubrication of food by saliva
- Salivary glands
- Saliva

Deglutition (swallowing)
- Phases of deglutition
  - Oral phase
  - Pharyngeal phase
  - Oesophageal phase
- Disorders of swallowing

ANATOMY OF MOUTH, PHARYNX AND OESOPHAGUS

MOUTH

Mouth is loosely used term to denote the external opening and for the cavity it leads to. The cavity containing anterior two-thirds of tongue and teeth the mouth cavity or oral cavity or buccal cavity (Figs. 8.2.1 and 8.2.2). The oral cavity extends from the lips to the oropharyngeal isthmus, i.e. junction of the mouth with the pharynx. Oral cavity is subdivided into two parts: the vestibule and oral cavity proper (Fig. 8.2-2).

- *Vestibule* lies between the lips and cheeks externally and the gums and teeth internally.

- *Oral cavity proper* lies within the alveolar arches, gums and teeth. The roof of the oral cavity is formed by the hard and soft palate.

- *The floor* is mainly formed by tongue and sublingual region of lower jaw.

The palate

The palate consists of hard and soft palate.

Hard palate, the anterior part of palate, is formed by processes of the maxillae and palatine bones, which are covered by mucous membrane.

Soft palate forms a muscular arch that extends posteriorly. Hanging from the middle of posterior margin of soft palate is a conical structure called the *uvula.*

Tongue

The tongue is a freely movable thick muscular organ covered by mucous membrane. It occupies the floor of the mouth and fills the oral cavity proper when the mouth is closed. The tongue presents following anatomical features:

Tip of the tongue is its free anterior end which is directed forwards and comes in contact with the incisor teeth.

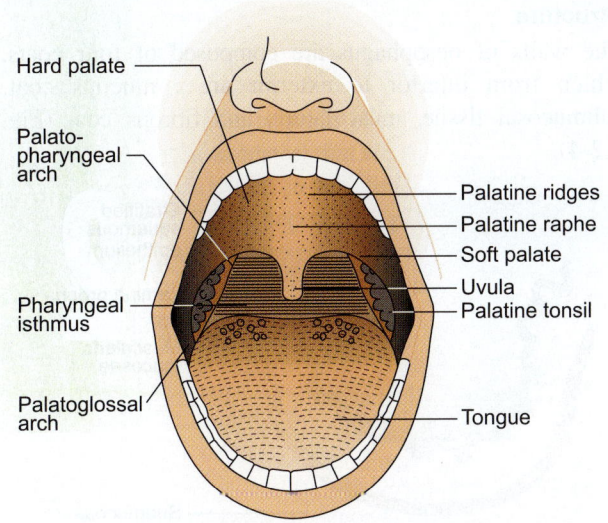

Fig. 8.2-1. Widely open oral fissure to show the mouth cavity.

Labels (top figure):
Hard palate
Palato-pharyngeal arch
Pharyngeal isthmus
Palatoglossal arch
Palatine ridges
Palatine raphe
Soft palate
Uvula
Palatine tonsil
Tongue

Fig. 8.2-2. Schematic coronal section through oral cavity.

Labels (second figure):
Nasal cavity
Nasal septum
Maxillary sinus
Palate
Tongue
Oral cavity proper
Vestibule
Buccinator muscle in cheeks
Tooth
Mylohyoid muscle
Lip

Body of the tongue is mainly composed of muscles covered by thick mucosa.

- *Dorsal surface* of the tongue is marked by rough projection called *papillae*. These provide friction that is useful in handling the food. These papillae contain taste buds (for details see page 500).

- *Ventral surface* of the tongue has a smooth mucosal covering. In the midline it presents a fold of mucous membrane called *frenulum* by which the tongue is anchored to the floor of mouth.

Root of the tongue or the posterior region of tongue is attached to the hyoid bone. The surface of this part of tongue is characterized by presence of rounded masses of lymphatic tissue called *lingual tonsils*.

Nerve supply of tongue : see page 500.

Functions of tongue include :

- Tells the taste of food (special organ of sense of taste) (see page 500) ,

- Helps in chewing and swallowing of food.

- Helps in speech.

Gums and teeth

Gums

Gums refer to dense fibrous tissue, covered by a vascular stratified squamous epithelium, which surrounds the necks of teeth and is attached to the alveolar margins of the jaws. The fibrous tissue forming the gums is continuous with the periodontal membrane which attaches the teeth to their sockets.

The teeth

The teeth develop in the sockets present in the alveolar processes of the mandible (forming lower jaw) and part of maxillary bone forming upper jaw.

Sets of teeth and time of eruption. There are two sets of teeth.

- *Deciduous set* (primary or milk teeth) comprises of 20 teeth (10 in each jaw). The eruption of milk teeth begins 6 months after birth and is completed by the second year. They start shedding round about 6-7 years.

- *Permanent set* comprises of 32 teeth that is 8 in each quadrant : 2 incisors, 2 canine, 2 premolar and 3 molar. The dental formula is written as below :

				midline					
3	2	1	2		2	1	2	3	(Maxilla)
3	2	1	2		2	1	2	3	(Mandible)

Parts of a tooth. Each tooth has three parts (Fig. 8.2-3):

- *Root* consists of one to three fangs contained in the socket.

- *Crown* is the part which projects beyond the level of gums, and

- *Neck* is the constricted portion between the root and crown.

Structure of a tooth. Each tooth consists of following regions (Fig. 8.2-3) :

- *Pulp cavity* occupies the centre of a tooth and extends from the root into the crown of the tooth. The cavity is filled by dental pulp consisting of loose fibrous tissue containing nerves, blood vessels and lymphatics, all of which gain access to pulp through the apical foramen.

- *Dentine* or ivory surrounds the pulp cavity and forms the bulk of tooth. It is hard avascular calcified tissue penetrated by minute canals called dentinal tubules. These tubules function as sensory receptors and account for the extreme sensitiveness of dentine to cold, heat, acid and drilling.

- *Enamel* is the external layer covering only the dentine of the crown of tooth. It is the hardest substance in the body.

- *Cementum* is bone-like material which surrounds the dentine in the area of root of tooth. It fastens the tooth into its bony socket.

C H A P T E R 8.2

Fig. 8.2-3. *Structure and parts of tooth.*

Functions of different types of teeth in chewing are:

- *Incisors* provide strong cutting action,
- *Canines* are responsible for tearing action.
- *Premolars and molars* have grinding action.

Fauces

The fauces is the name given to the aperture connecting mouth with the pharynx. The fauces include two arches and palatine tonsils :

- *Glossopalatine arch* (anterior pillar of fauces) extends from the side of uvula to the side of root of tongue.
- *Pharyngopalatine arch* (posterior pillar of fauces) extends from the side of uvula to the side of pharynx.
- *Palatine tonsils* are two masses of lymphoid tissue situated, one on either side, in the triangular space between the two arches. The tonsils function as lymph nodes.

PHARYNX

The pharynx is a median passage that is common to the gastrointestinal tract and respiratory system. It is divisible from above downwards into three parts :

- *Nasopharynx* or nasal part into which open the nasal cavities,
- *Oropharynx* or oral part which is continuous with the posterior end of oral cavity, and
- *Laryngopharynx* or laryngeal part which is continuous in front with larynx and below with the oesophagus.
  For detail see page 219, Fig. 7.1-5.

OESOPHAGUS

The oesophagus is a fibromuscular tube, about 25-30 cm long and 25-30 mm wide. It begins at the lower end of the pharynx, behind the trachea and descends in the mediastinum in front of the vertebral column. It passes through the diaphragm at the level of tenth thoracic vertebra, and terminates in the upper or cardiac end of the stomach, about the level of xiphoid process (Fig. 8.2-4).

Structure

The walls of oesophagus are composed of four coats, which from interior to exterior are : mucous coat, submucosal tissue, musculature, and fibrous coat (Fig. 8.2-4).

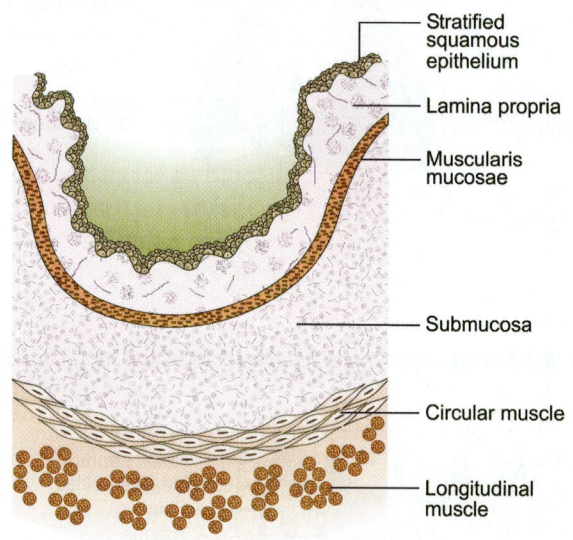

Fig. 8.2-4. *Microscopic structure of oesophagus.*

1. *Mucous coat* is formed by stratified squamous epithelium. It is arranged in longitudinal folds which disappear when the oesophagus is distended by the passage of food. It is studded with minute papillae and small glands which secrete mucus to lubricate the canal.

2. *Submucous coat* is formed by areolar tissue which serves to connect the mucous coat with the muscular coat and to carry the larger blood vessels and lymph vessels.

3. *Musculature of oesophagus* has following characterisitics :

- *Upper one-third of oesophagus* including the upper oesophageal sphincter is made up of striated muscle that is under the control of vagal fibres emerging from the nucleus ambiguus.
- *Lower two-thirds of oesophagus* including the lower oesophageal sphincter is composed of smooth muscle.

Upper oesophageal sphincter

Upper oesophageal sphincter (UES) is a true sphincter formed by the cricopharyngeal muscle. The UES is normally contracted tonically and serves to prevent the entry of air into the oesophagus during normal respiration. Its tone is maintained by the continual firing of vagal fibres originating from the nucleus ambiguus. The neurotransmitter released by these fibres is acetylcholine (ACh).

The UES opens during swallowing when a rapid

peristaltic wave starting in the pharyngeal muscles passes on to oesophagus.

Lower oesophageal sphincter

Lower oesophageal sphincter (LES) also known as cardiac sphincter refers to distal 2 cm of oesophagus. Its contractile characteristics are quite different from the rest of oesophageal smooth muscle (that is why it is called physiological sphincter).

The principal function of LES is to prevent regurgitation of gastric contents (food, gastric juice and air) into the oesophagus. When the intragastric pressure is markedly raised (e.g. after a heavy meal or ingestion of carbonated drinks), the resistance of LES is overcome and air escapes into the mouth (belching). The local hormone, gastrin, increases the tone of LES and helps to keep the sphincter more tightly closed during digestion.

4. Fibrous coat, the external layer of oesophagus, is made of thin layer of fibrous tissue which covers the muscular layer.

PHYSIOLOGICAL ACTIVITIES IN MOUTH, PHARYNX AND OESOPHAGUS

The functioning of digestive system starts from the mouth (oral cavity) and ends at the anus.

Ingestion of food, a function of mouth, pharynx and oesophagus, involves following processes:

- Placing of food into the mouth,
- Mastication, i.e. chewing the food into smaller pieces,
- Lubrication of the food with saliva, and
- Swallowing, i.e. deglutition.

MASTICATION

Mastication or chewing refers to the process by which the food placed in the mouth is cut and grounded into smaller pieces. It involves:

- Movements of the jaws,
- Action of teeth (the incisors provide a strong cutting action, whereas the molars have a grinding action), and
- Coordinated movements of the tongue and muscles of the oral cavity.

Chewing reflex. Mastication or chewing, though a voluntary act, is coordinated by chewing reflex that facilitates the opening and closing of the jaw. The cycle of opening and closing of the jaw leads to mastication.

Role of tongue. The tongue contributes to the grinding process by positioning the food between the upper and lower teeth.

Muscles of mastication include masseter, temporalis, and internal and external pterygoids. Buccinator is an accessory muscle of mastication which prevents accumulation of food between the cheek and teeth.

Net effect of mastication. The bolus of food becomes a homogenized mixture of small food particles, saliva and mucus, which is easy to swallow and digest.

LUBRICATION OF FOOD BY SALIVA

SALIVARY GLANDS

In addition to the chewing, another important physiological activity which takes place in the mouth is lubrication of food by saliva. The saliva is secreted by three pairs of major salivary glands (Fig. 8.2-5).

Fig. 8.2-5. Salivary glands and their ducts.

1. Parotid glands

Location. Parotid glands are the largest salivary glands (each weighing 20-30 gm), located near the angles of jaw.

Acini. The parotid glands are purely serous glands which secrete watery saliva containing more than 90% water. Parotid glands secrete 25% of the total salivary secretion (which is about 1500 ml/day).

Ducts. Ducts of the parotid glands open on the inner side of the right and left cheek and pour their secretions in the vestibule.

2. Sublingual glands

Location. The sublingual gland is the smallest of the three main salivary glands. It lies just below the mucosa on the floor of mouth. Each gland raises a ridge of mucosa which starts at the sublingual papilla and runs laterally and backwards. The ridge is called the sublingual fold.

Acini. The sublingual gland contains both serous and mucous acini, the latter predominating.

Ducts of sublingual gland are 8 to 20 in number. Most open into the mouth on the summit of sublingual fold but a few may open into the submandibular duct.

3. Submandibular glands

Location. The submandibular glands are large salivary glands which lie (one on each side) partly under cover of the body of the mandible.

Acini. The submandibular gland is composed of a mixture of serous and mucous acini, the former predominating.

Ducts. S-shaped duct of each submandibular gland opens on the sublingual papilla located just lateral to the frenulum lingua.

Note. The sublingual and submandibular glands secrete a fluid that contains a higher concentration of proteins and so is more viscous as compared to watery secretion of parotid glands.

Smaller salivary glands

In addition to the three pairs of salivary glands described above, several smaller glands are located throughout the oral cavity. Those in the tongue secrete lingual lipase.

SALIVA

Secretion and composition

Amount. Under normal circumstances the salivary glands secrete about 500 to 1500 ml of saliva every day. pH of saliva varies from 6 to 7.4.

Composition. Saliva is composed of *water* 99%, and *solids* 1%, which include:

Organic substances such as α-amylase (ptyalin), lingual lipase, kallikrein, lysozyme, small amounts of urea, uric acid, cholesterol and mucin. Inorganic substances are Na^+, Cl^-, K^+ and HCO_3^-.

Note. Composition of saliva varies with the salivary flow rate.

Phases of salivary secretion

1. *Cephalic phase* refers to secretion of saliva before entering of food into the mouth. It is caused by a conditioned reflex initiated by the mere sight or smell of food.

2. *Buccal phase* refers to secretion of saliva caused by stimulation of buccal receptors by the presence of food in the mouth.

3. *Oesophageal phase* occurs due to stimulation of salivary glands to a slight degree by the food passing through oesophagus.

4. *Gastric phase* refers to secretion of saliva by the presence of food in the stomach. It specially occurs when irritant food is present in the stomach (e.g. increased salivation before vomiting).

5. *Intestinal phase* refers to salivary secretion caused by presence of irritant food in the upper intestine.

Control of salivary secretion

- Salivary secretion is controlled entirely by autonomic nervous system (ANS) reflexes.
- Salivary secretion production is increased by both parasympathetic and sympathetic activity, however the activity of former is more important.

Functions of saliva

1. *Protective functions of saliva :*
- *Dilutes hot and irritant food substances* thus preventing injury to buccal mucosa.
- *Washes away food particles* that remain in the oral cavity at the end of meal and thus cleans the oral cavity.
- *Destroys harmful bacteria* in the mouth and thus minimizes risk of buccal infection and dental caries.
- *Dilutes any hydrochloric acid (HCl) and bile* which regurgitate into oesophagus and mouth.

2. *Role in mastication and deglutition is :*
- Salivary mucus lubricates the food and buccal mucosa and thus aids in mastication and swallowing.
- Helps bolus formation by acting as a glue.

3. *Digestive functions are :*
- *Initial starch digestion* starts by α-amylase (ptyalin) present in the saliva.
- *Initial triglyceride digestion* is caused by lingual lipase present in the saliva.

4. *Role in taste sensation.* Saliva acts as a solvent for various foodstuffs. As taste is a chemical sense, the taste receptors respond only to dissolved substances.

5. *Role in speech.* Salivary mucus lubricates the oral mucosa and thus aids speech by facilitating movements of lips and tongue.

6. *Excretory function.* Saliva acts as a vehicle for excretion of certain heavy metals, thiocyanate ions, alcohol and morphine.

7. *Role in temperature regulation is as below :*
- During state of dehydration, the salivary secretion is reduced which induces thirst.
- Panting mechanism. In dogs, saliva is evaporated from the surface of tongue to cause evaporative heat loss.

DEGLUTITION (SWALLOWING)

PHASES OF SWALLOWING

Deglutition or swallowing refers to passage of food from the oral cavity into the stomach. It comprises three phases:
- Oral phase (voluntary),
- Pharyngeal phase (reflex or involuntary), and
- Oesophageal phase (reflex or involuntary).

Oral phase

- Oral phase or the first stage of swallowing is a voluntary phase.
- During this phase the bolus of food formed after mastication is put over the dorsum of tongue. The tongue forces the bolus into the oropharynx by pushing up and back against the hard palate (Fig. 8.2-6A).

Pharyngeal phase

Pharyngeal phase or second stage of swallowing is an involuntary phase i.e. caused by reflex contraction of muscles of pharynx. Deglutition centre coordinating the reflex activity is located in the medulla oblongata and lower pons, i.e. in the nucleus of the tractus solitarius (NTS) and the nucleus ambiguus.

Events during pharyngeal phase

Events which take place during movement of bolus from the pharynx into the oesophagus occur in following sequence (Fig. 8.2-6B, C and D).

- *Oral cavity is shut off* from the pharynx by the approximation of posterior pillars of the fauces.
- *Nasopharynx is closed* by the upward movement of soft palate, preventing regurgitation of food into the nasal cavities.
- *Palatopharyngeal folds are pulled medially*, to make a slit-like opening for food, allowing only properly masticated food to pass through (selective action).
- *Vocal cords* strongly approximate stopping the breathing temporarily (*deglutition apnoea*), *larynx* is pulled upward and anteriorly by neck muscles enlarging the opening of oesophagus which is normally a slit and *epiglottis* swings backwards to close laryngeal opening. All this guides the food towards the oesophagus and prevents its entry into the trachea.
- *Upper oesophageal sphincter* (UES) which normally remains contracted tonically opens up and allows the

bolus of food to be pushed into the upper part of oesophagus by the rapid peristaltic contraction wave of pharynx which also continues in the oesophagus.

- Once the bolus of food has passed into the oesophagus, cricopharyngeus contracts, vocal cords open up allowing normal breathing to be resumed and the upper oesophageal sphincter (UES) once again goes into tonic contraction. The entire process of pharyngeal phase is completed in 1-2 seconds.

Oesophageal phase

During oesophageal phase the food bolus is propelled from the upper part of oesophagus to the stomach by the oesophageal peristalsis and aided by gravity.

Note. After the food enters the stomach, the LES contracts to prevent regurgitation of food into the oesophagus. With this the oesophageal phase of deglutition is completed.

DISORDERS OF SWALLOWING

1. Abolition of deglutition reflex

Abolition of deglutition reflex causes regurgitation of food into the nose or aspiration into the larynx and trachea. It may occur:

- When IX or X nerve is paralysed in lesions of medulla, and
- When pharynx is anaesthetized with cocaine (deglutition reflex is abolished temporarily).

2. Aerophagia

- Aerophagia refers to unavoidable swallowing of air along with the swallowing of food bolus and liquids.
- It usually occurs in nervous individuals having low tone of the upper oesophageal sphincter (UES).
- Some of the gases present in the air swallowed are absorbed, partly the air is regurgitated into the oral cavity and out in the atmosphere (belching), and majority of it passes on to the colon and is then expelled as flatus through the anus.

C H A P T E R 8.2

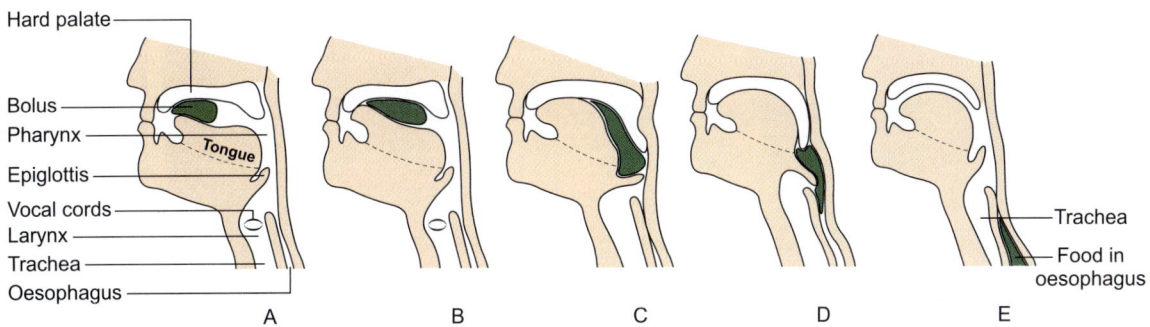

Hard palate
Bolus
Pharynx
Tongue
Epiglottis
Vocal cords
Larynx
Trachea
Oesophagus
Trachea
Food in oesophagus

A   B   C   D   E

Fig. 8.2-6. *Phases of swallowing: A, oral phase; B, C and D, early, middle and late pharyngeal phases; and E, oesophageal phase.*

3. Dysphagia

Dysphagia is a term used to denote difficulty in swallowing due to any cause.

4. Cardiac achalasia

- Cardiac achalasia is a neuromuscular disorder of the lower two-thirds of oesophagus characterized by absence of oesophageal peristalsis and failure of the lower oesophageal sphincter (LES) to relax during swallowing.
- Because of this, food transmission to stomach is impeded. In severe cases, oesophagus fails to empty the swallowed food into stomach for several hours.
- Over months and years oesophagus becomes enlarged and infected due to long-standing stasis of food.

5. Gastroesophageal reflux disease

Gastroesophageal reflux disease (GRD) refers to a condition in which incompetence of lower oesophageal sphincter (LES) causes reflux of acidic gastric contents into oesophagus. Reflux of stomach acid causes oesophageal pain (heartburn) and may lead to irritation of oesophagus or bronchioles (due to aspiration).

The Stomach

8.3

ANATOMY OF STOMACH

GROSS ANATOMY

General features

- Stomach is a J-shaped hollow muscular bag connected to the oesophagus at its upper end and to the duodenum at the lower end.

- The *volume* of stomach is 1200-1500 ml, but its *capacity* is greater than 3000 ml.

- The stomach has two curvatures. The concavity of the right inner curve is called *lesser curvature*, and the convexity of the left outer curve is the *greater curvature*. An angle along the lesser curvature, the *incisura angularis* (Fig. 8.3-1).

Anatomical relations of stomach (Fig. 8.3-1)

1. *Anteriorly* the stomach is related to left lobe of liver and anterior abdominal wall.

2. *Posteriorly* the structures related to stomach include: abdominal aorta, pancreas, spleen, left kidney and left adrenal gland.

3. *Superiorly* the stomach is related to diaphragm, oesophagus and left lobe of liver.

4. *Inferiorly* the stomach lies on transverse colon and small intestine (Fig. 8.3-1).

5. *To the left side* of stomach lie diaphragm and spleen.

6. *To the right side* of stomach are situated liver and duodenum (Fig. 8.3-1).

Parts of stomach

The stomach can be divided into five anatomic regions (Fig. 8.3-2):

Fig. 8.3-1. *Stomach and its associated structures.* **Note :** The greater omentum has been removed and liver turned up and to the right to show lesser omentum. The dotted lines show the normal position of liver.

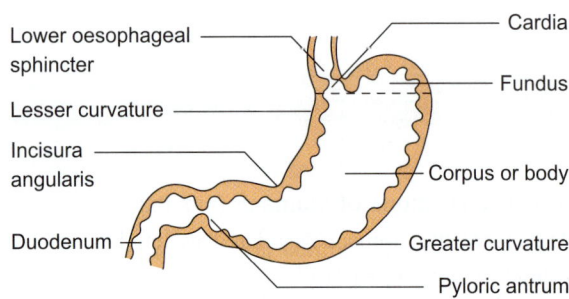

Fig. 8.3-2. *Schematic section to depict gross anatomy of stomach.*

- *Cardia* is the narrow conical portion of the stomach immediately distal to the gastroesophageal junction.
- *Fundus* is the dome-shaped proximal portion of the stomach.
- *Body or corpus* is the main part of the stomach that extends upto the incisura angularis.
- *Pyloric antrum* extends from the incisura angularis to the pyloric canal.
- *Pyloric canal or pylorus* is the distal-most one inch long tubular part of stomach.

Note. Anatomically the antrum and pylorus are continuous and respond to nervous control as a unit. Functionally,

first part of duodenum is associated with the pyloric part of stomach.

STRUCTURAL CHARACTERISTICS

The gastric wall consists of mucosa, submucosa, muscular coat, and serosa (serous layer).

1. Gastric mucosa

Gross features

- The inner surface of stomach exhibits coarse *rugae*. These infoldings of mucosa and submucosa are most prominent in the proximal stomach.
- The delicate texture of the mucosa is punctured by millions of gastric foveolae or pits, leading to the mucosal glands.

Histological features

Gastric mucosa comprises (Fig. 8.3-3):

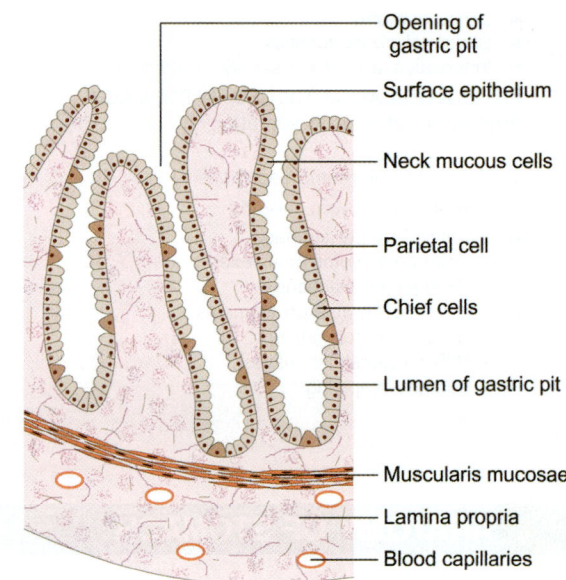

Fig. 8.3-3. *Histological features of gastric mucosa.*

Surface foveolar cells are tall columnar mucin-secreting cells which line the entire gastric mucosa as well as the gastric pits.

Mucous neck cells are present deeper in the gastric pits. These cells are thought to be the progenitors of both the surface epithelium and the cells of gastric glands.

Glandular cells form the gastric glands. There are three types of gastric glands—main gastric glands, cardiac tubular glands, and pyloric (antral) glands.

i. Main gastric glands, found in the body and fundus of stomach. These are simple tubular glands (Fig. 8.3-3). The alveoli of main gastric glands contain two types of cells:

- *Chief cells*, also known as peptic or zymogen cells, are

basophilic and secrete proteolytic proenzymes, pepsinogen I and II.

- *Parietal cells* (oxyntic cells) are acidophilic. These secrete *hydrochloric acid* (HCl) and the *intrinsic factor*.

ii. Cardiac tubular glands are found in the mucosa of cardia (a small conical part of the stomach) just around the distal end of oesophagus. These secrete *soluble mucus*.

iii. Pyloric (antral) glands are found in the antrum and pylorus region of the stomach. These glands contain two types of cells:

- *Mucus cells*, which secrete *soluble mucus,* and
- *G-cells*, responsible for release of the hormone gastrin.

2. Submucous coat
The submucous coat consists of loose areolar connective tissue connecting the muscular and mucous coats of the stomach.

3. Musculature of stomach
Characteristic features of gastric musculature are:

- The muscle coat of stomach has three layers, an outer longitudinal, middle circular, and an inner oblique (Fig. 8.3-4).
- The stomach and duodenum are divided by a thickened circular smooth muscle layer called *pyloric sphincter*.

Fig. 8.3-4. Three layers of gastric mucosa.

4. Serous coat
The serous coat of stomach is part of the peritoneum which covers the organ.

INNERVATION AND BLOOD SUPPLY OF STOMACH

Innervation of stomach
The stomach is supplied by an intrinsic and an extrinsic system.

1. Intrinsic innervation comprises two interconnected plexuses:

- *Myenteric (Auerbach's) plexus*, located between the layers of circular and longitudinal muscles of the stomach, and
- *Submucosal (Meissner's) plexus*, located in the submucosal layer.

The intrinsic innervation is directly responsible for peristalsis and other contractions. Because this system is continuous between the stomach and duodenum, peristalsis in the antrum influences the duodenal bulb.

2. Extrinsic innervation modifies the coordinated motor activity that arises independently in the intrinsic nervous system. It consists of the two components of autonomic nervous system:

- *Sympathetic innervation* comes via coeliac plexus and *inhibits motility,* and
- *Parasympathetic innervation* comes via the vagus nerve and *stimulates motility.*

Blood supply of stomach
The arteries supplying the stomach are derived from the coeliac artery and include :

1. *Left gastric artery.* It courses along the lesser curvature of the stomach from left to right, distributing branches to both surfaces. It anastomoses with the oesophageal arteries and branches of right gastric artery.

2. *Right and left gastroepiploic arteries.* They course, respectively, from the right and left side along the greater curvature of the stomach, anaestomose with branches of splenic artery and supply blood to the stomach.

The veins draining blood from the stomach include right and left gastroepiploic veins, and several short gastric veins. All of these eventually join the portal vein. A small quantity of the blood is returned to azygos veins instead of portal vein.

PHYSIOLOGICAL ACTIVITIES IN STOMACH

PHYSIOLOGY OF GASTRIC SECRETION

GASTRIC JUICE

Composition
Gastric glands secrete about 2-2.5 L of gastric juice in the lumen of stomach per day. It is acidic with a pH varying from 1 to 2. Important constituents of gastric juice are:

Water – 99.45%
Solids – 0.55%, which include:

Electrolytes such as Na^+, K^+, Mg^{2+}, Cl^-, HCO_3^-, HPO_4^{-2} and SO_4^{-2}. The electrolyte content of gastric juice varies with the rate of secretions. At low secretory rates, Na^+ concentration is high and H^+ concentration is low, but as acid secretion increases Na^+ concentration falls.

Enzymes present in the gastric juice are:

Pepsin, *Gastric lipase*, *Gastric gelatinase*, *Gastric amylase*, *Lysozyme* and *Carbonic anhydrase*.

Mucin or mucus is of two types:

- *Soluble mucus* secreted by mucous cells of pyloric and cardiac glands, and
- *Insoluble mucus* secreted by surface foveolar cells (tall columnar mucin-secreting cells) lining the entire gastric mucosa.

Intrinsic factor is secreted by parietal cells of gastric glands.

Secretion of gastric juice

Secretion of HCl

Hydrochloric acid (HCl) is secreted by the *parietal cells* (also called oxyntic cells). Gastric glands secrete about 2.5 L of HCl in a day having a pH of approximately 1.0.

Mechanism of HCl secretion. Various theories have been put forward to explain the origin of H⁺ of HCl. The hypothesis more widely accepted is shown in Fig. 8.3-5. Hydrochloric acid is made up of hydrogen (H^+) and chloride ions (Cl^-).

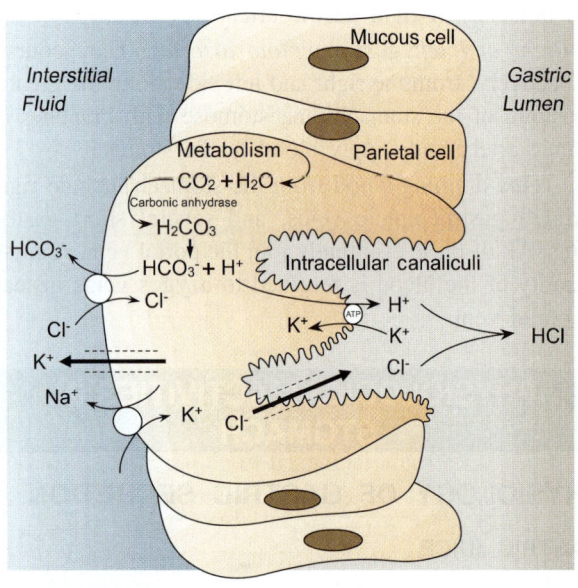

Fig. 8.3-5. *Mechanism of HCl secretion in the parietal cells of the stomach.*

- The H⁺ ions are believed to be generated inside the parietal cell from metabolic CO_2 and H_2O present in the cell. The enzyme carbonic anhydrase present in abundance in the parietal cells is essential for the secretion.

$$CO_2 + H_2O \xrightarrow[\text{anhydrase}]{\text{carbonic}} H_2CO_3 \longrightarrow H^+ + HCO_3^-$$

Because of the high intracellular negativity, the Cl⁻ present in the parietal cell is forced out into the lumen of gland through the Cl⁻ channels located on the apical membrane of the cell.

Functions of HCl

- HCl participates in the breakdown of proteins.
- It provides an optimal pH for the action of pepsin.
- It hinders the growth of pathogenic bacteria.

Pepsinogen secretion

- Pepsinogen is an inactive precursor (proenzyme) of pepsin. It is mainly secreted by *chief cells* of the main gastric glands. A small amount of pepsinogen is also secreted by pyloric glands.
- Pepsinogen is synthesized and stored as zymogen granules in the apical region of chief cells.
- Pepsinogen secretion is stimulated by vagal stimulation, gastrin, and histamine.
- Pepsinogen is converted to pepsin (the active form) by the action of HCl or preformed pepsin.

$$\text{Pepsinogen} \xrightarrow{\text{HCl}} \text{Pepsin}$$

$$\text{Pepsinogen} \xrightarrow{\text{Pepsin}} \text{Pepsin}$$

Function of pepsinogen. Pepsin, the active form of pepsinogen, is a proteolytic enzyme that begins the process of protein digestion.

Secretion of mucus

Mucus is of two types—insoluble and soluble.

Insoluble mucus is secreted by the mucus-secreting cells lining the entire gastric mucosa. The insoluble mucus is so viscid in nature that it forms a gel-like coat over the mucosa. These cells also secrete bicarbonate ions which make the mucus alkaline with pH of 7, that forms an extremely important protective layer saving the stomach from the destruction by HCl.

Soluble mucus is secreted by mucous cells of pylorus and cardiac glands.

Secretion of intrinsic factor

Intrinsic factor (IF), a glycoprotein, is secreted by the parietal cells of gastric mucosa, chiefly by those in the fundus.

Functions. The intrinsic factor is essential for the absorption of vitamin B_{12}. It forms a complex with B_{12} which is carried to the terminal ileum where the vitamin is absorbed.

Deficiency of intrinsic factor in some patients with idiopathic atrophy of gastric mucosa may cause a serious disorder called pernicious anaemia.

REGULATION OF GASTRIC SECRETION

Mechanisms regulating the gastric secretion include neural control and chemical control.

I. Neural control

Neural control over the gastric glands is exerted by local enteric plexus involving cholinergic neurons and impulses from the CNS via vagal (extrinsic) innervation.

Vagal stimulation increases the secretion of HCl by parietal cells and pepsin by chief cells. Vagal stimulation increases H^+ secretion by a direct path and an indirect path.

II. Chemical control

Chemical control on gastric glands is exerted mainly through:

1. **Role of gastrin.** Gastrin, a hormone, is secreted by the G-cells into the blood circulation (and not into gastric juice). It reaches the stomach through the arterial circulation and stimulates secretory activity of the parietal cells and chief cells.

2. **Role of histamine.** Histamine is released from the enterochromaffin-like (ECL) cells found in the base of the gastric gland. ECL cells bear both gastrin receptors and ACh receptors. They release histamine in response to both circulating gastrin as well as ACh released by vagal fibres. The histamine released stimulates *HCl secretion* from parietal cells by acting on H_2 receptors. H_2 receptor-blocking drugs, such as *cimetidine* and *ranitidine*, inhibit H^+ secretion by blocking the stimulatory effect of histamine.

3. **Role of somatostatin.** Somatostatin is secreted by D-cells located adjacent to G-cells or the parietal cells in the gastric glands. Somatostatin inhibits HCl secretion.

4. **Role of low pH (<3) in stomach.** Low pH (<3) in the stomach inhibits the secretion of H^+ by parietal cells by a negative feedback mechanism.

5. **Intestinal influences.** Chyme containing acid, fats and products of protein digestion when reaches the duodenum causes the release of several intestinal hormones like secretin, cholecystokinin (CCK), and gastric inhibitory peptide (GIP).

Phases of gastric secretion and their regulation

Meal-related gastric secretion can be divided into three phases (Fig. 8.3-6) :
- Cephalic phase,
- Gastric phase, and
- Intestinal phase.

1. Cephalic phase
- Cephalic phase of gastric secretion occurs before the entry of food into the stomach.
- The secretion is *initiated* by the thought, sight, smell or taste of food. Neurogenic signals originate in the cerebral cortex and appetite centres of amygdala or hypothalamus. The impulses are transmitted to dorsal vagal nuclei and from there through vagii to the stomach (Fig. 8.3-6).
- Emotions also influence this vagally-mediated gastric secretion. *Anger and hostility* are associated with increased gastric secretion and motility. *Fear and depression* decrease the gastric secretion and motility.

2. Gastric phase
- Gastric phase of gastric secretion occurs when food enters the stomach.
- The presence of food in the stomach induces gastric secretion by following *mechanisms:*
  - *Distension of the body of stomach,*
  - *Distension of the antrum* initiates vagally, mediated and local reflexes that result in gastrin release from the antral G-cells. Gastrin release is inhibited when pH becomes low (<3).
  - *Products of partial protein digestion* also stimulate gastrin secretion and this increases secretion of gastric acid mainly.
  - *Low pH* causes increased pepsinogen secretion through local reflexes.

3. Intestinal phase
- Intestinal phase of gastric secretion begins as the chyme begins to empty from the stomach into the duodenum.
- In contrast to the excitatory cephalic and gastric influences the intestinal influence on the gastric secretion is chiefly inhibitory in nature. Intestinal factor inhibits gastric secretion *by Enterogastric reflex* and through several hormones such as secretin, cholecystokinin (CCK), gastric inhibitory peptide (GIP), vasoactive intestinal polypeptide (VIP) and somatostatin which inhibit gastric secretion. The inhibitory influences discussed above help to terminate the gastric secretion when all the food has left stomach.

PHYSIOLOGY OF GASTRIC MOTILITY

The peristaltic activity of the gastric musculature has been given various names depending upon its features and motor function subserved by it. Gastric motility can be described as:
- Motility of the empty stomach, which includes:
  - Migrating motor complex, and
  - Hunger contractions.
- Gastric motility related to meal, includes:
  - Receptive relaxation,

S E C T I O N 8

CEPHALIC PHASE

Sight, smell, taste and thought of food

Emotion

→ Cerebral cortex
→ Hypothalamus
→ Vagal nuclei in medulla

To stomach
• Parietal cells
• Peptic cells
• G cells

Vagus ←

GASTRIC PHASE

Food in stomach

Distension — Partially digested protein products

Vagovagal reflex — Local reflex ←

G cells activation to secrete gastrin ←

Stimulate acid secretion

Gastrin in blood

Inhibit gastrin secretion

INTESTINAL PHASE

Enterogastric reflex

• Distension
• Low pH
• Protein breakdown products

Irritation of upper intestine mucosa

Hormonal secretion

Sympathetic nerve   Vagus nerve

Secretin
Enterogastron
Somatostatin
VIP
GIP

→ Circulation

Fig. 8.3-6. *Phases and regulation of gastric secretion.*

– Mixing peristaltic waves, and
– Gastric emptying.

Motility of empty stomach

1. Migrating motor complex (MMC) is the name given to the peristaltic wave that begins in the oesophagus and travels through the entire gastrointestinal tract (migratory motor activity) during interdigestive period.

- The MMCs remove any food remaining in the stomach and intestines during interdigestive period in preparation for the next meal; because of this they have been called the *interdigestive housekeepers*.

- The MMC are abolished immediately after the entry of food in the stomach.

2. Hunger contractions. Mild peristaltic contractions occur in the empty stomach, which over a period of hours increase in intensity and are called hunger contractions. MMCs are probably responsible for hunger contractions.

Gastric motility related to meals

1. Receptive relaxation and accommodation. Storage function of stomach is accomplished by receptive relaxation and accommodation.

- The passage of each bolus of food stimulates the stretch *receptors of oral region* and produces relaxation. By the end of meal about 1 to 2 L of food can be accommodated.

- Receptive relaxation is a *vagovagal reflex* initiated by distension of stomach and is synchronized with the primary peristaltic waves in the oesophagus.

2. Mixing peristaltic waves. The presence of food in the caudal region (distal body and antral part) of stomach increases the contractile activity of this part of stomach. This enhanced contractile activity (a combination of peristalsis and retropulsion) is called mixing waves which mix the food with stomach acid and enzymes and break it into smaller and smaller pieces. When the food is mixed into a pasty consistency it is called *chyme*.

3. Gastric emptying. Gastric emptying occurs when the chyme is decomposed into enough small pieces (typically less than 1 mm^3) to fit through the pyloric sphincter.

- Gastric emptying results from a progressive wave of forceful contraction which sequentially involves antrum, pylorus (pyloric sphincter) and proximal duodenum; thus all the three function as a unit.

FUNCTIONS OF STOMACH

After studying the physiological activities of stomach, its functions can be summarized as:

1. Mechanical or motor functions include:

- *Storage of food.*
- *Mixing of food.*
- *Slow emptying of food* into duodenum occurs to provide proper time for digestion and absorption by small intestine.

2. Digestive functions. Only small amounts of foods are digested in stomach as:

- *Carbohydrate digestion* in the stomach depends on the action of salivary amylase, which remains active until halted by the low pH of stomach.
- *Protein digestion.* About 10% of ingested protein is broken down completely in the stomach. *Gastric pepsin* facilitates later digestion of protein by breaking protein into peptone.
- *Fat digestion* in stomach is minimal due to the restriction of gastric lipase activity to triglycerides containing short chain (< 10 carbon) fatty acids.

3. Absorptive function. Stomach contributes little in absorption function.

4. Reflex functions. Various reflexes initiated from the stomach are:

- Gastro-salivary reflex,
- Gastro-ileal reflex,
- Gastro-colic reflex, and

- Presence of food in the stomach reflexly stimulates secretion of pancreatic juice and expulsion of bile.

5. Antiseptic action. HCl present in the gastric juice kills the bacteria and other harmful substances.

APPLIED ASPECTS

Important applied aspects of stomach which need special attention are:

- Gastric mucosal barrier and pathophysiology of peptic ulcer,
- Physiology of vomiting,
- Gastrectomy, and
- Gastric function tests.

GASTRIC MUCOSAL BARRIER AND PATHOPHYSIOLOGY OF PEPTIC ULCER

Gastric mucosal barrier

The gastric mucosal barrier protects the gastric mucosa from damage by intraluminal HCl, i.e. autodigestion. It is created by the following:

- *Mucin secretion.* The thin layer of surface mucus in the stomach and duodenum prevents the direct contact of acid and pepsin-containing fluid with surface epithelial cells.
- *Bicarbonate secretion.* Surface epithelial cells in both the stomach and the duodenum secrete bicarbonate which create an essentially pH neutral micro-environment immediately adjacent to the cell surface.
- *Epithelial barrier.* Intercellular tight junctions provide a barrier to the back-diffusion of H$^+$.
- *High mucosal blood flow.* It rapidly carries away any acid that penetrates the cellular lining, and also provides oxygen, bicarbonate, and nutrients to epithelial cells.
- *Prostaglandins* are responsible for maintaining the gastric mucosal barrier.

Pathophysiology of peptic ulcer

Peptic ulcer refers to excavation of mucosa of duodenum or pyloric part of stomach caused by the digestive action of gastric juice. Peptic ulcer can be caused by either of two ways:

1. Diminished ability of the gastroduodenal mucosal barrier to protect against the digestive properties of the acid-pepsin complex. Factors that disturb mucosal barrier include:

- *Bacterial infection by Helicobacter pylori.* At least 75% patients with peptic ulcer have recently been found to have chronic infection by *H. pylori.* The bacterium releases digestive enzymes that liquefy the barrier, which allows gastric secretion to digest the epithelial cells leading to peptic ulceration.

- *Other factors* which can disrupt the mucosal barrier are ethyl alcohol, vinegar, bile salts, cigarette smoking and non-steroidal anti-inflammatory drugs (NSAIDs), such as aspirin and ibuprofen.

2. *Excessive secretion of gastric acid.* Hyperacidity leads to ulcer formation in duodenum and pyloric part of stomach. Hyperacidity may occur due to:

- Increased parietal cell mass,
- Increased sensitivity for secretory stimuli,
- Excess gastrin secretion, as seen in Zollinger-Ellison syndrome in which patients are having *gastrinomas* (tumours that secrete gastrin).

Physiologic basis of management of peptic ulcer

Commonly employed measures for treatment of peptic ulcer are:

- *Antacids.* These form a gel that coats the mucosa and neutralizes the acid.
- *H₂-receptor blocking drugs* such as cimetidine.
- *M₁-muscarinic receptor blocking drugs* such as atropine.
- *Gastric H⁺-K⁺-ATPase inhibiting drugs* such as omeprazole.
- *Bilateral vagotomy combined with resection of gastrin-producing pyloric part of stomach* is performed in very severe cases of duodenal and pyloric ulcers.

PHYSIOLOGY OF VOMITING

Vomiting refers to forceful expulsion of contents from stomach and intestine.

Initiation of vomiting

Vomiting may be initiated by either activation of vomiting centre or by activation of the chemoreceptor trigger zone.

1. *Activation of vomiting centre*

Vomiting centre is situated in the reticular formation of medulla oblongata near the vagal nucleus. It may be activated directly or through afferents:

i. *Direct activation of the vomiting centre* occurs due to injury to the area or by raised intracranial pressure.

ii. *Afferent impulses* activating vomiting centre include (Fig. 8.3-7):

- *Visceral afferent pathway* in the sympathetic and vagi relay impulses arising due to irritation of mucosa of upper GIT.
- *Afferent impulses from the vestibular nuclei* mediate nausea and vomiting of motion sickness.
- *Afferents from higher centres* (diencephalon and limbic system) mediate emetic response to stimuli such as nauseating smell, sickening sights, and memory etc.

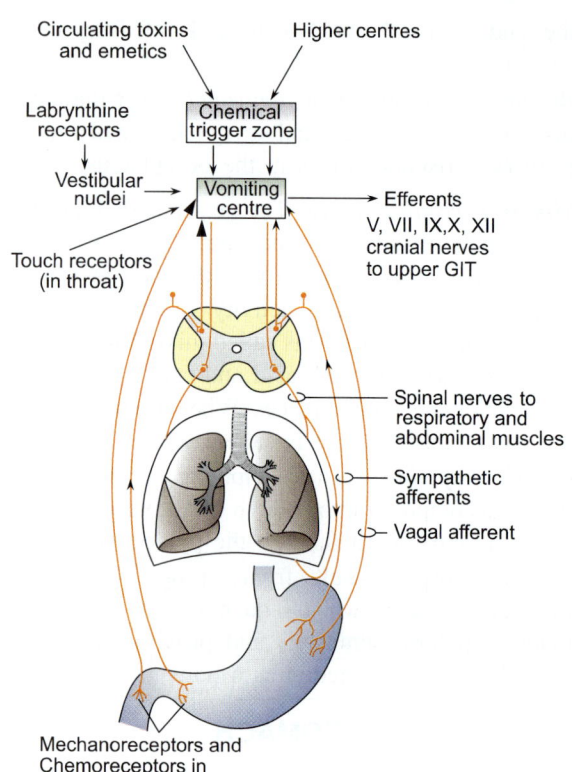

Fig. 8.3-7. *Pathway for vomiting reflex.*

2. Activation of chemoreceptor trigger zone

Chemoreceptor trigger zone (CTZ) is located in the area *postrema* (a V-shaped band of tissue on the lateral walls of fourth ventricle near the obex) which is outside the blood-brain barrier and is thus more permeable to many substances.

Efferent impulses from vomiting centre and CTZ

Efferent impulses from the vomiting centre and CTZ, which give effect to act of vomiting, are transmitted via V, VII, IX, X and XII cranial nerves to upper GIT and through spinal nerves to the muscles of respiration.

Sequence of mechanical events of vomiting

Vomiting is a complex process and consists of following phases:

1. *Pre-ejection phase.* It is characterized by feeling of nausea, excessive salivation and deep, rapid and irregular breathing.

2. *Retching phase* may precede in many cases. It is characterized by:

- *Closure of glottis* and
- *Rhythmic action of respiratory muscles.*

3. *Ejection phase* during which the GIT contents are actually expelled out.

Pancreas, Liver and Gall Bladder

8.4

Pancreas, liver and gall bladder are accessory organs of digestive system. It will be worthwhile to know about the physiological role of pancreas, liver and gall bladder in digestive system at this level, because secretions of these organs affect the digestive activities of small intestine.

PANCREAS

ANATOMY OF PANCREAS

Gross anatomy

The pancreas—an elongated, accessory digestive gland— lies retroperitoneally and transversely across the posterior abdominal wall, posterior to the stomach between the duodenum on the right and spleen on the left (Fig. 8.4-1).

Anatomically, pancreas is divided into four parts: head, neck, body, and tail.

- *Head* refers to right enlarged end of pancreas. It lies in the C-shaped space bounded by the duodenum. A projection arising from the lower left part of head is called *uncinate process.*

- *Neck.* Next to the head there is a short somewhat constricted part called the neck.

- *Body.* The neck is continuous with the main part of the pancreas - the body. The neck and body of pancreas are separated from the stomach by lesser sac.

- *Tail* refers to the left thin extremity of the pancreas.

Physiologically, on the basis of functions performed, the pancreas consists of two parts:

- *Exocrine part*, which produces a secretion called pancreatic juice that contains enzymes capable of hydrolyzing proteins, fats and carbohydrates.

- *Endocrine part* of the pancreas, the islets of Langerhans, produce the hormones insulin and glucagon, which play

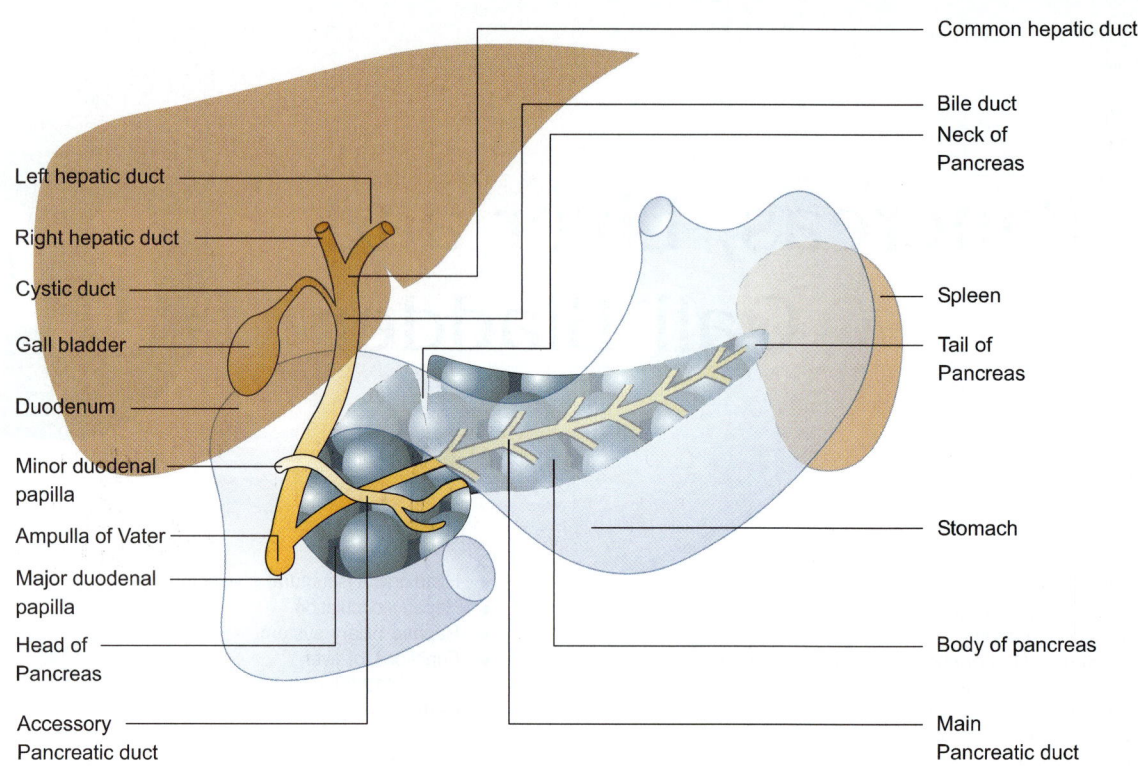

Fig. 8.4-1. *Anatomical relations of pancreas, pancreatic duct and extrahepatic biliary system.*

a key role in the carbohydrate metabolism. The endocrine part is discussed elsewhere (page 369).

Histological structural characteristics of exocrine part of pancreas

The exocrine part of the pancreas is in the form of a serous, compound tubuloalveolar gland, very similar to parotid gland in general structure (Fig. 8.4-2).

Fig. 8.4-2. *Histology of functional unit of exocrine pancreas.*

Acinar cells lining the alveoli appear triangular in section. Numerous secretory (or zymogen) granules can be demonstrated in the cytoplasm, especially in the apical part of cells.

The acinar cells produce thick secretion containing numerous enzymes (listed in composition of pancreatic juice).

Centroacinar cells. The centroacinar cells that are so called because they appear to be located near the centre of the acinus (alveolus). These cells really belong to the intercalated ducts which are invaginated into the acinus (Fig. 8.4-2).

Pancreatic ducts

The intercalated ducts, which receive secretions produced by acini, pass it on to *interlobular ducts*. Ultimately the pancreatic secretion passes into duodenum through the main pancreatic duct and accessory pancreatic duct.

Main pancreatic duct, also known as duct of Wirsung, begins in the tail and runs the length of the gland, receiving numerous tributaries on the way. It joins the common bile duct to form the ampulla of Vater, which opens into the second part of the duodenum at about its middle on the major duodenal papilla (Fig. 8.4-1). Ampulla of Vater is guarded by the sphincter of Oddi.

Accessory pancreatic duct, also called a duct of Santorini, when present, drains the upper part of the head and then opens into the duodenum about 2 mm above the main duct on the minor duodenal papilla.

Vessels and nerves of pancreas

Arterial supply to the pancreas comes from splenic and superior as well as inferior pancreaticoduodenal arteries.

Veins, corresponding to arteries, drain into the portal system.

Lymphatics drain into the lymph nodes situated along the arteries that supply the gland. The efferent vessels ultimately drain into the coeliac and superior mesenteric lymph nodes.

Nerve supply comes from both sympathetic and parasympathetic (vagi) nerves. Preganglionic vagal fibres synapse with ganglionic cells embedded in the pancreatic tissue; the postganglionic fibres innervate both the acinar cells and smooth muscles of the ducts. Vagal stimulation increases pancreatic juice secretion.

PANCREATIC JUICE (SECRETION)

Properties

- Pancreatic juice is a transparent colourless fluid isotonic with plasma.
- About 1200-1500 ml of pancreatic juice is secreted per day.
- Its specific gravity varies from 1.010 to 1.018.
- Pancreatic juice is markedly alkaline (pH 7.8 to 8.4), due to very high concentration of HCO_3^- (about 4-5 times that of plasma).

Composition

Pancreatic juice is composed of 99.5% water and 0.5% solids which include organic and inorganic substances.

Organic constituents of pancreatic juice are certain enzymes amylase, lipase, protease and trypsin inhibitor and other organic substances present in traces are albumin and globulin. Pancreatic enzymes are described with the functions of pancreas.

Inorganic substances present in the pancreatic juice are cations like Na^+, K^+, Ca^{2+}, Mg^{2+}, and Zn^{2+}; and anions such as HCO_3^-, Cl^- and traces of SO_4^{2-} and HPO_4^{2-}. Electrolyte composition varies with rate of secretion.

FUNCTIONS OF PANCREATIC JUICE

I. Digestive functions

The pancreatic juice is the major source of digestive enzymes which include :

1. *Pancreatic α amylase*. It is secreted in its active form. Its action on the carbohydrates is like that of salivary amylase (see page 266).

2. *Pancreatic lipases* or lipolytic enzymes include pancreatic lipase, cholesterol ester hydrolase and phospholipase A_2.

3. *Pancreatic proteases* or proteolytic enzymes include three endopeptidases (trypsin, chymotrypsin and elastase) and two exopeptidases (carboxypeptidase A and B).

- *Trypsin*. It is the most powerful proteolytic enzyme of the pancreatic juice.
  - It hydrolyses proteins into proteoses and to polypeptides.
  - It activates trypsinogen and other pancreatic enzymes.
- *Chymotrypsin*. It hydrolyses the proteins into small polypeptides.
- *Elastase*. It digests elastin.
- *Carboxypeptidase A* cleaves the carboxyl-terminal amino acid that have aromatic or branched aliphatic side chains.
- *Carboxypeptidase B* cleaves the carboxy-terminal amino acids that have basic side chains.
- *Nucleases* (ribonuclease and deoxyribonuclease). They split nucleic acids of ribose and deoxyribose type into nucleotides.

4. *Trypsin inhibitor*. If even a small amount of trypsin is released into the pancreas, the resulting chain reaction would produce active enzymes that could digest the pancreas. It is, therefore, not surprising that the pancreas normally contains a trypsin inhibitor which is secreted by the same cells and at the same time as the pancreatic proenzymes. Trypsin inhibitor protects the pancreas from autodigestion.

II. Neutralizing function

Pancreatic juice is highly alkaline due to high concentration of HCO_3^- and neutralizes the gastric HCl in the chyme that enters the duodenum.

REGULATION OF PANCREATIC SECRETION

Both, neural and hormonal, mechanisms are involved in the regulation of pancreatic secretion, with the latter playing the predominant role.

Neural regulation is through vagal efferents supplying the exocrine gland of pancreas.

Hormonal regulation is through secretin, cholecystokinin (CCK), gastrin and somatostatin.

The exact role of these regulatory mechanisms in regulation of different phases of pancreatic secretion viz. cephalic phase, gastric phase and intestinal phase is summarized below :

1. Regulation of cephalic phase

Cephalic phase of pancreatic secretion like that of gastric secretion occurs before the entry of food into the stomach.

Regulation of this phase is mainly through the reflex vagal stimulation.

2. Regulation of gastric phase

Gastric phase of pancreatic secretion occurs when stomach is distended by the food. This phase is regulated by *neural control* exerted through vagus and *hormonal control* executed through the hormone gastrin.

3. Regulation of intestinal phase

The intestinal phase of pancreatic secretion begins when

the chyme enters the duodenum and jejunum. It is characterized by marked increase in the secretion of both enzymes and aqueous component of pancreatic juice. This phase is regulated by the hormones secretin and cholecystokinin (CCK).

Interaction of nervous and humoral regulation

A vago-vagal reflex is initiated during intestinal phase of digestion which greatly potentiates the effects of secretin and CCK through the acetylcholine. Thus, vagus stimulation is much more potent in stimulating pancreatic secretions when CCK and secretin are present in the plasma.

DISORDERS OF PANCREAS

Common disorders of pancreas are:

1. Acute pancreatitis. It is an acute inflammatory disease of pancreas, thought to result from autodigestion of pancreatic tissue by the proteolytic enzymes which leak out of the acini and are activated within the pancreas.

2. Chronic pancreatitis is a chronic inflammation of pancreas which results in slow destruction of the tissue resulting in the deficiency of pancreatic secretions. Patients with extensive destruction of pancreas may develop:

- *Diabetes mellitus* due to pancreatic endocrine deficiency of insulin.
- *Digestive disturbances* due to deficiency of pancreatic enzymes mainly affect the fat metabolism resulting in *steatorrhoea* which is characterized by bulky, foul smelling, pale and greasy stools (due to increase in faecal fat content).

3. Cystic fibrosis is a disorder of pancreatic secretion. It is caused by a mutation in the cystic fibrosis transmembrane conductance regulator (CFTR) gene. It is associated with a deficiency of pancreatic enzymes resulting in steatorrhoea.

LIVER AND GALL BLADDER

THE LIVER

GROSS ANATOMY OF LIVER

Size and weight. Liver, the largest gland in the body, weighs approximately 1500 gms.

Location. It is located in the right hypochondric and epigastric regions and frequently extends in the left hypochondric area.

Surfaces. The liver has two surfaces. The upper convex surface fits closely into the under surface of the diaphragm. Below the *visceral surface* is concave and fits over the right kidney, the upper portion of the ascending colon, and the pyloric end of stomach.

Ligaments. The liver is connected to the undersurface of

diaphragm and the anterior walls by the ligaments. The falciform ligament, the coronary ligament and right and left triangular ligaments are formed by folds of peritoneum. The ligamentum teres and ligamentum venosum are fibrous cords resulting from the atrophy of left umbilical vein and ductus venosus (which exist in fetal life), respectively.

Lobes. Anatomically, the liver has been divided into *right and left lobes*. Right lobe is much larger and includes caudate lobe and quadrate lobe. Left lobe is much smaller. In current terminology, the liver consists of right and left functionally independent parts called the *portal lobes*, that are approximately equal in size (Fig. 8.4-3).

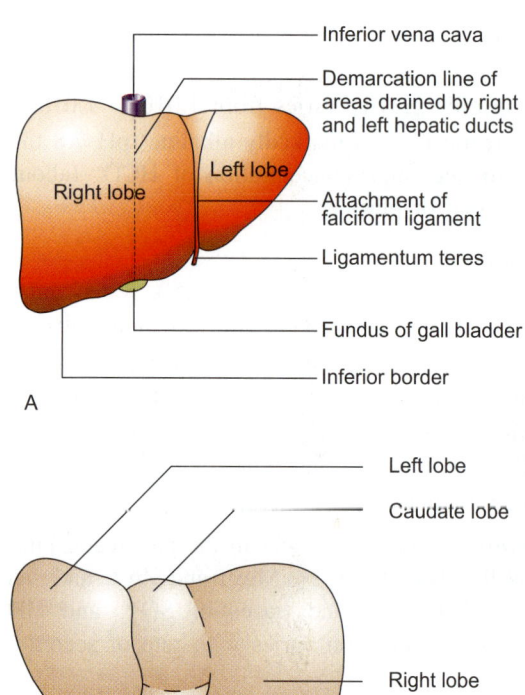

Fig. 8.4-3. *Gross anatomy of the liver : A, viewed from front; B, viewed from behind.*

The right and left functional parts of the liver have their own blood supply from the hepatic artery and portal vein and their own venous and biliary drainage.

Liver has got considerable physiological reserve. Even after removal of 80% of liver tissues, all *physiological* functions of liver can be accomplished normally.

The liver possesses considerable *regeneration power*. Original liver mass is restored within 6-8 weeks of removal of upto 3/4th of liver. This occurs due to active mitotic division of the cells.

HISTOLOGICAL STRUCTURAL CHARACTERISTICS

The liver tissue comprises about one lac hexagonal areas that constitute the *hepatic lobules* (Fig. 8.4-4A).

- Each hepatic lobule is made of ramifying columns of hepatic cells (*hepatocytes*) that are arranged in the form of one cell thick plates. In between the cells are present bile canaliculi. These hepatic cell plates are tunelled by a communicating system of lacunae called *blood sinusoids*. The sinusoids open into a central vein present in the centre of each lobule (Fig. 8.4-4B).

A

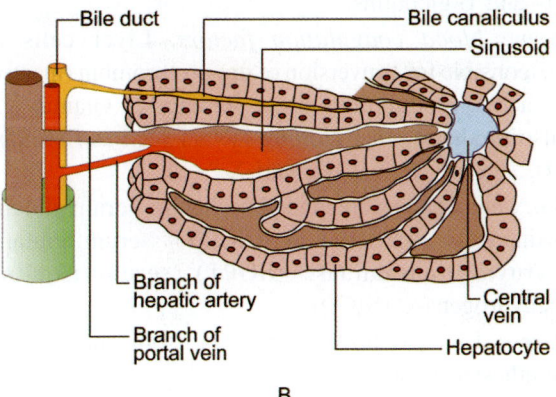

B

Fig. 8.4-4. Histological characteristics of the liver: A, hexagonal lobule with portal triad; and B, hepatocyte, sinusoid and biliary canaliculi seen under high magnification.

- Blood sinusoids are lined by endothelial cells. Few tissue macrophages called *Kupffer cells* are found at regular intervals in between the endothelial cells.
- *Portal triads* are present along the periphery of each lobule.
- *Portal triads* consist of a branch of portal vein, branch of hepatic artery and an interlobular bile duct. Blood from the branch of portal vein and hepatic artery enters the sinusoids which drain into central vein.
- *Concept of portal lobule,* instead of hepatic lobule, has been suggested by some workers. It has been described to consist of adjoining part of three hepatic lobules centred on a portal triad.

HEPATIC CIRCULATION

Liver receives about 1500 ml blood/min from two sources:
Hepatic artery, which is a branch of coeliac trunk, supplies about 20 to 25% (300 to 400 ml/min) of total blood which caters to metabolic requirement of the liver tissue.

Portal vein, which collects blood from the mesenteric and splenic vascular bed, supplies about 75 to 80% (1100-1200 ml/min) of the total blood.

Hepatic vein. The hepatic and portal streams of blood meet in the sinusoids. The various substances produced by liver cells, the waste products and CO_2 are discharged into the sinusoids. The sinusoids drain into the central vein of the lobule. The central veins from different lobules unite to form bigger veins. These veins ultimately form the right and left hepatic veins which open into the inferior vena cava.

HEPATIC BILIARY SYSTEM

Intrahepatic biliary system

The bile is secreted by liver cells into *bile canaliculi.* These canaliculi have no walls of their own. In fact, the bile canaliculi are the spaces bounded by canalicular surfaces of adjacent hepatic cells. These canaliculi form hexagonal network around the liver cells. At the periphery of a lobule the canaliculi become continuous with delicate *intralobular ductules,* which in turn become continuous with larger interlobular ductules of portal triads. The *interlobular ductules* are lined by cuboidal epithelium. Some smooth muscle is present in the wall of larger ducts. Ultimately, the larger ducts join to form the *right and left hepatic ducts* which leave the right and left parts of the liver and form part of extrahepatic biliary system.

Extrahepatic biliary apparatus

The extrahepatic biliary apparatus consists of gall bladder and the extrahepatic bile ducts (Fig. 8.4-1).

Gall bladder
(For details see page 283).

Extrahepatic ducts
Hepatic ducts. The right and left hepatic ducts emerge from the right and left lobes of the liver and after a short course join to form *common hepatic duct* which is about 4 cm long (Figs. 8.4-1 and 8.4-5).

Cystic duct. It is also about 4 cm long and connects the neck of gall bladder to the common hepatic duct to form the common bile duct.

Common bile duct (CBD) is about 8 cm long. It joins the pancreatic duct to form the common hepatopancreatic duct which is otherwise called the ampulla of Vater (Fig. 8.4-1). Ampulla of Vater opens into the duodenum at

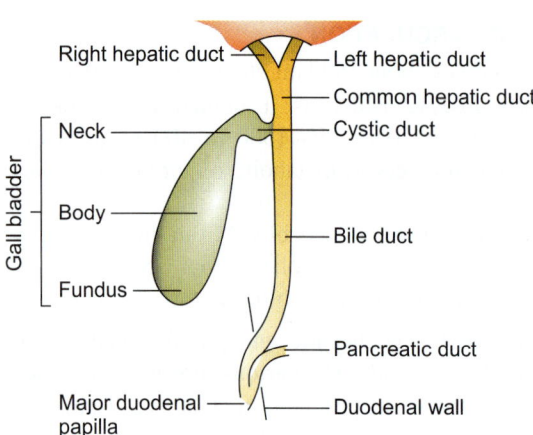

Right hepatic duct — Left hepatic duct
— Common hepatic duct
Neck — — Cystic duct
Body
— Bile duct
Fundus
— Pancreatic duct
Major duodenal — — Duodenal wall
papilla
Gall bladder

Fig. 8.4-5. *Scheme to show the parts of extrahepatic biliary system.*

major duodenal papilla. The terminal parts of bile ducts and ampulla of Vater are surrounded by circular muscle fibres known as sphincter of Oddi, which plays an important role in the storage and release of bile from the gall bladder.

FUNCTIONS OF LIVER

Various functions performed by liver are summarized here briefly.

I. Secretory functions

Liver cells act as exocrine gland and continuously secrete bile which is important for digestion and absorption of fats.

II. Metabolic functions

Liver is the key organ and the principal site where the metabolism of carbohydrates, lipids and proteins takes place. Liver is also involved in the metabolism of vitamins and minerals to certain extent.

1. Role in carbohydrate metabolism includes:

i. Liver acts as a glucostat in three ways:

- *Glycogenesis,* i.e. glycogen is formed from glucose and stored in liver.

- *Glycogenolysis*, i.e. breaking down of liver glycogen to glucose.

- *Glucogenesis*, i.e. formation of glucose from non-carbohydrate sources such as non-nitrogenous residues of amino acids.

2. Role in fat metabolism. Both degradation and synthesis of fats take place in liver.

3. Role in protein metabolism. In man, the protein turnover involves breakdown and resynthesis of 80-100 gm of tissue protein per day, and its 50% part (i.e. 40-50 gm) occurs in liver.

III. Detoxicating and protective functions

- Kupffer cells efficiently remove bacteria and other foreign bodies from portal circulation. This is the blood cleansing action of liver.

- Liver detoxifies certain drugs by either oxidation, or hydrolysis, or reduction or conjugation, and excretes out through bile.

IV. Storage functions

- Liver stores glucose (in the form of glycogen), vitamin B_{12}, and vitamin A.

- Liver acts as a blood-iron buffer and iron storage medium. It stores 60% of excess of iron mainly in the form of ferritin and partly as haemosiderin.

V. Excretory functions

Certain exogenous dyes like bromsulphthalein (BSP) and rose Bengal dye are exclusively excreted through liver cells.

VI. Synthesis function

Liver is the site for synthesis of:

- *Plasma proteins*, especially albumin and to some extent α- and β-globulins.

- *Some blood coagulation factors*. Liver cells are responsible for conversion of pre-prothrombin (inactive) to active prothrombin in the presence of vitamin K. It also produces other clotting factors such as fibrinogen (I), factors V, VII, IX and X.

- *Enzymes*, such as alkaline phosphatase, serum glutamic oxaloacetic transaminase (SGOT), serum glutamic pyruvic transaminase (SGPT), serum isocitrate dehydrogenase (SICD).

- *Urea*. Liver removes ammonia from the body to synthesize urea.

- *Cholesterol*. It is synthesized from the active acetate.

VII. Miscellaneous functions

- *Reservoir of blood*. Liver acts as reservoir of blood and it stores about 650 ml of blood. Also helps in regulation of blood volume.

- *Erythropoiesis*. Liver is an important site of erythropoiesis in fetal life.

- *Hormone metabolism*. Liver causes:
  - *Inactivation* of some hormones such as insulin, glucagon and vasopressin.
  - *Reduction and conjugation* of adrenal and gonadal steroid hormones such as cortisol, aldosterone, oestrogen and testosterone.
  - *Conversion of thyroid hormone*, i.e. tetra-iodothyronine (T_4) into tri-iodothyronine (T_3).

- *Destruction of RBCs* also occurs in liver.

- *Thermal regulation*. Liver also helps in thermo-regulation, as it produces large amount of heat.

GALL BLADDER AND BILE

GALL BLADDER

Gall bladder is a pear-shaped sac lying in gall bladder fossa on the undersurface of liver, where it is held in place by peritoneum which covers its inferior (or posterior) surface (Figs. 8.4.1 and 8.4-5). It is about 7 to 10 cm long, 2.5 cm wide and has a capacity to store about 30 to 50 ml of bile.

Parts. For descriptive purposes the gall bladder is divided into three parts (Fig. 8.4-5) :

- *Fundus* is the lowest globular part which projects beyond the inferior border of liver (Fig. 8.4-1A), and is surrounded all round by peritoneum.
- *Body* is the central part of gall bladder. Its superior (or anterior) surface is in direct contact with the liver.
- *Neck* is the narrow part succeeding the body of gall bladder. The neck becomes continuous with the cystic duct, through which the gall bladder drains into the bile duct.

Functions of gall bladder

Gall bladder subserves following functions :

1. Storage of bile. The bile secreted during interdigestive period is stored in the gall bladder. The gall bladder typically stores 30-50 ml of bile. During meals, the gall bladder contracts and releases its contents into the duodenum.

2. Concentration of bile. The mucosa of gall bladder is extensively folded and can actively absorb fluid and electrolytes. In this way, the gall bladder bile, in comparison to liver bile, becomes thicker, viscous and darker in colour.

3. Effect on the pH of bile. In the gall bladder, due to rapid absorption of HCO_3^- (mainly), Na^+ and Cl^-, the pH of bile is decreased from 8-8.6 to 7-7.6.

4. Secretion of mucus. Gall bladder secretes mucin which is added to the bile stored in it. The mucin acts as a lubricant in the intestine for the chyme.

THE BILE

Formation and storage of bile

Bile is a digestive juice formed continuously in the liver. It is formed by the hepatocytes and ductal cells lining the hepatic ducts.

- It is poured into the bile canaliculi from where it ultimately goes to common hepatic duct which joins with cystic duct to form common bile duct. During interdigestive period when the sphincter of Oddi is closed, the bile is directed via cystic duct to the gall bladder, where it is stored and concentrated.
- During meals, the sphincter of Oddi is relaxed, and when food reaches the duodenum, there occurs release

of CCK which causes contraction of gall bladder. Then the bile is released into the duodenum along with the pancreatic juice through the common opening ampulla of Vater.

Composition of bile

The bile is an alkaline juice composed of:

- Water and solids,
- Solids include organic and inorganic substances,
- Organic substances are bile salts, bile pigments, cholesterol, lecithin, fatty acids and enzyme alkaline phosphatase,
- Inorganic substances are Na^+, K^+, Ca^{2+}, HCO_3^- and Cl.

Since the bile is concentrated in the gall bladder, so the concentration of its ingredients in the liver bile and gall bladder bile is bound to differ.

Salient features of the some of the ingredients of bile are described here:

1. Bile salts

Bile salts are sodium and potassium salts of bile acids conjugated with either taurine or glycine.

Enterohepatic circulation of bile salts. Enterohepatic circulation is the recirculation of bile salts from the liver to small intestine and back again (Fig. 8.4-6).

- When the bile salts reach *terminal ileum*, 90 to 95% of bile salts are reabsorbed into the portal circulation. The

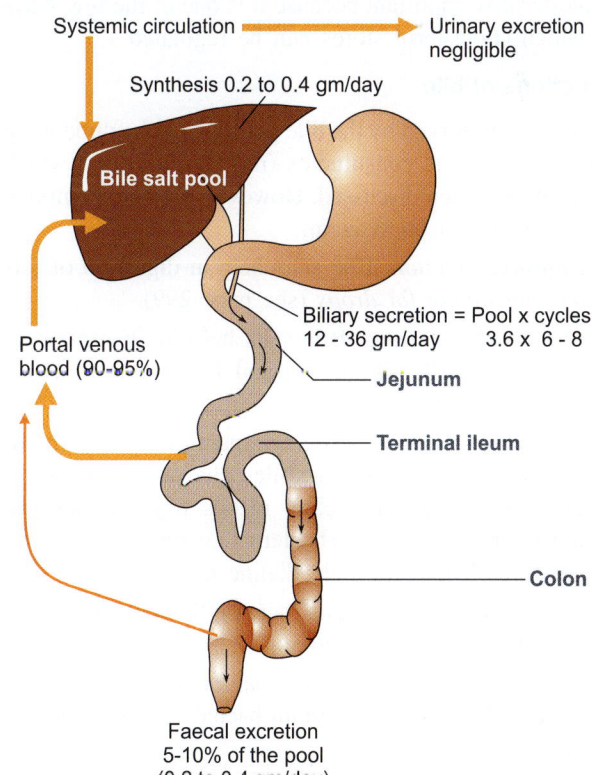

Fig. 8.4-6. Enterohepatic circulation of bile salts.

liver then extracts the bile salts from the portal blood and secretes them once again into the bile.

- The remaining 5-10% of bile salts are excreted into the faeces.

Circulating pool. The total circulating pool of bile salts is approximately 3.6 gm. About 4-8 gm of bile salts are required (more if the meal is high in fat) for digestion of fats during each meal; as the total content of bile salts in the body is only 3.6 gm, thus most circulate twice during each meal for proper digestion of fats. Consequently, the bile salts usually circulate 6-8 times daily.

2. Bile pigments

- The two principal bile pigments, *bilirubin* and *biliverdin*, are the other major constituents of bile which have no digestive function.
- Bile pigments are metabolites of haemoglobin formed in the liver.
- Intestinal bacteria metabolize bilirubin further to urobilinogen, which is responsible for the brown colour of stools.

3. Phospholipids

The phospholipids (primarily lecithins) are, after bile salts, the most abundant organic compound in bile.

4. Cholesterol

Cholesterol is an other important constituent of bile that does not have digestive function. Biliary secretion of cholesterol is important because it is one of the few ways in which cholesterol stores can be regulated.

Functions of bile

Functions subserved by the bile poured into the duodenum are because of its constituents (mainly bile salts) which have already been discussed. However, they are compiled and summarized once again:

1. *Digestive function.* Bile salts help in digestion of fats by *emulsifying fat drops* (see page 299).
2. *Absorptive functions.* Bile salts help in absorption of fats (by micelle formation) and fat soluble vitamins (see page 301).
3. *Excretory function.* Bile pigments are the major excretory products of the bile. The other substances excreted in bile are heavy metals (e.g. copper and iron), some toxins, some bacteria (e.g. typhoid bacteria), cholesterol, lecithin and alkaline phosphatase.
4. *Laxative action.* Bile salts increase the gastrointestinal motility and act as laxative.
5. *Protective action.* Bile is a natural detergent. So, it inhibits the growth of certain bacteria in the lumen of intestine.
6. *Choleretic action,* i.e. bile salts stimulate the liver to secrete bile.

7. *Maintenance of pH of GIT.* Being highly alkaline the bile juice neutralizes the gastric HCl present in the chyme entering the small intestine. Thus, an optimum pH is maintained for the action of digestive enzymes.
8. *Prevention of gall stone formation.* Bile salts keep the cholesterol and lecithin in solution and thus prevents the formation of gall stones. In the absence of bile salts the cholesterol precipitates along with lecithin and may form gall stones.
9. *Lubricating function.* The mucin secreted by gall bladder mucosa into the bile lubricates the chyme in the intestine.
10. *Cholagogue function.* Cholagogue is an agent, which increases the release of bile from gall bladder into the intestine. The bile salts perform this function indirectly. The bile salts stimulate the secretion of hormone CCK, which has got cholagogue action.

Regulation of bile

The regulation of bile juice released into the duodenum, after the meals, is performed at two levels:

- Regulation of biliary secretion, and
- Regulation of release of bile from the gall bladder.

A. Regulation of biliary secretion

Secretion of the bile juice is controlled by secretin and vagal stimulation.

B. Regulation of release of bile juice from gall bladder

1. *Hormonal control.* The hormone *cholecystokinin* (CCK) is the major stimulus for gall bladder contraction and sphincter of Oddi relaxation. When chyme enters the small intestine, *fat and protein digestion products* directly stimulate the secretion of CCK.

2. *Neural control.* Vagal stimulation also causes contraction of gall bladder and relaxation of sphincter of Oddi. Vagal stimulation occurs directly during the cephalic phase of digestion and indirectly via a vagovagal reflex during the gastric phase of digestion.

APPLIED ASPECTS

DISORDERS OF LIVER AND GALL BLADDER

Jaundice or icterus

Jaundice or icterus refers to yellow discoloration of skin and mucous membrane due to raised levels of bilirubin in the blood.

- *Normal values* of serum bilirubin range between 0.3 and 1 mg%,
- *Jaundice* manifests when serum bilirubin becomes more than 2 mg%.

Types of jaundice. Jaundice is of three types:

- *Haemolytic jaundice* (pre-hepatic jaundice).
- *Hepatocellular jaundice* occurs due to damage to hepatocytes, as seen in viral hepatitis, cirrhosis and drug-induced hepatitis.
- *Obstructive jaundice*, also called post-hepatic jaundice, occurs due to blockage in bile duct either due to stone or any growth (e.g. in carcinoma of head of pancreas).

Cirrhosis of liver

Cirrhosis of liver refers to an irreversible chronic damage to liver with extensive fibrosis.

Viral hepatitis

Aetiology. Viral hepatitis (inflammation of liver) is caused by hepatitis virus A, B, C, D, E, F or G.

Hepatitis-B is more popular.

Cholecystitis

Cholecystitis refers to inflammation of gall bladder.

Gall stones

Gall stones are formed due to precipitation of cholesterol. Normally, cholesterol is present in soluble form due to a proper ratio of cholesterol and bile salts (1:20 to 1:30). When, this ratio falls below 1:13, the cholesterol is precipitated forming many small crystals.

LIVER FUNCTION TESTS

The liver function tests (LFTs) are the investigations to assess the capacity of the liver to carry any of the functions it performs. Thus, LFTs help in:

- Assessing the extent of functional damage to the liver,
- Diagnosing the cause of hepatic insufficiency, and
- Assessing the progress/regress of the disease.

I. Tests to assess secretory functions of liver

1. Serum bilirubin. The *normal values* are:

- Total serum bilirubin: 0.3-1.0 mg%,
- Conjugated bilirubin: 0.1-0.3 mg%, and
- Unconjugated bilirubin: 0.2-0.7 mg%.

Van den Bergh test is specific to identify the increase in serum bilirubin (above reference level). The results of test are interpreted as:

- Normal serum: Negative reaction,
- Haemolytic jaundice: Indirect positive reaction,
- Obstructive jaundice: Direct positive reaction, and
- Hepatic jaundice: Biphasic reaction.

2. Urine bilirubin and bile salts. Normally urine does not contain bilirubin and bile salts. In liver insufficiency, when the serum bilirubin levels increase above 2 mg% the bilirubin is excreted in the urine (*bilirubinuria*).

3. Urine urobilinogen. In normal individuals, less than 4 mg of urobilinogen is excreted in the urine. In liver insufficiency, initially there occurs mild increase in the daily excretion of urine urobilinogen. However, in later stages urobilinogen is absent in the urine. This occurs because of the fact that the swollen liver cells block bile canaliculi and prevent excretion of conjugated bilirubin in the bile.

4. Faecal stercobilinogen.

- Normal levels 20-25 mg%.
- Increased initially in liver insufficiency producing dark brown stools.
- Decreased in later stages of liver insufficiency producing pale-coloured stool.

5. Faecal fat levels.

- Normally 5-6% of total fat intake per day in excreted in the faeces.
- In liver insufficiency fat excretion in faeces increases upto 40-50% of total intake (steatorrhoa).

II. Tests to assess metabolic functions of liver

1. Galactose tolerance test. This test is based on the principle that galactose after absorption from the gut gets converted into glycogen in the liver. Therefore, in liver insufficiency its level in the blood rises.

2. Blood glucose level. The normal fasting blood glucose level is 70-90 mg%. In hepatic insufficiency its level decreases.

3. Blood and urine amino acid levels. Blood and urine amino acid levels are estimated to assess protein metabolism. In liver damage blood amino acid levels (normal 30-65 mg%) and urine amino acid levels are increased.

4. Lipid profile. In hepatic insufficiency lipid profile is affected as:

Abnormalities of serum lipid levels are sensitive but nonspecific indicators.

III. Tests to assess synthesis functions of liver

1. Estimation of plasma proteins

- *Albumin.* Liver cell damage causes hypoalbuminaemia (normal 6.4-8.3 gm%).
- *Globulins.* Hyperglobulinaemia is usually associated with hypoalbuminaemia.
- *A:G ratio.* In liver disorder there occurs reversal of A:G ratio (normal 1.7:1).

2. Serum levels of liver enzymes.

- *Transaminases.* The activity of transaminase like SGPT and SGOT increases in hepatic insufficiency.
- *Alkaline phosphatase.* Alkaline phosphatase is not a liver-specific enzyme, but secreted into the bile. In

obstructive jaundice its level is markedly increased (>30 KA units).

3. Blood urea. Liver is the main site for urea formation from ammonia. Decreased level of blood urea (normal 20-40 mg%) and raised blood ammonia level (normal 20-80 mg%) occur in liver insufficiency.

4. Coagulation factors. Factors II, V, VII, IX and X and vitamin K needed to activate these factors are synthesized by the liver. The integrity and activity of these factors is determined by prothrombin time test (PTT). Prolonged prothrombin time (PT) (normal 10-16 sec) indicates severe liver disease.

IV. Tests to assess detoxication functions of liver

1. Bromsulphthalein (BSP) excretion test. BSP is taken up by the liver cells from the blood and detoxified and excreted in the bile. The rate of removal of BSP from the blood depends on the functional efficiency of liver and rate of hepatic blood flow.

V. Tests to assess hepatic cellular integrity

1. Ultrasonography is done to detect diffuse disease of parenchyma of the liver (cirrhosis liver, fatty liver), abscess, cysts, tumours, gall stones and dilatation of biliary system proximal to site of obstruction.

2. Computed tomography (CT). CT scan has the same diagnostic significance as the ultrasonography except that it can also detect even smaller lesions.

3. Liver biopsy. This is performed by a special needle passed through intercostal space under local anaesthesia to obtain tissue for histopathological examination.

4. Fine needle aspiration (FNA). Very fine needle is usually guided by ultrasound and material is aspirated for cytological, histopathological and bacteriological examination.

5. Cholecystography is done to assess the functions and diseases of gall bladder. Nowadays this test is less commonly performed than ultrasonography.

The Small Intestine

8.5

ANATOMY OF SMALL INTESTINE

GROSS ANATOMY

The small intestine is convoluted tube which extends from the pylorus of stomach to the ileocaecal valve, where it joins with caecum, the first part of large intestine. It is about 6-7 metres in length.

Parts of small intestine

It is divided into three parts: the duodenum, the jejunum and the ileum (see Fig. 8.1-1.).

Duodenum. The first and *shortest* part (25 cm long) of the small intestine is also the *widest* and most fixed part. It is C-shaped and for descriptive purposes is divided into four parts: superior (1st) part, descending (2nd) part, horizontal (3rd) part, and ascending (4th part). Superior part of duodenum is also called *duodenal cap* or bulb. It is the region which is struck by acidic gastric contents when they pass through pylorus and is a *common site for peptic ulcer*. The bile and pancreatic ducts open by a common hepatopancreatic ampulla of Vater on the posteromedial wall of descending (2nd) part of duodenum.

Fig. 8.5-1. *The mucosal surface of jejunum (A) and ileum (B).*

Jejunum and ileum. Jejunum and ileum form, respectively, the proximal 2/5th and distal 3/5th of the remaining part of small intestine. There is no sharp demarcation between jejunum and ileum. The inner mucosal surfaces of jejunum and ileum, however, can be differentiated from each other.

STRUCTURAL CHARACTERISTICS OF SMALL INTESTINE

Histologically the wall of small intestine is made up of 4 layers, which from within to outwards consist of: mucosa, submucosa, muscle coat, and serosa (Fig. 8.5-2).

Fig. 8.5-2. *Histological structure of small intestine. Note features of plica circularis and villi.*

Features of mucosal surface of small intestine

Although the small intestine is about 6 metres long, it has an absorptive area of over 250 square metres. This larger surface is created by certain characteristic features of the interior i.e. mucosal surface of the small intestine, which include:

Plica circulares

The mucosal surface shows numerous circular folds (plicae circulares or valvulae conniventes) (Fig. 8.5-1). Each fold is made up of all layers of the mucosa (lining epithelium, lamina propria, and muscularis mucosa). The submucosa also extends into the fold. The circular folds increase surface area for absorption, and also slow down the passage of contents through small intestine which facilitate absorption.

Villi

Villi are finger-like projections of mucous membrane seen throughout the length of small intestine (Fig. 8.5-2).

Structure. Each villus is covered by a single layer of columnar epithelial cells called enterocytes. The *microvilli* protrude from the surface of intestinal cells. The core of each villus contains (Fig. 8.5-3):

- An *arteriole and venule* and
- A fine network of *nerves* which has connections with submucosal and myenteric plexus.

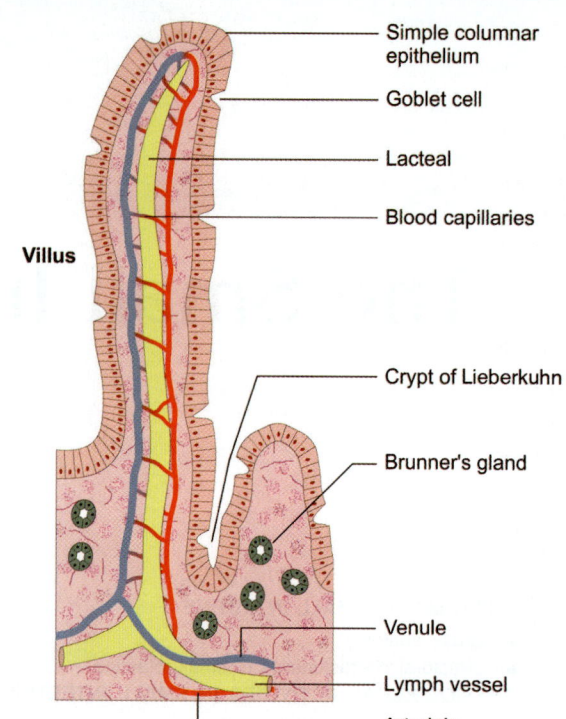

Fig. 8.5-3. *Structure of an intestinal villus, crypts of Lieberkuhn and an enterocyte.*

Activity. During digestion and absorption, the villi contract quickly with an irregular rhythm and relax slowly. Their muscular fibres serve to pump the lymph from core of villi towards the submucosal lacteals.

The crypts of Lieberkuhn

The crypts of Lieberkuhn are single tubular intestinal glands which invaginate deep into the lamina propria, present between the villi throughout the length of small intestine (Fig. 8.5-3). These glands are lined by undifferentiated columnar cells and also contain goblet cells, argentaffin cells and Paneth cells.

Duodenal glands of Brunner are limited only to the duodenum. These are compound tubulo-alveolar glands present in submucosa of duodenum. Their ducts pass through the muscularis mucosa to open into the crypts of Lieberkuhn. They are situated mostly near the pylorus; beyond pylorus their number greatly diminishes. Secretion of these glands contain *mucus and HCO_3^-* which neutralizes gastric acid entering the duodenum and thus protects its mucosa.

PHYSIOLOGICAL ACTIVITIES IN SMALL INTESTINE

SMALL INTESTINAL SECRETIONS
Composition and formation

The intestinal juice also called *succus entericus* comprises the intestinal secretions which include:

1. *Aqueous component of intestinal juice.* Aqueous component of intestinal juice primarily refers to water and electrolytes secreted by the epithelial cells of small intestine, especially those present in the crypts of Lieberkuhn.

Functions. The watery secretion provides a solvent into which the products of digestion are dissolved. This fluid is rapidly reabsorbed by the intestinal villi. Thus, circulation of this fluid from the crypts to the villi supplies a watery vehicle for absorption of foodstuffs from the small intestine.

2. *Intestinal enzymes.* Brush border of epithelial cells covering the villi contains a large number of intracellular digestive enzymes. The enzymes which have been identified in the brush border are:

1. *Peptidases* (proteolytic enzymes).
2. *Disaccharidases* such as sucrase, maltase and lactase.
3. *Intestinal lipases*.
4. *Enterokinase* or enteropeptidase.

3. *Mucus.* Mucus in the small intestine is secreted by:

1. *Brunner's glands*, which secrete thick alkaline mucoid secretion that serves a protective role, preventing HCl and chyme from damaging the duodenal mucosa.

2. *Goblet cells* also secrete lot of mucus which protects the intestinal mucosa and lubricates the chyme.

Regulation of small intestinal secretions

1. *Local stimuli.* Mechanical distension of intestinal mucosa by the food or irritation by chemicals, via local myenteric reflexes, increase the volume and total enzyme output of the small intestine; that is why, the greater is the chyme, greater is the secretion of intestinal secretion.

2. *Role of vasoactive intestinal polypeptide (VIP).* Though the secretion of the crypts of Lieberkuhn is mainly regulated by the local stimuli, but the local hormone VIP is also reported to increase its secretion.

3. *Secretion of Brunner's gland* is increased by:

- Vagus stimulation,
- Direct tactile stimulation or irritation of the duodenal mucosa, and
- Secretin.

Functions of intestinal juice

See functions of small intestine (page 290).

MOTILITY OF SMALL INTESTINE

Motility of small intestine includes :

- Mixing movements such as segmentation contractions and pendular movements,
- Propulsive movements such as peristaltic contractions and peristaltic rush, and
- Movements of villi, and

- Motility reflexes.

MIXING MOVEMENTS

The mixing movements of small intestine are responsible for proper mixing of chyme with digestive juices like pancreatic juice, bile juice and intestinal juice. The mixing movements of small intestine include:

- Segmentation contractions, and
- Pendular movements.

1. Segmentation contractions

During segmentation contraction, a section of the small intestine (about 2-5 cm) contracts, sending the intestinal contents (chyme) in both oral and caudal directions. That section of the small intestine then relaxes, and the contents move back into that segment. At the same time, the adjoining segment which was relaxed, now contracts (Fig. 8.5-4).

— Chyme

Fig. 8.5-4. *Segmentation contractions of small intestine.*

The alternate contracted and relaxed segments give a ring-like appearance resembling the chain of sausages.

2. Pendular movements

These are small constrictive waves which sweep forward and backward or upward and downward in pendular fashion. These mixing movements can be noticed only by close observation.

PROPULSIVE MOVEMENTS

The propulsive movements of small intestine are involved in pushing the chyme towards the aboral end of intestine. These include:

- Peristaltic contractions, and
- Peristaltic rush.

1. Peristaltic contractions

Characteristic features. Peristalsis refers to a wave of contraction preceded by a wave of relaxation.

The peristaltic contractions are highly coordinated and typically a peristaltic contraction involves contraction of a segment behind the bolus, and simultaneous relaxation of the segment in front of the bolus, causing the chyme to be propelled caudally (Fig. 8.5-5).

Fig. 8.5-5. *Peristaltic contraction moves the food through intestine by pushing bolus ahead of muscle contraction.*

Law of intestine. The peristaltic waves always travel from the oral end towards the aboral end of the intestine. This phenomenon has been labelled as the *Law of the intestine* by Starling in 1901.

2. Peristaltic rush
Peristaltic rush refers to a very powerful peristaltic contraction which occurs when intestinal mucosa is irritated intensely as in some infectious processes.

MOVEMENTS OF VILLI
Movements of villi consist of alternate shortening and elongation of the villi caused by contraction and relaxation of the muscle. *Villikinin*, a hormone secreted from small intestinal mucosa, play an important role in increasing the movements of villi.

Functions. The surface area of villi is increased during elongation. This helps in absorption of digested foodstuffs from the lumen of intestine.

Initiation. Local nervous reflexes, which occur in response to the presence of chyme in small intestine, initiate the movements of villi.

MOTILITY REFLEXES
1. *Gastroileal reflex.* Gastroileal reflex refers to marked increase in the peristaltic contractions of ileum associated with relaxation of ileocaecal sphincter which occur immediately after the meals. As a result, the intestinal contents are delivered to the large intestine.

2. *Intestinointestinal reflex.* Intestinointestinal reflex refers to relaxation of smooth muscles of the rest of the small intestine in response to overdistension of one segment of the intestine.

FUNCTIONS OF SMALL INTESTINE
The functions of small intestine can be summarized as:

1. *Mechanical functions.* The mixing and propulsive movements of the small intestine help in thorough mixing of chyme with the digestive juices (pancreatic juice, bile juice and succus entericus) and propel it towards the large intestine.

2. *Digestive functions* of small intestine are carried out by the digestive enzymes present in the :
- Succus entericus (see page 289),
- Pancreatic enzymes (see page 279), and
- Bile (see page 283).

3. *Absorptive function* is accomplished by the huge surface area created by the presence of plicae circulares, villi and microvilli. The end products of digestion of carbohydrates, proteins and fats are absorbed through portal system or through the lymph. For details of absorption, see page 299.

4. *Hormonal functions.* The small intestine secretes certain hormones which exert their effect on the secretions and motility of gastrointestinal tract. These hormones include *enterogastrone, secretin* and *cholecystokinin.*

5. *Activator function.* The enzyme enterokinase secreted by small intestine activates trypsinogen into trypsin which in turn activates other enzymes.

6. *Protective function.* The mucus secreted into the succus entericus protects the intestinal wall from the gastric acid chyme.

7. *Hydrolytic function.* The aqueous component of the succus entericus provides water and thus helps in all the hydrolytic processes of enzymatic reactions of digestion of various food particles.

The Large Intestine

ANATOMY OF LARGE INTESTINE

GROSS ANATOMY

The large intestine is a tube about 6 cm in diameter and 150 cm in length. It normally arches around and encloses the coils of small intestine and tends to be more fixed than the small intestine. It extends from the ileum to the anus and is divided into following parts (Fig. 8.6-1):

Caecum with appendix. *Caecum* is a blind-ended sac into which opens the lower end of ileum. The ileocaecal junction is guarded by the ileocaecal valve which allows inflow but prevents backflow of intestinal contents.

- *Appendix* is worm-shaped tube that arises from the medial side of caecum which in human being is a vestigial organ.

Colon. The colon, major part of large intestine, can be differentiated from the small intestine by the presence of *haustrations* (a series of sacculations) and *taenia coli* (three bands of thickenings in muscular layer) which run

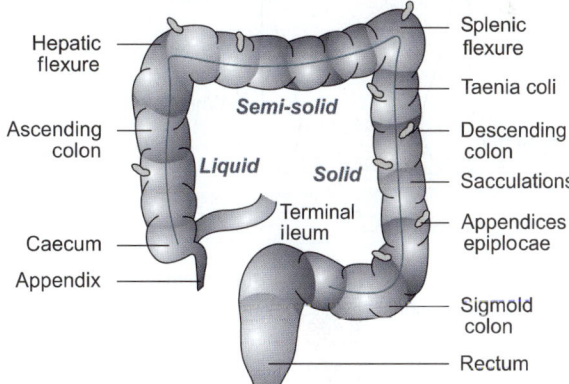

Fig. 8.6-1. *Functional organization of the large intestine.*
Note : *The labelling of the figure also depicts consistency of faecal contents in its different segments.*

along the length of the colon, approximately equidistant from each other. The colon, although one continuous tube, is subdivided into the ascending, transverse, descending and sigmoid colon.

- *Ascending colon* extends upward from the caecum along the right side of abdomen upto the liver. On reaching the liver it bends to the left, forming the right hepatic flexure.

- *Transverse colon* extends from the right hepatic flexure to the left splenic flexure and is about 50 cm in length. It is covered by peritoneum all round and is suspended from the posterior abdominal wall by the transverse mesocolon.

- *Descending colon* extends from the left splenic flexure to the pelvic inlet. It is about 25 cm long and ends by becoming continuous with sigmoid colon.

- *Sigmoid colon* begins at the pelvic inlet as continuation of the descending colon and joins the rectum in front of the sacrum.

Rectum descends in front of the sacrum to leave the pelvis by piercing the pelvic floor. Here it becomes continuous with anal canal in the perineum. Anteriorly, the rectum is related in the male to the urinary bladder and prostate, and in the female to the lower part of uterus and the vagina.

It opens to the exterior through the anus, the opening which is guarded by two sphincters (see page 293).

Interior of the anal canal is divided into three parts (Fig. 8.6-2) :

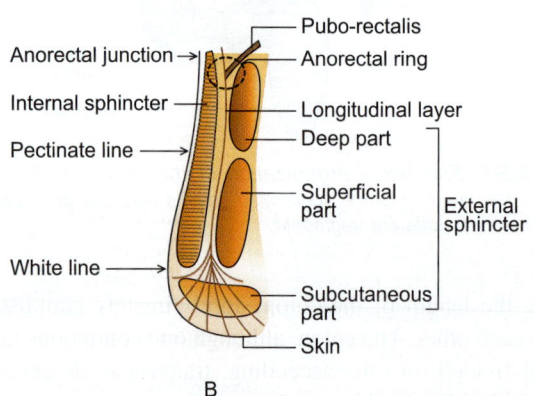

Fig. 8.6-2. Schematic interior view of the anal canal (A), and longitudinal section through the anal canal wall to show the anal sphincters and their relation to interior of anal canal (B).

- *Upper part,* about 15 mm in length, is characterized by presence of longitudinal mucosal folds, the anal columns.

- *Middle part,* about 15 mm in length, is lined by smooth mucosa. It is separated above from the upper part by a wavy line of mucosa the *pectinate* line and below from the lower part by the *white line.*

- *Lower part,* about 10 mm in length, is lined by skin.

STRUCTURAL CHARACTERISTICS

Histological structure of large intestines is similar to that described in general (see page 258) with following special characteristics.

Mucosa of large intestine is characterized by:

- Absence of plica circulares and villi (as seen in small intestine).

- A large number of simple tubular glands (crypts of Lieberkuhn) lined by simple columnar epithelial cells with large number of goblet cells which secrete mucus (Fig. 8.6-3).

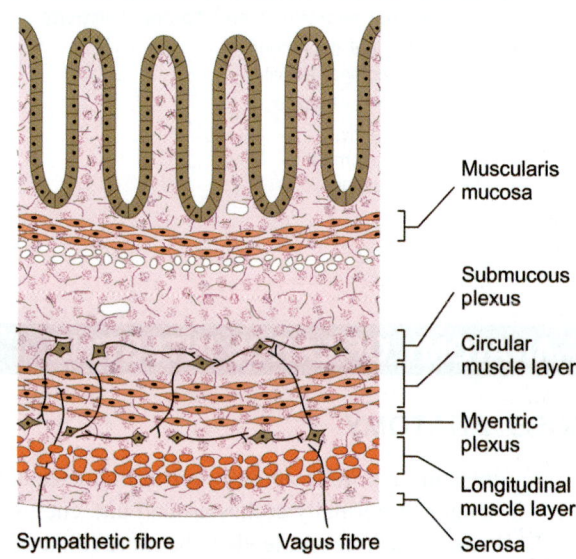

Fig. 8.6-3. Histological structure of the colon.

Longitudinal layer of muscle coat of colon is unusual

- Most of the fibres in it are collected to form three thick bands, the taenia coli which can be seen through the serous layer (Fig. 7.6-1). A thin layer of longitudinal fibres is present in the intestines between the taenia.

- The taenia coli are shorter in length than other layers of the wall of colon. This results in the production of *sacculations* (also called *haustrations*) on the wall of colon.

Serous layer is missing over the posterior aspect of the ascending and descending colon. At places small peritoneal bags of fat, called *appendices epiploicae,* project from the colonic serosa.

PHYSIOLOGICAL ACTIVITIES IN LARGE INTESTINE

LARGE INTESTINAL SECRETIONS AND BACTERIAL ACTIVITY

LARGE INTESTINAL SECRETIONS

- The large intestinal secretions mainly comprise mucus secreted by the goblet cells, and some water and lot of HCO_3^- secreted by glands of Lieberkuhn.
- The mucus lubricates the faecal matter and also protects the mucous membrane of large intestine by preventing the damage caused by mechanical injury or chemical substances.
- The alkaline nature (pH 8.0) of the mucoid secretions of the large intestine is due to the presence of HCO_3^-. It serves to neutralize the acids formed by bacterial action on the faecal matter.

INTESTINAL BACTERIAL ACTIVITY

Bacterial flora. At birth, the colon is sterile, but the colonic bacterial flora becomes established early in life and includes:

- *Harmless bacteria* such as *E. coli* and *Enterobacter aerogenes;* and
- *Potentially dangerous bacteria* such as *Bacteroides fragilis*, various types of cocci and gas gangrene bacilli. These bacteria can cause serious disease in tissues outside the colon.

Intestinal bacterial activities include:

- *Synthesis of vitamins* such as vitamin C, a number of B-complex vitamins and folic acid.
- *Trophic effects on colonic mucosa.* Unabsorbed carbohydrates are converted to short-chain fatty acids by colonic bacteria. Some of the short-chain fatty acids produced have a trophic effect on colonic mucosa.
- *Play a role in cholesterol metabolism* by decreasing plasma cholesterol and LDL levels.

MOTILITY OF LARGE INTESTINE

MOVEMENTS OF LARGE INTESTINE

Types of movements

The different types of movements (most accepted nomenclature) of colon are:

1. Haustral shuttling

The haustral shuttling or haustral contractions are similar to the segmentation contractions of small intestine, which vigorously mix the contents of colon and by exposing more of the contents to mucosa facilitate absorption.

2. Peristalsis

Peristalsis is a progressive contractile wave preceded by a wave of relaxation. In the colon, the peristalsis waves are very small pressure waves of prolonged duration.

Function. They propel the contents towards rectum very slowly (5 cm/hr). It can take upto 48 hours for the chyme to traverse the colon.

3. Mass movements

- The mass movements are special type of peristaltic contractions which are observed in the colon only.
- These occur 3-4 times a day generally after meals and each contraction lasts for about 3 minutes.
- The mass movements force the faecal material rapidly in mass down the colon. They also move material into the rectum, and rectal distension initiates the defaecation reflex.

Gastrocolic reflex

Gastrocolic reflex refers to contraction of colon induced by entry of food into the stomach. This reflex results in an urge to defaecate after a meal. Because of this defaecation after meals is a rule in children. However in adults, the bowel training suppresses this reflex.

DEFAECATION

Functional anatomy

A brief description of functional anatomy of the anal sphincters which play most important role in the process of defaecation needs special emphasis.

1. *Internal or involuntary anal sphincter* consists of thickened circular smooth muscles at the pelvic-rectal flexure. It extends from the upper end of anal canal upto the white line. This sphincter relaxes reflexly in response to stimulation of stretch receptors when the rectum is distended.

Innervation of internal anal sphincter is by:

- *Parasympathetic pelvic splanchnic nerves* which are inhibitory, and
- *Sympathetic nerves* which are excitatory.

2. *External or voluntary anal sphincter* consists of somatic skeletal muscle fibres innervated by the pudendal nerves. It is divided into deep, superficial and subcutaneous parts (Fig. 8.6-2). Characterstic features are:

- It is maintained in a state of tonic contraction.
- Mild to moderate distension of the rectum increases its force of contraction.
- Moderately severe distension of rectum initiates a reflex which inhibits the discharge of somatic pudendal nerves (which cause tonic contraction) and thus relaxes the internal anal sphincter.

- The external anal sphincter can be voluntarily relaxed, the action which aids the reflex emptying of the distended rectum.

The act of defaecation

Defaecation, the process of excretion of faecal material, involves both voluntary and reflex activity. The events associated with process of defaecation proceed as follows:

1. *Distension of rectum.* Usually, once or twice a day gastrocolic reflex drives the faeces into the rectum which increase the intrarectal pressure passively.

2. *Defaecation reflexes.* As the rectum starts filling, the resultant rise in the intra-rectal pressure stimulates the stretch receptors, and sets up defaecation reflexes. As a result there occurs:

- Intensification of colonic peristaltic contraction further raising the intra-rectal pressure.
- When the rectal pressure reaches to about 55 mmHg there occurs further relaxation of internal and external anal sphincters.

3. *Role of voluntary control on defaecation.* Once the above described reflex effects are obtained, the voluntary control mechanism depending upon the convenience may or may not allow the act of defaecation to occur:

When defaecation is not allowed, the voluntary control mechanism maintains the contraction of external anal sphincter (which is composed of skeletal muscle innervated by the pudendal nerves). Soon, the internal anal sphincter also closes, and the rectum relaxes to accommodate the faecal matter within it. Once the defaecation reflex dies out, it recurs after some hours.

When it is convenient to defaecate:

- The external anal sphincter is relaxed voluntarily. Thus both internal and external sphincters are relaxed.
- The intra-abdominal pressure is increased by contraction of abdominal and diaphragmatic muscles (a process of expiring against closed glottis, i.e. Valsalva manoeuvre).
- The smooth muscles of the distal colon and rectum contract forcibly, propelling the faecal matter out of the body through the anal canal.

Faeces

Composition. Faeces or the faecal matter is derived mainly from the intestinal secretion and partly from the undigested material. The faecal matter consists of: *water*, forms the main bulk of faeces (75%), and *solids*, contribute 25% to total faecal matter weight. These include: inorganic material, mostly calcium and phosphate, undigested plant fibres, epithelial cells, dead bacteria, constituents of intestinal secretions including bile pigments, fats and proteins.

pH of stools is slightly acidic (5-7) due to the organic acids formed from carbohydrates by colonic bacteria.

Brown colour of stools is due to the pigment *urobilin* which is formed from oxidation of urobilinogen which is colourless.

Odour of stools is due to the presence of substances like indole, skatole, mercaptans and hydrogen sulphide. These substances are formed by the action of colonic bacteria on the food.

FUNCTIONS OF LARGE INTESTINE

The functions of large intestine thus can be summarized as:

1. *Secretory functions.* The large intestinal secretion mainly comprise mucin which helps to lubricate the faecal matter. The alkaline nature (pH 8) of the secretion serves to neutralize the acids formed by bacterial action on the faecal matter.

2. *Synthesis functions.* The bacterial flora of the large intestine synthesize folic acid, vitamin B_{12} and vitamin K.

3. *Absorptive functions.* Absorption of water and electrolytes is the chief function of proximal part of the colon. Organic substances like glucose, alcohol, and some drugs like anaesthetic agents, sedatives and steroids can also be absorbed in large intestine. The vitamin K and a number of B complex vitamins which are synthesized in colon by bacterial flora are also absorbed in the large intestine.

4. *Excretory functions.* Heavy metals like mercury, lead, bismuth and arsenic are excreted by large intestine through the faeces.

APPLIED ASPECTS

Applied aspects of defaecation

Defaecation in infants. In infants, defaecation reflex causes automatic emptying of lower bowel without normal voluntary control on external anal sphincter. The voluntary control of the reflex by higher centres is attained by social training as the child grows.

Defaecation in individuals with spinal cord transection. In individuals with spinal cord transection, initially there occurs retention of faeces. But defaecation reflex returns quickly. However, reflex evacuation occurs automatically, without voluntary control, when the rectal pressure increases to about 55 mmHg.

Role of dietary fibres. Dietary fibres increase bulk of faeces: this plays a role in defaecation reflex by distending the rectum.

Role of dietary fibres in prevention of diseases. Epidemiological evidences indicate that groups of people who consume a diet which contains large amounts of vegetable fibres have a low incidence of diverticulitis, cancer of colon, diabetes mellitus, and coronary artery disease.

Therapeutic role of dietary fibres. The daily recommended intake of dietary fibres is about 25 to 35 gm/day. High fibre supplements have therapeutic role in following conditions:

- In constipation,
- In spastic colon and diverticular disease,
- In diabetes and high cholesterol levels.

Disorders of large intestine motility

1. *Hirschsprung's disease.* Hirschsprung's disease, or the aganglionic megacolon refers to congenital absence of Auerbach's plexus in the wall of rectosigmoid region. This leads to blockage of both the peristalsis and mass contractions at the aganglionic segment. Therefore, the faeces pass the aganglionic segment with difficulty and accumulate in the large intestine leading to dilatation of the colon (megacolon).

2. *Constipation.* Constipation refers to failure of voiding of faeces which produces discomfort. It results from infrequent mass movement in the colon. As a result the faecal matter remains in the colon for longer time, so large amount of fluid is absorbed and the faeces become hard and dry.

3. *Diarrhoea.* Diarrhaea is a condition which is characterized by increased frequency of daefecation with increased water content of the faeces.

Digestion and Absorption

8.7

DIGESTION AND ABSORPTION OF CARBOHYDRATES

Dietary carbohydrates

Dietary intake of carbohydrates is 250-850 gm/day, which represents 50 to 60 per cent of the diet. Major carbohydrates in the human diet are present in following forms:

1. Polysaccharides. These may be present in following forms:

- *Starch* is the carbohydrate reserve of plants.
- *Glycogen*. It is available in non-vegetarian diet and so often referred to as animal starch.
- *Cellulose* (plant polysaccharide), which is present in diet in large amounts. But there is no enzyme in the human GIT to digest it.

2. Oligosaccharides. Based on the number of monosaccharide units present, oligosaccharides are further subdivided into di-, tri-, tetra- and pentasaccharide.

Disaccharides include:

- Sucrose (glucose + fructose) also known as table sugar (cane or beet sugar).
- Lactose (glucose + galactose) also called milk sugar.
- Maltose (glucose + glucose). It is a product of starch hydrolysis. It is present in germinating seeds.

3. Monosaccharides. Monosaccharides consumed mostly in human diet are : *hexoses* such as glucose (in fruits, vegetables and honey), and fructose in fruits.

Pentoses do not occur in free form, but are found in nucleic acid and in certain polysaccharides such as pentosans of fruits and gums.

Digestion of carbohydrates

The digestion of carbohydrates begins in mouth, continues in stomach but occurs mainly (almost all) in the small intestine.

1. *Digestion of carbohydrates in the mouth.* Initial starch digestion starts in the mouth by the enzyme α-amylase (ptyalin) present in the saliva which digests cooked starch to maltose.

2. *Digestion of carbohydrates in the stomach.* In the stomach there occurs minimal carbohydrates digestive activity: The enzyme α-amylase (which enters the stomach with food) activity continues in the stomach for 20-30 minutes till the highly acidic gastric juice mixes with the food and makes it inactive. *The HCl of the gastric juice may hydrolyse some sucrose.*

3. *Digestion of carbohydrates in the small intestine* is by:

- *Pancreatic α-amylase* which is present in the pancreatic juice poured into the duodenum. Its actions on the carbohydrates are much powerful and so it acts on boiled as well as unboiled starch and variety of other carbohydrates except cellulose.

- *Brush border enzymes of small intestine.* The carbohydrate splitting brush border enzymes of small intestine include *dextrinase, maltase, sucrase* and *lactase.* These brush border enzymes digest the oligosaccharides into monosaccharides on the surface of epithelial cells of villi.

End products of carbohydrate digestion

- The end products of carbohydrates are monosaccharides such as glucose, fructose and galactose.
- A little amount of pentoses are the end products of digestion of nucleic acids and partial digestion of pentosans.

Absorption of carbohydrates

Carbohydrates are absorbed from the GIT in the form of monosaccharides.

Site of absorption. Most of the monosaccharides are absorbed from the mucosal surface of jejunum and upper ileum.

Mechanism of absorption. Various monosaccharides are absorbed by following mechanisms:

- *Glucose* and *galactose* are absorbed by a common *Na⁺-dependent active transport* system,
- *Fructose* is absorbed by *facilitated diffusion*, and
- *Pentoses* are absorbed by simple diffusion.

Rate of absorption of monosaccharides is variable, being:

- Fastest with glucose and galactose,
- Intermediate with fructose, and
- Slowest with mannose or pentoses.

Fate of glucose in the body

1. *Storage as glycogen.* About 5% of the total glucose absorbed is stored as glycogen in the liver and muscles.
2. *Catabolism to produce energy.* About 50-60% of the glucose absorbed is catabolised in the body tissues to produce energy.
3. *Conversion into fat.* About 30-40% of glucose is converted into fat and is stored in the fat depot.

Abnormalities of carbohydrate digestion and absorption

1. *Congenital lactose intolerance.* It refers to a condition in which lactose (milk sugar) cannot be digested due to congenital deficiency of enzyme lactase.

- The undigested lactose acts as osmotic particles and draws excessive fluids into intestine resulting in *diarrhoea.*
- The diarrhoea so produced can lead to life-threatening dehydration and electrolyte imbalance.
- Avoidance of milk and milk products prevents the symptoms from developing if the infant can be fed by synthetic milk containing sucrose instead of lactose.

2. *Secondary lactase deficiency* occurring in adults is very common. It produces intestinal distension, diarrhoea and flatulence. For adults, it is usually not a problem, as they can easily avoid milk and milk products.

DIGESTION AND ABSORPTION OF PROTEINS

Sources of proteins

The proteins that are digested and absorbed in the GIT come from two sources: exogenous and endogenous.

1. Exogenous (dietary) proteins

- *Daily requirement* of dietary proteins for adults is 0.5-0.7 gm/kg body weight and for children (1-3 years) it is 4 gm/kg.
- *Sources of dietary proteins* with high biological value are meat, fish, eggs, cheese and other milk products. Soyabeans, wheat and various types of pulses are also rich source of proteins.
- *Structure of dietary proteins.* The dietary proteins are made of long chains of amino acids bound together by peptide linkages.

2. Endogenous proteins

Endogenous proteins, totaling 30-50 gm/day, are the proteins which reach the intestine through various gastrointestinal secretions and those which are present in the desquamated epithelial cells of the gut.

Digestion of proteins

Proteins are digested by the proteolytic enzymes to amino acids and small polypeptides before they are absorbed. Digestion of proteins does not occur in the mouth, as there are no proteolytic enzymes in the saliva. Digestion of proteins, thus, begins in the stomach and is completed in the small intestine.

Digestion of proteins in the stomach

Pepsin, secreted by chief cells of the main gastric glands in an inactive form (pepsinogen), is responsible for digesting about 10-15% proteins entering the gastrointestinal tract.

- Pepsinogen is converted into pepsin (active form) by the action of HCl or preformed pepsin.
- Pepsin splits proteins into proteoses, peptones and polypeptides (Fig. 8.7-1).

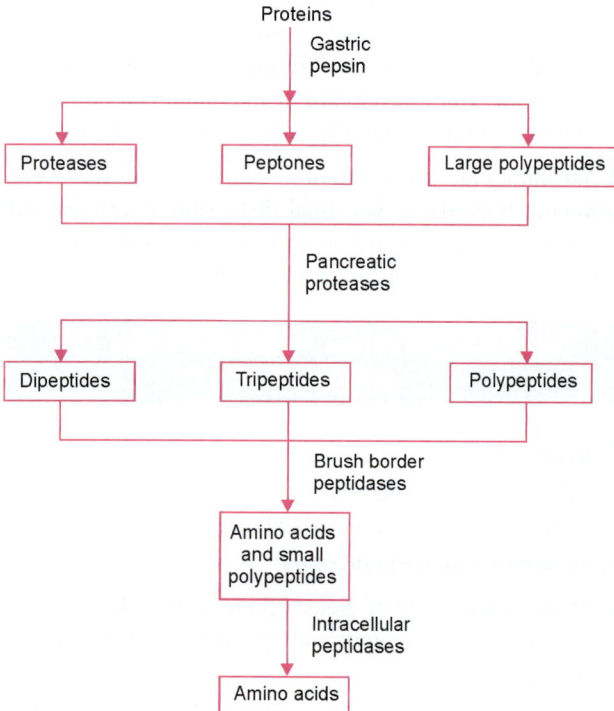

Fig. 8.7-1. *Steps of digestion of proteins.*

Digestion of proteins in the small intestine

In the small intestine the proteins are digested by the pancreatic proteases, brush border peptidases and intracellular peptidases.

Pancreatic proteases or proteolytic enzymes of pancreas play a major role in protein digestion.

- *Various types of proteases* along with their functions are described on page 279.
- *Pancreatic proteases* digest the proteins and split them into dipeptides, tripeptides and small polypeptides, which are further digested by brush border peptidases (Fig. 8.7-1).
- Some of the dipeptides and tripeptides are absorbed directly into the epithelial cells of mucosa of small

intestine and are further digested by intracellular enzymes into amino acids.

Brush border peptidases include aminopeptidases, dipeptidases, tripeptidases, nuclease and related enzymes. These enzymes continue the digestive process begun by the pancreatic proteases, eventually converting the proteins to small polypeptides and amino acids (Fig. 8.7-1).

Intracellular peptidases are the proteolytic enzymes present in the cytosol of epithelial cells of small intestine. Within minutes, these digest the last dipeptides and tripeptides into amino acids which then enter the blood.

Digestion of nucleic acid and nucleoproteins

Nucleic acid and nucleoproteins are found in abundance in the foodstuffs which are rich in nuclei such as liver, kidney, pancreas, yeast, etc.

In the stomach, HCl hydrolyses the nucleoproteins, removing proteins which are digested together with other proteins as described above.

In the small intestine, the free nucleic acids are digested by the pancreatic enzymes and brush border enzymes.

- *Pancreatic enzymes* such as ribonuclease and deoxyribonuclease in the duodenum digest free nucleic acids into nucleotides and nucleosides
- *Brush border enzymes* such as nucleases, nucleotidases and nucleosidases convert nucleotides and nucleosides into pentoses (purine and pyrimidine).

End products of protein digestion

The protein digestion which starts in the stomach is completed in the enterocyte of small intestine. The end products of protein digestion are amino acids.

Absorption of proteins

Mechanisms of absorption into the intestinal epithelial cells

The end products of protein digestion (amino acids, dipeptides and tripeptides) are absorbed through the luminal membrane of the epithelial cells of small intestine. Following mechanisms of absorption are known:

1. Na^+-dependent active transport mechanism. The levo amino acids, dipeptides and tripeptides are absorbed by a Na^+-dependent active transport mechanism.

2. Simple diffusion. The dextro amino acids are absorbed solely by passive diffusion.

3. Endocytosis. Small amounts of larger polypeptides are absorbed by endocytosis. Proteins absorbed by endocytosis usually excite immunological/allergic reaction. In newborn infants, immunoglobulins present in the colostrum are absorbed in the intestinal mucosa by endocytosis and impart passive immunity to child.

Further digestion in the epithelial cells

Once amino acids and polypeptides are absorbed into the intestinal epithelial cells, the intracellular peptidases break the remaining linkages of tripeptides, and dipeptides causing release of amino acids.

Transport of amino acids into blood capillaries

From inside the epithelial cells the amino acids are transported into the interstitial space across the basolateral membrane of the cells by facilitated or simple diffusion. From the interstitium the amino acids enter the capillaries of villus by simple diffusion, and then via portal vein they reach the liver and general circulation.

DIGESTION AND ABSORPTION OF FATS

Dietary fats

Dietary fat is of both vegetable and animal origin. Mostly it is in the form of neutral fat (triglycerides). It also includes small amounts of phospholipids, cholesterol, some free fatty acids, lecithin and cholesterol esters.

Daily intake of fats in the diet varies widely, from about 25 to 160 gm.

Digestion of fats

Site of digestion. Although lipolytic enzymes are secreted in the mouth (*lingual lipase*) and stomach (*gastric lipase*), their action is so insignificant that practically digestion of all the dietary fats occurs in the small intestine. Under normal conditions gastric lipase is soon inactivated by gastric juice (at pH 2.5).

Mechanism of digestion of fats. The digestion of fat includes three steps:

- Emulsification of fat by bile salts,
- Hydrolysis of fat by pancreatic and intestinal lipolytic enzymes, and
- Acceleration of fat digestion by micelle formation.

Absorption of fats

Most of the fat absorption occurs in the duodenum; almost all the digested lipids are totally absorbed by the time the chyme reaches the mid jejunum. Absorption of fats is accomplished by following steps.

1. *Transportation as micelles to the brush border membrane.* The bile salt micelle acts as a transport vehicle for the products of fat digestion.

2. *Diffusion of lipids across the enterocyte cell membrane.* Once the micelle comes in contact with the cell membrane, the monoglycerides, free fatty acids, cholesterol and fat soluble vitamins (being soluble in the cell membrane) diffuse passively at a rapid speed through the enterocyte cell membrane to the interior of the cell, leaving bile salts in the intestinal lumen.

The bile salts released from micelle after diffusion of their associated lipids are absorbed in the terminal ileum by a Na^+-dependent active transport process.

3. *Transport of lipids from inside the enterocytes to the interstitial space.* Once inside the cell, the end products of fat digestion enter the interstitium by two mechanisms:

i. Diffusion across the basal border of enterocyte. The small chain fatty acids are able to diffuse across the basal border of enterocytes to enter the interstitium.

ii. Formation and excretion of chylomicrons from enterocytes by exocytosis. The large chain fatty acids, cholesterol and lysophosphatides enter the smooth endoplasmic reticulum, where they are reconstituted.

The re-formed lipids coalesce to form small lipid droplets (about 1 nm in diameter) called chylomicrons. The chylomicrons are then excreted into the interstitium by *exocytosis* from the basolateral membrane of enterocyte. Covering of β-lipoproteins is essential for the exocytosis to occur.

4. *Transport of lipids into circulation.* After exiting the enterocytes (i.e. in the interstitium), the chylomicrons merge into larger droplets. From the interstitium the lipids diffuse into the *lacteals*, from which they enter the lymphatic circulation and via thoracic duct gain access into the blood circulation.

Applied aspects

Lipid malabsorption

Lipid malabsorption is much more common than carbohydrate and protein malabsorption.

- *Causes* of lipid malabsorption include:
  - Deficiency of pancreatic lipase in certain pancreatic diseases,
  - Bile deficiency in disorders of liver and gall bladder.
- *Steatorrhoea*, i.e. increased amount of fat in the stools is common manifestation of fat malabsorption.

Serum lipid profile

Lipids are present as lipoprotein complexes. Depending upon the density the lipoproteins are of following types:

- Very low density lipoproteins (VLDL). Density is <1.060.
- Low density lipoproteins (LDL).
- High density lipoproteins (HDL). Density is 1.060-1.200).

Normal values

- Serum triglycerides: 30-150 mg%
- Serum cholesterol: 150-240 mg%
- Serum phospholipids: 150-300 mg%
- Serum free fatty acids (FFA or NEFA = 10-30 mg%).

ABSORPTION OF WATER, ELECTROLYTES, MINERALS AND VITAMINS

WATER ABSORPTION

Water balance in the GIT
- The gastrointestinal tract receives about 9 litres of water per day which includes about 2 L of ingested water and about 7 L contained in salivary, gastric, biliary, pancreatic and intestinal secretions (Table 8.7-1).
- The gastrointestinal tract absorbs about 8.8 litres of water (about 95% of total water received) per day. About 60% of absorption occurs in jejunum, 20-25% in ileum and 10-15% in colon (Table 8.7-1).
- The gastrointestinal tract excretes about 0.2 litres of water in the faeces per day.

Table 8.7-1. Daily water balance in GIT

Input (in litres)	Absorption (in litres)	Faecal excretion (in litres)
WATER INGESTED : 2	Jejunum (60%) : 5.5	0.2
WATER IN GIT SECRETIONS : 7 • Saliva : 1.5 • Gastric juice : 2.5 • Bile : 0.75 • Pancreatic juice : 0.75 • Intestinal juice : 1.5	Ileum (25%) : 2.0 Colon (10-15%) : 1.3	
TOTAL 9	8.8	0.2

Mechanism of water absorption
In general water is absorbed passively and iso-osmotically across the gastrointestinal mucosa following the osmotic gradient created by the active absorption of electrolytes and nutrients.

ABSORPTION OF SODIUM

Sodium balance in GIT. Gastrointestinal tract receives about 40 gm of sodium per day, out of which about 10 gm is ingested with food and about 30 gm is contained in the gastrointestinal secretions. All of it is reabsorbed.
Site of absorption. Though sodium can be reabsorbed in the entire length of the intestine but maximum absorption occurs in the jejunum.

ABSORPTION OF CALCIUM

Body calcium. Calcium is the most abundant among the minerals in the body. The total content of calcium in an adult man is about 1 to 1.5 kg of which about 99% is present in the bones and teeth. A small amount (10%)

found outside the skeletal tissue performs a wide variety of functions.

Dietary calcium. Best sources of dietary calcium are milk and milk products. Good sources of calcium are beans, leafy vegetables, fish, cabbage and egg yolk.

Dietary requirements of calcium are:
- Infants (<1 year): 300-500 mg/day
- Children (1-18 years): 800-1200 mg/day
- Adult men and women: 800 mg/day
- Women during pregnancy, lactation and postmenopause: 1500 mg/day

Site of absorption. Most of the ingested calcium is absorbed in the upper small intestine (duodenum and jejunum).

Mechanism of absorption. Normally, about 75-80% of the daily intake (about 1000 mg) of calcium is absorbed from the upper small intestine. Most of the calcium is absorbed by an active transport mechanism.

Regulation of calcium absorption. Calcium absorption from the small intestine is well regulated to maintain the plasma calcium (*homeostasis of calcium*) levels within a narrow range (9-11 mg%). Vitamin D and parathyroid hormone (PTH) play main role in the regulation of calcium absorption.

ABSORPTION OF IRON
- Absorption occurs mainly in the duodenum and upper jejunum.
- Normally about 10% of the 15-20 mg iron ingested each day is actually absorbed in heathy adult male. This absorption is more in menstruating women.

Mechanism of iron absorption
Mechanism of iron absorption for the purpose of understanding can be described under three headings:

A. Transport of iron across brush border of enterocyte

In the diet iron may be present as haem (derived from meat) or non-haem iron.

1. *Absorption of haem iron.* Haem iron is the iron present in myoglobin, haemoglobin and related compounds. From these compounds, the haem is released by proteolytic enzymes in the gut. From the lumen the haem is transported inside the enterocyte across the brush border membrane by a *haem transport* protein. Inside the cell, the ferrous iron (Fe^{2+}) is released from the haem by the enzyme haemoxygenase.

2. *Absorption of non-haem iron.* Most of the dietary non-haem iron is present in ferric form (Fe^{3+}) whereas iron can be absorbed more efficiently in ferrous form (Fe^{2+}).

- Iron has got tendency to form insoluble complexes with dietary phytates, phosphates and dietary fibres. Gastric HCl tends to break insoluble iron complex apart and thus facilitates iron absorption.
- Ferrous iron (Fe^{2+}) is transported across the brush border by the *iron transport protein* or *receptors* present on the cell membrane (Fig. 8.7-2). Once inside the enterocyte, fate of non-haem ferrous iron is same as that of haem iron.

Fig. 8.7-2. *Absorption of iron. Haem is carried across brush border of enterocyte by haem transport protein (HT) and Fe^{2+} of non-haem iron by iron transport protein (IT). Inside the enterocyte some iron binds to ferritin and some across basolateral membrane by active transport process. In the blood iron binds to the transport protein transferrin (TF).*

B. Fate of iron in the enterocyte

As shown in Fig. 8.7-2, in the cytosol of enterocyte the free ferrous iron (Fe^{2+}) has two fates:

- A part of Fe^{2+}, depending upon the body's requirement, is actively transported across the basolateral membranes of the enterocytes into the interstitium, from where it enters the blood.
- Rest of the ferrous iron is oxidized to ferric form and bound to apoferritin forming ferritin. It is difficult to release iron from this storage form, and in general the ferritin stays in the enterocyte until the cell is sloughed off at the tip of villus.

C. Transport of iron in the blood

Normally, the iron absorbed into the blood binds with a *apotransferrin* to form the *transferrin* and is transported in this form in the plasma.

Mucosal block theory of absorption

This theory states that, iron absorption is increased when body iron stores are depleted or when erythropoiesis is increased, and decreased under the reverse conditions.

- As compared to normal conditions, in iron deficiency states a larger percentage of dietary iron enters the circulation and smaller amount forms ferritin in the epithelial cells.
- In the presence of iron overload, more ferritin is formed in the enterocytes and shed with these cells in the stools.

ABSORPTION OF VITAMINS

Absorption of fat soluble vitamins

Fat soluble vitamins (A, D, E and K) become part of micelle formed by bile salts and are absorbed along with other lipids in the upper part of small intestine.

The absorption of fat soluble vitamins is deficient if fat absorption is depressed because of lack of pancreatic enzymes or if bile is excluded from the intestine by obstruction of bile duct.

Absorption of water soluble vitamins

- Most vitamins are absorbed in the upper part of small intestine (jejunum) except vitamin B_{12} which is absorbed in the ileum.

Excretory System

Anatomy of Excretory System

9.1

INTRODUCTION

Literally, the word excretion means elimination of any matter from the body of an organism. The organs which are involved in the process of excretion include:

- *Kidneys*, which excrete water and water-soluble waste products,
- *Lungs*, which excrete carbon dioxide, water vapours and other volatile substances such as acetone,
- *Skin*, which excretes water and salts mainly in the form of sweat, and
- *Gastrointestinal tract*, which excretes faeces (excreta).

However, *sensu stricto*, the term excretion refers to elimination of principal products of metabolism except carbon dioxide. The principal products of metabolism, other than carbon dioxide, are ammonia, urea, uric acid, creatinine, various pigments and inorganic salts.

Excretory organs. Thus, in strictest sense, kidneys are the excretory organs. Together with a pair of ureters and a urinary bladder, kidneys constitute the excretory system (Fig. 9.1-1).

THE KIDNEYS

GROSS ANATOMY

External features

Gross anatomical features of a human kidney, illustrated in Fig. 9.1-2A, are:

Location. The kidneys are bean-shaped organs that lie retroperitoneally on the posterior abdominal wall, one on each side of the vertebral column at the level of T_{12} to L_1 vertebrae. The right kidney lies slightly inferior to the left kidney.

Size and shape. During life the kidneys are reddish-brown in colour. Each kidney in an adult human weighs about 150 gm and measures approximately 10 cm in length, 5 cm in width and 2.5 cm in thickness.

Renal hilum and sinus. The renal hilum is a vertical cleft present on the concave medial margin. It is the entrance

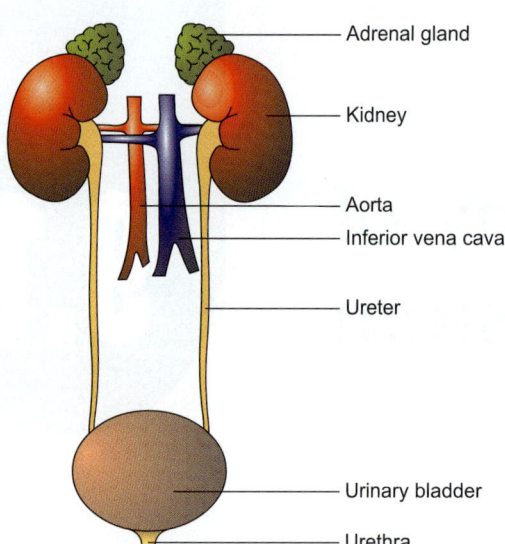

Fig. 9.1-1. *The urinary organs.*

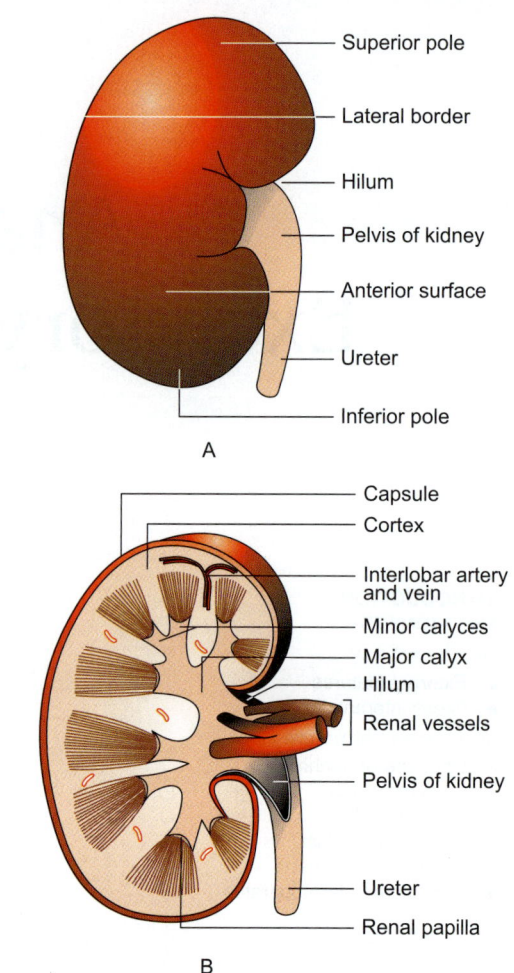

Fig. 9.1-2. *Anatomical features of human kidney.*

to space within the kidney—the renal sinus. Through renal hilum the renal artery enters, and the renal vein and renal pelvis leave the renal sinus. The *renal sinus* is thus occupied by the renal pelvis, calyces, vessels, nerves, and a variable amount of fat.

Renal pelvis and calyces. The renal pelvis is the flattened, funnel-shaped expansion of the superior end of ureter. Within the renal sinus the pelvis divides into two (or three) parts called *major calyces*. Each major calyx divides into a number of *minor calyces*. The end of each minor calyx is shaped like a cup into which fits a projection of kidney tissue called renal papilla (the apex of renal pyramid).

Gross internal structure

Gross internal structure of the kidney, as seen in coronal section through the organ, exhibits that kidney tissue consists of an outer region called the cortex and an inner region called the medulla (Fig. 9.1-2B).

Medulla. It is made up of triangular areas of renal tissue, that are called the renal pyramids. Pyramids are 4 to 14 in number and separated from each other by cortical columns of Bertin. Each pyramid has a base directed towards the cortex; and an apex (or renal papilla) which is directed towards the renal pelvis and fits into the minor calyx. The medulla can be subdivided into two parts:

- *Outer medulla*, that is further subdivided into the outer stripe, and the inner stripe.
- *Inner medulla* is also called papillary zone.

Cortex. The renal cortex can be divided into two parts which are continuous with each other:

- *Cortical arches* or cortical lobules refer to the tissue lying between the bases of pyramids and surface of the kidney.

- *Renal columns* refer to the cortical tissue that lies in between the pyramids.
- *Lobe of kidney.* Each pyramid, surrounded by a shell of cortex, constitutes a lobe of the kidney.

MICROSCOPIC STRUCTURE OF KIDNEY

Microscopically, the cortex and medulla of the kidney are composed of nephrons, blood vessels, lymphatics, and nerves.

Nephron is a structural and functional unit of the kidney. Each kidney contains approximately 1.2 million nephrons. Each nephron is capable of forming urine.

Structure of the nephron

A nephron consists of two major parts (Fig. 9.1-3):
- Renal corpuscle, and
- Renal tubule.

Renal corpuscle

Renal corpuscle or Malpighian corpuscle is a rounded structure comprising glomerulus surrounded by glomerular capsule (Fig. 9.1-4A).

Fig. 9.1-3. *Parts of a typical nephron. Organization of cortical and juxtamedullary nephrons showing different parts. Note differences between two types of nephrons.*

Glomerulus. Glomerulus refers to a rounded tuft of anastomosing capillaries. Blood enters the glomerulus through an *afferent arteriole* and leaves it through an *efferent arteriole* (note that the efferent vessel is an arteriole, and not a venule).

Glomerular capsule. Glomerular capsule, also known as Bowman's capsule, encloses the glomerulus and is formed of two layers: the inner layer covers the glomerular capillaries and is called *visceral layer*; and the outer layer is called *parietal layer*. In fact, the Bowman's capsule represents the cup-shaped blind beginning of the renal tubule. Space between the visceral and parietal layer of the capsule (called Bowman's space or urinary space) is continuous with the lumen of the renal tubule.

Ultrastructure of glomerular membrane

Glomerular membrane refers to the membrane that separates blood of glomerular capillaries from the fluid present in the Bowman's space. It is also called *filtration barrier* and consists of three major layers (Fig. 9.1.4B):
- Capillary endothelium.
- Basement membrane.
- Bowman's visceral epithelium or the inner layer of Bowman's capsule which forms the third layer of

glomerular membrane, is formed by special cells called *podocytes.*

Renal tubule

Renal tubule is a long complicated tubule that is divisible into following main parts (Fig. 9.1-3):

1. ***Proximal tubule.*** The proximal tubule initially forms several coils, *proximal convoluted tubule* (PCT), followed by a straight segment, *proximal straight tubule* (PST) or *pars recta* that descends towards the medulla.

2. ***Intermediate tubule or loop of Henle*** that consists of:
- Descending thin segment (DTS),
- Ascending thin segment (ATS), and
- Thick ascending limb (TAL).

In *juxtamedullary nephrons*, the DTS joins ATS to form the hair-pin band (loop). Near the end of thick ascending limb (TAL), the nephron passes between its afferent and efferent arterioles. This short segment of the thick ascending limb is called the *macula densa.*

3. ***Distal convoluted tubule.*** It begins a short distance beyond the macula densa and extends to a point in the cortex where the connecting tubules (CNT) of two or more nephrons join to form the cortical collecting ducts.

Fig. 9.1-4. *Structure of a glomerulus (A) and glomerular membrane (B).*

4. *Collecting duct*. The collecting duct is divisible into three parts:

- *Cortical collecting duct* (CCD), i.e. the portion present in the cortex,
- *Outer medullary collecting duct* (OMCD), i.e. the portion present in the outer medulla, and
- *Inner medullary collecting duct* (IMCD), i.e. the portion present in the inner medulla. Several IMCDs coalesce together before finally opening at the tip of the renal papilla.

Characteristics of epithelium lining the renal tubule

The epithelium lining the different segments of renal tubule has some special characteristic features which are suited to perform specific transport functions.

Type of cells. The cells lining the renal tubule are mostly cuboidal except in the thin segment where these are flat or squamous type.

Cortical collecting duct is composed of two cell types:

- *Principal cells*,
- *Intercalated cells*

Inner medullary collecting duct is composed of a single layer of cells that have poorly developed apical and basolateral surfaces and a few mitochondria.

Types of nephrons

There are two types of nephrons: cortical (superficial) and juxtamedullary. Differences between the cortical and juxtamedullary nephrons are depicted in Fig. 9.1-3.

Juxtaglomerular apparatus

Juxtaglomerular apparatus as the name indicates (juxta – near) refers to collection of specialised cells located very near to the glomerulus. It forms the major component of renin-angiotensin-aldosterone system. The juxtaglomerular apparatus comprises three types of cells (Fig. 9.1-5):

Fig. 9.1-5. *Juxtaglomerular apparatus.*

1. *Juxtaglomerular cells*. Juxtaglomerular (JG) cells are specialised *myoepithelial* (modified vascular smooth muscle) cells located in the media of the *afferent arteriole* in the region of juxtaglomerular apparatus. They act as *baroreceptors* (tension receptors) and respond to changes in the transmural pressure gradient between the afferent arterioles and the interstitium.

2. *Macula densa cells*. Macula densa cells refer to the specialised renal tubular epithelial cells of a short segment of the thick ascending limb of loop of Henle which passes between the afferent and efferent arterioles supplying its glomerulus of origin. They act as *chemoreceptors* and are stimulated by decreased NaCl concentration and thereby causing increased renin release.

3. *Mesangial cells*. Mesangial cells or *lacis* cells are the interstitial cells of the juxtaglomerular apparatus.

Functionally, these cells possibly relay the signals from macula densa to granular cells after modulating the signals. In this way, a decreased intraluminal Na⁺ load, Cl⁻ load, or both in the region of macula densa stimulates the juxtaglomerular cells to secrete renin.

RENAL BLOOD VESSELS
Arrangement of arterial vessels (renal artery and its branches) in the kidney (Fig. 9.1-6)

Renal artery (one for each kidney), a major branch from the aorta, divides into a number of lobular arteries at the hilum of kidney.

Lobular artery (one for each pyramid), divides into two or more interlobar arteries.

Interlobar arteries enter the tissue of the renal columns and run towards the surface of kidney. Reaching the level of the bases of the pyramids, the interlobar arteries divide into arcuate arteries.

Arcuate arteries run at right angles to the parent interlobar arteries. They lie parallel to the renal surface at the junction of pyramid and cortex. They give a series of interlobular arteries.

Interlobular arteries run through the cortex at right angles to the renal surface to end in a subcapsular plexus. It has

been held that interlobular arteries divide the renal cortex into small lobules. Each interlobular artery gives off a series of afferent arterioles.

Afferent arterioles. Each afferent arteriole enters the Bowman's capsule and divides into a rounded tuft of anastomosing capillaries called *glomerulus*. The glomerular capillaries join to form the efferent arteriole.

Efferent arterioles leaving the glomeruli of two types of nephrons exhibit different behaviour:

- *Efferent arterioles arising from the cortical nephrons* divide into *peritubular capillaries* that surround the proximal and distal convoluted tubule forming a rich meshwork of microvessels. These capillaries drain into interlobular veins.

- *Efferent arterioles arising from the juxtamedullary nephrons* give rise to *vasa recta*. The *vasa recta* descend with the long loops of Henle into renal medulla and return to the area of the glomerulus, and drain into interlobular or arcuate vein.

Side branches arising from the vasa recti form capillary network at different levels along the loop of Henle (Fig. 9.1.7).

Fig. 9.1-6. Scheme to show arrangement of arteries within the kidney.

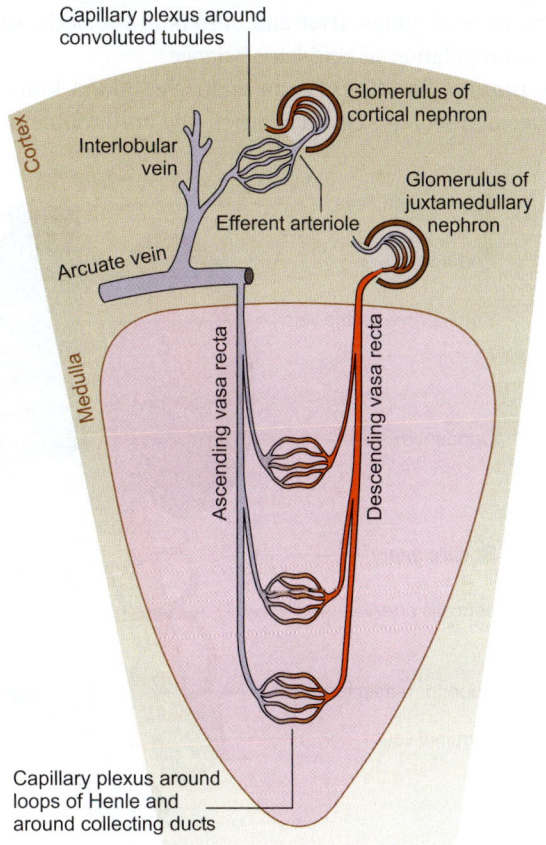

Fig. 9.1-7. Scheme to show behaviour of efferent arterioles arising from the glomeruli of cortical and juxtamedullary nephrons.

Arrangement of venous vessels (renal veins)

The pattern of renal venous system is similar to that found in the end arterial system, except for the presence of multiple anastomoses between veins at all levels of the venous circulation. The corresponding veins which run parallel to the arterial vessels are the interlobular veins, the arcuate veins, the interlobar veins, and the renal veins which exit the kidney at hilus.

FUNCTIONS OF KIDNEYS

The kidneys serve several major functions:

1. *Excretory function*. The kidneys excrete a number of end products of metabolism in urine. Thus, formation of urine is the major function of kidneys. The kidneys eliminate these substances from the body at a rate that matches their production. In addition to the metabolic wastes, the kidneys also excrete foreign substances from the body, such as drugs, pesticides, and other chemicals ingested in food.

2. *Regulation of water and inorganic ion balance*. Control of volume of body fluids and their inorganic ion balance is an important homeostatic role of kidneys.

3. *Regulation of acid-base balance*. Kidneys, in co-ordination with lungs, liver and buffers in the body, play a role in regulation of acid-base balance.

4. *Hormonal function*. As an endocrine gland kidneys produce and secrete renin, calcitriol, and erythropoietin.

URETERS, BLADDER AND URETHRA

THE URETERS

The ureters (right and left) are long tubes which convey the urine from the renal pelvis to urinary bladder (Fig. 9.1-1). Each ureter is about 25-30 cm long and about 4-5 mm in diameter.

***Parts*.** For the purpose of description only, the ureter can be divided into three parts :

- *Abdominal part* extends from the renal pelvis to the brim of bony pelvis (Fig. 9.1-8). This part of the ureter lies behind the peritoneum in front of the psoas muscle along the posterior abdominal wall.
- *Pelvic part*. At the brim of pelvis the ureter crosses the upper end of the external iliac artery and vein, and comes to lie on the lateral wall of pelvis (Figs. 9.1-8 and 9.1-9). Finally it leaves the pelvis wall and runs forwards to reach the urinary bladder.
- *Intracystic part* is the small part of the ureter which passes obliquely through the posterior wall of urinary bladder (Fig. 9.1-10). Because of this oblique intra-cystic course of the ureter, when urine accumulates and the pressure in the bladder rises, the ureters are compressed and the openings occluded. This prevents reflux of urine into the ureters (towards the kidneys) as the bladder fills and also during micturition when

Fig. 9.1-8. *Relations of abdominal part of ureter.*

Inferior vena cava — Aorta
Portal vein — Splenic vein
Superior mesentric vein — Lt renal vein
Rt kidney — Lt kidney
Renal pelvis
Duodenum — Lt colic artery
Rt colic artery — Psoas major
Ileocolic artery — Lt ureter
Inferior mesenteric vessels
Superior mesenteric artery — Testicular artery
Terminal ileum — Genitofemoral nerve
Sigmoid colon
Rt external iliac vessels — Lt external iliac vessels
Rt internal iliac vessels — Lt internal iliac vessels

Fig. 9.1-9. *Diagrammatic depiction of course and relations of pelvic part of ureter.*

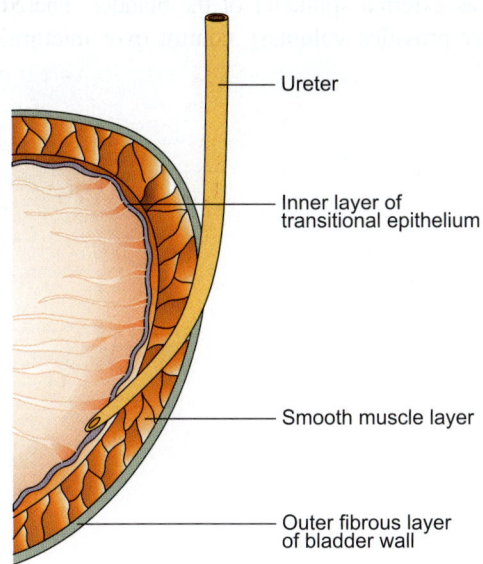

Fig. 9.1-10. *Intracystic part of ureter.*

pressure increases due to contraction of the muscular wall of the bladder.

Structure. Uretric wall consists of three coats (Fig. 9.1-11):

- *Outer fibrous coat* of the ureter becomes continuous with the fibrous capsule of the kidney.
- *Middle muscular coat* consists of an inner longitudinal layer and an outer circular layer of smooth muscle.
- *Inner mucous coat* consists of the lining transitional epithelium and the underlying connective tissue.

Function. The ureters propel the urine from the kidneys into the urinary bladder by peristaltic contractions of the smooth muscular coat.

THE URINARY BLADDER AND URETHRA

Gross anatomy of urinary bladder

Location. The urinary bladder, a hollow muscular viscus,

Fig. 9.1-11. *Microscopic structure of ureter.*

is a temporary reservoir for urine. It is situated in the pelvic cavity behind the pubis, in front of the rectum in the male and in front of the anterior wall of the vagina and the neck of the uterus in the females (Fig.11.3-1A). It is a freely movable organ but is held in position by folds of peritoneum and fascia.

External features. The main body of empty bladder is pyramidal, having an apex and a base. The lowest part of the bladder is called neck, which continues as urethra.

Interior of the bladder. In an empty bladder, the greater part of the mucosa shows irregular folds due to its loose attachments to the muscular coat. The interior of the base (posterior surface) of the bladder presents a triangular area, the trigone where the mucosa is smooth due to its firm attachment (Fig. 9.1-12).

Fig. 9.1-12. *Coronal section through the bladder and prostate to show the interior of the bladder, internal urethral sphincter and external urethral sphincter.*

Internal urethral orifice is located at the apex (inferior angle) of the trigone. The ureters open into the bladder at superior angles of the trigone (Fig. 9.1-12). The ureters pierce the bladder wall obliquely, and this provides a valve-like action, which prevents a reverse flow of urine towards the kidneys as the bladder fills.

Structure of the bladder

The wall of the urinary bladder consists of three layers: an outer serous layer, a thick coat of smooth muscle, and the inner mucous membrane (Fig. 9.1-12).

Mucous membrane is lined by transitional epithelium.

Muscular coat is formed by smooth muscle fibres which are arranged in three layers: inner longitudinal, middle circular and outer longitudinal. The fibres of outer layer, at the sides of bladder, are arranged obliquely and intersect one another. These fibres constitute the detrusor muscle. Contraction of this muscle coat is responsible for emptying of the bladder.

Serous coat is a reflection of the peritoneum and covers only the superior surface and the upper part of lateral surfaces of the bladder.

Urethra and its sphincters

Male urethra, about 20 cm in length, is divided into three parts: prostatic urethra (3 cm), membranous urethra (1.25 cm), and penile urethra (15.75 cm). Membranous urethra is surrounded by the external sphincter.

Female urethra is about 3.8 cm long. It extends from the neck of the bladder to the external meatus. It traverses the external sphincter and lies immediately in front of the vagina.

Sphincters of the urethra

1. *Internal sphincter.* The circular smooth muscle fibres in the area of the neck of bladder are thickened to form the internal sphincter (sphincter vesicae). The natural tone of the internal sphincter prevents emptying of the bladder until the pressure in the body of bladder rises above a threshold level.

2. *External sphincter.* Beyond the bladder neck, it is encircled by a ring of voluntary (skeletal type) muscle known as external sphincter of the bladder. The external sphincter provides voluntary control over micturition.

Physiology of Excretory System

URINE FORMATION

Processes concerned with urine formation

The main function of the kidneys is to clear waste products from blood and excrete them in the urine. The kidneys accomplish their excretory function by formation of urine.

Three processes are involved in urine formation (Fig. 9.2-1):

Fig. 9.2-1. *Steps involved in the formation of urine :*
1, filtration; 2, reabsorption; 3, secretion; and 4, excretion.

- Glomerular filtration,
- Tubular reabsorption,
- Tubular secretion

GLOMERULAR FILTRATION

Glomerular filtration refers to the process of ultrafiltration of plasma from the glomerular capillaries into the Bowman's capsule.

Composition of glomerular filtrate

The unique characteristic features of the glomerular filtration membrane determines the composition of glomerular filtrate, in that it is like that of plasma except for absence of proteins (colloids) and cells. Filtration membrane permeability alteration in diseases, however, may alter diffusibility of colloids and cells. As a result filtration of proteins is increased, and albumin appears in the urine in significant amount (*albuminuria* or *proteinuria*).

Dynamics of glomerular filtration

The forces which determine the bulk flow or ultrafiltration of protein-free plasma across the glomerular membrane are the same which determine formation of tissue fluid.

The glomerular filtration rate (GFR) will depend upon the balance of Starling forces (Fig. 9.2-2). According to Starling hypothesis the GFR can be expressed as:

$$GFR = K_f [(P_{GC} - P_{BS}) = (\pi_{GC} - \pi_{BS})]$$

where:

GFR is the filtration across the glomerular membrane.

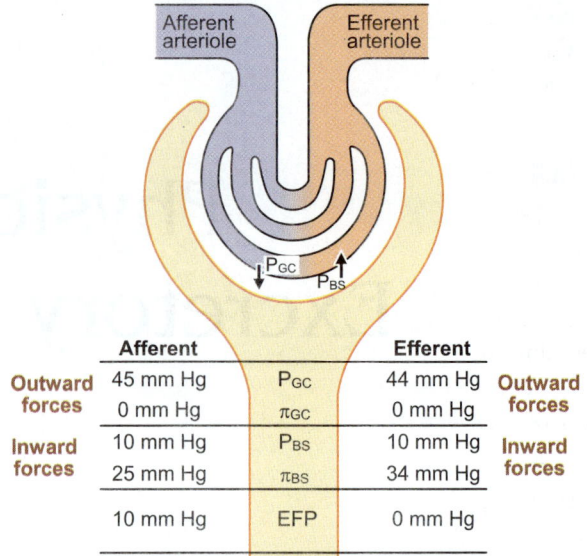

Fig. 9.2-2. *Depiction of Starling forces across the glomerular filtration membrane.*

	Afferent			Efferent	
Outward forces	45 mm Hg	P_{GC}	44 mm Hg		**Outward forces**
	0 mm Hg	π_{GC}	0 mm Hg		
Inward forces	10 mm Hg	P_{BS}	10 mm Hg		**Inward forces**
	25 mm Hg	π_{BS}	34 mm Hg		
	10 mm Hg	EFP	0 mm Hg		

K_f or the filtration coefficient of the glomerular membrane.
P_{GC} is glomerular capillary hydrostatic pressure. Its normal value is about 45 mmHg.
P_{BS} is the Bowman's space hydrostatic pressure. Its normal value is about 10 mmHg.
π_{GC} is the glomerular capillary oncotic pressure. Its normal value is 25 mmHg.
π_{BS} is the Bowman's space oncotic pressure. Its normal value is zero, because glomerular filtrate contains no proteins.

Normal glomerular filtration rate

The normal glomerular filtration rate (GFR) in an average-sized man is about 125 ml/min (range 90-140 ml/min). The values in women are 10% lower than those in men.

Factors affecting glomerular filtration rate

1. Filtration coefficient (K_f). Increased K_f raises GFR and decreased K_f reduces GFR as K_f is the product of permeability and filtration area of the glomerular capillary membrane.

2. Hydrostatic pressure in Bowman's space fluid (P_{BS}) opposes filtration and therefore GFR is inversely related to it. It is increased in acute obstruction of urinary tract (e.g. a ureteric obstruction by stone).

3. Glomerular capillary hydrostatic pressure (P_{GC}). GFR is mainly dependent on arterial pressure, renal blood flow, afferent arteriolar resistance, and efferent arteriolar resistance.

4. Glomerular capillary oncotic pressure (π_{GC}). GFR is inversely proportional to π_{GC}. In hyperproteinaemia and in haemoconcentration, the π_{GC} is raised leading to decrease in GFR. Conversely in hypoproteinaemia and haemodilution the π_{GC} is reduced leading to increased GFR.

TUBULAR REABSORPTION AND SECRETION

Of the 180 L glomerular filtrate formed per day, about 1.5 L (i.e. less than 1%) per day is excreted as urine. The different segments of the renal tubule viz. proximal tubule, loop of Henle, distal tubule, and collecting duct determine the composition and volume of the urine by process of *selective reabsorption* of solutes and water and *selective secretion* of solutes.

Tubular reabsorption denotes the active transport of solutes and passive movement of water from the tubular lumen into peritubular capillaries. In other words, reabsorption is the removal of substances of nutritive value such as glucose, amino acids, electrolytes (Na$^+$, K$^+$, Cl$^-$, HCO$_3^-$) and vitamins from the glomerular filtrate. Small proteins and peptide hormones are reabsorbed in the proximal tubules by endocytosis.

Tubular secretion refers to the transport of solutes from the peritubular capillaries into the tubular lumen, i.e. it is the addition of a substance to the glomerular filtrate.

Active secretion of substances occurs into the tubular fluid with the help of certain non-selective carriers. The carrier which secretes para-aminohippuric (PAH) acid can also secrete uric acid, bile acids, oxalic acid, penicillin, probenecid, cephalothin and furosemide.

TRANSPORT ACROSS DIFFERENT SEGMENTS OF RENAL TUBULE

The substances transported across the different segments of renal tubules are described below and enlisted in Table 9.2-1.

TRANSPORT ACROSS PROXIMAL TUBULE

The proximal tubule reabsorbs:

- Approximately 67% of the filtered water, Na$^+$, Cl$^-$, K$^+$ and other solutes, and
- Almost all the glucose and amino acids filtered by the glomerulus.

The proximal tubule does not reabsorb inulin, creatinine, sucrose and mannitol.

The proximal tubule secretes H$^+$, PAH, urate, penicillin, sulphonamides, and creatinine.

Sodium reabsorption

The process of sodium reabsorption in proximal tubule is *isosmotic*, i.e. the reabsorption of sodium and water are exactly proportional.

Table 9.2-1. Transport of substances across different segments of renal tubule

Reabsorbtion		Non-	Secretion
Active	Passive	reabsorbtion	
Proximal tubule			
Na$^+$	Cl$^-$	Inulin	H$^+$
K$^+$	HCO$_3^-$	Creatinine	Water
Ca^{2+}	HPO$_4^-$	Sucrose	Penicillin
Mg^{2+}	Water	Mannitol	Sulphonamide
HPO$_4^{2-}$	Urea		Creatinine
SO$_4^{2-}$			
NO$_3^-$			
Glucose			
Amino acids			
Protein			
Urate			
Vitamins			
Acetoacetate			
β-hydroxybutyrate			
Henle's loop			
Na$^+$	Cl$^-$		
K$^+$	HCO$_3^-$		
Ca^{2+}	Water		
Distal tubule and collecting duct			
Na$^+$	Cl$^-$		K$^+$
Ca^{2+}	HCO$_3^-$		H$^+$
Mg^{2+}	Water		
Water			

Mechanisms of Na$^+$ reabsorption

Na$^+$ is reabsorbed by *cotransport with H$^+$ or organic solutes (glucose, amino acids, phosphate and lactate)*. The Na$^+$ absorption is a two-step process (Fig. 9.2-3A):

Across the basolateral membrane, Na$^+$ moves against an electrochemical gradient via Na$^+$-K$^+$-ATPase pump, which pumps Na$^+$ into the paracellular spaces and lowers the intracellular Na$^+$ concentration.

Across the apical membrane, the sodium moves down an electrochemical gradient as above. The entry of Na$^+$ is mediated by specific antiporter and symporter proteins, and not by diffusion through channels.

Water reabsorption

Approximately 67% of the filtered water is absorbed in the proximal tubule by osmosis in response to a transtubular osmotic gradient established by the solute reabsorption (i.e. Na$^+$-Cl$^-$, Na$^+$-glucose, and so forth). The osmotic water absorption is termed as *obligatory water absorption* as it cannot be changed according to the needs of the body.

Fig. 9.2-3. *Mechanism of reabsorption of sodium and other solutes in proximal tubule : A, early proximal tubule; and B, late proximal tubule.*

Protein reabsorption

Normally, only a small amount of proteins is filtered by the glomerulus (40 mg/L). However, because of high GFR (180 L/day) the total amount of protein filtered per day is significant (180 L/day × 40 mg/L = 7.2 gm/day). Normally, the proteins are completely taken into the cells of proximal tubules by the process of *endocytosis*. Once inside the cells, enzymes digest the proteins and peptides into their constituent amino acids which exit across the basolateral membrane and return to the blood in the peritubular capillaries.

When the amount of filtered proteins increases (due to disruption of glomerular filtration barrier in kidney diseases), the reabsorbing mechanisms saturate and the proteins may appear in the urine (*proteinuria*).

Glucose reabsorption.

Glucose is freely filtered into the glomerular filtrate. Filtration load of glucose increases in direct proportion to the plasma glucose concentration (P glucose). Filtered load of glucose = GFR × P glucose (P_G).

Mechanism of tubular reabsorption

All the filtered glucose is completely reabsorbed into the proximal tubule by an active transport mechanism (Fig. 9.2-4):

Carrier mediated Na⁺-glucose cotransport. Carrier protein located at the apical membrane in the proximal tubule reabsorbs glucose from tubular fluid into the blood.

- The carrier protein for glucose in early and late proximal tubule is called SGLT-2 and SGLT-1, respectively (SGLT= sodium-dependent glucose transporter).

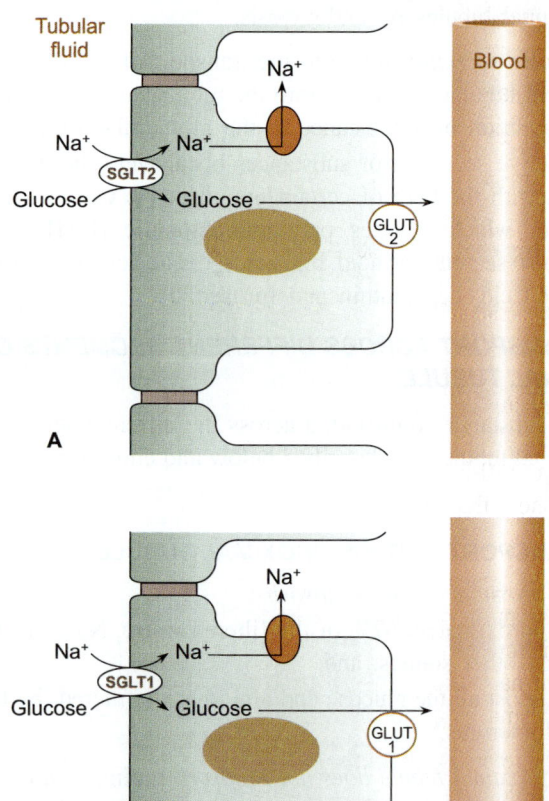

Fig. 9.2-4. *Mechanism of glucose reabsorption in: A, early proximal tubule; and B, late proximal tubule.*

Facilitated diffusion moves the glucose out of the cell through the basolateral membrane. The carrier for facilitated diffusion across the basolateral membrane in early and late proximal tubule is called GLUT-2 and GLUT-1, respectively (GLUT = glucose transporter).

Characteristics of glucose transport and glucose excretion

Glucose is reabsorbed by a transport maximum process, i.e. there are limited number of Na^+-glucose carriers. The characteristics of glucose transport and glucose excretion can be elicited from the glucose titration curve.

Glucose titration curve (Fig. 9.2-5) depicts that:

Filtered load increases with the plasma glucose concentration (P_G).

Fig. 9.2-5. *Glucose titration curve (for details see text).*

Renal threshold, i.e. the plasma glucose concentration at which glucose first appears in the urine (glycosuria) is about 180-200 mg%. At plasma levels below renal threshold the reabsorption of glucose is complete (100%).

Transport maximum As shown in Fig. 9.2-5, beyond plasma glucose concentration of 350 mg% (T_{mG}) the reabsorption rate does not increase, i.e. becomes constant and is independent of P_G. Therefore, as the T_{mG} is reached, the urinary excretion rate increases linearly with increase in plasma glucose concentration.

Splay refers to the region of the glucose curve between threshold and T_{mG}, i.e. between P_G 180 mg% and 350 mg%. It represents the excretion of glucose in urine before the T_{mG} is fully achieved. Note that in the region of splay the reabsorption curve is rounded indicating that though the reabsorption rate is increasing with increase in P_G, but reabsorption is less than filtration. Similarly, the excretion curve is also rounded in the region of splay, indicating that though the urinary excretion is increasing with increase in P_G, but there is no linear relation.

Causes of splay are:

- *Heterogenicity in glomerular size,* proximal tubular length, and number of carrier proteins for glucose reabsorption.
- *Variability in* T_{mG} *of the nephron.*

TRANSPORT ACROSS LOOP OF HENLE

About 20% of filtered Na^+ and Cl^-, 15% of filtered water and cations such as K^+, Ca^{2+} and Mg^{2+} are reabsorbed in the loop of Henle. Reabsorption occurring in different parts of loop of Henle is:

Thin descending limb of loop of Henle

Water absorption occurs passively (because of hypertonic interstitial fluid) in this part of loop of Henle. It is accompanied by diffusion of sodium ions from interstitial fluid into tubular lumen.

Thick ascending limb of loop of Henle

This limb is impermeable to water but is involved in the reabsorption of 20% of the filtered Na^+, and Cl^- and other cations.

Note. Thick ascending limb is *impermeable* to water. Thus, NaCl and other solutes are reabsorbed without water. As a result, tubular fluid Na^+ and tubular fluid osmolarity decreases to less than their concentration in plasma. This segment is therefore called the *diluting segment*. Further, Na^+ reabsorbed from this segment is the main driving force behind the counter-current multiplier system which concentrates Na^+ and urea in medullary interstitium.

TRANSPORT ACROSS DISTAL TUBULES AND COLLECTING DUCT

Approximately 7% of the filtered NaCl, and about 8-17% of water is reabsorbed and K^+ and H^+ are secreted in these segments.

Early distal tubule

Early distal tubule (initial segment of distal tubule) reabsorbs Na^+, Cl^- and Ca^{2+}, and is impermeable to water.

Late distal tubule and collecting duct

Late distal tubule and collecting duct have two cell types (principal cells and intercalated cells) which perform both reabsorption and secretory functions:

Role of antidiuretic hormone. H_2O absorption occurs in response to the effect of antidiuretic hormone (ADH) on the principal cells. ADH increases H_2O permeability by directing the insertion of H_2O channels in the luminal membrane. In the absence of ADH, the principal cells are virtually impermeable to water.

Role of aldosterone. Aldosterone by its effect on principal cell increases Na⁺ reabsorption and increases K⁺ secretion. About 2% of overall Na⁺ absorption is affected by aldosterone (Fig. 9.2-6).

Fig. 9.2-6. *Mechanism of transport in principal cells and intercalated cells of the late distal tubule and collecting duct. CA = Carbonic anhydrase.*

Intercalated cells reabsorb K⁺ and secrete H⁺

Aldosterone also increases H⁺ secretion by intercalated cells by stimulating the K^+_- H⁺-ATPase (in addition to its actions on the principal cells).

CONCENTRATION AND DILUTION OF URINE

The kidneys possess unique property of regulating the volume and osmolality of the urine by concentrating and diluting it as per needs of the body.

Purpose of concentration and dilution of urine. The main purpose is to maintain the osmolality and volume of the body fluids within a narrow range which is accomplished by kidneys in concert with other systems by regulating the excretion of water and NaCl, respectively.

The kidney can produce urine with osmolality as low as 30 mOsm/kg H_2O to as high as 1400 mOsm/kg H_2O by changing the water excretion as high as 23.3 L/day to as low as 0.5 L/day, respectively.

Principal factors. Principal factors responsible for mechanism of concentration and dilution of urine are:

- Antidiuretic hormones (see page 348), and
- Hyperosmolality and osmolality gradient in medullary interstitium of kidneys.

MEDULLARY HYPEROSMOLALITY AND MEDULLARY GRADIENT

The interstitial fluid of the medulla is critically important in concentrating the urine, because the osmotic pressure of this fluid provides the driving force for reabsorbing water from both the descending thin segment (DTS) and the collecting duct.

Normal osmolality of plasma and other body fluids is about 300 mOsm/kg H_2O. The interstitial fluid of the renal cortex has the same osmolality as that of plasma, and virtually all osmoles attributable to NaCl. The osmolality of the renal medulla is higher than the plasma (i.e. *hyperosmolar*) and that it goes on increasing progressively from about 300 mOsm/kg H_2O at corticomedullary junction to about 1200 mOsm/kg H_2O at papilla (medullary gradient) where a maximally concentrated urine is excreted (Fig. 9.2-7). This hyperosmolality and medullary gradient is generated, and maintained by the so-called countercurrent system.

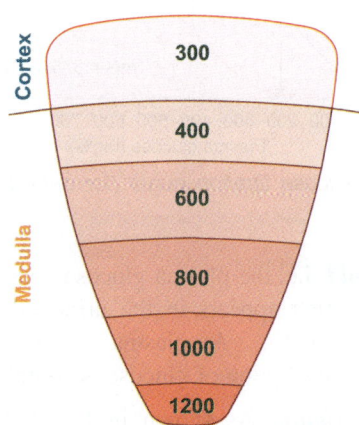

Fig. 9.2-7. *Osmolality gradient of renal medullary interstitium (values are in mOsm/kg H_2O).*

COUNTERCURRENT SYSTEM

A countercurrent system refers to a system in which the inflow runs parallel to, counter to, and in close proximity to the outflow for some distance. The countercurrent flow system is formed by U-shaped tubules.

In the kidney, the structures which form the counter-current system are loop of Henle and the vasa recta. The countercurrent system of kidney consists of two components:

- *Countercurrent multiplier*, which is formed by the operation of loop of Henle and is responsible for production of hyperosmolality and a gradient in renal medulla, and

- *Countercurrent exchanger* which is formed by the operation of vasa recta and is responsible for maintenance of the medullary gradient and hyperosmolality.

Countercurrent multipliers

The working of countercurrent multiplier, that operates in the loop of Henle and generates hyperosmolarity and medullary gradient, can be best understood by describing it as two processes:

- Origin of single effect, and
- Multiplication of the single effect.

Origin of single effect in inner medulla

The origin of single effect for the Development of medullary gradient and hyperosmolality occurs in the inner medullary interstitium due to .

- Passive transport of sodium ions from ascending thin segment into the interstitium,
- Active transport of sodium from inner medullary collecting duct, and
- Diffusion of urea from the collecting duct into medullary interstitium.

Role of urea. Urea plays an important role in the development of medullary osmotic gradient, especially when concentration of ADH is high in the blood. Under such circumstances, inner medullary collecting duct

(IMCD) absorbs large amount of urea, which plays an important role in the countercurrent system.

Multiplication of the single effect

The hyperosmolality and medullary gradient is in fact generated by the multiplication of the single effect by the countercurrent multiplier. The main characteristics of the components of countercurrent multiplier which play role in multiplication of single effect are :

- High permeability of descending thin segment to water.
- Impermeability to water and ability to actively absorb solutes by thick ascending limb (TAL).
- In renal medulla all other tubular structures (except ascending limb) are in osmotic equilibrium. The descending limb therefore acquires the increased osmolality of the surrounding fluid. The effect is multiplied as new iso-osmolar filtrate arrives at the descending limb and forces the concentrated tubular contents towards the tip of loop of Henle (hair-pin band).

Countercurrent exchanger

Vasa recta (the countercurrent exchanger). If the vasa recta would have been a straight blood vessel, the osmotic gradient in the medullary pyramid would not last long, as the Na+ and urea in the interstitial spaces would have been removed by the circulation (Fig. 9.2-8). However, because of the hair-pin (U-shaped) anatomical arrangement of the vasa recta operates as countercurrent exchanger and retains these solutes in the medullary interstitium. Thus,

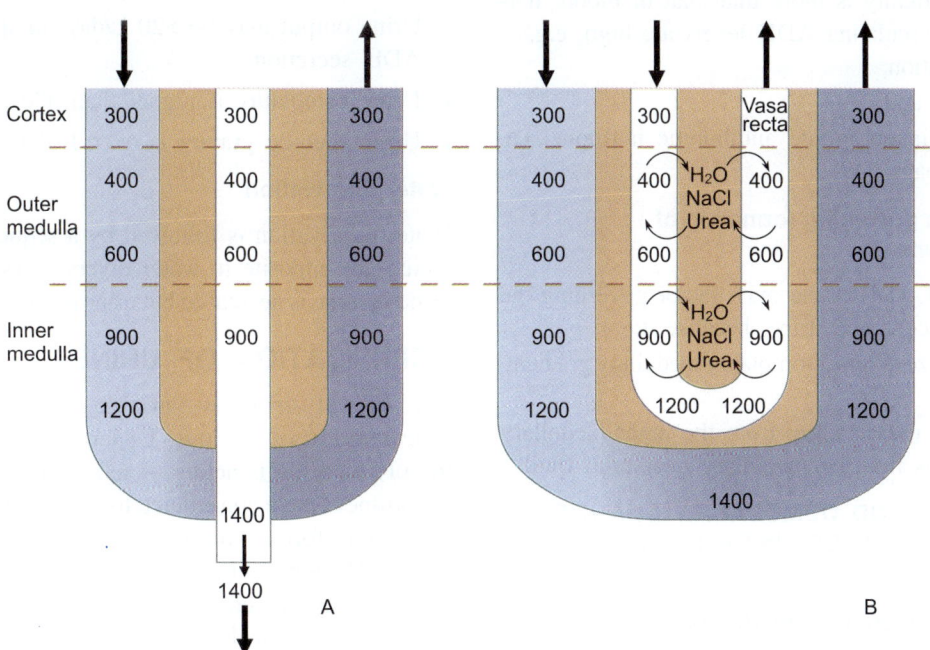

Fig. 9.2-8. Operation of vasa recta as countercurrent exchanger in the kidney : A, effect on medullary osmolality if vasa recta would be straight tube; and B, as vasa recta a 'U' shaped structure.

the countercurrent exchanger formed by the vasa recta is responsible for the maintenance of the hyperosmolality medullary gradient generated by the countercurrent multiplier.

MECHANISM OF URINE DILUTION AND CONCENTRATION

PRODUCTION OF DILUTED URINE

Conditions in which dilute urine is formed

Dilute urine is called *hyposmotic urine*, in which urine osmolality is less than blood osmolality. It is produced under following circumstances:

- When circulating levels of ADH are low (e.g. after water drinking), central diabetes insipidus (see page 349), or
- When ADH is ineffective (e.g. nephrogenic diabetes insipidus.

Principal factors governing formation of dilute urine

As mentioned earlier, the principal factors governing formation of dilute and concentrated urine are hyperosmolality medullary gradient and the presence or absence of ADH. The renal medullary osmotic gradient is smaller in the absence of ADH. This is because ADH stimulates both countercurrent multiplication and urea cycling.

PRODUCTION OF CONCENTRATED URINE

Conditions in which concentrated urine is formed

Concentrated urine is also called *hyperosmotic urine*, in which urine osmolality is more than that of blood. It is produced when circulating ADH levels are high, e.g.

- Water deprivation,
- Haemorrhage, and
- Syndrome of inappropriate antidiuretic hormone, i.e. SIADH (see page 349).

Principal factors governing formation of concentrated urine

The high level of ADH is the main factor governing the formation of concentrated urine, because it:

- Increases the size of hypersomolality medullary gradient, and
- Augments the urea cycling from the inner medullary collecting ducts into the medullary interstitial fluid.

URINE VOLUME AND OSMOLALITY CHANGES IN RESPONSE TO WATER INTAKE AND WATER DEPRIVATION

Water diuresis versus osmotic diuresis

Water diuresis

Water diuresis refers to increased urinary output following excessive intake of water or hypotonic solution.

Pathophysiology. It occurs due to absence of ADH in the plasma.

Characteristic features

- Water diuresis begins about 15 minutes after ingestion of water and reaches its maximum in 40 minutes.
- Urine output may be increased to 20 L/day.
- Urine formed is diluted, osmolality is always below 30 mOsm/kg H_2O and may be as low as 50 mOsm/kg H_2O.
- Specific gravity of urine is always below 1.010.

Osmotic diuresis

Osmotic diuresis refers to increased urine output because of an osmotic effect.

Pathophysiology

Presence of large quantities of unreabsorbed solutes in the proximal tubules exert an appreciable osmotic effect. Osmotic diuresis may occur under following circumstances:

- When the filtered load of naturally occurring substances such as Na^+, glucose, (e.g. in diabetes mellitus), urea, etc. exceeds the maximum capacity of the tubules to reabsorb (Tm).
- Following administration of compounds such as mannitol and related polysaccharides that are filtered but not reabsorbed.
- Following infusion of large amounts of sodium chloride and urea.

Characteristic features

- Urine output may be >20 L/day, in spite of maximal ADH secretion.
- Urine osmolality is higher than 300 mOsm/kg H_2O.
- Urine specific gravity is over 1.010.

Water deprivation

Water deprivation is followed by a sequence of changes which are opposite to water diversis. As a consequence urine volume is decreased but urine osmolality is increased.

ACIDIFICATION OF URINE

The pH of urine is variable depending upon the concentration of H^+ ions. Under normal circumstances, the pH of urine is acidic (~ 6.0). This clearly indicates that kidneys have contributed to the *acidification of urine*, when it is formed from the plasma (pH 7.4). In other words, H^+ ions generated in the body in the normal circumstances are eliminated by acidified urine. Thus, the role of kidneys in the maintenance of acid-base balance of the body (blood pH) is highly significant.

The kidneys regulate the blood pH by three main mechanisms:

- Reabsorption of the filtered HCO_3^-, and
- Generation of $NaHCO_3^-$ of the alkali reserve of the body, and
- Excretion of acid in the form of titrable acid and ammonium ions.

All these mechanisms are accomplished through process of H^+ secretion by the nephron.

Hydrogen ion secretion

The tubular cells of proximal tubule, distal tubule, and collecting ducts are capable of secreting H^+. The kidney is the only organ which can eliminate the fixed acids by active secretion of H^+.

Mechanism of H^+ secretion by proximal tubule

Steps involved are (Fig. 9.2-9):

- *Formation of carbonic acid.* Carbonic acid (H_2CO_3) is first formed in the cells of proximal tubules from CO_2 and H_2O by a reaction that is catalyzed by the intracellular *carbonic anhydrase*.
- *Dissociation of carbonic acid* (H_2CO_3) then occurs in H^+ and HCO_3^-.
- Secretion of H^+ into the lumen occurs via *Na$^+$-H$^+$ exchange mechanism* in the luminal membrane by *Na$^+$-H$^+$-antiporter* (Fig. 9.2-9).
- The secreted H^+, in the lumen, combines with the filtered HCO_3^- and helps its reabsorption (as described below). Therefore, this process does not result in net secretion of H^+
- *HCO_3^- formed in the cell* (from dissociation of H_2CO_3) diffuses into the interstitial fluid. Thus, for each H^+ secreted one Na^+ ion and one HCO_3^- ion enter the interstitial fluid. The latter adds up to the alkali reserve of the body.

Mechanism of H^+ secretion by distal tubules and collecting ducts.
In the distal tubule and collecting ducts, H^+ secretion occurs independent of Na^+.

- H^+, K^+-ATPase is responsible for secretion of some of the H^+ coupled with reabsorption of K^+ in these parts of renal tubules.

Fate of H^+ secreted in the renal tubule.
The secretion of H^+ in the renal tubule can continue only if the H^+ is immediately buffered in the luminal fluid.

- In proximal tubule, the secreted H^+ is buffered by the filtered HCO_3^- (i.e. consumed in reabsorption of filtered HCO_3^-, vide infra), and
- In distal tubule and connecting ducts the secreted H^+ ions are buffered by Na_2HPO_4 and NH_3 and are excreted as titrable acid and ammonium ion (NH_4^+, vide infra).

Reabsorption of filtered HCO_3^-

Proximal tubule reabsorbs approximately 80% of the filtered HCO_3^-.

Loop of Henle reabsorbs 15% of the filtered HCO_3^-, mainly in the region of thick ascending limb (TAL).

Generation of new HCO_3^-

As discussed above, the kidneys play an important role in the maintenance of acid-base balance of the body by completely reabsorbing the filtered HCO_3^-. However, in reality, HCO_3^- reabsorption alone does not replenish the HCO_3^- lost during the titration of non-volatile acids which are daily added to the plasma from the diet and produced by metabolism. Therefore, to maintain acid-base balance, the kidneys replace this lost HCO_3^- with new HCO_3^- by following processes:

- Excretion of H^+ as titrable acid, and
- Excretion of H^+ as NH_4.

Excretion of H^+ as titrable acid

Excretion of H^+ as titrable acid refers to the excretion of secreted H^+ along with the primary urinary buffer, the dibasic phosphate (HPO_4^{-2}). This reaction occurs in the distal tubules and collecting ducts (9.2-10).

Fig. 9.2-9. *Cellular mechanism for secretion of H^+ by proximal tubular cell (A) and intercalated cells of late tubule (B).*

Fig. 9.2-10. *Mechanism for excretion of H⁺ as titrable acid and synthesis of new HCO₃⁻.*

As a result of H⁺ excretion in the form of titrable acid, the pH of urine is progressively decreased (from 7.4, that of blood). The *acidification of the urine* may lower its pH to a minimum of 4.5.

Excretion of H⁺ as ammonium ion

Excretion of H⁺ as NH_4^+ is another mechanism of excretion of secreted H⁺ and formation of new HCO_3^-. The amount of H⁺ excreted as NH_4^+ depends upon both the amount of NH_3 synthesized by renal cells and the urine pH. *NH_4^+ is a major urine acid.* It is estimated that about half to two-thirds of body acid load is eliminated in the form of NH_4^+ ions. The process by which the kidneys excrete NH_4^+ is complex.

PHYSIOLOGY OF MICTURITION

Micturition is the process by which urinary bladder empties when filled. Before discussing the physiological events in micturation it will be worthwhile to revise anatomy (see page 311) and innervation of urinary bladder.

INNERVATION OF THE URINARY BLADDER (Fig. 9.2-11)

Motor innervation

Parasympathetic innervation. The parasympathetic efferent fibres (nervi erigentes) are derived from the second, third and fourth sacral segments (mainly S_2 and S_3). These fibres carry motor impulses to the urinary bladder causing contraction of detrusor muscle and emptying of the bladder. These fibres are inhibitory to the internal sphincter.

Sympathetic innervation. These nerves arise in the 11th thoracic to the second lumbar segments (T_{11} to L_2). These fibres are said to be inhibitory to detrusor muscle and motor to the sphincter vesicae.

Somatic motor innervation. The somatic pudendal nerve (S_2, S_3 and S_4) supplies the external sphincter which is voluntary.

Sensory innervation

Sensation of bladder distension. Afferents from the detrusor stretch receptors travel to the spinal cord via the pelvic splanchnic nerve (nervi erigentes). From the region of the bladder neck and trigone, the afferents travel via the hypogastric plexus to spinal cord segments T_{11} to L_2.

In the spinal cord, the fibres of awareness of bladder distension run in the posterior column (fasciculus gracilis) to reach the spinal, pontine and suprapontine micturition centres.

Sensation of bladder pain. The pain fibres are stimulated by excessive distension or spasm of the bladder wall, or by stone, inflammation or malignant disease irritating the bladder. The pain fibres run predominantly in the hypogastric plexus but are also present in the nervi erigentes.

In the spinal cord, the fibres carrying pain sensation run in the lateral spinothalamic tract.

Urethral sensations, including sensation of imminent voiding associated with maximal bladder filling, reach the spinal cord via the pudendal nerve.

In the spinal cord, fibres carrying urethral sensations travel in the dorsal column.

The main physiological events in the process of micturition are:

- Filling of urinary bladder, and
- Emptying of urinary bladder.

FILLING OF URINARY BLADDER

Transport of urine into urinary bladder through ureters

As urine collects in the renal pelvis, the pressure in the pelvis increases and initiates a peristaltic contraction beginning in the pelvis and spreading along the ureter to force urine towards the bladder.

Capacity of the bladder

Physiological capacity of the bladder varies with age, being 20 to 50 ml at birth, about 200 ml at 1 year, and can be as high as 600 ml in young adult males. In all cases, the physiological capacity is about twice that at which the first desire to void is felt.

EMPTYING OF THE BLADDER

Emptying of the bladder is basically a reflex action called the micturition reflex, which is controlled by supraspinal centres and is assisted by contraction of perineal and abdominal muscles.

MOTOR INNERVATION   **SENSORY INNERVATION**

Fig. 9.2-11. *Innervation of urinary bladder.*

Micturition reflex

Initiation. Micturition reflex is initiated by stimulation of the stretch receptors located in the wall of urinary bladder.

Stimulus. Filling of bladder by 300 to 400 ml of urine in adults constitutes the adequate stimulus for the micturition reflex to occur.

Afferents. The afferents from the stretch receptors in the detrusor muscle and urethra travel along the pelvic splanchnic nerves and enter the spinal cord through dorsal roots to S_2, S_3 and S_4 segments to reach the sacral micturition centre (Fig. 9.2-12).

Sacral micturition centre is formed by the sacral detrusor nucleus and sacral pudendal nucleus.

Efferents. Efferents arising from the sacral detrusor nucleus are the pregnanglionic parasympathetic fibres which relay

in the ganglia near or within bladder and urethra (Fig. 9.2-12). The postganglionic parasympathetic fibres are excitatory to the detrusor muscle and inhibitory to the internal sphincter.

Response. Once micturition reflex is initiated, it is self-regenerative, i.e. initial contraction of the bladder wall further activates the receptors to increase sensory impulses (afferents) from the bladder and urethra which cause further increase in reflex contraction of detrusor muscle of the bladder. The cycle thus keeps on repeating itself again and again until the bladder has reached a strong degree of contraction.

Voluntary control of micturition

Role of supraspinal centres

The micturition reflex is fundamentally a *spinal reflex* facilitated and inhibited by higher brain centres (*supraspinal*

***Fig. 9.2-12.** Pathway and supraspinal control of micturition reflex.*

centres) and, like defaecation, is subjected to voluntary facilitation and inhibition. In infants and young children, micturition is purely a reflex action. *Voluntary control* is gradually acquired as a learned ability of the toilet training. *Supraspinal control centres* which control the micturition reflex (a completely automatic cord reflex) include the pontine micturition centre (PMC) and suprapontine centres.

Role of perineal and abdominal muscles in micturition
Certain muscular movements, which aid the emptying of bladder, but are not the essential component of micturition process are:

- At the onset of micturition, the levator ani and perineal muscles are relaxed,

- The diaphragm descends, and
- The abdominal muscles contract, accelerating the flow of urine by raising intra-abdominal pressure which in turn secondarily increase the intravesical pressure thereby increasing the flow of urine.

APPLIED ASPECTS

PATHOPHYSIOLOGY OF COMMON RENAL DISORDERS

The applied aspects of common renal disorders which need some elaboration are:

- Common urinary symptoms, and
- Renal failure.

COMMON URINARY SYMPTOMS

Polyuria, nocturia and urinary frequency. Normal urine output per day is 800 to 2500 ml. Therefore, a reasonable criterion to satisfy the definition of polyuria is excretion of 3.0 L of urine daily, provided the patient is not on high fluid diet.

Nocturia means excessive amount of urine passed at night.

Urinary frequency means the increase in the number of times the patient goes for urination. Polyuria is differentiated from increased frequency by measuring the 24-hour urine output.

Dysuria and urgency of micturition. *Dysuria* refers to pain or burning during micturition. *Urgency of micturition* is the exaggerated sense or urge to micturate. It is due to either irritative or inflammatory disorders of urinary bladder. This is often associated with increased frequency of urination.

Incontinence. This refers to inability to retain urine in the bladder. It results from neurological or mechanical disorders of the complicated system that controls normal micturition.

Enuresis refers to the involuntary passage of urine at night or during sleep. It is also called night bedwetting or nocturnal enuresis. It is normal in children upto 2-3 years of age. In some children it continues for long.

Oliguria refers to urine output less than 500 ml/day in an average adult. It invariably occurs in acute on chronic renal failure or acute renal failure.

Anuria is said to occur when patient does not pass any urine or passes less than 50 ml of urine/day. In physiological sense the term anuria means less formation or absence of formation of urine by the kidney.

RENAL FAILURE

Renal failure refers to the deterioration of renal functions resulting in decline in glomerular filtration rate (GFR) and rise in urea and non-nitrogenous substances in the blood.

Acute renal failure

Acute renal failure refers to sudden decrease in GFR, associated with rapid rise in blood urea.

Common causes of acute renal failure are :
- Severe haemorrhage,
- Shock,
- Acute glomerulonephritis, and
- Urinary tract obstruction.

Chronic renal failure

Chronic renal failure refers to slow insiduous deterioration of kidney functions resulting in uraemia.

Common causes of chronic renal failure are mainly due to kidney diseases : polycystic kidney, pyelonephritis.

RENAL FUNCTION TESTS

Renal function tests are carried out to assess the functional capacity of the kidneys. Renal function tests can be divided into following groups:
- Analysis of urine,
- Analysis of blood,
- Renal clearance tests,
- Tests for tubular functions,
- Radiology and renal imaging, and
- Renal biopsy.

Anylysis of urine

Analysis of urine helps, of course, to a limited degree, to assess kidney functioning. In patients with suspected renal disorder, the urine analysis should be performed for volume, specific gravity, osmolality, pH, abnormal constituents, microscopic examination, and bacterio-logical finding.

1. *Volume.* Normal urine output per day is 800-2500 ml. Abnormalities of urine volume include: polyuria, oliguria and anuria.

2. *Colour.* The normal light yellow colour of the urine is due to the presence of urochrome pigment (a compound of urobilin and urobilinogen with peptide). On standing, the colour deepens due to oxidation of uribilinogen into urobilin. Abnormalities of urine colour include:
- *Brownish yellow*, due to presence of conjugated bilirubin in patients with hepatic and post-hepatic jaundice.
- *Cloudy appearance* is seen in strongly alkaline urine due to precipitation of calcium phosphate, and due to precipitation of urates.
- *Frothy appearance* is indicative of proteinuria.
- *Red-dark brown* tinge of urine is seen in porphyria.

3. *Osmolality and specific gravity.* Normal urinary osmolality varies from 50 mOsm/kg to 1200 mOsm/kg and specific gravity from 1.003 to 1.030, depending upon the state of hydration of the body. If the early morning urine sample after an overnight fast has an osmolality of > 600 mOsm/kg H_2O (and sp. gravity > 1.018), then the patient has a normal urine concentrating ability. Certain abnormalities are:
- Fixed urinary osmolality of 300 mOsm/kg H_2O (sp. gr. 1.010) is an evidence of fairly advanced urinary failure.
- Persistently low urinary osmolality (less than 100 mOsm/kg H_2O) even after eight hours of fluid deprivation is diagnostic of diabetes insipidus.

4. *Urine pH*. Normal pH of urine varies from 4.5 to 8.0. Urine is normally slightly acidic, except for a short post-prandial alkaline tide. Intake of high protein non-vegetarian diet shifts the urinary pH towards acidic side while vegetarian diet shifts it towards alkaline side.

5. *Chemical analysis for abnormal urinary constituents* may reveal:

i. *Proteinuria.* Normally, upto 150 mg of proteins are excreted daily in urine. Excretion of > 150 mg/day of protein is called proteinuria. It occurs in following conditions :

- In congestive heart failure,
- After prolonged standing, and
- Renal diseases and in toxaemia of pregnancy.

ii. *Glycosuria* refers to presence of glucose in the urine. Glycosuria may be due to diabetes mellitus, renal disorders (renal glycosuria), GIT disorders (alimentary glycosuria). Other sugars like galactose and fructose may also be present in urine in certain inborn errors of metabolism.

iii. *Ketonuria* refers to presence of ketone bodies (acetoacetic acid, β-hydroxybutyric acid, and acetone) in the urine. Ketonuria occurs in patients suffering from ketosis due to severe diabetes mellitus or prolonged starvation.

iv. *Bilirubinuria* refers to appearance of bilirubin in the urine in patients with elevated conjugated bilirubin levels, in hepatic or post-hepatic jaundice. Normally, 1-3.5 mg of urobilinogen is excreted daily in the urine. Its excessive excretion in the urine is one of the characteristic features of haemolytic jaundice.

v. *Haemoglobinuria*, i.e. presence of haemoglobin in the urine, indicates intravascular haemolysis, as seen in black-water fever due to falciparum malarial infection.

vi. *Haematuria*, i.e. presence of blood in the urine is seen in acute glomerulonephritis, and renal stone disease.

6. *Microscopic examination*. Examination of a centrifuged sediment of urine may show casts, cells and crystals.

i. *Casts* are proteinaceous plugs formed by coagulation of Tamm-Horsfall protein within the renal tubules and washed out by the flow of tubular fluid.

ii. *Crystals* are usually present in normal urine and thus have no pathological significance. Commonly seen are crystals of calcium oxalate, calcium phosphate, calcium-ammonium-magnesium phosphate (triple phosphate) or uric acid.

iii. *Cells* found on microscopic examination may be RBCs, leucocytes, tubular epithelial cells, and squamous epithelial cells.

7. *Bacteriological examination of urine*. The mid-stream sample of urine is examined for pus cells and bacteria. Bacteriuria and pyuria indicate urinary tract infection.

Analysis of blood

Estimation of blood levels of the substances that are excreted by the kidneys throw some light on the functional status of kidney, although these tests are less sensitive than clearance tests.

1. *Blood urea level* (normal 20-40 mg%) is an index of glomerular function. The blood urea levels begin to rise after about 50% glomerular damage has occurred.

2. *Plasma creatinine concentration* (normal 0.6-1.5 mg%) is more reliable than blood urea, as the latter is subjected to variations by dietary proteins, hydration, and tissue breakdown.

3. *Serum proteins levels* (Normal: total protein, 6.7-8 gm%; albumin, 3-5 gm%; globulins, 2-3 gm%; and A/G ratio, 1.7:1) are reduced if there is significant proteinuria with renal failure. In nephrotic syndrome the albumin levels decrease and globulin levels increase, leading to reversal of A/G ratio.

4. *Serum cholesterol levels* (normal 150-200 mg%) are increased in nephrotic syndrome.

5. *Serum electrolyte* levels (normal: Na^+, 152 mEq/L; K^+, 5 mEq/L; Ca^{2+}, 9-11 mg%; PO_4^{3-}, 3-4.5 mg%; SO_4^{2-}, 0.5-1.5 mEq/L; and Mg^{2+}, 1.5-2.5 mEq/L) are of value in variety of renal disorders. For example, chronic renal failure is mostly accompanied by high potassium and phosphate but low sodium and calcium levels in blood.

Renal clearance tests

The renal clearance can be defined as the volume of plasma that is cleared of a substance in one minute by excretion of the substance in the urine. It is a 'virtual volume'. The unit of renal clearance (C) is ml/min, and is calculated from the following formula:

$$C = \frac{UV}{P},$$

where C = renal clearance, U = urine concentration of the substance, V = rate of flow of urine, and P = plasma concentration of the substance.

Renal clearance as kidney function test. Renal clearance of a substance is correlated more directly with the status of kidney function. It shows a deviation from normal (earlier) in the course of renal damage.

Renal clearance tests, therefore, can be employed to assess the different functions of a nephron, e.g.

- To assess glomerular filtration,
- To assess tubular secretory capacity, and

- To assess renal plasma flow (RPF) and renal blood flow (RBF).

Tests for tubular functions

The reabsorptive and secretory functions of renal tubules can be tested by following tests:

- Urine concentration test.
- Urine dilution test.
- Urine acidification test.
- Other methods of study of tubular function

Radiology and renal imaging

Though, not, strictly speaking, kidney function tests but are quite useful investigations in present day clinical practice to assess anatomical and physiological abnormalities of the kidneys.

1. *Plain radiograph of abdomen* is useful in detecting calcium-containing (radiopaque) renal stones.

2. *Intravenous pyelography* (IVP) is performed by injecting a radiopaque dye like urographin intravenously and taking radiographs of the abdomen at short intervals (1, 5, 10, and 30 minutes) (Fig. 9.2-13).

Fig. 9.2-13. *Intravenous pyelogram.*

3. *Ultrasonography* is a quick, non-invasive, inexpensive and harmless method to evaluate size, shape, position of kidney and to detect tumour, stones, cysts, etc. of the kidneys, ureter, prostate and urinary bladder.

4. *Computed tomography (CT)* is performed to detect abnormalities in and around the kidneys as mentioned above in ultrasonography.

5. *Radionuclide studies* are carried out by injecting radioactive compounds which are concentrated and excreted by the kidneys. Radioactivity of the kidneys is recorded by gamma camera.

Renal biopsy

Renal biopsy is performed percutaneously with the help of needle. The biopsy specimen is subjected to light, electron and immunofluorescence microscopic studies. This technique has increased knowledge and better understanding of glomerular and tubular diseases.

DIALYSIS AND RENAL TRANSPLANTATION

DIALYSIS

The term dialysis in physiological sense refers to the diffusion of solutes from an area of higher concentration to the area of lower concentration through a semipermeable membrane. This principle has been used to dialyse the blood of patients with renal failure especially those developing uraemia.

Uraemia develops when more than 75% of nephrons are damaged and is characterized by:

- Accumulation of nitrogenous waste products in the blood,
- Metabolic acidosis, and
- Hyperkalaemia.

Types of dialysis. By dialysis the dissolved crystalloids of the plasma pass through a semipermeable membrane so that their levels are brought down to lower levels. Two types of dialysis procedures are available:

- Haemodialysis or artificial kidney, and
- Peritoneal dialysis.

RENAL TRANSPLANTATION

Renal transplantation is the final answer to all the problems in cases with chronic renal failure. It reverses metabolic and excretory abnormalities.

Physiology of Acid-Base Balance

GENERAL CONSIDERATIONS

ACIDS AND BASES

Acids and bases. Acid refers to a substance that acts as proton (H⁺) donor while base refers to a substance that accepts proton (H⁺). Examples of a few acids and their corresponding bases are:

Acid	Base
HCl	$H^+ + Cl^-$
H_2CO_3	$H^+ + HCO_3^-$

Alkalies refer to metallic hydroxides, e.g. NaOH and KOH. These compounds do not directly satisfy the criteria of bases. However, they dissociate to form metallic ion and OH⁻ which being the base accepts H⁺ ions. Therefore, for all practical purposes, alkalies are considered bases.

Strong acid and bases. Acid or base having strong tendency to dissociate into ions is called strong acid or strong base; and the acid or base having weak tendency to dissociate into ions is called weak acid or weak base.

In general a strong acid has a weak base, while a weak acid has a strong base. For example, strong acid HCl has weak base Cl⁻, and weak acid HCN has a strong base CN⁻. *Ampholytes* refer to the substances that can act both as acids and bases. Water is the best example of ampholyte.

Concept of pH and H⁺ concentration

H⁺ ion concentration. The acidic or basic nature of a solution is measured by H⁺ ion concentration. Since the concentration of H⁺ions in biological fluids is exceedingly low, the conventional units such as mEq/L or moles/L etc. Therefore,

pH is the term suggested to express H⁺ ion concentration. pH is defined as the negative logarithm of H⁺ concentration.

$$pH = -\log [H^+]$$

It is important to note that pH and (H⁺) are inversely related. For example, pH of plasma with a H⁺ ion concentration of 0.00004 mEq/L is 7.4, while pH of HCl with H⁺ ion concentration of 150 mEq/L is 0.8.

Neutral pH, acidic pH and alkaline pH. Pure water has an equal concentration of H$^+$ and OH$^-$ ions, i.e. 10^{-7} M each. Thus pure water has pH of 7 which is neutral. Therefore, solutions with pH less than 7 are considered acidic and those with more than 7 are considered alkaline.

H$^+$ CONCENTRATION AND pH OF BIOLOGIC FLUIDS

The H$^+$ concentration and pH of some biologic fluids is depicted in Table 9.3-1.

Table 9.3-1 : H$^+$ concentration and pH of biologic fluids

Fluid	H$^+$ concentration		
	nEq/L	mol/L	pH
1. Pure water	100	1×10^{-7}	7.0
2. Blood			
Normal mean	40	3.98×10^{-8}	7.4
Normal range	44-36	4.36×10^{-8}	7.36-7.44
		to 3.6×10^{-7}	
Acidosis (severe)	126	1.26×10^{-7}	6.9
Alkalosis (severe)	20	2.00×10^{-8}	7.7
3. Cerebrospinal fluid CSF (Normal range)	44-36	4.36×10^{-8}	7.36-7.44
		to 3.6×10^{-7}	
4. Gastric juice (pure)	100,000,000	1×10^{-1}	1.0
5. Pancreatic juice	10	1×10^{-8}	8.0
6. Urine			
Normal average	1000	1×10^{-6}	6.0
Maximum acidity	31,600	3.16×10^{-5}	4.5
Maximum alkalinity	10	1×10^{-8}	6.0
7. Intracellular fluid (ICF)	158	1.58×10^{-7}	6.8

MAINTENANCE OF BLOOD pH

GENERAL CONSIDERATIONS

BLOOD AND PLASMA pH

- The term blood pH always refers to plasma pH.
- Normal plasma pH is 7.4 (H$^+$ concentration ~40 nEq/L), which is higher than the intracellular pH of the erythrocyte (7.2).
- Plasma pH compatible with life varies from 7.7 to 6.9 (H$^+$ concentration is 20 to 120 nEq/L).
- Normally, the pH of ECF is maintained between a narrow range of 7.35 and 7.45.

DIETARY AND METABOLIC PRODUCTION OF ACIDS AND BASES

The daily consumed diet contains many acids and alkalies. In addition, cellular metabolism produces a number of acidic and alkaline substances that have an impact on the body pH.

Acid production by the body

The metabolic activities of the body are accompanied by production of two types of acids:

1. *Volatile acids*. CO_2 is the volatile acid produced from the aerobic metabolism of cells. It is also major end product in oxidation of carbohydrates, fats and amino acids. CO_2 accounts for over 12,000 mEq/L of H$^+$ per day. It is considered acid, because CO_2 combines with H_2O (by a reaction catalyzed by carbonic anhydrase, i.e. CA) to form weak acid H_2CO_3, which dissociates into H$^+$ and HCO_3^- by the following reaction:

$$CO_2 + H_2O \rightleftharpoons H_2CO_3 \rightleftharpoons H^+ + HCO_3^-$$

It is called volatile, because it is a gas, and under normal circumstances almost all the CO_2 is excreted by lungs.

2. *Non-volatile acids*, also called fixed acids, contribute about 50 to 100 mEq H$^+$ per day, depending upon the diet. *These include*:

- Sulphuric acid,
- Phosphoric acid,
- Hydrochloric acid,
- Organic acids like lactic acid, acetic acid and β-hydroxybutyric acid, and
- Uric acid produced in metabolism of nucleoproteins.

Production of bases by the body

In normal circumstance, a negligible amount of bases is formed in the body, because

- HCO_3^- produced by the metabolism of organic anions (e.g. citrate) offsets non-volatile acid production to some degree.
- *Ammonia* produced in the amino acid metabolism is converted to urea, hence its contribution as a base in the body is insignificant.

DEFENCES AGAINST CHANGES IN H$^+$ CONCENTRATION

There are three lines of defence to regulate the body's acid-base balance and maintain the blood pH (around 7.4):

I. *Buffer systems of body fluid*. These:

- Form first line of defence,
- Act instantaneously in ECF, and
- Immediately combine with H$^+$ to prevent changes in H$^+$ concentration and form a temporary measure to control changes in H$^+$ concentration.

II. *Respiratory mechanism* to regulate acid-base balance:

- Forms second line of defence,
- Acts within a few minutes,

- Acts via respiratory centre to regulate removal of CO_2 (and therefore H_2CO_3), and
- Forms a short-term measure to regulate changes in H^+ concentration.

III. *Renal mechanism* to regulate acid-base balance:
- Forms third line of defence,
- Takes days or weeks,
- Slow, but most powerful and effective in regulating pH,
- Acts by reabsorbing filtered HCO_3^-, generating new HCO_3^- and excreting H^+ as titrable acid and ammonium ion, and thus
- Provides a permanent solution to acid-base balance.

I. BUFFER SYSTEM : PRIMARY DEFENCE

Buffers. A buffer is a solution, consisting of a weak acid and its salt with strong base, that prevents a change in pH when H^+ ions are added to or removed from a solution. It must be borne in mind that a buffer cannot remove H^+ ions from the body. It temporarily acts as a shock absorbant to reduce the free H^+ ions. The H^+ have to be ultimately eliminated by the renal mechanism.

When acid is added to a buffer solution, its H^+ ion concentration is increased and the reaction is forced towards right leading to increase in undissociated molecules, therefore, increase in H^+ concentration is less.

When base is added to buffer, reaction shifts towards left; more H^+ ions are released from the buffer to combine with base, thereby limiting the decrease in H^+ concentration.

Henderson-Hasselbalch equation which is used to calculate the pH in a buffer system can be derived as:
The general equation for a buffer is

$$HA \rightleftharpoons H^+ + A^-$$

A^- represents any anion from a buffer (i.e. H^+ acceptor) and HA the undissociated acid from a buffer (i.e. H^+ donor). By the law of mass action, at equilibrium

$$K = \frac{[H^+][A^-]}{[HA]} \qquad ...(1)$$

(K = Dissociation constant of the acid HA)
The equation, to represent free H^+ ion in a solution, can be rewritten as:

$$[H^+] = K = \frac{[HA]}{[A^-]} \qquad ...(2)$$

we know that $pH = \log \dfrac{1}{[H^+]}$

By taking the reciprocals and logarithms (for log, multiplication becomes addition).

$$\log \frac{1}{[H^+]} = \log \frac{1}{K} + \log \frac{[A^-]}{[HA]} \qquad ...(3)$$

As $\log \dfrac{1}{K} = pK$, the equation (3) may be rewritten as:

$$pH = pK + \log \frac{[A^-]}{[HA]}$$

From this equation, it is evident that buffering capacity of a buffer system is greatest when amount of anions $[A^-]$ and undissociated acid [HA] is same, i.e.

$$\frac{[A^-]}{[HA]} = 1, \ or \ \log \frac{A^-}{HA}$$

Thus, pH = pK. Therefore, most effective buffers in the body are those with pK close to the pH in which they operate.

CLASSIFICATION OF THE BUFFER SYSTEMS

Buffer systems in the body can be classified by different methods:

A. *Bicarbonate versus non-bicarbonate buffers*
1. *Bicarbonate buffer* forms 53% of the buffering in the whole body. Out of it:
- Plasma HCO_3^- contributes 35%, and
- Erythrocyte HCO_3^- contributes 18%.

2. *Non-bicarbonate buffers* form remaining 47% of the buffering in the whole body. With a contribution from:
- Haemoglobin and oxyhaemoglobin   35%
- Plasma proteins   7%
- Organic phosphate   3%
- Inorganic phosphate   2%

B. *Extracellular versus intracellular buffers*
Extracellular buffers
1. *Bicarbonate* (HCO_3^-) is the major extracellular buffer, which is produced from CO_2 and H_2O.
2. *Phosphate* is a minor extracellular buffer. Phosphate is most important as urinary buffer; excretion of H^+ as $H_2PO_4^-$ is called titrable acid.
3. *Plasma proteins* form the non-bicarbonate buffer in the blood and is responsible for 7% of the total buffering of blood.
4. *Haemoglobin*, though found intracellularly, is more conventionally regarded as part of extracellular system (as described later).

Intracellular buffers
1. *Organic phosphate*, e.g. AMP, ADP, ATP, and 2,3-diphosphoglycerate (DPG).
2. *Proteins* of the skeletal muscles.
3. *HCO_3^-* present in intracellular fluid of skeletal and cardiac muscles.

MAJOR BUFFER SYSTEMS OF THE BODY

The major buffer systems involved in the maintenance of body pH are:
- Bicarbonate buffer,

- Phosphate buffer, and
- Protein buffer.

1. Bicarbonate buffer system

The carbonic acid-sodium bicarbonate (H_2CO_3-$NaHCO_3$) is the most predominant buffer system of the extracellular fluid; particularly the plasma H_2CO_3 in the body is formed by CO_2 and H_2O:

$$CO_2 + H_2O \xrightarrow[\text{anhydrase}]{\text{carbonic}} H_2CO_3$$

This reaction is catalyzed by the enzyme carbonic anhydrase, which is present in the RBCs, walls of the lungs, alveoli, and epithelial cells of renal tubules.

Dynamics of bicarbonate buffer system

Carbonic acid dissociates into hydrogen and bicarbonate ions:

$$H_2CO_3 \rightleftharpoons H^+ + HCO_3^-$$

According to Henderson-Hasselbalch equation for this system:

$$pH = pK + \log \frac{[HCO_3^-]}{[H_2CO_3]} \qquad (1)$$

The pK^1 of this system (6.1) is still low relative to the pH of the blood (7.4), but the system is one of the most effective buffer systems in the body because the amount of dissolved CO_2 is controlled by respiration, and plasma concentration of HCO_3^- is regulated by the kidney. Therefore, pH of ECF can be precisely controlled.

2. Phosphate buffer system

Inorganic orthophosphate buffer system

Inorganic orthophosphate buffer system is formed by sodium dihydrogen phosphate and disodium hydrogen phosphate ($NaH_2PO_4 \sim Na_3HPO_4$), which exist at a plasma pH of 7.4 in a concentration ratio of 1:4.

Sites of operation of $NaH_2PO_4 – Na_2HPO_4$ buffer

1. In ECF (plasma and interstitial fluid), the HPO_4^{2-} / $H_2PO_4^-$ buffer exists in small concentration (0.66 mmol/L) and thus contributes little to the buffering capacity of plasma.

2. In intracellular fluid (ICF), the HPO_4^{2-} / $H_2PO_4^-$ forms an important buffer pair because:

- Its concentration in ICF is high (6 mmol/L), and
- Its pK (6.8) is much closer to pH of ICF (6.9).

3. In renal tubules, the HPO_4^{2-} / $H_2PO_4^-$ forms an effective extracellular buffer because:

- Phosphate becomes greatly concentrated in the tubular fluid due to reabsorption of H_2O, and
- pH of tubular fluid and urine is more acidic than the pH of ECF, i.e. it is close to pK of phosphate buffer.

The HPO_4^{2-} / $H_2PO_4^-$ system is a major elimination route for H^+ via the urine (see page 321).

Organic phosphate buffer system

Organic phosphates such as AMP, ADP, ATP and 2,3-diphosphoglycerate (2,3-DPG) exist in quantitatively significant amount in ICF (8.4 mmol/L), giving this compartment the capacity to effectively buffer both non-carbonic and carbonic acid, as well as alkali.

3. Protein buffer system

The protein buffer system of the blood is constituted by the plasma proteins and haemoglobin combinedly.

Plasma proteins buffer system

Plasma proteins buffer system accounts for 15% of the buffering capacity of the whole blood. Plasma proteins are effective buffers because both their free carboxyl and free amino groups dissociate:

$$RCOOH \rightleftharpoons RCOO^- + H^+;$$

$$pH = pK^1 RCOOH + \log \frac{[RCOO^-]}{[RCOOH]};$$

$$RNH_3^+ \rightleftharpoons RNH_2^+ + H^+;$$

$$pH = pK^1 RNH_3 + \log (RNH_2) / (RNH_3)$$

Because of their amphoteric nature plasma proteins can combine with acids and bases as:

- *In acidic pH*, the NH_2 group of the proteins acts as base and accept proton and is converted to NH_3.
- *In alkaline pH*, the –COOH group of the proteins acts as acid and can donate a proton and thus becomes COO^-.
- *At normal pH* of blood, proteins act as acids and combine with cations (mainly sodium).

Haemoglobin buffer system

Haemoglobin buffer system (Hb / HHb and HbO_2^-/$HHbO_2$) account for 35% of the total buffering capacity of the whole blood. It mainly buffers the fixed acids, besides being involved in the transport of gases (O_2 and CO_2).

Deoxyhaemoglobin (Hb) is better buffer than oxyhaemoglobin (HbO_2), because the imidazole groups of Hb dissociate less than those of HbO_2, making Hb a weaker acid.

II. RESPIRATORY MECHANISM FOR pH REGULATION

Second line of defence against acid-base disorders is formed by the respiratory mechanism, which provides a short-term but rapid control. It acts via respiratory centre, located in the medulla to regulate removal of CO_2 and therefore carbonic acid (H_2CO_3) concentration in the blood.

Role of respiratory centres

Respiratory centres are influenced by both CO_2 as well as H^+ concentration through central and peripheral chemoreceptors.

Respiratory response occurs in response to metabolic acid-base disorders only and consists of:

1. *Hyperventilation*. It occurs in response to metabolic acidosis and results in lowering of pCO_2 to match the decreased HCO_3^-.

2. *Hypoventilation* occurs in response to metabolic alkalosis and results in raising the pCO_2 to match the increased HCO_3^-.

III. RENAL MECHANISM FOR pH REGULATION

The kidneys regulate pH through three main processes (see page 320):

ACID-BASE DISORDERS

Acidosis refers to decline in blood pH, while *alkalosis* refers to rise in blood pH. As described above, our body has been provided with an efficient system for the maintenance of acid-base equilibrium with a result that the pH of blood is almost constant (7.4). The blood pH compatible to life is 6.8-7.8, beyond which life cannot exist.

SIMPLE ACID-BASE DISORDERS

The physiological aspects of simple acid-base disorders are summarized in Table 9.3-2 and described:

Metabolic acidosis

Physiological disturbance that produces metabolic acidosis is either increased net non-volatile acid load or loss of base (HCO_3^-).

Primary disturbance in metabolic acidosis is *decreased plasma HCO_3^-* producing a *low plasma pH*.

Causes of metabolic acidosis include:

- Diabetic ketoacidosis.
- Lactic acidosis in hypoxia.
- Diarrhoea (GI loss of HCO_3^-).
- Chronic renal failure (failure to excrete H^+ as titrable acid and NH_4).

Compensatory mechanisms

When metabolic acidosis is produced by non-renal factors, the respiratory and renal compensatory mechanisms tend to minimize the change in pH of blood. In renal failure, only respiratory compensation is possible.

1. *Respiratory compensation*. Increased H^+ stimulates the respiratory centre through peripheral chemoreceptors and produces *hyperventilation* (*Kussmaul breathing*) which in turn decreases the arterial pCO_2 value and minimizes the degree of acidosis.

2. *Renal compensation* is slow, but an effective, it consists of:

- *Increased excretion of fixed H^+ as titrable acid and NH_4.*
- *Increased reabsorption of 'new' HCO_3^-*, which replenishes the HCO_3^- used in buffering the added fixed H^+.
- *In chronic metabolic acidosis*, an adaptive increase in NH_3 synthesis helps in the excretion of excess H^+.

Metabolic alkalosis

Physiological disturbance that produces metabolic alkalosis is either addition of non-volatile alkali or loss of H^+ from the body.

Primary disturbance in metabolic alkalosis is *increased plasma HCO_3^-* producing a high plasma pH.

Causes of metabolic alkalosis include:

Table 9.3-2. Summary of characteristics of simple acid-base disorders

Disorder	Primary disturbance (approximate values)	Arterial plasma			Defence mechanism		
		pH (Normal 7.4)	HCO_3^- (mEq/L) (Normal 24)	pCO_2 (mmHg) (Normal 40)	Buffering	Respiratory compensation	Renal compensation
Metabolic acidosis	↓Plasma HCO_3^-	↓ (7.28)	↓ (18)	→ (40)	ECF & ICF	Hyperventilation (↓pCO_2)	↑H^+ excretion ↑New HCO_3^- reabsorption
Metabolic alkalosis	↑Plasma HCO_3^-	↑ (7.5)	↑ (30)	→ (40)	ECF & ICF	Hypoventilation (↑pCO_2)	↓H^+ excretion ↓New HCO_3^- reabsorption
Respiratory acidosis	↑pCO_2	↓ (7.34)	↑ (25)	↑ (48)	ICF	None	↑H^+ excretion ↑New HCO_3^- reabsorption
Respiratory alkalosis	↓pCO_2	↑ (7.53)	↓ (22)	↓ (27)	ICF	None	↓H^+ excretion ↓New HCO_3^- reabsorption

ICF : Intracellular fluid; ECF: extracellular fluid; ↑ increased; ↓ decreased; and → normal

- Haemorrhage,
- Vomiting (H^+ is lost from the stomach), and
- Hyperaldosteronism (increased H^+ secretion by distal tubule).

Compensatory mechanisms

1. **Respiratory compensation**. Increased pH (or decreased H^+) inhibits the respiratory centre through peripheral chemoreceptors and produces *hypoventilation* which in turn elevates pCO_2 and thus normalizes plasma pH.

Note. It is important to note that the magnitude of respiratory compensation is limited by the fact that hypoventilation results in decreased arterial pO_2 which stimulates the respiratory centres via peripheral chemo-receptors.

2. **Renal compensation** for metabolic alkalosis consists of:

- *Decreased H^+ secretion* by the renal tubules, and
- *Increased HCO_3^- excretion*, as the filtered load of HCO_3^- exceeds the ability of renal tubule to reabsorb it. The urinary loss of HCO_3^- decreases the plasma level of HCO_3^- thereby restoring the pH of blood to near normal.

Respiratory acidosis

Primary disturbance in respiratory acidosis is *increased pCO_2*, which by mass action causes an increase in H^+ and thus lowers the blood pH.

Causes. The pCO_2 is increased due to decreased gas exchange across the alveoli because of following causes:

1. *Inadequate ventilation* (Airway obstruction).
2. *Impaired gas diffusion*.

Compensatory mechanism

Note. There is no respiratory compensation for respiratory acidosis only renel composition is there.

Respiratory alkalosis

Primary disturbance in respiratory alkalosis is decreased pCO_2 associated with low H^+ and thus an elevated plasma pH.

Causes. The pCO_2 is decreased due to increased gas exchange in the lungs because of increased ventilation.

Compensatory mechanisms

Note. There is no respiratory compensation for respiratory alkalosis.

Renal compensation. Decreased pCO_2 causes a deficit of H^+ in the renal cells for secretion which leads to:

- Decreased excretion of H^+ as titrable acid and NH_4^+,
- Decreased reabsorption of new HCO_3^-, and
- Decreased reabsorption of the filtered HCO_3^-.

The resulting decrease in serum HCO_3^- helps to normalize the pH. In this way the alkalosis is mostly, but not completely, compensated by the renal mechanism.

Endocrine Systems

Organization and General Principles of Endocrinal System

10.1

ORGANIZATION OF ENDOCRINAL SYSTEM

The biological functions of the multicellular living organisms are very well coordinated. This coordination is achieved by two main control systems—nervous system and the endocrinal system. Nervous system is principally related with functions of the body in external and internal environment. The nervous system co-ordinates the body functions through transmission of impulses via nerve fibres. Endocrinal system is mainly concerned with different metabolic functions of the body especially the chemical reactions and transport of various substances. The endocrinal functions are accomplished through a wide range of chemical messengers, the hormones.

The endocrinal system consists of various endocrine glands and neurosecretory cells located in the hypothalamus. The various endocrine glands present in the body (Fig. 10.1-1) are :

1. *Pituitary gland (hypophysis).* Pituitary gland is also known as hypophysis which in Greek means undergrowth of the brain. It has two main parts: adenohypophysis and neurohypophysis. *Adenohypophysis* secretes growth hormone (GH) or somatotropins, follicle-stimulating hormone (FSH), luteinizing hormone (LH), prolactin, thyrotropin or thyroid-stimulating hormone (TSH), and corticotropin or adrenocorticotropic hormone (ACTH). The *neurohypophysis* stores the antidiuretic hormone (ADH) or vasopressin and oxytocin synthesised by the hypothalamus.

2. *Thyroid gland.* The thyroid gland is present in the neck in front of trachea. It secretes thyroxine (T_4) and triiodothyronine (T_3). The C cells or parafollicular cells secrete calcitonin.

3. *Parathyroid glands.* These are four in number, very small glands situated behind the lobes of the thyroid gland and secrete parathormone.

4. *Adrenal glands.* These are situated on the upper poles of the two kidneys, hence also called suprarenal glands. The outer cortex region of the adrenal glands secretes cortisol, aldosterone and sex steroids and the inner medullary region secretes catecholamines (adrenaline and noradrenaline).

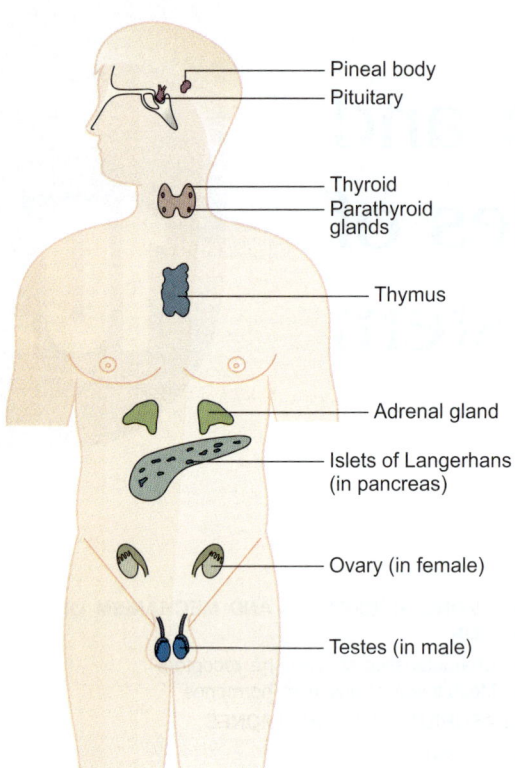

Fig. 10.1-1. *Positions of the endocrine glands in the body.*

Labels in figure: Pineal body; Pituitary; Thyroid; Parathyroid glands; Thymus; Adrenal gland; Islets of Langerhans (in pancreas); Ovary (in female); Testes (in male)

5. *Pancreatic islets (islets of Langerhans).* These are small groups of cells, which secrete insulin, glucagon and somatostatin.

6. *Gonads.* These include ovaries in females and testes in males. The ovaries secrete oestrogens and progesterone (female sex steroids) and testes secrete male sex hormone (testosterone).

7. *Pineal gland.* It is a small gland present in the roof of third ventricle in the brain. It secretes melatonin and other biogenic amines.

8. *Placenta.* During pregnancy placenta secretes various hormones like human chorionic gonadotropin (HCG), oestrogen, progesterone, somatotropins and relaxin.

9. *Gastrointestinal mucosa* also secretes various hormones collectively known as gastrointestinal (GIT) hormones, e.g. gastrin, secretin, cholecystokinin-pancreozymin (CCK-PZ), etc.

10. *Kidneys.* In addition to their renal functions, the kidneys secrete erythropoietin, prostaglandins and 1,25-dihydroxycholecalciferol, and also help in activation of angiotensin production.

11. *Atrial muscle cells.* These secrete atrial natriuretic peptides (ANP) and many other peptides.

12. *Skin.* This is also considered to act as an endocrine structure by producing vitamin D, which is now considered to be a hormone.

HORMONES : GENERAL CONSIDERATIONS

DEFINITION

The word hormone is derived from the Greek word *hormon* which means to execute or to arouse. In the classic definition hormones are secretory products of the ductless glands which are released in catalytic amounts into blood stream and transported to specific target cells (or organs), where they elicit physiologic, morphologic and biochemical responses.

HORMONE TRANSPORT, PLASMA CONCENTRATION AND HALF-LIFE

Hormone transport

After secretion into blood stream, the hormones may circulate in two forms:

Unbound form. Some hormones circulate as free molecule, e.g. catecholamines and most peptide and protein hormones circulate unbound.

Bound form. Some hormones, such as steroids, thyroid hormones, and vitamin D circulate bound to specific globulins that are synthesized in the liver. The binding of hormones to proteins is advantageous as it:

- Protects the hormone against clearance by the kidney,
- Slows down the rate of degradation by the liver, and
- Provides circulating reserve of the hormone.

Plasma concentration and half-time

Hormones are usually secreted into the circulation in extremely low concentrations.

Half-life

Most hormones are metabolized rapidly after secretion. In general:

- Peptide hormones have short half-life,
- Steroids and thyroid hormones have significantly longer half-life because they are bound to plasma proteins.

FUNCTIONS OF HORMONES

Hormones regulate existing fundamental processes but do not initiate reactions de novo.

1. *Regulation of biochemical reactions.* Hormones regulate the metabolic functions in a variety of ways:

- They stimulate or inhibit the rate and magnitude of biochemical reactions by controlling enzymes and thereby cause morphologic, biochemical, and functional changes in target tissues.
- They modulate energy producing processes and regulate the circulating levels of energy-yielding substances (e.g. glucose, fatty acids). However, they are not used as energy sources in biochemical reactions.

2. Regulation of bodily processes. Hormones regulate different bodily processes such as growth, maturation, differentiation, regeneration, reproduction and behaviour.

Thus, main function of endocrine glands is to maintain homeostasis in internal environment.

REGULATION OF HORMONE SECRETION

The quantity of hormones secreted is regulated in accordance with their requirement. General mechanisms that govern the secretion of hormones include:

- Feedback control,
- Neural control, and
- Chronotropic control.

1. Feedback control

Feedback control is of two types:

- Negative feedback control, and
- Positive feedback control.

Negative feedback control. Generally the influence of blood concentration of the hormone concerned or its effect is to inhibit further secretion of the hormone and is called negative feedback control (Fig. 10.1-2A).

Positive feedback control, which is less common, acts to amplify the initial biological effects of the hormone (Fig. 10.1-2B).

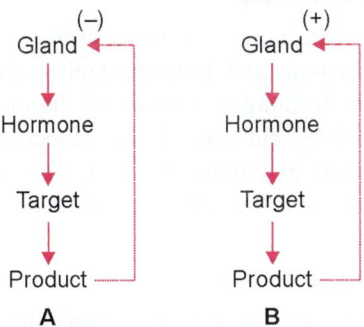

Fig. 10.1-2. *Hormonal regulation by feedback control mechanism: A, negative feedback; and B, positive feedback.*

2. Neural control

Neural control acts to evoke or suppress hormone secretion in response to both external and internal stimuli.

External stimuli which can modulate hormone release through neural mechanisms may be visual, auditory, olfactory, gustatory and tactile.

Internal stimuli which influence hormonal release through neural mechanism include pain, emotion, sexual excitement, fright, stress and changes in blood volume.

3. Chronotropic control

Chronotropic control of hormone secretion accounts for:

- Oscillating and pulsatile release of certain hormones,
- Diurnal variation in hormonal levels,
- Menstrual rhythm,
- Seasonal rhythm, and
- Developmental rhythm.

The source of regular oscillatory cycles is a pulse generator(s) located in the suprachiasmatic nucleus (SCN) of the hypothalamus (Fig. 10.1-3).

The intrinsic circadian clock is also located in the SCN, which is responsible for endocrinal, metabolic and behavioural coordinated rhythms.

Fig. 10.1-3. *The origin of circadian rhythms in endocrine gland secretion, metabolic process and behavioral activity.*

HORMONE: RECEPTORS AND MECHANISM OF ACTION

Characteristics of hormone receptors

All hormones act through specific receptors. Almost all hormone receptors are large proteins present in hormone sensitive target cells.

Receptor specificity. There are specific receptors for each hormone. This is the reason that all hormones circulate to all parts of the body, yet each hormone has specific target tissue for its action (Fig. 10.1-4).

Mechanism of action of hormones

The main mechanisms of hormone actions are:

- Action through change in membrane permeability,
- Action through effect on gene expression by binding of hormones with intracellular receptors,

Fig. 10.1-4. *Specificity of hormone action is because of specific receptors.*

- Action through secondary messengers which activate intracellular enzymes when hormones combine with membrane receptors, and
- Action through tyrosin kinase activation.

MEASUREMENT OF HORMONES

Measurement of blood level of hormones is essential to confirm the endocrinal disorders associated with either deficiency or excess of a hormone. Since the hormones exist in the blood in very low concentration, the conventional methods of estimation such as colorimetry are not of much use. Therefore, they are measured by hormone assays and some special techniques which include:

1. Bioassay

In this method hormone levels were assessed by injecting the unknown sample of plasma in experimental animals and observing quantitatively the specific biological effect. The effect chosen was a characteristic action of the hormone for which a clear dose-response relationship existed.

2. Immunoassay

The immunoassay methods, frequently employed for estimation of hormone levels, include:

- Radioimmunoassay (RIA), and
- Enzyme-linked immunosorbent assay (ELISA).

i. *Radioimmunoassay.* The radioimmunoassay is performed as:

- An unknown sample of plasma in which the concentration of a particular hormone (H) to be estimated is mixed with commercially available purified specific antibody (anti-H) and an appropriate amount of the purified hormone tagged with radioactive isotope (H+). The mixture is incubated in the cold.
- The antibodies have high affinity for the hormone. There occurs a competition between the free hormone (H) present in the unknown sample of plasma and the tagged hormone (H+) for binding to the specific antibody (anti-H).

ii. *Enzyme-linked immunosorbent method.* Enzyme-linked immunosorbent (ELISA) method is principally similar to RIA, i.e. it is also based on the principle of antigen-antibody reaction. Any antigen that is protein can be measured by this technique. In this method, radioactivity is not measured, instead specific antibody hormone (antigen) complex is stained with suitable dye, and the intensity of colour is measured by spectrophotometer. This technique is useful in estimating peptide and steroid hormones.

3. Cytochemical assay

This test is much more sensitive than the immunoassay, but is cumbersome and time-consuming and so rarely used. In this technique, genesis of hormone can be detected in slices cut out of the endocrine gland by incubating them in culture medium. This test is very useful in measuring the minute basal levels of hormone secretion.

4. Dynamic tests

Dynamic tests are needed in certain situations when simple blood hormone level estimation is not enough. Two types of dynamic tests are:

i. *Suppression type of dynamic tests* are useful in certain conditions, e.g. to know whether a lung cancer is secreting ACTH.

ii. *Stimulation type of dynamic tests* are useful in certain other conditions, e.g. metyrapone test is performed to know whether the corticotrophs of the pituitary (which secrete ACTH) are normally functioning or not.

Hypothalamus and Pituitary Gland

10.2

INTRODUCTION AND FUNCTIONAL ANATOMY

The hypothalamic-pituitary unit forms a unique component of the entire endocrine system that regulates growth, lactation, fluid homeostasis, and the functions of thyroid gland, adrenal glands, and gonads.

GROSS ANATOMY AND DEVELOPMENT OF PITUITARY GLAND

Pituitary gland, also called hypophysis cerebri, is a small gland, weighs about 0.5 gm and is approximately 1 cm in diameter. It is situated in the hypophyseal fossa (sella turcica) of the sphenoid bone.

Physiologically, the pituitary gland consists of three distinct parts or lobes (Fig. 10.2-1):

- Anterior lobe or adenohypophysis,
- Posterior lobe or neurohypophysis, and
- Intermediate lobe or pars intermedia.

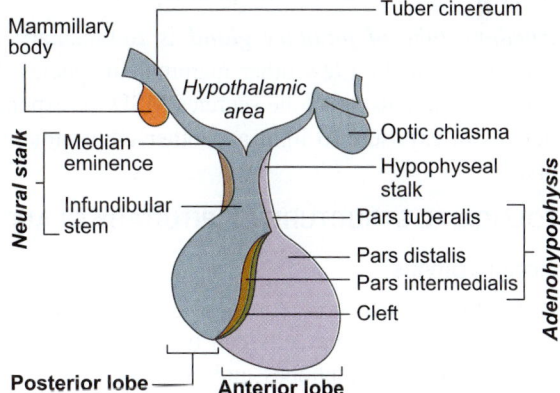

Fig. 10.2-1. *Anatomical subdivisions of pituitary gland.*

Development of pituitary gland

Anterior pituitary is ectodermal in origin. It develops from *Rathke's pouch* which is an embryonic upward outpouching from the roof of the primitive oral cavity.

Posterior pituitary or neurohypophysis develops from a lowered outpouching of neuroectodermal tissue from the central areas of hypothalamus (tuber cinereum and median eminence).

From the above, it is quite clear that the anterior and posterior pituitary develop independently from widely different origins, and it is only a coincidence that when fully formed, they happen to lie so close together that they are considered parts of the same organ.

Parts of pituitary gland

Adenohypophysis. The glandular anterior lobe of pituitary gland is called adenohypophysis. It constitutes about 80% of the pituitary gland. It can be further divided into three parts (Fig. 10.2-1):
- *Pars distalis*
- *Pars intermedia*
- *Pars tuberalis*

Neurohypophysis. The posterior lobe of pituitary is a neural structure and hence called neurohypophysis. It consists of three parts (Fig. 10.2-1):
- *Pars posterior.*
- *Infundibular stem.*
- *Median eminence.*

Pituitary stalk. The median eminence and infundibulum constitute the neural stalk. The posterior pituitary maintains its neural connection with hypothalamus by this neural stalk. The neural stalk surrounded by pars tuberalis of adenohypophysis constitutes the pituitary stalk.

Intermediate lobe of pituitary gland is rudimentary in humans as well as in a few other mammalian species. In certain lower animals, this lobe secretes MSH in response to changes in exposure to light and other environmental factors.

HISTOLOGICAL STRUCTURE OF PITUITARY GLAND

Adenohypophysis

Pars Distalis consists of cords of cells separated by fenestrated sinusoids. The cells can be divided into two main types: the chromophobes and chromophils.

1. Chromophobes. These are agranular cells and it is considered that the chromophils are derived from the chromophobes.

2. Chromophils. These are granular cells, constitute 50% of the cells of anterior pituitary. Chromophils are further classified as: acidophils (35%), and basophils (15%).

i. *Acidophilic cells (α cells).* The granules of these cells are acidophilic.

ii. *Basophilic cells (β cells).* The granules of these cells and basophilic.

3. Folliculostellate cells. These cells send processes between the secretory cells. Recently it has been demonstrated that these contain and secrete the cytokine 1L-6, but their physiological role is still not clear.

Pars Tuberalis. It mainly consists of undifferentiated cells with few acidophils and basophils.

Pars Intermedia. It contains β cells, few secretory cells and chromophobe cells.

Neurohypophysis

Histologically posterior pituitary contains following structures;

1. Unmyelinated nerve fibres. These are the axons of the neurons located in the supraoptic and paraventricular nuclei of hypothalamus. These carry precursor of posterior pituitary hormones and end as close terminals near the blood capillaries (Fig. 10.2-2).

2. Pituicytes are the special type of supporting cells, having long dendritic processes. These are present in between the axons.

3. Glial cells like astrocytes and oligodendrocytes are also seen.

BLOOD SUPPLY OF PITUITARY GLAND

Arterial supply

The arterial blood to the pituitary gland is supplied by the branches of:
- Internal carotid arteries (superior and inferior hypophyseal branches),
- Anterior cerebral artery, and
- Posterior cerebral artery.

Hypothalamohypophyseal portal system (Figs. 10.2-2 and 10.2-3).

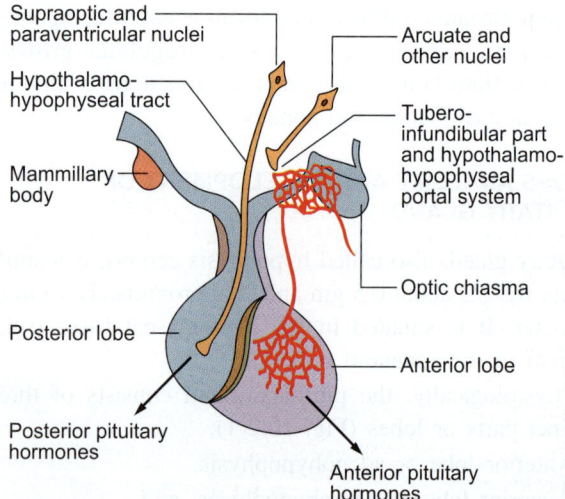

Fig. 10.2-2. *Anatomical and functional relationship between hypothalamus and pituitary gland through hypothalamo-hypophyseal tract and hypothalamohypophyseal portal system.*

Fig. 10.2-3. *Schematic diagram to explain anatomical and functional relationship between hypothalamus and pituitary gland.*

- The branches from superior hypophyseal artery form a ring around the upper part of the pituitary stalk and further branched to form a *capillary network*.

- The blood from this capillary network is drained by *long portal veins* in the infundibulum.

- Then in the anterior lobe, these long portal veins break up into another set of capillary network and represented as *sinusoids of pars anterior*. This arrangement is called *hypothalamo-hypophyseal portal system*.

- The inferior hypophyseal (branch of internal carotid artery) branches to form a capillary network at the lower end of infundibulum stem.

- The short portal vessels arise from this capillary network and supply blood mainly to posterior pituitary and some part of anterior pituitary.

- The short portal vessels provide link between the anterior and posterior pituitary.

Venous drainage

The blood from anterior pituitary is drained to cavernous sinus and then into jugular vein.

Note : The anterior pituitary lies outside the blood-brain barrier, hence it is accessible to influences from general circulation (hormones and neurotransmitter by the brain and hormones secreted in the general circulation).

HYPOTHALAMIC-PITUITARY RELATIONSHIP

The influences from the hypothalamus are conveyed to pituitary gland by two different tracts:

1. *Hypothalamo-hypophyseal tract.* It is composed of axons of the large neurosecretory cells of the supraoptic and paraventricular nuclei of hypothalamus. These fibres pass to neurohypophysis through the infundibular stem and form a series of dilated terminals known as Herring bodies (Fig. 10.2-2). The neurosecretory cells of supraoptic and paraventricular nuclei secrete peptide hormones (vasopressin and oxytocin), which travel down their axons in neurosecretory granules to be stored in the nerve terminals lying the neurohypophysis. Upon stimulation of the cell bodies, the granules are released from the axonal terminals by exocytosis.

2. *Tubero-infundibular tract and hypothalamo-hypophyseal portal system.* It consists of fibres arising from the arcuate nuclei of the tuberal region of the hypothalamus, and extend to the median eminence (Fig. 10.2-2). The cell bodies of these hypothalamic neurons synthesize certain releasing and inhibiting hormones which are conveyed by the tubero-infundibular tract to the median eminence region where they are stored in the nerve terminals. When hypothalamic neurons are stimulated by nerve impulses, the releasing or inhibiting hormones are discharged into the median eminence and enter the capillary plexus of superior hypophyseal artery. From here they are transported down the portal vessels (long portal veins) and then exit from the secondary capillary plexus to reach the specific endocrine target cells in the adenohypophysis where they regulate the secretion of tropic hormones of anterior pituitary (Fig. 10.2-3).

ENDOCRINAL ASPECTS OF HYPOTHALAMUS

FUNCTIONAL ANATOMY

Hypothalamus is a specialized centre in the brain that functions as a master coordinator of hormonal action. It is a part of the brain situated below the thalamus and is very closely connected to pituitary gland as described above. Thus hypothalamus provides an important link between the endocrine system and the nervous system. Before proceeding further see details of functional anatomy of hypothalamus at page 437.

ENDOCRINAL FUNCTIONS OF HYPOTHALAMUS

The hypothalamus serves its endocrinal functions through the neurosecretory cells which are arranged in different nuclei of hypothalamus.

The main endocrinal functions of hypothalamus are:

1. Control of anterior pituitary function

Hypothalamus controls the functioning of anterior pituitary through various hypothalamic-hypophysiotropic hormones, i.e. various hypothalamic-releasing and -inhibiting hormones. The hypothalamic-releasing and -inhibiting hormones are released in response to neural stimuli.

Various hypothalamic-releasing and -inhibiting hormones include:

- Growth hormone releasing hormone (GHRH),
- Growth hormone inhibiting hormone (GRIH), also called somatostatin,
- Corticotropin releasing hormone (CRH),
- Thyrotropin releasing hormone (TRH),
- Gonadotropin releasing hormone (GnRH),
- Prolactin releasing hormone (PRH), and
- Prolactin inhibiting hormone (PIH).

Functions of hypothalamic-releasing and -inhibiting hormones. In general they control the release of various tropic hormones from anterior pituitary. However, now it has known that besides regulating the secretion of specific tropic hormone, a hypothalamic hormone may also influence the secretion of another anterior pituitary hormone. For example:

- TRH, besides promoting secretion of TSH, also stimulates the secretion of prolactin.
- Somatostatin, discovered as a growth hormone inhibiting hormone (GHIH), also inhibits the secretion of TSH.
- Growth hormone releasing hormone (GHRH) also stimulates the secretion of ACTH and prolactin.
- GnRH promotes the release of both LH and FSH.

2. Control of posterior pituitary function

The large (magnocellular) neurosecretory cells forming the supraoptic and paraventricular nuclei of hypothalamus are responsible for synthesis of the two posterior pituitary peptide hormones (oxytocin and ADH). These hormones reach the posterior pituitary through hypothalamic-hypophyseal tract described above (Figs. 10.2-2 and 10.2-3).

ANTERIOR PITUITARY HORMONES

The hormones of adenohypophysis are broadly classified into three categories:

I. *Hormones of growth hormone family* include :

- Growth hormone (GH), and
- Prolactin (PRL)

II. *Glycoprotein hormone family.* The hormones of glycoprotein family secreted by anterior pituitary include:

- Thyroid stimulating hormone (TSH),
- Luteinizing hormone (LH), and
- Follicular stimulating hormone (FSH).

III. *Pro-opiomelanocortin peptides (POMC).* The hormones of this group are:

- Adrenocorticotropic hormone (ACTH),
- Melanocyte stimulating hormone (MSH), α-MSH and β-MSH are produced in the intermediary lobe (which is rudimentary in humans),
- β-lipotropin, and
- β-endorphin.

Physiological aspects of growth hormone are discussed in detail in this chapter. Other hormones are discussed in different chapters e.g. TSH with thyroid hormone, (see page 351) and ACTH with adrenal gland and prolactin in reproductive system (see page 409).

GROWTH HORMONE

Growth hormone (GH), also called *somatotropin*, is the most important hormone for postnatal growth and development to adult size. It also helps to maintain lean body mass and bone mass in adults.

STRUCTURE, SYNTHESIS, SECRETION, PLASMA LEVEL AND METABOLISM

Structure. GH consists of a single unbranched chain containing 191 amino acids. Its molecular weight is 2000.

Synthesis. GH is synthesized by acidophilic cells called *somatotrophs* of anterior pituitary.

Plasma levels. The basal plasma GH level varies from 2-4 ng/ml.

Secretion. GH is released in *pulsatile* fashion.

- *Secretion is increased* by sleep, stress, hormones related to puberty, starvation, exercise, and hypoglycaemia.
- *Secretion of GH is decreased* by somatostatin, somatomedins, obesity, hyperglycaemia, and pregnancy.

Circulation. Circulating GH is bound to a plasma protein (GH binding protein).

Metabolism. Growth hormone is rapidly metabolized, probably at least in part, in the liver. Metabolic clearance and daily urinary GH excretion correlates well with the integrated 24-hour plasma GH profile.

REGULATION OF GH SECRETION

1. Hypothalamic control

Hypothalamus controls GH secretion by releasing two hormones, growth hormone releasing hormone (GHRH) and growth hormone release inhibiting hormone (GRIH) (Fig. 10.2-4).

Growth hormone releasing hormone (GHRH). It stimulates the secretion of GH from the anterior pituitary.

Growth hormone release inhibiting hormone (GRIH), also called somatostatin, is a polypeptide. It inhibits the release of GH from the anterior pituitary.

2. Negative feedback control of GH secretion

The negative feedback control mechanism for GH involves the role of somatomedins, GH and GHRH (Fig. 10.2-4).

i. *Negative feedback control by somatomedins.* Somatomedins are insulin-like growth factor (IGF) that are produced when growth hormone acts on target tissues. Somatomedins inhibit the secretion of GH directly or by stimulating the secretion of somatostatin from the hypothalamus.

ii. *Negative feedback control by GH.* Growth hormone also inhibits its own secretion by stimulating the secretion of somatostatin from the hypothalamus.

Fig. 10.2-4. *Control of growth hormone secretion. GHRH (growth hormone releasing hormone), and GRIH (growth hormone release inhibiting hormone).*

iii. *Negative feedback control by GHRH.* GHRH inhibits its own secretion from the hypothalamus. This mechanism is called *ultrashort feedback loop.*

ACTIONS OF GROWTH HORMONE

Growth hormone promotes growth and also influences the normal metabolism, therefore, besides acting on one specific organ, its actions are generalized.

1. Growth promoting actions of GH

Growth hormone promotes linear growth of an individual by its effects on the bone, cartilage and other connective tissues.

Effects on cartilage. GH stimulates the proliferation of chondrocytes (cartilage cells) present in the epiphyseal end plates of long bones.

Effects on bone. GH stimulates osteoblastic activity which converts cartilage into bone. This process continues upto adolescence till there is fusion of epiphyseal end plate with shaft of the bone. The bone mass also increases during this period.

2. Metabolic actions of GH

i. *Effects on protein metabolism.* Growth hormone has an

anabolic effect on protein metabolism. It promotes the protein deposition in the tissues by following effects:
- Increases the rate of amino acid uptake into the cells.
- Increases protein synthesis in ribosomes.
- Stimulates transcription (RNA synthesis from DNA).

ii. *Effects on fat metabolism.* GH promotes lipolysis in adipose tissue (catabolic effect) and then increases fat utilization for energy.

iii. *Effects on carbohydrate metabolism.* GH is antagonistic to insulin and produces hyperglycaemia by following effects:
- Decreases the uptake as well as utilization of glucose by the tissues for energy production, and
- Inhibits glycolysis and thus glycogen stores tend to increase.

iv. *Effects on mineral metabolism*. Growth hormone promotes bone mineralization in growing children.

APPLIED ASPECTS: ABNORMALITIES OF ANTERIOR PITUITARY HORMONES

The abnormalities related to pituitary hormones occur either due to excess or deficiency of the hormones secreted. The most common causes of pituitary hormone disturbances are pituitary tumours which may cause symptoms of excess of one or more hormones and simultaneous deficiency of other hormones, hence a mixed picture may evolve. The various hormones of pituitary, their site of action and diseases produced by them are given in Table 10.2-1.

Pituitary disorders seen in clinical practice are:
- Hypopituitarism,
- Abnormalities of growth hormone,
- Prolactin deficiency, and
- Cushing's syndrome (see page 367).

HYPOPITUITARISM

Hypopituitarism is a clinical condition of hyposecretion of one or more pituitary hormones. Hypopituitarism can be due to hypothalamic causes or pituitary causes. Since anterior pituitary has a large reserve, the endocrine abnormalities are produced only when large part of pituitary is destroyed.

ABNORMALITIES OF GROWTH HORMONE SECRETION

The abnormalities of growth hormone secretion include:
- Hypersecretion of GH, and
- Hyposecretion of GH.

Hypersecretion of GH

Hypersecretion of GH occurs in tumours of acidophilic cells of anterior pituitary. Depending upon the age of an individual, excess of GH may cause:
- Gigantism,
- Acromegaly.

1. Gigantism

It is a clinical condition resulting from hypersecretion of GH in growing children before the closure of epiphysis of long bones. The main feature of gigantism is *abnormal height* (7-8 feet due to excessive growth of long bones) with huge status and the person becomes 'giant' (Fig. 10.2-5).

2. Acromegaly

It is a clinical condition that occurs due to excess of GH in adults (after epiphyseal closure of long bones has occurred) and causes excessive growth in those areas where cartilage persists.

Clinical features are (Fig. 10.2-6) :
- *Acromegalic face*, which is characterized by thick lips, macroglossia, broad and thick nose, prominent eyebrows, thickened skin, and coarse facial features.

Table 10.2-1. Pituitary hormones: site of action and diseases associated with their deficiency and excess.

Hormone	Site of action	Diseases	
		Excess	Deficiency
Anterior pituitary			
Growth hormone (GH)	All somatic cells	Gigantism in adolescents	Dwarfism
Adrenocorticotropic hormone (ACTH)	Adrenal cortex	ACTH-dependent Cushing's syndrome	Hypoadrenalism (rare)
Thyroid stimulating hormone (TSH)	Thyroid	Hyperthyroidism	Hypothyroidism
Prolactin	Breast	Hyperprolactinaemia	—
Gonadotropins	Gonads	Hypergonadism	Hypogonadism
Melanocytic stimulating hormone (MSH)	Skin	Hyperpigmentation	—
Posterior pituitary			
Antidiuretic hormone	Kidneys	—	Diabetes insipidus

Fig. 10.2-5. *Photograph showing tall stature in a patient with gigantism as compared to a man of average size.*

A   B

Fig. 10.2-6. *Clinical features of acromegaly: A, note coarse facial features, broad thick nose, prognathism, prominent eyebrows and thickened skin; and B, large spade-like hand with short thick wide fingers.*

- *Prognathism,* i.e. protrusion of the lower jaw due to elongation and widening of mandible associated with increased spacing of the teeth.
- *Acral part abnormalities* include large spade-like hands, thick wide fingers, large feet with increase in size of the shoes. Height is normal, build is stout and stocky.

- *Kyphosis* may occur due to improper vertebral growth.
- *Excessive growth of internal organs,* i.e. cardiomegaly, hepatomegaly, splenomegaly and renomegaly may be associated.
- *Increased sympathetic activity* may cause increased sweating and hypertension.

Hyposecretion of GH

Deficiency of GH in childhood leads to stunted growth or *dwarfism.*

Deficiency of GH in adulthood results in *mild anaemia* which is refractory to usual treatment with haematinics like iron.

- Reduction in muscle mass, and
- Hypoglycaemia may also occur.

Dwarfism

Short stature may be due to endocrinal or non-endocrinal causes.

Endocrinal causes of dwarfism are:

- Growth hormone deficiency (pituitary dwarf)
- Panhypopituitarism
- Hypothyroid dwarf (see page 355)
- Cushing's syndrome (see page 367).

Non-endocrinal causes of dwarfism include:

- Familial dwarfism
- Achondroplasia
- Nutritional (malnutrition or malabsorption)
- Chromosomal abnormalities, e.g. Turner's syndrome.

Growth hormone related dwarfism (Pituitary dwarfism) occurs due to deficiency of GH in early childhood.

Characteristic features. Deficiency of GH causes retardation of growth in all parts of the body proportionately. Consequently, a pituitary dwarf with a chronological age of 20 years has the body structure like that of a normal child of 7-10 years of age. Thus a pituitary dwarf has following features (Fig. 10.2-7):

- Shortness of stature (dwarf),
- Normal mental activity,
- Plumpness (fatness),
- Immature faces,
- Delicate extremities, and
- Sexual maturity does not occur when associated with gonadotropin deficiency.

POSTERIOR PITUITARY HORMONES

The two important hormones released from posterior pituitary are:

Fig. 10.2-7. *Clinical features of pituitary dwarf.*

- Antidiuretic hormone, and
- Oxytocin (see page 407).

ANTIDIURETIC HORMONE

Antidiuretic hormone (ADH), as the name indicates, prevents diuresis and is chiefly concerned with conservation of body water. Since it also causes vasoconstriction, it is also called vasopressin or more precisely arginine vasopressin (AVP).

STRUCTURE, SYNTHESIS, STORAGE, RELEASE, TRANSPORT AND METABOLISM

Structure. ADH and OTC both are homologous neurohormones, polypeptide in nature.

Synthesis. ADH as well as OTC are synthesized in the cell bodies of magnocellular neurons of both paraventricular and supraoptic nuclei of hypothalamus. The secretory granules containing hormone precursors, known as Herring bodies, are transported down the axons by axoplasmic flow to the nerve endings in the posterior pituitary.

Secretion. ADH and OTC are released when a nerve impulse is transmitted from the cell body in the hypothalamus down the axon, where it depolarizes the neurosecretory vesicles.

Transport. The hormone and other secreted products separately enter the closely adjacent capillary. The hormone

then reaches the target cells and by circulatory interconnections to the anterior pituitary also.

Metabolism. The circulating vasopressin is rapidly inactivated in the liver and kidney.

ACTIONS OF ADH

1. *Action on kidney.* The main role of ADH is regulation of water balance in the body by acting on the distal convoluted tubules and collecting ducts of the renal nephron. ADH increases the permeability of these cells to water.

2. *Vasoconstrictor effect.* ADH in large doses causes vasoconstriction and leads to rise in blood pressure. Haemorrhage is a potent stimulus to ADH secretion (see page 202).

3. *Action on anterior pituitary.* ADH travels to the anterior pituitary via the portal veins and causes increased ACTH secretion.

REGULATION OF ADH SECRETION

The main factors which regulate the ADH secretion are:

1. Effective osmotic pressure of plasma or plasma osmolality

Plasma osmolality in normal individuals is maintained very close to 285 mOsm/L by ADH. Change in plasma osmolality is a very potent regulator of ADH secretion. Thus, water deprivation (which increases plasma osmolality) stimulates ADH secretion. On the other hand, a water load (which decreases plasma osmolality) decreases ADH secretion.

Mechanism of action. Changes in plasma osmolality affect the osmoreceptors.

- *Osmoreceptors* refer to group of neurons located in the anterior hypothalamus.
- The rise in plasma osmolality even by 1-2% results in shrinkage of osmoreceptors causing reflex increase of ADH secretion.

2. Changes in blood volume

Changes in circulating blood volume, central blood volume, cardiac output and blood pressure affect the secretion of ADH.

3. Other factors affecting ADH secretion

Factors, other than the two major stimuli (i.e. hypovolaemia and plasma osmolality), which affect ADH secretion are:
- *Stress* of pain, chronic emotional stress, and surgical procedures cause increase in ADH secretion.
- *Adrenaline* decreases the ADH.

ABNORMALITIES OF ADH SECRETION

Abnormalities of ADH secretion include:

- Syndrome of inappropriate hypersecretion of ADH, and
- Diabetes insipidus.

Syndrome of inappropriate hypersecretion of ADH

Syndrome of inappropriate hypersecretion of antidiuretic hormone (SIADH) refers to a condition in which ADH secretion is increased despite the presence of hypo-osmolality. Excessive ADH secretion leads to water intoxication, i.e. overhydration, and because of this SIADH is also called *dilution syndrome*.

Diabetes insipidus

Diabetes insipidus refers to a clinical condition of polyuria that occurs either due to deficiency of ADH (vasopressin) release or failure of renal response to ADH.

Characteristic features

The diabetes insipidus is characterized by decreased renal absorption of water leading to following features:

1. *Polyuria*, i.e. passage of large amount of urine, upto 3-20 liters, is the most important single feature of diabetes insipidus.

2. *Polydypsia*. Polyuria is followed by obligatory poly-dypsia (drinking of large amount of water). It occurs due to stimulation of thirst mechanism.

3. *Dehydration* may occur in severe cases. Its signs and symptoms include dry tongue and dry mouth. Fall of blood pressure and loss of consciousness may be seen in acute severe cases.

Thyroid Gland, Parathyroid Glands and Thymus

10.3

THYROID GLAND

ANATOMY OF THYROID GLAND

Gross anatomy

Thyroid gland is the largest endocrine gland in the body (weighing about 15-25 gm in adults). It consists of two lobes joined together by a narrow isthmus and is located on either side of trachea just below the larynx at the level of 5th to 7th cervical and 1st thoracic vertebra. The lobes are conical in shape. Each lobe is about 5 cm long and 3 cm wide (Fig. 10.3-1). Structures in relation to thyroid gland are :

- Two parathyroid glands are present on the posterior surface of each lobe.
- Recurrent laryngeal nerve lies close to the lobes.

Blood supply

Arterial blood supply. Superior thyroid artery (a branch of external carotid artery), and inferior thyroid artery (a branch of subclavian artery) supply the blood to the thyroid gland. It receives high blood supply (400-600 ml/ 100 gm/min).

Venous drainage occurs through thyroid veins which ultimately drain the blood into internal jugular vein.

Histological structure

Histologically each *lobe* of thyroid gland is divided into various *lobules* by fibrous tissue septa. Each lobule is made up of an aggregation of several *follicles*. Each follicle is lined by *follicular cells*.

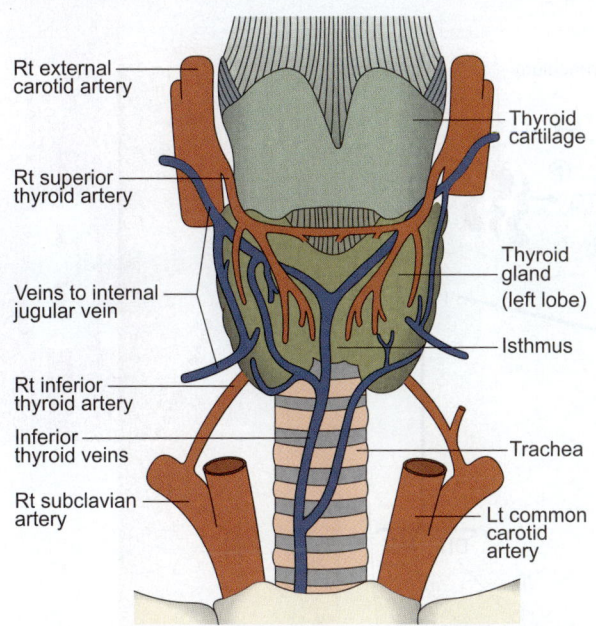

Rt external
carotid artery

Rt superior
thyroid artery

Veins to internal
jugular vein

Rt inferior
thyroid artery

Inferior
thyroid veins

Rt subclavian
artery

Thyroid
cartilage

Thyroid
gland
(left lobe)

Isthmus

Trachea

Lt common
carotid
artery

Fig. 10.3-1. *Location of thyroid gland and its relations.*

Follicular cells. These vary in shape with the degree of glandular activity. Normally (at an average level of activity) the cells are *cuboidal* and the colloid in the follicles is moderate in amount. During high degree of activity the cells become columnar and flat when inactive (Fig. 10.3-2B). These cells secrete thyroid hormones.

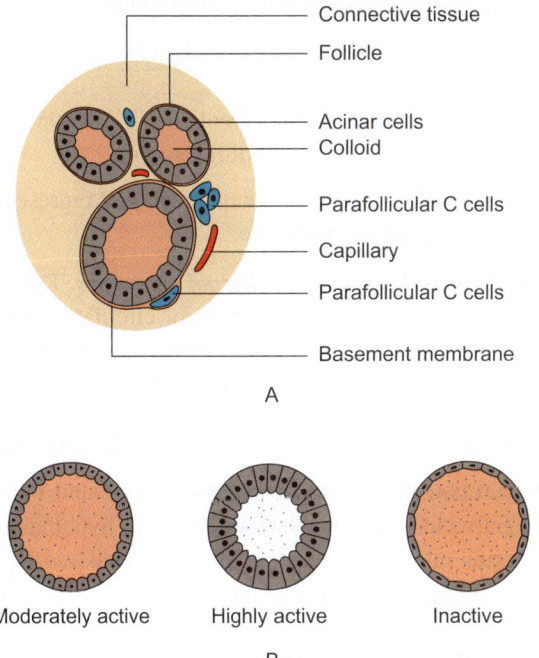

Connective tissue

Follicle

Acinar cells

Colloid

Parafollicular C cells

Capillary

Parafollicular C cells

Basement membrane

A

Moderately active   Highly active   Inactive

B

Fig. 10.3-2. *Histological structure of thyroid gland (A) and variations in follicular cell size with activity (B).*

Parafollicular cells or *C cells* are scattered between follicular cells and basement membrane (Fig. 10.3-2A). and secrete calcitonin.

Colloid. This is a homogeneous material that fills the cavity of each follicle. The major constituent of the colloid is thyroglobulin, a glycoprotein with a molecular weight of 660,000. During active state the follicles are depleted of colloid; and in resting state when unstimulated, the follicles accumulate colloid.

THYROID HORMONES

INTRODUCTION

The two principal thyroid hormones include thyroxine (T_4) and triiodothyronine (T_3).

- *Thyroxine* or T_4 (tetraiodothyronine) constitutes 90% of thyroid output.
- *Triiodothyronine* or T_3 (triiodothyronine) constitutes 10% of thyroid output; however, it is responsible for most of the tissue actions of thyroid hormone.
- *Calcitonin* is a hormone secreted by parafollicular cells of thyroid gland. It is concerned with calcium homeostasis.

BIOSYNTHESIS AND STORAGE OF THYROID HORMONES

Iodine is essential for the synthesis of thyroid hormones. It is ingested in the form of iodides. Sources of iodine are sea fish (richest), bread, milk and vegetables. Iodine is added to the table salt to prevent iodine deficiency.

- Daily average intake of iodine is 500 μg.
- Daily requirement of iodine is 100-200 μg.

Most, 80% (i.e. 400 μg/day), of the iodides absorbed from gastrointestinal tract into the circulation are selectively removed from circulation by cells of thyroid gland. Plasma iodide level is 0.15 to 0.3 μg %.

Thyroxine (T_4) and triiodothyronine (T_3) are synthesized from tyrosine and iodide by the enzyme complex peroxidase. The steps involved in the synthesis of thyroid hormones are (Fig. 10.3-3):

1. Iodine trapping. The first step in the synthesis of thyroid hormones is *uptake of iodide* by the thyroid gland and is called iodine trapping.

2. Synthesis and secretion of thyroglobulin. Thyroglobulin is a large glycoprotein that is synthesized in the thyroid epithelial cells as peptide units. These units move to the apical plasma membrane and release into the lumen of follicle (Fig. 10.3-3).

It is also the storage site of the two hormones within the thyroid gland.

3. Oxidation of iodide. Then iodine is transported into the lumen of the follicles.

Fig. 10.3-3. *Steps in synthesis and release of thyroid hormones: 1, iodine trapping; 2, synthesis of thyroglobulin; 3, oxidation of iodine; 4, organification of thyroglobulin; 5, coupling reaction; 6, storage of thyroid hormone in colloid; 7, take up of colloid by epithelial cell by endocytosis; 8, colloid vesicle; 9, release of T_3 and T_4 after proteolysis; and 10, diffusion of T_3 and T_4 into the capillary.*

Thyroid is the only tissue that can oxidise iodide to iodine. TSH promotes this reaction while antithyroid drugs (thiourea, thiouracil, methimazole) inhibit.

4. *Organification of thyroglobulin* refers to iodination of tyrosine residues present in the thyroglobulin molecule to form monoiodotyrosine (MIT) and diiodotyrosine (DIT).

5. *Coupling reaction*. Two molecules of DIT couple to form thyroxine (T_4). One molecule of MIT, when coupled with one molecule of DIT, produces triiodothyronine (T_3). The enzyme peroxidase is required during coupling.

6. *Storage*. Once thyroglobulin has been iodinated, it is stored in the lumen of the follicle as colloid for several months. It is estimated that the stored thyroid hormones can meet the body requirement for 1-3 months.

TRANSPORT AND METABOLISM OF THYROID HORMONES

Transport of T_4 and T_3. Secreted T_4 and T_3 circulate in the blood stream in two forms : bound and free.

1. *Bound form*. Most of the circulating T_4 (99.95%) and T_3 is bound to specific binding protein.

2. *Free form*. These free, unbound hormones represent the biologically active hormone.

Metabolism and excretion of thyroid hormones. The major pathways of peripheral matabolism of circulating thyroid hormone include deiodination, deamination (decarboxylation), and conjugation with glucuronic acid.

REGULATION OF THYROID HORMONE SECRETION

The secretion of thyroid hormones is regulated by:
- Negative feedback mechanism (through hypothalamus-anterior pituitary-thyroid gland axis), and
- Autoregulation of thyroid gland.

A. Regulation through negative feedback mechanism

The negative feedback mechanism operating through hypothalamus-anterior pituitary-thyroid gland axis (Fig.

10.3-4) plays an essential role in controlling secretion of thyroid hormones by :

Role of thyroid stimulating hormone (TSH). It is a glycoprotein which increases the secretion of thyroid hormones. TSH production is in turn regulated through:

1. *Feedback control by plasma T_4 and T_3.* (Fig. 10.3-4). A fall in T_4 and T_3 levels stimulates TSH secretion from anterior pituitary, while a rise in T_4 and T_3 levels inhibits TSH secretion.

2. *Hypothalamic control of TSH.* Hypothalamus adjusts TSH secretion by secreting thyrotropin-releasing hormone (TRH).

Role of thyrotropin-releasing hormone. Thyrotropin-releasing hormone (TRH) is a tripeptide secreted by arcuate nucleus of hypothalamus and stored in median eminence from where it is released into the hypothalamo-hypophyseal portal vessels to reach the anterior pituitary. TRH acts on the basophils in the anterior pituitary, and controls the release of TSH. Secretion of TRH by hypothalamus is controlled by:

- *Nervous stimuli* like emotion, stress, exposure to cold etc. and also by
- *Negative feedback control* exerted by plasma T_3 and T_4 levels on the hypothalamus (Fig. 10.3-4).

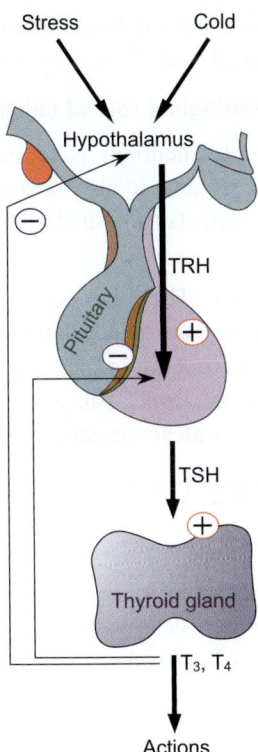

Fig. 10.3-4. *Regulation of thyroid hormone secretion by negative feedback control mechanism through hypothalamus-anterior pituitary-thyroid gland axis.*

B. Autoregulation of thyroid gland

The secretion of thyroid gland is regulated by food iodine contents. If there is deficiency of iodine content in the diet then the *iodine trapping* mechanism of the follicular cells becomes super-efficient and vice versa is also true, i.e. when there is excess of iodine content in the food then iodine trapping becomes less efficient. In this way iodine availability for thyroxine synthesis remains constant and this phenomenon is called autoregulation of thyroid gland.

ACTIONS OF THYROID HORMONE

The thyroid hormones do not have any discrete target organ. They effect cellular activity of almost all the tissues of the body. The biochemical functions attributed to thyroid hormones are summarized:

1. Effects on growth and tissue development

Thyroid hormones are important for normal body growth and development. Some important effects are on:

- Development of nervous tissue,
- Bone development,
- Teeth development,
- Normal cycle of growth and maturation, and
- Subcutaneous tissues.

2. Effect on the metabolic rate in general

The thyroid hormone in general stimulates the metabolic activities and increases the basal rate of oxygen consumption and heat production in most tissues of the body except the brain, retina, gonads, lungs and spleen.

3. Effects on metabolism

i. *Effect on carbohydrate metabolism.* T_4 and T_3 lead on to increased almost all aspects of glucose metabolism, i.e. rapid uptake of glucose by the cells, enhanced glycolysis, enhanced gluconeogenesis, and increased insulin secretion and its effects on carbohydrate metabolism.

ii. *Effect on fat metabolism.* Thyroid hormones cause increase in the levels of fatty acids and a decrease in the quantity of cholesterol, phospholipids and triglycerides in plasma.

iii. *Effect on protein metabolism.* In physiological amounts, the thyroid hormones function as anabolic hormone leading to positive nitrogen balance, and

iv. *Metabolic effects through other hormones.* T_4 and T_3 potentiate the respective stimulatory effects of epinephrine, norepinephrine, glucagon, cortisol and growth hormone on gluconeogenesis, lipolysis, ketogenesis, and proteolysis of the labile protein pool.

v. *Effect on vitamin metabolism.* Thyroid hormones cause increased need for vitamins leading to relative vitamin deficiency in hyperthyroidism.

vi. *Effect on water and electrolyte balance.* Thyroid hormones play role in regulation of water and electrolyte balance.

4. Respiratory effects

Thyroid hormones stimulate O_2 utilization, which is accomplished by following effects :

i. *Increase in the resting respiratory rate, minute ventilation, and ventilatory responses* to hypercapnia and hypoxia.

ii. *Increase in oxygen carrying capacity of blood* by slightly increasing the red blood cell mass.

5. Cardiovascular effects

In general, the thyroid hormones have the following effects on cardiovascular system:

i. *Tachycardia*, i.e. increased heart rate (at rest, even during sleep) is an important physical sign.

ii. *Force of cardiac contraction* is increased by inotropic effects via adrenergic stimulation.

iii. *Cardiac output* is increased as a result of increased blood volume, increased heart rate and increased force of contraction.

6. Effects on nervous system

a. Effect on development of nervous system

T_3 seems to be necessary for proper axonal and dendritic development as well as normal myelination in the nervous system. Critical period for development of nervous system is up to 1 year of life.

b. Effect on functioning of nervous tissue in adults

T_4 enhances wakefulness, alertness, responsiveness to various stimuli, auditory sense, awareness of hunger, memory, and learning capacity.

7. Effects on gastrointestinal tract

Effects of thyroid hormones on gastrointestinal tract (GIT) include:

- Increase in appetite and therefore increase in food intake, and

- Increase in motility of gastrointestinal tract.

    Excess of thyroid hormone often causes diarrhoea.

8. Effects on reproductive system

In males, lack of thyroid hormones causes complete loss of libido, and excess of hormones causes impotence.

In females, lack of thyroid has varying effects:

- Menorrhagia and polymenorrhagia,

- Irregular periods or even amenorrhoea occurs in some women.

CALCITONIN

Synthesis and structure

Synthesis. Calcitonin is synthesized in the C-cells or parafollicular cells of the thyroid gland. These cells are of neural crest origin which during development migrate to the developing thyroid gland.

Regulation of secretion

The secretion of calcitonin is regulated by following factors:

1. *Increase in plasma calcium concentration* is the major regulator of calcitonin secretion. Normal plasma calcium level is 9-11 mg%. Concentration reaches to 9.5 mg% and that above this calcium level, plasma calcitonin is directly proportional to plasma calcium.

2. *Gastrointestinal hormones* such as gastrin, CCK, glucagon, and secretin have all been reported to stimulate calcitonin secretion, with gastrin being the most potent stimulus.

3. *Other factors* like β-adrenergic agonist, dopamine, and oestrogen also stimulate calcitonin secretion.

Plasma levels, half-life and degradation

Plasma levels of circulating calcitonin range from 10 to 20 pg/ml.

Degradation. Circulating calcitonin is heterogeneous, and it is largely degraded and cleared by the kidney.

Actions and physiological role of calcitonin

The major effect of calcitonin is to rapidly lower the plasma calcium level and it also decreases the plasma phosphate. These effects of calcitonin are due to its following actions:

1. *Action on the bone.* The main action of calcitonin on the bone is to oppose the bone resorptive action of PTH.
2. *Action on kidney.* Calcitonin increases loss of calcium and phosphate in the urine. This effect also contributes in producing hypocalcaemia and hypophosphataemia.

ABNORMALITIES OF THYROID GLAND

HYPERTHYROIDISM

Hyperthyroidism refers to increased secretion of thyroid hormones. Its common causes are:
- Graves' disease (described below), and
- Toxic nodular goitre.

Graves' disease

Graves' disease is an autoimmune disease characterized by development of thyroid stimulating antibodies (TSAb) against the TSH receptors, also called long-acting thyroid stimulator (LATS). These antibodies bind to TSH receptors and mimic TSH action on thyroid growth and hormone synthesis.

Symptoms and signs (Fig. 10.3-5)

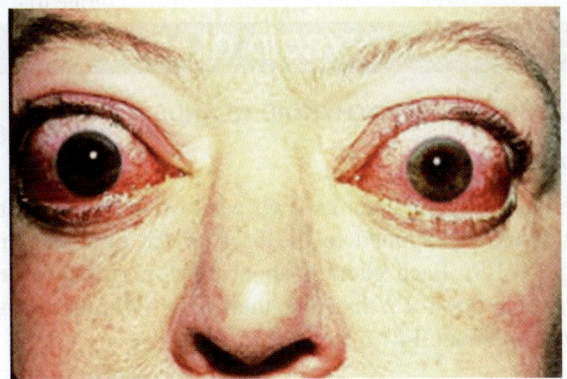

Fig. 10.3-5. *Graves' disease.*

1. *General features* include marked increase in basal metabolic rate (BMR), weight loss despite an increased intake of food, and increased heat production causing discomfort in warm environments, excessive sweating and a greater intake of water.

2. *Goitre.* Goitre refers to swelling of thyroid gland. Graves' disease is characterized by diffuse goitre, while a single or more nodules indicate toxic nodular goitre.

3. *Cardiovascular features* are:
- Increased pulse rate or sinus tachycardia, and
- Arrhythmias (atrial fibrillation is commonest).

4. *Neuromuscular features* are nervousness, irritability, restlessness, psychosis, tremors of hand, muscular weakness, and exaggerated tendon reflexes.

5. *Gastrointestinal features* are diarrhoea or steatorrhoea and vomiting.

6. *Dermatological features* are perspiration (increased sweating or hyperhidrosis), loss of hair, redness of palm.

7. *Reproductive features* are impotence in males and oligomenorrhoea or amenorrhoea, abortions and infertility in females.

8. *Ophthalmological signs* are lid retraction producing staring look and lid lag, and exophthalmos, i.e. bulging out of eyeball.

HYPOTHYROIDISM

Hypothyroidism is a clinical syndrome caused by low levels of circulating thyroid hormones. Depending upon the aetiology, hypothyroidism can be primary or secondary.

Primary hypothyroidism is caused by disorder of thyroid gland, and

Secondary hypothyroidism is caused by diseases of anterior pituitary and hypothalamus.

Clinical features

Clinical features depend upon the age at which deficiency manifests and duration and severity of the disease. Two different clinical entities are:
- Infantile hypothyroidism (cretinism).
- Adult hypothyroidism (myxoedema).

1. *Infantile hypothyroidism (cretinism).* It occurs when thyroid deficiency occurs during first year of life and is characterized by (Fig. 10.3-6) mental retardation, marked retardation of growth (drawf), delayed milestones of development, potbelly, protruding tongue, flat nose, dry skin and sparse hairs.

Treatment should be prompt otherwise mental deficiency will persist.

2. *Adult hypothyroidism* is also called myxoedema because of characteristic infiltration of skin by myxoedematous tissue (Fig. 10.3-7). Symptoms and signs include:

Fig. 10.3-6. *Clinical features of cretinism. Note short stature, potbelly and idiotic look.*

C H A P T E R   1 0 . 3

Fig. 10.3-7. *Photograph of a patient with myxoedema showing puffy face, thick lips and periorbital oedema.*

- *General features*: Tiredness and weight gain without an appreciable increase in caloric intake (due to lower than normal metabolic rate). Decreased heat production, lower body temperature causing intolerance to cold, and decreased sweating.
- *Cardiovascular features.* Adrenergic activity is decreased causing bradycardia. Other features include pericardial effusion and precipitation of angina.
- *Neuromuscular features.* Movement, speech and thought are all slowed, and lethargy, sleepiness, delayed relaxation of ankle jerks, aches and pain are common.
- *Dermatological features.* Dry thick skin (toad skin), sparse hair, non-pitting oedema due to infiltration by myxoedematous tissue (myxoedema).
- *Reproductive features.* Menorrhagia and infertility (common), galactorrhoea and impotence (less common).
- *Gastrointestinal features.* Constipation (common) and adynamic ileus (less common).
- *Haematological features* include anaemia.

GOITRE

Goitre refers to any abnormal increase in the size of the thyroid gland. The term goitre does not denote the functional status of thyroid gland, because it may be associated with:
- *Euthyroid*, i.e. normal thyroid hormone level,
- *Hypothyroidism,* i.e. low thyroid hormone level, and
- *Hyperthyroidism,* i.e. high thyroid hormone levels as seen in Graves' disease and toxic nodular goitre.

Iodine deficiency goitre or endemic goitre occurs when the daily dietary intake of iodine falls below 10 μg (normal requirement 100-200 μg/day). It decreases the synthesis and secretion of thyroid hormone leading to increased TSH levels and proliferation of thyroid gland tissue (goitre). It is mostly found in the geographic regions away from the sea coast where the water and soil are low in iodine content. Consumption of iodized salt is advocated to overcome the problem of endemic goitre. In certain cases administration of thyroid hormone is also indicated.

PARATHYROID GLANDS

ANATOMY OF PARATHYROID GLANDS

Gross anatomy

The parathyroid glands are two pairs of small endocrine glands closely applied to the back of the thyroid gland (Fig. 10.3-8). Each gland is about the size of a split pea, measuring 6 × 4 × 2 mm. The total weight of four normal glands is about 140 mg.

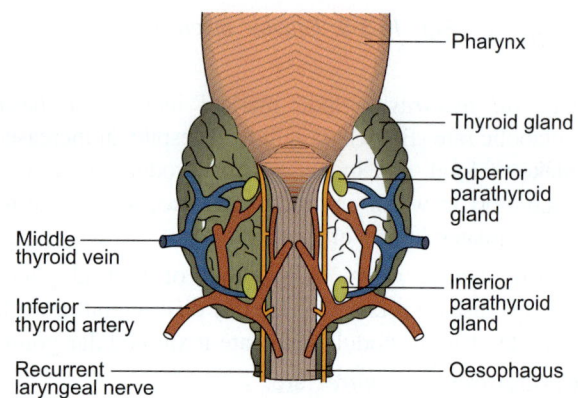

Fig. 10.3-8. *Location of parathyroid glands (viewed from behind).*

Histological structure

The parenchyma of the parathyroid gland is made up of cells that are arranged in cords. The cells of the parathyroid glands are of two main types: chief cells and oxyphil cells.

Chief cells, also called as principal cells, are much more numerous. Chief cells secrete the parathyroid hormone (PTH) or parathormone.

Oxyphil cells. These cells first appear at puberty and their function is still not clear.

PARATHYROID HORMONE (PTH)

Structure, synthesis and secretion of PTH

Structure. Parathyroid hormone (PTH) is a single chain polypeptide, containing 84 amino acids and having molecular weight 9500.

Synthesis. PTH is synthesized from a precursor molecule called prepro-PTH. PTH is released from chief cells by exocytosis in response to decrease in plasma ionized calcium concentration.

Regulation of PTH secretion

1. *Role of plasma ionized calcium.* The secretion of PTH is mainly regulated by circulating levels of ionized calcium. The secretion of PTH is inversely related to the plasma calcium concentration. Maximum secretion occurs when plasma ionized calcium levels fall below 3.5 mg%.

2. *Role of serum magnesium concentration*

- *Mild decrease* in serum Mg^{2+} concentration stimulates PTH secretion, while
- *Severe decrease* in serum Mg^{2+} concentration inhibits PTH secretion and produces symptoms of hypoparathyroidism (e.g. hypocalcaemia).

3. *Role of plasma phosphate concentration.* A rise in plasma concentration of phosphate causes an immediate fall in ionized calcium concentration, which in turn stimulates PTH secretion.

4. *Role of vitamin $1,25-(OH)_2D_3$.* It decreases PTH secretion.

Plasma levels, and degradation of PTH

Plasma level of PTH is about 130 pg/ml.

Degradation of PTH occurs rapidly in the peripheral tissues. PTH is predominantly split in the liver.

Actions of PTH

The prime function of PTH is to maintain plasma calcium level by acting on three major target organs: directly on bone and kidney, and indirectly on the gastrointestinal tract (Fig. 10.3-9).

1. *Actions on the bone.* PTH stimulates calcium and phosphate resorption from bones, i.e. causes decalcification or demineralization of bone.

2. *Actions on kidney.* The actions of PTH on kidney are:

i. *Increase in calcium reabsorption.* PTH increases the reabsorption of calcium from the ascending limb of loop of Henle and the distal tubules of kidney and helps to prevent hypocalcaemia.

ii. *Inhibition of phosphate reabsorption in the proximal tubule* is the most dramatic effect of PTH on the kidney. This effect produces phosphaturia and hypophosphataemia.

iii. *Stimulation of reabsorption of Mg^{2+} by the renal tubules.*

iv. *Stimulation of synthesis of 1,25-dihydroxycholecalciferol* is a very important action of PTH in the kidney.

3. *Actions on intestines.* Parathormone greatly enhances both calcium and phosphate absorption from intestine indirectly by increasing synthesis of 1,25-dihydroxycholecalciferol in the kidney.

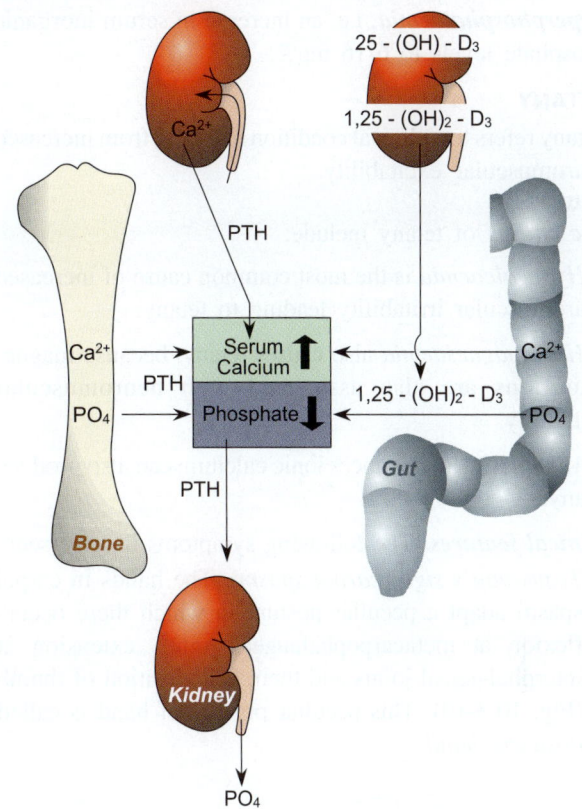

Fig. 10.3-9. *Action of parathyroid hormone (PTH) on bone, kidney and intestine.*

ABNORMALITIES OF PARATHYROID GLANDS

Hyperparathyroidism and hypercalcaemia

Hyperparathyroidism is a clinical condition characterized by excessive secretion of parathyroid hormone (PTH).

Clinicobiochemical features. The main characteristic feature of hyperparathyroidism is involvement of bones which may present as hypercalcaemia, hypercalciuria and renal calculi (renal stones). Hypercalcaemia may produce muscle weakness, lethargy, constipation, peptic ulceration. Hypercalcaemia is also responsible for hypertension and cardiac arrhythmia.

Hypoparathyroidism and hypocalcaemia

Hypoparathyroidism refers to a clinical condition characterized by low level of plasma calcium either due to deficient production of PTH or its unresponsiveness.

Characteristic features of hypoparathyroidism

Characteristic features of hypoparathyroidism are:

Hypocalcaemia. Total serum calcium may be decreased to 4-8 mg% and the ionized calcium to 3 mg%. Fall in the levels of ionized calcium leads to a clinical condition called *tetany* (described below):

Hyperphosphataemia, i.e. an increase in serum inorganic phosphate levels to 6-16 mg%.

TETANY

Tetany refers to a clinical condition resulting from increased neuromuscular excitability.

Causes

The causes of tetany include:

1. *Hypocalcaemia* is the most common cause of increased neuromuscular irritability leading to tetany.

2. *Hypomagnesaemia* also causes tetany, because magnesium ions are also associated with neuromuscular irritability.

3. *Alkalosis*, which reduces ionic calcium, can also produce tetany.

Clinical features. The following symptoms may be seen:

- *Trousseau's sign (carpal spasm).* The hands in carpal spasm adapt a peculiar posture in which there occurs flexion at metacarpophalangeal joints, extension at interphalangeal joints and there is apposition of thumb (Fig. 10.3-10). This peculiar posture of hand is called *obstetric hand.*

Fig. 10.3-10. Carpal spasm (Trousseau's sign) in a patient with tetany.

- *Laryngeal stridor* (loud sound) results from spasm of laryngeal muscles. It may produce asphyxia.

Management of tetany includes treatment of hypocalcaemia—an intravenous injection of 20 ml of 10% calcium gluconate is given to correct hypocalcaemia and relieve tetany.

THYMUS

ANATOMY

Gross anatomy

Thymus is a small lymphoid structure located in the lower part of neck in front of the trachea, below the thyroid gland (Fig. 10.3-11). The thymus consists of two lobes connected by areolar tissue. The lobes are covered by a fibrous capsule which sends septa. At birth, it is small (weighing 10-12 gm), gradually enlarges till puberty when it weighs 20-30 gm, and then it starts decreasing in size and in old age weighs about 3-6 gm. The sex glands exert a depressant effect on the thymus, therefore, castration (removal of gonads) prolongs the period of persistence of the thymus.

Fig. 10.3-11. Location of thymus gland in an adult.

Histological structure

Histologically, thymus consists of the inner medulla and outer cortex.

- *Medulla.* It comprises reticular epithelial cells, a few lymphocytes and concentric corpuscles of Hassall.
- *Cortex.* It includes actively multiplying, closely packed lymphocytes and contains no Hassall's corpuscles.

Functions

Thymus has two functions:

- Immunological functions (see page 54) and
- Endocrinal functions.

Endocrine function of thymus. Thymus tissue secretes two hormones, thymosin and thymin.

i. *Thymosin.* It is a peptide which promotes proliferation of T-lymphocytes in the thymus and peripheral lymphoid tissue.

ii. *Thymin*, also called thymopoietin, inhibits acetylcholine release at motor nerve endings and thus suppresses neuromuscular activity.

Adrenal Glands

10.4

- **ANATOMY OF ADRENAL GLANDS**
  - Gross anatomy
  - Histological structure
  - Blood supply
- **HORMONES OF ADRENAL CORTEX**
- **Glucocorticoids**
  - Synthesis
  - Plasma levels, transport, metabolism and excretion
  - Actions of glucocorticoids
  - Regulation of glucocorticoid secretion
- **Mineralocorticoids**
  - Synthesis
  - Plasma levels, transport, metabolism and excretion

- Actions of aldosterone
- Regulation of aldosterone secretion
- **Adrenal sex steroids**
  - Synthesis
  - Plasma levels, contribution
- **HORMONES OF ADRENAL MEDULLA**
  - Synthesis, storage and secretion of catecholamine hormones
  - Actions of catecholamines
- **APPLIED ASPECTS**
  - An integrated response to stress
  - Hyperactivity of adrenal cortex
  - Hypoactivity of adrenal cortex
  - Diseases of adrenal medulla

ANATOMY OF ADRENAL GLAND

Gross anatomy

There are two adrenal glands, situated one on either side, at the upper pole of kidney, hence also called 'suprarenal gland' (Fig. 10.4-1). Normally, each gland weighs about 5 gm and consists of two parts, the adrenal cortex and the medulla.

Histological structure

Adrenal cortex. The adrenal gland is covered by a connective tissue capsule from which septa extend into the gland substance. The mature human adrenal cortex consists of three distinct layers or zones of cells (Fig. 10.4-2).

1. *Zona glomerulosa,* constituting outer one-fifth of cortex, is a small zone present under the capsule. It consists of cells that secrete *aldosterone* and *corticosterone.*

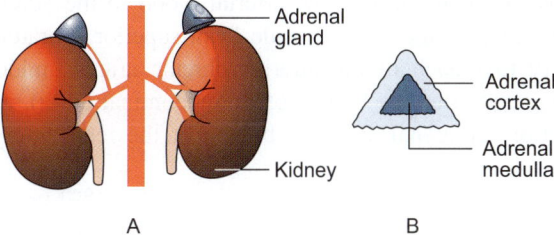

Fig. 10.4-1. *Location (A) and divisions (B) of adrenal gland.*

2. *Zona fasciculata* is the widest zone forming middle three-fifths of the cortex. It is made up of cells that are arranged in two cell thick straight columns. Sinusoids intervene between the columns.

3. *Zona reticularis* forms the inner one-fifth of the cortex. It is made up of a network of compactly arranged cords of cells (hence the name zona reticularis).

Fig. 10.4-2. *Histological structure of adrenal gland.*

Adrenal medulla. Histologically it is made up of chromaffin cells, innervated by preganglionic sympathetic neurons.

Functionally, these cells are considered to be modified postganglionic neurons which do not have axons. Catacholomines are stored in the chromaffin granules. In addition to the catecholamines, the chromaffin granules also contain proteins, lipids, and adenine nucleotides (mainly ATP).

Nerve endings, present in the adrenal medulla, are the *cholinergic preganglionic* sympathetic fibres that synapse directly on chromaffin cells. These fibres traverse the splanchnic nerve and are myelinated emanating mainly from the lower thoracic segments (T_5 and T_9) of the ipsilateral intermediolateral grey column of the spinal cord (Fig. 10.4-3).

Blood supply (Fig. 10.4-4)

Arterial blood supply. The arterial blood to the adrenal gland reaches the outer capsule from superior suprarenal artery (a branch of the inferior phrenic artery), middle suprarenal artery (a branch of the abdominal aorta), and inferior suprarenal artery (a branch of the renal artery).

Fig. 10.4-3. *Preganglionic sympathetic fibres synapsing directly on chromaffin cells in the adrenal medulla.*

① Superior suprarenal artery	⑤ Sinusoidal capillaries in adrenal cortex
② Middle suprarenal artery	
③ Inferior suprarenal artery	⑥ Medullary veins supplying medulla (forms portal vascular system)
④ Suprarenal vein	

Fig. 10.4-4. *Schematic diagram to show arterial supply and venous drainage of adrenal gland.*

The arterial blood enters sinusoidal capillaries in the cortex and then drains into medullary veins which supply blood to medulla and thus form a *portal system*. This arrangement of portal circulation exposes the medulla to relatively high concentrations of corticos-teroids from the cortex.

Venous drainage. The venous blood drains via single central vein. The right suprarenal vein drains into the inferior vena cava and left suprarenal vein into the left renal vein.

HORMONES OF ADRENAL CORTEX

Hormones secreted by adrenal cortex, called *corticosteroids*, can be grouped as:

- *Glucocorticoids*, which include *cortisol* and *corticosterone*, have widespread effect on glucose and protein metabolism.
- *Mineralocorticoids*. Aldosterone is the chief mineralo-corticoid. It regulates sodium balance and ECF volume in the body.
- *Adrenal sex steroids*. These include dehydroepian-drosterone (DHEA) and its sulphate ester.

GLUCOCORTICOIDS

SYNTHESIS

The glucocorticoids are synthesized largely by the cells forming zona fasciculata with a small contribution by the cells of zona reticularis of adrenal cortex.

PLASMA LEVELS, TRANSPORT, METABOLISM, AND EXCRETION OF GLUCOCORTICOIDS

Plasma levels

Plasma levels of glucocorticoids and other corticosteroids

are shown in Table 10.4-1. The plasma levels of total cortisol show diurnal fluctuation and range from 10-25 μg% with an average of 14 μg%. The rate of secretion of cortisol, which is about 15 mg/day under normal condition, may increase to 300 to 400 mg/day under conditions of severe stress.

Table 10.4-1. Average 8 A.M. plasma levels and secretion rate of corticosteroids in adult humans

Corticosteroid (μg/dl)	Plasma concentration (mg/day)	Secretion rate
Cortisol	14.0	15
Corticosterone	1.0	03
Aldosterone	0.009	0.15
Dehydroepiandrosterone (DHEA) sulphate	115	15

Transport

In the plasma, cortisol circulates in two forms :

Bound form. Most of the plasma cortisol (5%) is bound to specific corticosteroid, binding α_2-globulin (CBG), which is a glycoprotein and is also called *transcortin*. A small amount (15%) is bound to albumin.

Free form of cortisol constitutes only 5-10% of the total plasma cortisol.

Metabolism and excretion

Corticosteroids are degraded in the liver and excreted in the urine and faeces.

ACTIONS OF GLUCOCORTICOIDS

Glucocorticoids are essential for survival. The actions of glucocorticoids are grouped as :

I. Metabolic effects of glucocorticoids

The different metabolic effects of glucocorticoids are:

1. *Effects on carbohydrate metabolism.* Glucocorticoids exert an anti-insulin effect, which leads to hyperglycaemia by following actions:

i. *Increased gluconeogenesis.* Glucocorticoids increase the rate of glucose production from non-carbohydrate sources by as much as 6-10 folds.

ii. *Decreased utilization of glucose in peripheral tissues.*

2. *Effects on protein metabolism* exerted by glucocorticoids are :

- *Catabolic effect.* Cortisol enhances the release of amino acids by proteolysis in skeletal muscle and other extrahepatic tissues.

- *Antianabolic effect.* It is the ability of the glucocorticoids to inhibit the synthesis of protein.

3. *Effects on fat metabolism* are complex and include:

i. *Lipolytic effects.* Although cortisol itself has only a slight lipolytic activity, its presence is necessary for epinephrine, growth hormone, and other lipolytic substances to stimulate hydrolysis of stored triglycerides at maximal rates.

- Fatty acid synthesis is inhibited in the liver by cortisol.

ii. *Lipogenic role.* Glucocorticoids stimulate lipogenesis.

4. *Effects on electrolyte and water metabolism.* Glucocorticoids control distribution of body water and electrolytes by following actions:

i. *Retention of sodium and water.*

ii. *Promotion of diuresis.*

II. Physiological actions on various organs and systems

In addition to the metabolic effects, the glucocorticoids affect various organs and systems throughout the body (Fig. 10.4-5):

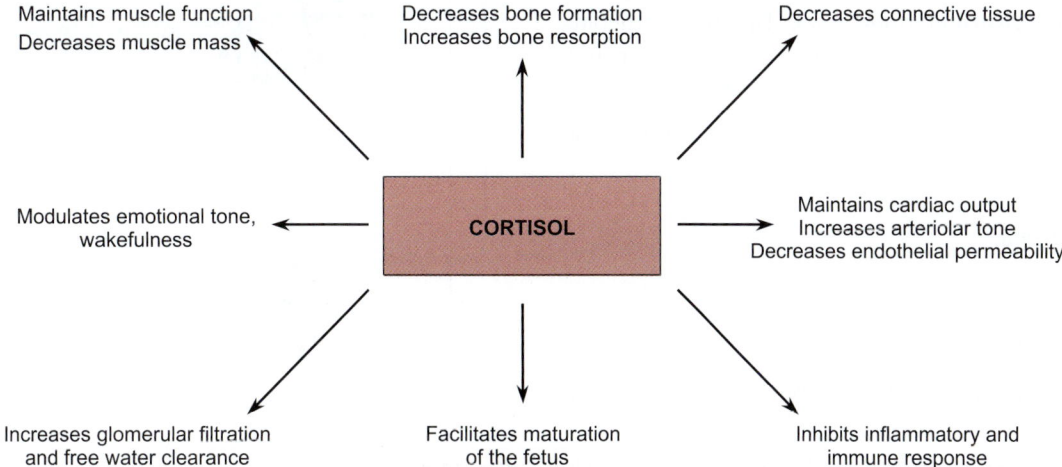

Fig. 10.4-5. *Effects of glucocorticoids on various tissues, organs and systems of the body.*

C H A P T E R   1 0 . 4

1. Effects on muscle

i. *Contractility and work performance* of skeletal and cardiac muscles is maintained by the cortisol.

ii. *Decrease in muscle mass and strength* is caused by an excess of cortisol. This occurs due to decrease in muscle protein synthesis and increase in muscle catabolism.

2. Effects on bone. The glucocorticoids cause:

i. *Increased bone resorption.*

ii. *Inhibition of bone formation.*

Note. Because of the above effects on bone, *osteoporosis* results in skeletal deformity.

3. Effects on connective tissue. Cortisol decreases collagen synthesis producing thereby:

- Thinning of the skin, and
- Thinning of walls of capillaries, which leads to their easy rupture and to intracutaneous haemorrhage.

4. Effects on vascular system. Cortisol is essential for maintaining normal blood pressure by:

- Sustaining myocardial performance,
- Enhancing the vasopressure effect of catecholamines (especially norepinephrine) and angiotensin II, and maintaining normal blood volume.

5. Effects on kidney are:

- Increase in glomerular filtration rate (GFR) by increasing glomerular plasma flow,
- Rapid excretion of water load, and
- Increase in calcium and phosphate excretion by decreasing their reabsorption in the proximal tubules.

6. Effects on central nervous system. Glucocorticoid receptors (GR) are present in various parts of the brain, especially in the limbic system. Through these receptors, the glucocorticoids modulate excitability behaviour and mood.

7. Effects on gastrointestinal tract. The glucocorticoids increase gastric acid secretion and can lead to peptic ulceration following long-term use of cortisol.

8. Effects on blood cells and lymphatic organs. The excess of glucocorticoids leads to:

- Eosinopenia and basopenia,
- Lymphopenia,
- Neutrophilia,
- Polycythemia, and
- Thrombocytosis.

III. Anti-inflammatory, anti-immunity and anti-allergic effects

These effects are not produced by the glucocorticoids which are normally secreted physiologically, but are produced by their large doses when administered therapeutically and are thus called the pharmacological actions of glucocorticoids.

IV. Role of glucocorticoids in fetal life

Maturation of CNS, retina, skin and lungs is facilitated by the cortisol in utero.

V. Role of glucocorticoids in stress

Various stresses, e.g. trauma, cold, illness, starvation are associated with activation of the hypothalamic-hypophyseal-adrenal axis. Increased secretion of glucocorticoids is one of the various mechanisms involved in adaptation to various stresses.

REGULATION OF GLUCOCORTICOID SECRETION

The glucocorticoid secretion is regulated by hypothalamic-anterior pituitary-adrenal cortex axis which exerts its effect through (Fig. 10.4-6):

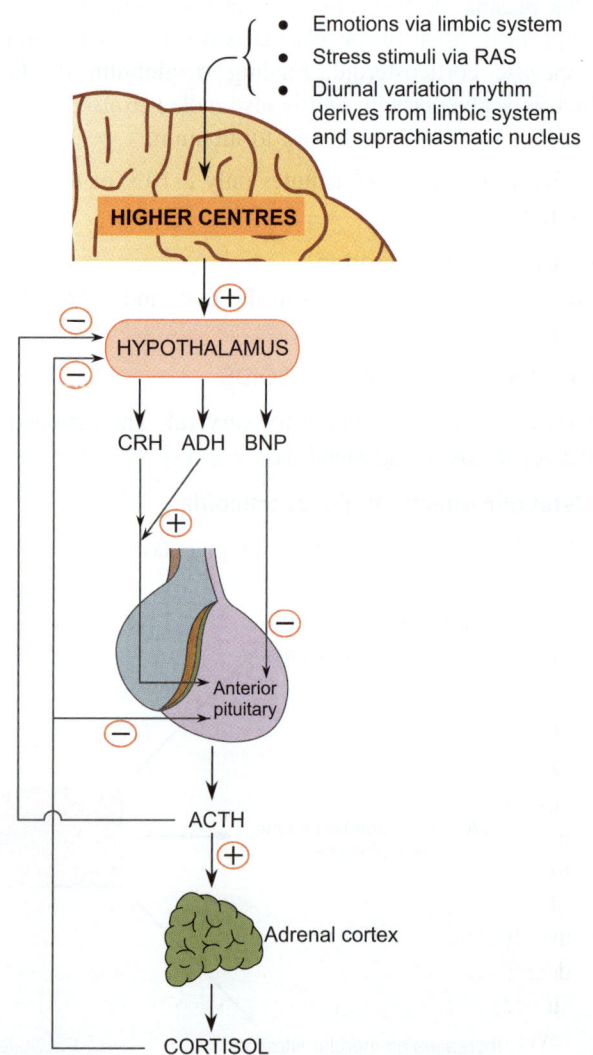

Fig. 10.4-6. *Hypothalamic-anterior pituitary-adrenal axis and negative feedback mechanism.*

- Corticotropin releasing hormone (CRH),
- Adrenocorticotropic hormone (ACTH), and
- Glucocorticoid negative feedback effect.

Note. Since CRH and ACTH are related to regulation of glucocorticoid release, they are described in detail here rather than along with other hormones of hypothalamus and anterior pituitary, respectively.

1. Role of corticotropin releasing hormone

Corticotropin releasing hormone (CRH) is secreted by the small cells of paraventricular nucleus of hypothalamus. CRH is a polypeptide with 41 amino acids.

Actions of CRH include:

i. *Stimulation of synthesis and release of ACTH* by acting on the *corticotrophs.*

ii. *Other actions of CRH* related to or independent of ACTH include:

- Central arousal,
- Increase in blood pressure,
- Diminution of reproductive function by decreasing synthesis of gonadotropin-releasing hormone (GnRH) and gonadotropins,
- Decrease in feeding activity and growth, and
- Stimulation of release of cytokines in immune cells.

2. Role of adrenocorticotropic hormone

Adrenocorticotropic hormone (ACTH) is secreted by *corticotrophs.*

Actions of ACTH

i. *Actions on adrenal cortex.* ACTH is primarily concerned with growth and functions of adrenal cortex.

ii. *Extra adrenal actions* of ACTH occur only with very high levels which are seen in abnormal conditions.

Regulation of ACTH secretion

i. *Hypothalamic control* on ACTH secretion is mainly exerted through CRH (see above). The hypothalamic control is responsible for following characteristics of ACTH secretion:

- *Diurnal variation* in the levels of ACTH (and thus of cortisol) is due to variation in CRH release. A large peak in the levels of ACTH and cortisol occurs in the morning (6 to 8 AM) during awakening (plasma level of ACTH range between 20 and 100 pg/ml with an average of 50 pg/ml). Thereafter the average level decreases markedly (5 pg/ml), just before or after the subject falls asleep. In night workers the rhythm is reversed.

- *Pulsatile release of ACTH* is also due to pulsatile release of CRH—upto three pulses per hour, and each

pulse lasts about 20 minutes. Cortisol pulses follow the ACTH pulses (Fig. 10.4-7).

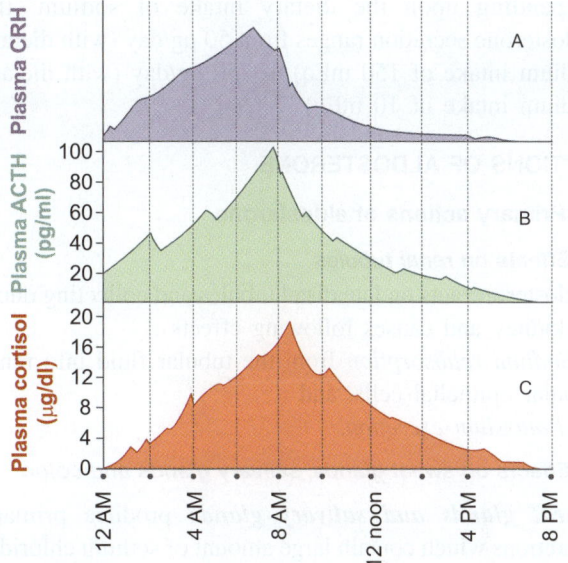

Fig. 10.4-7. *Diurnal variations and pulsatility in secretion of CRH (A), ACTH (B) and cortisol (C). Note the ACTH peak follows CRH peak and cortisol peak follows ACTH peak by 10 minutes.*

ii. *Negative feedback inhibition of ACTH* is caused by (Fig. 10.4-6):

- Plasma cortisol levels (long-loop negative feedback), and

- Plasma ACTH levels (short-loop negative feedback).

3. Negative feedback control of glucocorticoid secretion

Chronically elevated plasma levels of free cortisol exert a direct negative feedback action on its own secretion. This effect is exerted at two levels (Fig. 10.4-6):

- On hypothalamus to decrease formation of CRH, and
- On anterior pituitary to decrease formation of ACTH.

MINERALOCORTICOIDS

The mineralocorticoids include:

- Aldosterone. It is the chief mineralocorticoid,
- Deoxycorticosterone (DOC), and 18-hydroxy-deoxycorticosterone (18-OH-DOC) are secreted in small amount and have some mineralo-corticoid activity.

Since aldosterone is the major mineralocorticoid, so discussion in this section is limited to it.

SYNTHESIS

Aldosterone, the chief mineralocorticoid, is synthesized exclusively by the *zona glomerulosa cells.*

PLASMA LEVELS, TRANSPORT, METABOLISM AND EXCRETION

Plasma levels

Depending upon the dietary intake of sodium, the aldosterone secretion ranges from 50 µg/day (with dietary sodium intake of 150 mEq) to 250 µg/day (with dietary sodium intake of 10 mEq).

ACTIONS OF ALDOSTERONE

A. Primary actions of aldosterone

1. Effects on renal tubules

Aldosterone acts on late distal tubules and collecting ducts of kidney and causes following effects :
i. Sodium reabsorption from the tubular fluid into renal tubular epithelial cells, and
ii. Potassium excretion.

2. Effects on sweat glands, salivary glands and colon

Sweat glands and salivary glands produce primary secretions which contain large amount of sodium chloride. The sodium chloride is absorbed as the secretion passes through the ducts, and in turn K^+ and HCO_3^- are excreted. Thus aldosterone decreases the loss of Na^+ and Cl^- in sweat and salivary secretion.

Colon. The aldosterone stimulates sodium reabsorption from the colon while enhancing potassium excretion in the faeces.

B. Secondary effects of aldosterone

The secondary effects include:

i. *Hypokalaemia*, i.e. decrease in plasma K^+ levels may occur in aldosterone excess due to increased urinary excretion of K^+.

ii. *Hypernatraemia*.

REGULATION OF ALDOSTERONE SECRETION

Aldosterone secretion is controlled by following factors (Fig. 10.4-8):

1. Renin-angiotensin system

The secretion of aldosterone is influenced by changes in the circulating fluid volume which are sensed in the kidney. The signals arising from the kidney increase aldosterone secretion when ECF volume is decreased and vice versa.

Conditions associated with decreased ECF are:
- Sodium deprivation (e.g. dietary restriction),
- Haemorrhage,
- Upright posture for several hours, and
- Acute diuresis.

Fig. 10.4-8. *Regulation of aldosterone secretion.*

Steps involved in the secretion of aldosterone by renin-angiotensin system are:
- *Decrease in ECF volume* leads to decrease in renal arterial blood flow and pressure.
- *Decrease in renal perfusion pressure* causes the juxtaglomerular cells of the afferent arterioles to secrete renin.
- *Renin* catalyzes the conversion of angiotensinogen (alpha 2-globulin substrate present in the plasma) to angiotensin I.
- *Angiotensin I* is converted into angiotensin II by the action of angiotensin converting enzyme (ACE) present in the endothelium of blood vessels, especially in the lungs.
- *Angiotensin II* binds to specific plasma membrane receptors present on adrenal zona glomerulosa cells and increases the secretion of aldosterone.

Aldosterone secretion may be increased to 4- to 8-fold by renin-angiotensin system.

2. Plasma potassium concentration

There exists a vital negative feedback relationship between plasma potassium concentration and aldosterone secretion, i.e. *an increase in plasma concentration* by only 0.5 mEq/L immediately raises plasma aldosterone levels 3-fold.

3. Role of ACTH

ACTH also plays role in mineralocorticoid secretion.

ADRENAL SEX STEROIDS

Adrenal sex steroids include:

- *Dehydroepiandrosterone* (DHEA), its sulphate ester (DHEA-S) and *androstenedione* are the major androgenic precursor products of adrenal cortex.
- *Oestrogen and progesterone* are produced in very small amounts.

SYNTHESIS

The adrenal sex steroid precursors are synthesized in the *zona reticularis*.

The 17-hydroxylated derivatives of pregnenolone and progesterone are the starting points for synthesis of androgen precursors.

PLASMA LEVELS, CONTRIBUTION TOWARDS SEX STEROIDS

Plasma levels

Normal plasma level of DHEA is 150-200 μg% at 25 years of age in both sexes.

Contribution of adrenal glands towards sex steroids

During fetal life, adrenal cortex is hyperplastic and secretes large amount of DHEA which acts as the main precursor for synthesis of oestrogen by placenta.

In adult woman, the adrenal glands supply 50 to 60% of the androgenic hormone requirement. DHEA-S contributes to increased muscle mass, growth of pubic and axillary hair and libido.

In adult man, since testes produce a large quantity of testosterone, the adrenal androgen precursors are of little biological importance. However, they may be partly responsible for development of male sex organs in childhood.

HORMONES OF ADRENAL MEDULLA

The adrenal medulla secretes *catecholamines* which include epinephrine, norepinephrine and dopamine. About 80% of adrenal medullary catecholamine is epinephrine and rest is norepinephrine.

SYNTHESIS AND STORAGE OF CATECHOLAMINE HORMONES

Synthesis of catecholamines

Epinephrine and norepinephrine are synthesized in different cells from L-tyrosin.

Storage of catecholamines in storage granules

The epinephrine formed in the cytoplasm is then taken back up by the chromaffin granules, in which it is stored as the predominant adrenomedullary hormone.

Factors regulating catecholamine synthesis are :

- Acute sympathetic stimulation,
- Chronic stimulation of preganglionic fibres,
- ACTH,
- Cortisol, and
- Epinephrine.

REGULATION

Nervous control of secretion

The catecholamine secretion is entirely controlled by the splanchnic nerves supplying the medulla. These fibres, when stimulated, act by releasing acetylcholine close to the adrenal medullary chromaffin cells.

Physiological and psychological stimuli for release. The adrenal medullary activation occurs as a part of generalized sympathetic response to any emergency situation. Therefore, this has also been called *sympathetic alarm reaction*. The various sensory stimuli associated with rapid release of epinephrine (and probably norepinephrine) from adrenal medulla include:

- Perception or even anticipation of danger or harm (anxiety),
- Pain,
- Trauma,
- Hypovolaemia from haemorrhage or fluid loss,
- Hypotension,
- Anoxia,
- Exposure to extremes of temperature,
- Hypoglycaemia, and
- Severe exercise.

CIRCULATION, METABOLISM AND EXCRETION

Circulation

- *Secreted epinephrine* and norepinephrine from the adrenal medulla is in the ratio of 4:1.
- *Basal plasma levels* (in recumbent humans) of free epinephrine are 30 pg/ml and that of free norepinephrine are 300 pg/ml.
- *Variation in plasma levels* of catecholamines according to physiological or pathological states are quite common.

ADRENERGIC RECEPTORS AND ACTIONS OF CATECHOLAMINES

Adrenergic receptors

The adrenergic receptors are of two types:

Alpha (α) receptors. These are further of two types (α$_1$ and α$_2$). The alpha-adrenergic receptors are sensitive to both epinephrine and norepinephrine. These receptors are associated with most of the excitatory functions of the body but have one major inhibitory function (i.e. inhibition of intestinal motility).

Beta (β) receptors. These are further of three types β$_1$, β$_2$ and β$_3$. Beta-adrenergic receptors respond to epinephrine and in general are relatively insensitive to norepinephrine. These receptors are associated with most of the inhibitory functions of the body but have an important excitatory function (i.e. excitation of myocardium).

Actions of catecholamines

- The catecholamines exert their effects by binding with adrenergic receptors as described above.
- Actions of catecholamines on individual organs and systems are similar to those resulting from stimulation of sympathetic nervous system.
- In general, the effects produced by adrenomedullary stimulation last longer (about 10 times) than those produced by sympathetic stimulation.

I. Metabolic actions of catecholamines

1. *General metabolic effects of epinephrine*

- Increased O$_2$ consumption (by 20-40%) and increased CO$_2$ output.
- Raised basal metabolic rate (BMR) and respiratory quotient (RQ).
- Increased heat production due to stimulation of cellular oxidative processes.

2. *Effect on carbohydrate metabolism.* Epinephrine produces hyperglycaemia and makes the glucose available for the brain and other tissues to meet the emergency.

3. *Effects on fat metabolism.* Catecholamines cause increase in lipolysis by stimulating hormone-sensitive lipase in adipose tissue and muscles.

II. Physiological actions of catecholamines

1. *Effects on cardiovascular system.* The net effects of epinephrine and norepinephrine are (Table 10.4-2):

Table 10.4-2. Cardiovascular effects of catachalamine

Parameter	Epinephrine	Norepinephrine
• Heart rate	↑	↓
• Cardiac output	↑	↓
• Peripheral resistance	↓	↑
• Systolic blood pressure	↑	↑
• Diastolic blood pressure	↓	↑
• Mean arterial pressure	↓ or N	↑

2. *Effects on other systems include :*

On CNS catecholamines activate reticular activating system (RAS) thus leading to arousal and alerting responses producing anxiety, apprehension, and coarse tremors of extremities.

On GIT epinephrine causes contraction of sphincters of gut; the net result is production of constipation.

On urinary bladder. Epinephrine produces retention of urine.

On skin. Catecholamines act on pilomotor muscle producing piloerection of hair.

On skeletal muscle. During exercise epinephrine increases blood supply (by causing vasodilation).

On eyes. Epinephrine causes dilation of the pupil (mydriasis).

On respiration. Epinephrine via β$_2$ receptors relaxes smooth muscles of bronchioles producing broncho-dilation. It also increases rate and force of respiration

On blood. Epinephrine produces following effects:
- Increases RBC count, and
- Increases plasma protein concentration

APPLIED ASPECTS

The important applied aspects in relation to the adrenal gland which need mention include:
- An integrated response to stress,
- Hyperactivity of adrenal cortex,
- Hypoactivity of adrenal cortex, and
- Diseases of adrenal medulla.

AN INTEGRATED RESPONSE TO STRESS

Stress, may it be emotional, physical or biological, evokes an integrated response of sympathoadrenal medullary system and hypothalamic-pituitary-adrenal cortex axis.

STEPS INVOLVED IN STRESS ADAPTATION by an integrated response of the above system are:

Perception of stress signals. Stress is perceived by many areas of the brain, from the cortex down to brain stem including limbic system and reticular activating system (RAS).

Stimulation of hypothalamus. Major stresses activate the CRH and ADH neurons in the paraventricular nucleus and adrenergic neurons.

Activation of hypothalamic-pituitary-adrenal axis. CRH and ADH release stimulates ACTH release and ultimately elevates plasma cortisol levels.

Activation of sympathoadrenal medullary system. Sudden exposure to any type of stress initially produces the sympathetic alarm reaction. Stimulation of adrenergic neurons of hypothalamus ultimately leads to release of epinephrine from adrenal medulla and norepinephrine from the sympathetic ganglia.

Integrated role of hormones released by hypothalamic-pituitary-adrenal axis and sympathoadrenal medullary system in stress adaptation. Together these hormones help in adaptation to stress by their following actions (Fight and Flight):

- *Increase in glucose production* and shift glucose utilization towards the central nervous system away from peripheral tissues.
- *Free fatty acid supply* to heart and to the muscles.
- *Cardiovascular adjustments.* Catecholamines and cortisol raise blood pressure and cardiac output, and they improve the delivery of substrates to tissues.
- *Arousal, defensively useful behavioural activation* and *focussed attention* result from the adrenergic stimuli to the pertinent brain centres.
- *Inhibition of activities that are not useful during stress and divert individuals, and their resources, from defensive responses to danger* is an important part of adaptation to stress. For example, inhibition of growth hormone, gonadotropin release, and sexual activity.
- *Interaction with immune system.*

HYPERACTIVITY OF ADRENAL CORTEX

Disorders of hyperactivity of adrenal cortex include:
- Cushing's syndrome (hypercortisol state), and
- Conn's syndrome (hyperaldosteronism).

CUSHING'S SYNDROME

Cushing's syndrome refers to the group of clinical conditions occurring due to prolonged excessive levels of glucocorticoids.

Characteristic features of Cushing's syndrome are (Fig. 10.4-10):

1. *Truncal or centripetal obesity.* It occurs due to redistribution of body fat from extremities (which is in the abdominal wall, back and face) producing following characteristic features:
- Buffalo hump
- Moon face
- Purple striae or cutaneous abdominal striae or livid stretch marks. Causes rupture of subdermal tissues producing reddish purple striae.
2. *Muscle weakness* and backache due to protein catabolism.
3. *Sodium and water retention* may cause weight gain, oedema and hypertension.

Fig. 10.4-10. *Photograph of a patient with Cushing's syndrome showing: A, moon face; and B, truncal obesity and purple striae on the abdomen.*

4. *Hyperglycaemia* occurs due to gluconeogenesis and inhibition of peripheral utilization of glucose. It may lead to glycosuria and adrenal diabetes.
5. *Hirsutism and menstrual irregularity* may occur due to increased adrenal androgens.
6. *Susceptibility to osteoporosis and bone fracture* is increased due to protein depletion and bone resorption.
7. *Susceptibility to infections* is increased due to immunosuppression.
8. *Psychological, emotional and personality changes* may occur due to CNS effects of glucocorticoids.
9. *Blackening of skin* may occur due to pigmentation caused by MSH-like effects of excessive ACTH.
10. *Susceptibility to peptic ulceration* is increased.

HYPERALDOSTERONISM

Hyperaldosteronism (Conn's syndrome) refers to overproduction of the hormone aldosterone, a major sodium-retaining hormone.

Characteristic features of hyperaldosteronism are:
- *Sodium and water retention* leading to hypertension and oedema.
- *Hypokalaemia* may occur due to increased potassium excretion producing muscle weakness.
- *Metabolic alkalosis* may occur due to secretion of more amount of H$^+$ into renal tubules. Metabolic alkalosis may produce hypocalcaemia causing tetany.

HYPOACTIVITY OF ADRENAL CORTEX

Adrenocortical deficiency, depending upon the site of lesion, can be divided into two types:

I. *Primary adrenocortical deficiency* occurs due to involvement of adrenal cortex and is associated with high ACTH levels due to feedback mechanism. The conditions producing primary adrenocortical deficiency include:
- Addison's disease, and
- Congenital adrenal hyperplasia.

II. *Secondary adrenocortical deficiency* occurs due to involvement of either hypothalamus or pituitary or due to exogenous glucocorticoid administration and is associated with *low ACTH level* due to less production.

ADDISON'S DISEASE

Characteristic features occur due to chronic deficiency of hormones secreted by all the three zones of adrenal cortex:
1. *Glucocorticoid insufficiency* produces weight loss, malaise, anorexia, nausea, vomiting, weakness and diarrhoea. Since glucocorticoids are essential for adaptation to stress, therefore in Addison's disease exposure to any type of stress, e.g. even mild infection may be fatal.
2. *Mineralocorticoid deficiency* produces hyponatraemia, hyperkalaemia, acidosis and decreased ECF volume with hypotension.
3. *Loss of androgens* causes sparse hair in females.
4. *Increased ACTH secretion* occurs due to feedback mechanism and causes diffuse pigmentation of the skin

and mucous membranes (because of its MSH- like actions).

Addisonian crisis or adrenal crisis

It refers to acute adrenal insufficiency characterized by sudden collapse. The condition becomes fatal if not treated in time.

CONGENITAL ADRENAL HYPERPLASIA

Causes. Congenital adrenal hyperplasia is caused by congenital deficiency of one of the enzymes involved in the biosynthesis of glucocorticoids, particularly *21-hydroxylase deficiency* and deficiency of *11-hydroxylase*.

Characteristic features occurring because of above pathophysiological changes are virilism and excessive body growth.

In boys, adrenal hyperplasia leads to:
- Precocious body growth leading to stocky appearance called *infant hercules.*
- Precocious sexual development with enlarged penis even at age of 4 years.

In female fetus, high plasma androgen levels cause *masculinized pattern* of development (*virilism*). Sometime the female fetus may be born with male type external genitalia. This condition is called *pseudo-hermaphroditism.*

DISEASES OF ADRENAL MEDULLA

PHAEOCHROMOCYTOMA

Phaeochromocytoma is a rare benign tumour arising from the epinephrine- and norepinephrine-secreting chromaffin cells of adrenal medulla.

Clinical features, produced by the excess of epinephrine and norepinephrine, include:
- Episodic or non-episodic hypertension with postural drop.
- Attacks of tachycardia, palpitation, sweating, pallor, headache and chest discomfort.
- Abdominal pain, vomiting, constipation and glucose intolerance.
- Weight loss and weakness.

Pancreatic and Gastrointestinal Hormones of Other Organs and Local Hormones

10.5

ENDOCRINE PANCREAS

FUNCTIONAL ANATOMY

The endocrine part of the pancreas comprises numerous rounded collections of cells known as *pancreatic islets* or the *islets of Langerhans*. These are embedded within the exocrine part, and they constitute 1 to 1.5% of the human pancreatic mass.

Islets of Langerhans

Each islet contains four types of cells (Fig. 10.5-1):
- *Beta (β) cells* make up 60 to 70% of the total cells and constitute the central core of the islet. These cells secrete insulin.
- *Alpha (α) cells* form about 20% of the total cells and constitute the outer rim of the islet. These cells secrete glucagon.

Fig. 10.5-1. *Schematic histological structure of pancreas.*

- *Delta (δ) cells* form about 10% of total cells and are intermixed. These are source of somatostatin.

369

- *PP cells.* These are also peripherally placed scattered amongst the α cells. These are source of pancreatic peptide.

Gap junctions link beta cells to each other, alpha cells to each other, and beta cells to alpha cells for rapid communication.

INSULIN

Insulin is a polypeptide hormone secreted by the β cells of islets of Langerhans of pancreas. Historically, insulin is the first hormone to be isolated, purified, crystallized and synthesized.

Some of the important factors stimulating and inhibiting insulin secretion are depicted in Table 10.5-1.

Table 10.5-1. Factors stimulating and inhibiting insulin secretion

Factors stimulating insulin secretion	Factors inhibiting insulin secretion
• ↑ Blood glucose	• ↓ Blood glucose
• ↑ Amino acids	• Somatostatin
• ↑ Fatty acids	• Norepinephrine,
• Glucagon	epinephrine
• GIP	
• ACh	
• Growth hormones, cortisol	

Plasma levels of insulin

- Average basal peripheral plasma insulin level is 10 μU/ml.
- A 3- to 10-fold increase in plasma insulin level is noted after a typical meal. The peak occurs after 30 to 60 minutes of initiating the meal.

Actions of insulin

A. Metabolic effects
B. Effects on ion transport
C. Role in cell growth and development.

A. Metabolic effects of insulin

The insulin plays a key role in the metabolism of carbohydrates, lipids and proteins. The major targets for insulin actions are the muscle mass, the liver and adipose tissue.

1. *Effects on carbohydrate metabolism.* Insulin decreases blood glucose concentration by following mechanisms:

1. *Insulin increases uptake of glucose in target cells.*

2. *Insulin promotes glucose utilization by :*
- *Glycolysis* (oxidation of glucose) is increased in muscle and liver by insulin.
- *Glycogen* formation (glycogenesis) from glucose in muscle and liver is promoted by insulin.

3. *Insulin decreases glucose production* by inhibiting:
- Gluconeogenesis, and
- Glycogenolysis.

2. *Effects on lipid metabolism.* The metabolism of both endogenous and exogenous fat is profoundly influenced by insulin in target tissues—liver, adipose tissue and muscle.

  i. Insulin increases lipogenesis
 ii. Insulin decreases lipolysis
iii. Insulin reduces ketogenesis
 iv. Effect of insulin on lipoprotein metabolism. It appears that insulin is required for the utilization of VLDL and LDL.

From the effects of insulin on carbohydrate and fat metabolism described above, it is obvious that insulin regulates use of glucose and FFA for energy production.

3. *Effects of insulin on protein metabolism.* Insulin is an anabolic hormone; it stimulates protein synthesis and inhibits protein degradation.

B. Effects of insulin on ion transport

Insulin increases K^+, PO_4^{3-} and Mg^{2+} uptake into the skeletal muscle cells and of K^+ and PO_4^{3-} into hepatic cells from ECF by increasing membrane permeability.

Another effect of insulin on electrolytic balance is to increase reabsorption of K^+, PO_4^{3-} and Na^+ by the tubules of the kidney.

C. Role of insulin in cell growth and development

Insulin is an important factor for growth and development with following roles:

- *Anabolic action* of insulin is as important as growth hormone for promotion of normal growth.
- *Direct stimulatory effect on macromolecules.* Insulin also stimulates the synthesis of macromolecules in tissues such as cartilage and bone; and thereby directly contributes to body growth.
- *Stimulation of other growth factors* such as somatomedins (insulin-like growth factors 1 and 2, i.e. IGF-1 and IGF-2), epidermal growth factor (EGF), nerve growth factor (NGF), and relaxin.

GLUCAGON

Glucagon secreted by α-cells of islets of Langerhans Basal levels of glucagon in a normal fasting individual are 100-150 pg/ml.

Actions of glucagon

The actions of glucagon, in almost all respects, are exactly opposite to those of insulin. It promotes mobilization of stored nutrients such as glucose, fatty acids, and ketoacids and thus is a hormone of energy release. Its metabolic effects are as follows:

1. *Effects on carbohydrate metabolism.* Glucagon predominantly acts on the liver and increases the blood sugar level by following actions:

i. It increases glycogenolysis.

ii. It increases gluconeogenesis.

2. *Effects on lipid metabolism.* Glucagon is a powerful *lipolytic agent.* It activates lipase in adipose tissue which releases FFA and glycerol into the circulation. In the liver, excess of FFAs are oxidised resulting in energy production and ketone body synthesis (ketogenesis). Thus glucagon is a ketogenic as well as a hyperglycaemic hormone.

3. *Effects on protein metabolism.* Glucagon increases the amino acid uptake of liver, which in turn promotes gluconeogeneis. Thus, glucagon *lowers plasma amino acids*.

4. *Calorigenic effect.* Glucagon also has a calorigenic effect. This effect is probably related to increased hepatic deamination of amino acids.

5. *Other actions of glucagon.* Other miscellaneous actions of glucagon include:

- Inhibition of renal tubular sodium reabsorption, resulting in natriuresis.
- Modest increase in force of contraction of the heart.
- Stimulation of secretion of growth hormone, insulin and pancreatic somatostatin.
- Glucagon may act locally in the regulation of appetite.

Regulation of glucagon secretion

I. Role of blood levels of nutrients

There exists a feedback relationship between blood levels of glucagon and nutrients (Fig. 10.5-3).

1. *Blood glucose level.* Hypoglycaemia causes a 2- to 4-fold increase in plasma levels of glucagon (Fig. 10.5-3).

High blood glucose concentration inhibits glucagon secretion (Fig. 10.5-3).

2. *Plasma amino acids.* Secretion of glucagon is increased by a protein-rich meal.

3. *Free fatty acids and ketoacids.* Glucagon stimulates production and release of free fatty acids (FFA) and ketoacids, which in turn suppress glucagon secretion, i.e. there is a feedback relationship (Fig. 10.5-3).

II. Role of gastrointestinal hormones

Gastrointestinal (GT) hormones such as CCK-PZ, gastrin and GIP increase glucagon secretion.

Fig. 10.5-3. *Feedback relationship between glucagon and nutrients. Glucagon stimulates production and release of glucose, free fatty acids and ketoacids, which in turn suppress glucagon secretion, and glucagon in turn stimulates the conversion of amino acids to glucose.*

III. Role of nervous system

Sympathetic nerve stimulation to pancreas increases glucagon secretion. Various stresses, fasting, exercise and infection increase the glucagon secretion in part by their stimulatory effect on sympathetic nervous system and partly by release of glucocorticoids.

Vagal stimulation and acetylcholine also acutely increase glucagon secretion.

Neurohormone, somatostatin, inhibits the secretion of glucagon.

SOMATOSTATIN AND PANCREATIC POLYPEPTIDE

SOMATOSTATIN

Structure and synthesis. Pancreatic somatostatin is a neuropeptide, synthesized by δ cells.

Regulation of secretion. Somatostatin secretion is increased after ingestion of food, because increased blood glucose, amino acids, fatty acids and gastrointestinal tract hormones stimulate its secretion. Glucagon, β-adrenergic and cholinergic neurotransmitters also stimulate somatostatin secretion. Insulin and α-adrenergic neurotransmitters inhibit somatostatin secretion.

Actions. Somatostatin has following effects:

- Acts on the islets of Langerhans and inhibits secretion of insulin and glucagon.
- Increases the motility of stomach, duodenum and gall bladder.
- Decreases secretion of hydrochloric acid, pepsin, gastrin, secretin, intestinal juices and panceatic juice.
- Inhibits the absorption of glucose, xylose, and triglycerides across the mucosal membrane.

PANCREATIC POLYPEPTIDE

It is synthesized by PP cells of islets of Langerhans.

Its secretion is also stimulated by hypoglycaemia and inhibited by glucose administration.

Actions and physiological importance. Its best known action is to inhibit exocrine pancreatic secretion. Its true physiological importance is not known.

HORMONAL REGULATION OF BLOOD GLUCOSE LEVEL

A healthy individual is capable of maintaining the blood glucose level within a narrow range.

- Fasting blood glucose level in a postabsorptive state varies between 70-110 mg%.
- Postprandial blood glucose level, i.e. after a large carbohydrate meal or following oral administration of glucose in the dose of 1 gm/kg body weight, the blood glucose level increases to about 140 mg% (less than 150 mg%) in a period of less than 1 hr. However, this response to oral administration of carbohydrate, when plotted on a time scale, is called *glucose tolerance curve* (Fig. 10.5-4) and is used clinically as a test to study the maintenance of blood glucose levels.

Role of hormones in regulation of blood glucose

Under normal circumstances the various hormones play a significant role in maintaining the blood glucose levels within normal physiological range. This is accomplished by preventing the occurrence of hyperglycaemia and hypoglycaemia.

Prevention of occurrence of hyperglycaemia

The occurrence of hyperglycaemia after a pure carbohydrate load or a mixed meal in a healthy individual is prevented by a manifold (4-5 times) increase in insulin secretion (for details see actions of insulin).

Prevention of occurrence of hypoglycaemia

Hypoglycaemia, which may occur due to fasting or

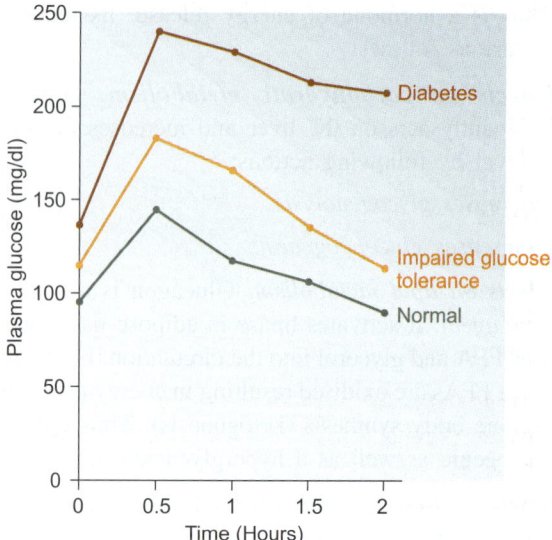

Fig. 10.5-4. *Glucose tolerence curve.*

prolonged exercise, is prevented in a healthy individual by a number of hormones, which include glucagon, epinephrine, growth hormone and glucocorticoids. It is obvious that there is only one hormone, insulin, which prevents hyperglycaemia, whereas at least four hormones are available for prevention of hypoglycaemia.

APPLIED ASPECTS

Important applied aspects of enodcrine pancreas which need mention are:

- Diabetes mellitus,
- Hypoglycaemia.

DIABETES MELLITUS

Diabetes mellitus is a clinical syndrome of hyperglycaemia occurring due to deficiency of insulin.

Types and stages of diabetes mellitus

Diabetes mellitus can be classified into following types:

1. *Primary diabetes mellitus* in which cause is not known. It is of further two types:

- Insulin-dependent diabetes mellitus (IDDM), and
- Non-insulin-dependent diabetes mellitus (NIDDM).

2. *Secondary diabetes mellitus.* It is associated with certain pathological conditions such as pancreatitis, cystic fibrosis, acromegaly, Cushing's syndrome, etc.

Insulin-dependent diabetes mellitus

Insulin-dependent diabetes mellitus (IDDM), or type I diabetes, is considered an autoimmune disorder in which antibodies destroy the β cells of islets causing an absolute deficiency of insulin.

Characteristic features of IDDM are:

- It manifests before 40 years of age (usually between 12-15 years) and is also called juvenile onset diabetes. It accounts for 10-20%.
- Patients are usually lean.
- Classical triad of presenting symptoms consisting of polyuria, polydipsia and polyphagia is associated with weight loss.
- Ketosis and acidosis are common complications of this diabetes mellitus.
- Plasma insulin levels are very low or undetectable.

Non-insulin-dependent diabetes mellitus

Non-insulin-dependent diabetes mellitus (NIDDM) or type II diabetes is also a genetic disorder. It is supposed to occur due to decrease in insulin receptors on the insulin responsive (target) cells.

Characteristic features of NIDDM are:

- It manifests after 40 years of age and so is also called as *adult onset diabetes*.
- It is most common and accounts for 80-90% of diabetic population.
- Most of the patients are obese.
- Symptoms begin gradually and may be ignored and many a time diagnosis is made on urine examination which shows glycosuria.
- Plasma insulin levels are often normal or even elevated.
- Ketoacidosis is not very common.

IDDM versus NIDDM

The comparison between IDDM and NIDDM is given in Table 10.5-2.

Pathophysiology of diabetes mellitus

Pathophysiology of diabetes mellitus revolves around the metabolic alterations associated with insulin deficiency. Most important among them are hyperglycaemia, ketoacidosis, hypertriglyceridaemia and protein catabolism.

Hyperglycemia and its consequences

Hyperglycaemia (elevation of blood glucose concentration) is the characteristic feature of uncontrolled diabetes mellitus. It occurs due to lack of insulin. The consequences of hyperglycaemia are :

- *Glycosuria*, i.e. excretion of glucose into the urine.
- *Polyuria*, i.e. passage of large amount of urine frequently.
- *Loss of electrolytes* (sodium, potassium and phosphate) in urine.
- *Cellular dehydration*. High glucose concentration increases osmotic pressure of extracellular fluid and osmotic transfer of water from cells to extracellular fluid leading to dehydration of cells.
- *Polydipsia*, i.e. excessive drinking of water, results from activation of thirst.
- *Increased caloric loss* is the result of loss of glucose in urine.

Table 10.5-2. IDDM versus NIDDM

Feature	IDDM	NIDDM
General features		
Defect	Insulin deficiency due to β-cell destruction	Resistance of target tissues to insulin
Prevalence	10-20% of diabetic population	80-90% of diabetic population
Age of onset	< 40 years	> 40 years
Body weight	Low (thin and lean)	High (obese or normal)
Gene locus	Chromosome 6	Chromosome 1
Family history	Mild or moderate	Very strong
Clinical features		
Duration of symptoms	Weeks (rapid)	Months to year (slow)
Presenting symptoms	Polyuria, polydypsia, polyphagia complications	Usually patients present with different
Complication at the time of diagnosis	Absent	Present (in 10-20% cases)
Acute complication	Ketoacidosis	Hyperosmolar coma
Biochemical features		
Plasma insulin	Decreased or absent	Normal or increased
Autoantibodies	Frequently found	Rare
Ketonuria	Present	Absent
Treatment		
Treatment of choice	Insulin (oral hypoglycaemics not useful) not required)	Oral hypoglycaemics (insulin usually
Mortality, if not treated	High	Low

C
H
A
P
T
E
R

10.5

- *Polyphagia*, i.e. excessive eating, occurs due to stimulation of satiety centre.
- *Loss of body weight* occurs because of loss of calories in the urine and mobilization of fats and proteins for energy production.

HYPOGLYCAEMIA

Hypoglycaemia refers to a clinical condition caused by blood glucose levels below 45 mg% (2.5 mmol/L).

Symptoms and signs of hypoglycaemia

Symptoms and signs of hypoglycaemia occur due to effects of low levels of glucose per se (mainly on nervous system especially brain) and because of sympathetic stimulation (mainly on CVS, GIT and skin).

1. *CNS* symptoms are called *neuroglycopenic symptoms*. Since metabolism of brain mainly depends on blood glucose level, it is depressed when glucose level falls below 50-70 mg%. CNS becomes quite excitable which results in hallucinations, extreme nervousness, tremors, confusion, difficulty in concentration, inco-ordination, convulsions, and drowsiness. When blood glucose levels fall further (<30 mg%) hypoglycaemic coma may develop, which needs to be differentiated from hyperglycaemic coma in diabetics, and needs an emergency treatment by immediate administration of large quantity of glucose intravenously.

2. *CVS* symptoms in hypoglycaemia are palpitation, tachycardia, and cardiac arrhythmias.

3. *GIT* symptoms include nausea and vomiting

4. *Skin* symptoms are sweating and hypothermia.

GASTROINTESTINAL HORMONES

GASTROINTESTINAL HORMONES

General consideration

Gastrointestinal hormones are secreted by the glandular cells scattered in the epithelium of the gastrointestinal tract, mainly stomach and small intestines. These hormones are released into the blood capillaries in response to stimulation by various chemicals (present in the chyme) or mechanically. Through portal circulation the hormone reaches its target region situated nearby in GIT. The gastrointestinal hormones are characterised by two main features.

- Each hormone may affect more than one target tissue, and
- Each target tissue responds to more than one hormone at a time.

For details (see page 261)

HORMONES OF OTHER ORGANS

In addition to main endocrine glands, other organs also have endocrinal functions, e.g. atrial natriuretic peptide (ANP) is secreted by heart, renin by kidney, melatonin by pineal gland and so on.

HORMONES OF THE HEART

The hormones of the heart include :

Atrial natriuretic peptide (ANP). It is the first natriuretic hormone isolated from the heart.

Brain natriuretic peptide (BNP). It is the second natriuretic hormone first isolated from the porcine brain and hence named as BNP. In human it is isolated from the heart.

Actions of ANP include :

i. It increases sodium excretion by increasing glomerular filtration rate, and inhibiting Na^+ reabsorption at the level of renal tubules.

ii. It lowers the blood pressure by :

- Relaxing vascular smooth muscles of arterioles and venules, and
- Increasing capillary permeability.

HORMONES OF THE KIDNEY

The main function of the kidney is excretion of waste products but it also secretes three hormones:
- Renin,
- 1,25 dihydroxycholecalciferol, and
- Erythropoietin.

Renin

Renin is a glycoprotein. In humans, renin is secreted by granular cells of *juxtaglomerular apparatus* of kidney into the blood stream. The only action of active renin is to convert angiotensinogen into angiotensin-1.

1,25-dihydroxycholecalciferol

1,25-dihydroxycholecalciferol or vitamin D, also called calcitriol, is now considered a hormone. 1,25-dihydroxy-cholecalciferol, the active form of vitamin D_3, is synthesized from its precursor called vitamin D_3. It reaches the blood from two different sources :

i. *Dietary sources* include fish, fish liver oil, egg's yolk. Its daily requirement is 400 IU or 10 μg.

ii. *Cutaneous source.* The keratinocytes located in the inner layer of epidermis synthesize vitamin D_3 by action of ultraviolet rays (from sunlight) on 7-dehydroxycholesterol.

The synthesis of 1,25-dihydroxycholecalciferol from vitamin D_3 occurs in the liver and in the kidney.

Functions of 1,25-dihydroxycholecalciferol (calcitriol) are :

i. The main function is to maintain plasma calcium and phosphate levels by acting at three different sites : intestine, bone and kidney.

- It helps in calcium absorption from gut,
- It helps in reabsorption of calcium from renal tubular fluid, and
- On bones it increases bone resorption.

ii. It also plays an important role in regulation of growth and development by production of growth factors.

Erythropoietin

Erythropoietin is a glycoprotein. In adults it is mainly (85%) secreted by juxtaglomerular cells of the kidney with some contribution (15%) from hepatocytes in the liver. The main role of erythropoietin is to stimulate bone marrow for erythropoiesis (for details see page 43).

PINEAL GLAND

Gross anatomy and location. The pineal gland, also known a epiphysis, is a small structure (5 mm × 7 mm) shaped like a pine cone. It is situated in the groove between two superior colliculi in the diencephalic area of brain above the hypothalamus (Fig. 10.5-5). It forms the posterior boundary of the third ventricle.

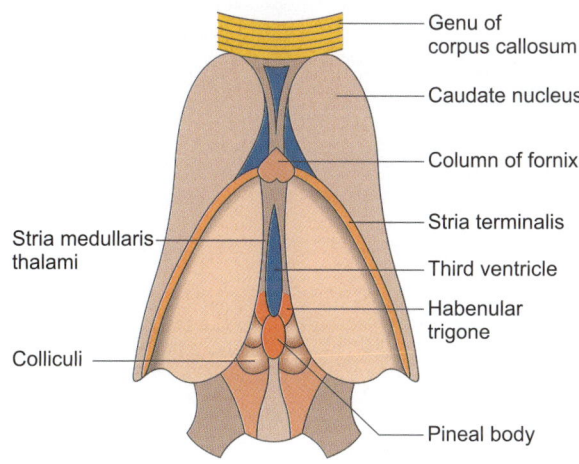

Stria medullaris thalami

Colliculi

Genu of corpus callosum

Caudate nucleus

Column of fornix

Stria terminalis

Third ventricle

Habenular trigone

Pineal body

Fig. 10.5-5. Location of pineal gland in the groove between two superior colliculi.

Structure. The stroma of pineal gland has two types of cells : neuroglial cells and parenchymal cells. The parenchymal cells possess the secretory function.

In infants the pineal gland is quite large and the cells are arranged in alveoli, but

In adults the size of pineal gland decreases and gets calcified i.e. small concretions of calcium phosphate and carbonate (pineal sand) appear in the tissues.

Melatonin

The hormone melatonin is synthesized by parenchymal cells of the pineal gland from tryptophan.

Functions of melatonin are :

i. *Role in circadian rhythm of the body.* The melatonin secretion shows diurnal variations i.e. it is secreted more in the dark period than in the light period of the day-night cycle. This correlates with various internal activities in different periods of the day, i.e. *circadian rhythm.*

ii. *Effect on the gonads.* Melatonin exerts both inhibitory and facilitatory effects on the gonads due to diurnal change in melatonin secretion. It inhibits onset of puberty.

iii. *Effect on MSH and ACTH secretion.* Melatonin decreases the secretion of these hormones.

iv. *Sleep.* Melatonin has role in induction of sleep.

LOCAL HORMONES

Local hormones are the substances which are produced in many tissues, and execute their actions in the same area or in immediate neighbourhood. Commonly produced local hormones are :

Prostaglandins and related substances

Prostaglandins and related substances such as thromboxanes, prostacyclins, leukotriens are lipid in nature and are synthesized from *arachidonic acid.* Prostaglandins are named so because first of all these were isolated from prostatic fluid of semen. However, now they are known to be synthesized in almost all the tissues of the body. Prostaglandins have multitudinous physiological effects in:

- Inflammatory response.
- Regulation of blood pressure.
- Initiates labour by stimulating ueterine contractions.
- Role in blood coagulation; prostaglandins inhibit platelet aggregation.
- Regulation of blood flow to kidneys.
- Potentiate pain during inflammation.
- Inhibit secretion of gastric HCl.

Thromboxane A$_2$ is synthesized by platelets. It promotes:

- Vasoconstriction, and
- Platelet aggregation.

Prostacyclin is produced in vascular endothelium. It produces vasodilatation.

Leukotrienes are mediators of allergic responses and inflammation. These are released when specific allergens combine with antibodies on the surface of mast cells. They produce bronchoconstriction, arteriolar constric-tion and increase vascular permeability.

Histamine

This hormone is synthesized by basophils in the blood and mast cells in the tissues. It is released during inflammatory response and is responsible for increasing capillary permeability. Histamine also causes:

- Contraction of smooth muscles of bronchi.
- Stimulation of gastric HCl secretion and gut motility.

Serotonin (5-HT)

Serotonin (5-Hydroxytryptamin, 5-HT) is present in blood platelets, in brain tissue and in intestinal wall. It plays important role in haemostasis (see page 65), in GIT secretions and motility.

Other local hormones

These include acetylcholine, ADP, AMP, plasma polypeptides (angiotensin, plasma kinins, e.g. bradykinin).

Reproductive Systems

Sexual Growth and Development

PREPUBERTAL SEXUAL GROWTH AND DEVELOPMENT

Reproduction is a multidimensional subject with physiological, biochemical, genetic, psychological, emotional, social, economic, moral and many other aspects. The physiology of reproductive system begins with sexual growth which involves two processes:
- Sex determination, and
- Sex differentiation.

SEX DETERMINATION

Sex determination, also known as genetic differentiation, refers to the genotype of the fetus, whether male or female. The genotype is determined by the presence of sex chromosomes, hence also known as *chromosomal sex differentiation*.

Human chromosomes. Each cell (except ovum and sperm) in a normal adult male and female possesses 46 chromo-

somes (44 autosomes + 2 sex chromosomes) usually arranged in an arbitrary pattern (karyotype).
- *Sex chromosomes* are called X and Y chromosomes.
- *The females* possess 44 autosomes plus 2 X chromosomes (44 + XX).
- *The males* possess 44 autosomes plus 1 X chromosome and 1 Y chromosome (44 + XY).

Human gametes. The mature male gametes are called sperms and mature female gametes are called ova. During gametogenesis there occurs meiosis (*reduction division*); therefore the mature sperm and ovum contain half the number of chromosomes, i.e. 23 (22 autosomes + one sex chromosome). This is called *haploid* number.
- Since, the primitive female germ cells (*oogonia*) from which mature ova are formed contain 44 + XX chromosomes, so each ovum will contain 22 + X chromosomes (Fig. 11.1-1).
- The primitive male germ cells (spermatogonia) from which mature sperms are formed contain 44 + XY

SECTION 11

chromosomes, so half of the normal sperms will contain 22 + X and other half will have 22 + Y chromosomes (Fig. 11.1-1).

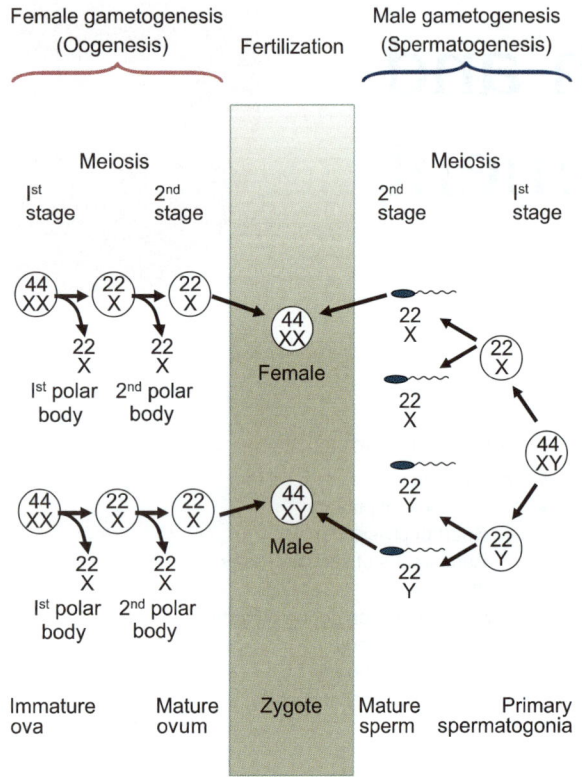

Fig. 11.1-1. Basis of genetic sex determination.

Genetic sex determination of the embryo occurs during fertilization, i.e. penetration of the ovum by the sperm as:

- When an ovum (22 + X) is fertilized by a sperm containing 22 + X chromosomes, the resultant zygote's chromosomal pattern will be 44 + XX (*female genotype*).
- When an ovum (22 + X) is fertilized by a sperm containing 22 + Y chromosomes, the resultant zygote's chromosomal pattern will be 44 + XY (*male genotype*).

SEX DIFFERENTIATION

After fertilization, the normal sex differentiation in the embryo proceeds sequentially. The stages of sex differentiation are:

- Gonadal differentiation,
- Genital differentiation, and
- Psychological differentiation.

Gonadal differentiation

Gonadal differentiation or *gonadogenesis* refers to formation of gonads, i.e. testes in males and ovaries in females. Gonadal sex differentiation is dependent on the genotype of the embryo.

Testicular differentiation. In genetic male (44 + XY) embryo, the bipotential gonads begin to differentiate into testes at approximately 6th week. The Y chromosome plays key role in the process of testicular differentiation. The gene responsible for testicular differentiation is called SRY gene (sex-determining region of Y-chromosome). The SRY gene encodes the *testis determining factor* (TDF) which triggers the testicular differentiation.

Ovarian differentiation. In genetic female (44 + XX) embryo, by about 10th week of gestation, ovarian differentiation occurs in the absence of testis determining factor (TDF). The ovaries develop on each side from the cortical region of the bipotential gonad.

Genital differentiation

Genital sex differentiation, also known as *phenotypic sex* differentiation, refers to the differentiation of internal, and external genitalia.

Differentiation of internal genitalia

The primordia of internal genitalia are a paired set of Wolffian (male) ducts and a paired set of Mullerian (female) ducts. By 7th week of gestation, the embryo has both male and female primordial ducts (Fig. 11.1-2A).

Differentiation of male internal genitalia. In the genetic male fetus (44 + XY) with functioning testes (Fig. 11.1-2B), the testosterone secreted by the Leydig cells stimulate the Wolffian ducts to form the epididymis, vas deferens and seminal vesicles. The Mullerian inhibiting substance (MIS) (encoded by gene present on Y chromosome) causes regression of the Mullerian ducts by apoptosis.

Differentiation of female internal genitalia (Fig. 11.1-2C). In the genetic female fetus (44 + XX), in the absence of MIS, the female ducts (Mullerian ducts) proliferate and form oviduct (uterine tubes), uterus and upper two-thirds of vagina. In the absence of testosterone Wolffian ducts degenerate.

Differentiation of external genitalia

The external genitalia in both sexes develop from *common anlagen*, which are the urogenital sinus, the genital sinus, the genital tubercle, the genital swelling, and the genital (urethral) folds (Fig. 11.1-3). The external genitalia derived from the common anlagen in male and female are shown in Table 11.1-1.

Psychological differentiation

Psychological sex differentiation refers to normal sexual behaviour in adult male and female. It is determined by the effect of androgens on the development of brain in the embryonic stage.

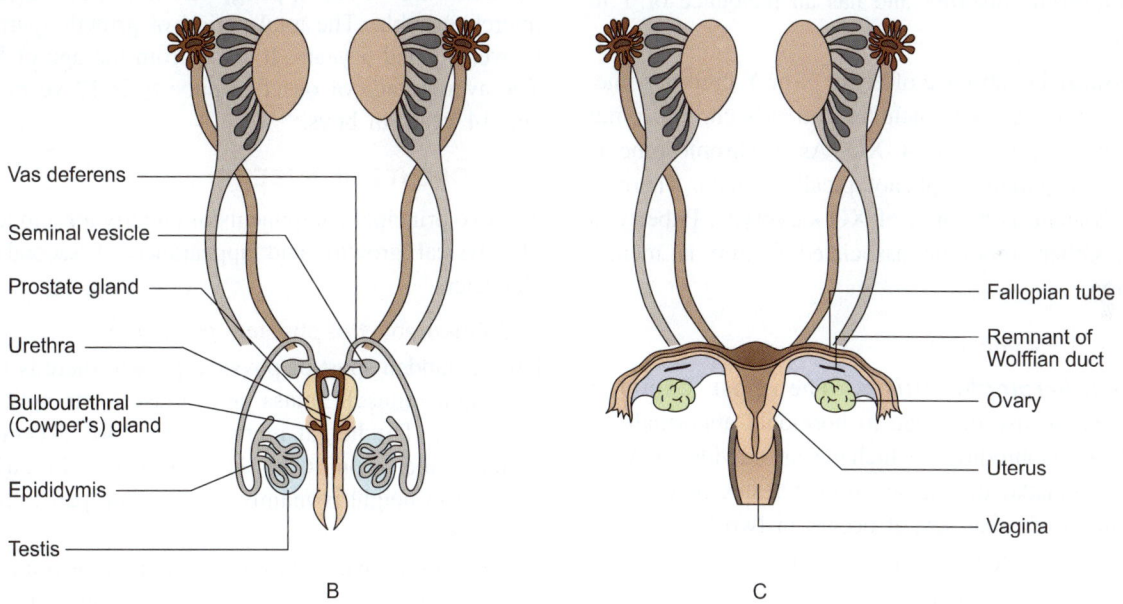

Fig. 11.1-2. *Development of male (B) and female (C) internal genitalia from primordial genital ducts (A).*

Table 11.1-1. The male and female external genitalia derived from the common anlagen

Anlagen part	Male derivative	Female derivative
Urogenital sinus	Prostate and prostatic urethra	Urethra
Urethral fold	Penile urethra and shaft of penis	Labia minora
Genital swelling	Scrotum	Labia majora
Genital tubercle	Glans penis	Clitoris

DISORDERS OF SEXUAL DEVELOPMENT

Abnormalities of sexual development occur due to:

- Defect in sex chromosomes leading to genetic abnormalities,
- Hormonal abnormalities leading to defect in gonadal and genital differentiation.

Chromosomal abnormalities

1. Trisomy. Chromosomal abnormalities usually arise during gametogenesis due to *nondisjunction* of sex

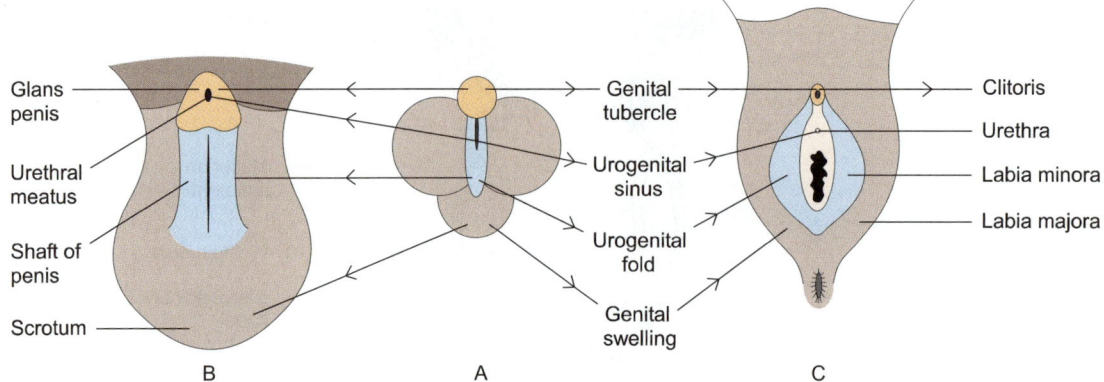

Fig. 11.1-3. *Differentiation of external genitalia in male (B) and female (C) from common anlagen (A).*

chromosomes. The presence of extra X or Y chromosome (trisomy) gives rise to many syndromes associated with abnormal development, mental retardation and abnormal growth. For example, individual with XXY pattern of chromosomes *(Klinefelter syndrome)* is an abnormal male due to presence of Y chromosome. It is the most common sex chromosome disorder and has an incidence of 1 in 500 males.

2. *Monosomy* i.e. absence of either X or Y chromosome, e.g., *Turner's syndrome* includes patient's chromosomal pattern (karyotype) as 44 + XO. As Y chromosome is absent hence patient is phenotypically female. There is ovarian dysgenesis because of XO karyotype. Puberty is delaycd. Other important associated feature is mental retardation.

Hormonal abnormalities

1. *Pseudohermaphroditism.* The most common developmental disorders due to hormonal abnormalities is pseudohermaphroditism, which means individual having genotype (gonads) of one sex (either testes or ovaries) and genitalia of other sex. It occurs in two forms:

- Female pseudohermaphroditism, and
- Male pseudohermaphroditism.

2. *True hermaphroditism.* It is a very rare condition, in which gonads of both sexes are present (an ovary on one side and testis on other side), thus resulting in numerous variations in phenotypic (internal and external genitalia) differentiation.

PUBERTY AND ADOLESCENCE

INTRODUCTION

Puberty and adolescence are the phases of growth between childhood and adulthood.

- *Puberty* refers to the stage of gonadal development and maturation to the point where reproduction is possible for the first time.
- *Adolescence* refers to the period of sudden spurt of physical growth between childhood and adulthood.

Since these two phases (adolescence and puberty) of growth are overlapping, hence the terms are interchangeable. The total period of growth spurt ranges between 3 and 5 years. It starts from the age of 8 years. The average age of onset of puberty is 12 years in girls and 14 years in boys.

COMPONENTS OF PUBERTY

The two principal components of puberty are sudden spurt of physical growth, and appearance of secondary sex characters.

1. Sudden spurt of physical growth

During sudden spurt of physical growth there is increase in height, muscle mass and muscle strength of an individual. The height increases by 7 to 12 centimetres in boys and about 6 to 11 centimetres in girls. The increase in height is mainly of the trunk part rather than of limbs.

The muscle mass and muscle strength also increase in both the sexes but the increase is far greater in boys as compared to girls.

2. Appearance of secondary sex characters

Stages of development of secondary sex characters. The sequence of events of puberty which occurs in 3 to 5 years period have been discussed in 5 stages (Table 11.1-2).

Types of secondary sex characters. The secondary sex characters are almost fully developed by the stage 5 of the puberty both in males and females. These can be grouped as (Table 11.1-3):

- Structural,
- Functional, and
- Psychological.

Table 11.1-2. Sequence of events during puberty in male and female

Stage of puberty	In females		In males	
	Bone age in years	Characteristics	Bone age in years	Characteristics
Stage 1	Upto 7½	Pre-adolescent age	7½ years	Pre-adolescent age
Stage 2	10½	Appearance of breast buds (thelarche)	12	Genital development begins (enlargement of testis)
Stage 3	11½	(i) Axillary and pubic hair appear (pubarche) (ii) Enlargement of breast (elevation) (iii) Sudden increase in height (height spurt)	14	(i) Axillary and pubic hairs start appearing (ii) Enlargement of penis
Stage 4	13	(i) Menstruation starts (menarche) (ii) Breast areola begins to elevate and project	15	(i) Further growth of testis, penis and genitalia (ii) Sudden increase in height (height spurt)
Stage 5	14	(i) Adult genitalia (ii) Secondary sex characters	16½	(i) Adult genitalia (ii) Secondary sex characters

Table 11.1-3. Secondary sex characters in female and male

Group	In female	In male
A. Structural:		
(i) Body configuration	Narrow shoulders, broad hips (broad pelvis) Thighs converge Arms diverge (wide carrying angle)	Shoulders are broader than pelvis
(ii) Skin	Skin is smooth and light	Skin is thick, dark and oily (sebaceous glands' secretion thickens and predisposing to acne)
(iii) Hair growth on:		
• Body	Body hair fine and scanty	Body hair rough and dark
• Face	—	Moustaches and beard appear
• Scalp	Thick growth, frontal hairline rounded	Frontal hairline indented at the side
• Pubic region	Concave	Convex and extends towards umbilicus (triangle with apex up)
(iv) Muscularity	Muscles are soft (+)	Muscle bulk and strength is far greater (+++)
(v) Subcutaneous fat	Female distribution of fat due to deposition of fat in breast and hips which gives characteristic curves and contours to the body	
(vi) Genitalia and accessory sex organs	Adult type : • Clitoris increases in size, labia majora and minora get enlarged • Breasts are developed • Uterus and vaginal growth increases and their activity starts	Adult type: • Penis and scrotum increase in size and become pigmented, scrotal skin thickens and rugal folds appear • Prostate, seminal vesicles, bulbourethral glands enlarge and their secretion begins
B. Functional		
(i) Voice	No change (remains soft and shrill)	Larynx enlarges and vocal cords get thickened, therefore, voice becomes loud, bass (low-pitched), deep and breaks
(ii) Basal metabolic rate (BMR)	Lower	5 to 10% higher than female
(iii) RBC count and Hb concentration	Lower	Higher
(iv) Menstrual cycle	Begins	Absent
C. Psychological	Girls are more emotional, shy, introvert and sexually attracted towards males	Behaviour is more aggressive, extrovert, competitive, and interested in opposite sex

HORMONAL CHANGES DURING PUBERTY

Besides ovaries and testes, other endocrinal glands (adrenal, thyroid and anterior pituitary), also grow in size and their activity increases at the onset of puberty. The hormonal changes noticed at the time of puberty are:

1. Gonadotropins. In both sexes the levels of gonadotropins—follicular stimulating hormone (FSH) and luteinizing hormone (LH) secreted from *anterior pituitary gland*—rise slowly from birth of the child upto pre-adolescent age, but at the time of puberty (early teen-age) their levels suddenly increase. In prepubertal stage the gonadrotropin secretion is not under the check of gonadal hormones (oestrogen and testosterone).

2. Adrenal androgens. There is increase in the secretion of adrenal androgens at puberty. The onset of this stage of increase or activation is called adrenarche.

Functions subserved by adrenal androgens at puberty are:

- Growth of pubic and axillary hair in both sexes, and
- Growth of muscle mass and its strength.

3. Growth hormone. Normally from birth upto prepubertal stage the growth hormone secretion is intermittent (a few peaks every 24 hours) but at the time of puberty, though basal level of growth hormone does not rise but there is increase in the frequency and amplitude of the peaks. It is responsible for generalised growth spurt at adolescence (see page 345).

4. Thyroid gland secretions (thyroxine) also increase during puberty. Thyroxine is necessary for normal growth and development (see page 353).

5. Gonadal hormones (sex hormones). There is slow increase in secretion of sex hormones in children between the age of 7 and 10 years. But, there is rapid rise in oestrogen secretion (in girls) and testosterone in boys in early teenage.

DISORDERS OF PUBERTY

Disorders of puberty are related to the time of its onset, e.g.

- Early onset of puberty (precocious puberty), and
- Late onset of puberty (delayed or absent puberty).

1. Precocious puberty

Precocious puberty refers to onset of puberty in a child before 8 years of age. It is more commonly seen in girls. There is early development of secondary sex characters and gametogenesis also starts earlier.

2. Delayed or absent puberty

Puberty is considered to be pathologically delayed in case of female, if menarche does not occur by 17 years of age, or in case of male, testicular development and maturation fails to occur by the age of 20 years.

Delayed puberty is more commonly observed in boys than in girls. Delayed or absent puberty is a matter of great concern when it occurs in following conditions:

- *Failure of hypothalamus/pituitary* to secrete gonadotropins, as in panhypopituitarism.
- *Primary gonadal failure*. It refers to developmental failure or gonadal dysgenesis which occurs in Klinefelter syndrome in males and Turner syndrome in females.

Male Reproductive System

ANATOMY OF MALE REPRODUCTIVE SYSTEM

INTERNAL AND EXTERNAL GENITALIA

The male reproductive system comprises the internal and external genital organs which can be functionally organized as (Fig. 11.2-1):

I. Gonads or primary male sex glands

Gonads or primary male sex glands are a pair of testes. The main functions of the testes are to produce sperms and secrete testosterone (male sex hormone).

II. Accessory sex glands of male reproductive system

1. Seminal vesicles

Seminal vesicles are two lobulated glands situated on either side of the prostate between the urinary bladder and rectum.

- They secrete a thick alkaline fluid that mixes with the sperms as they pass into the ejaculatory ducts and urethra.
- The duct of each seminal vesicle joins the ductus deferens to form the ejaculatory duct.

2. Bulbourethral (Cowper's) glands

Bulbourethral (Cowper's) glands are two pea-sized glands situated on either side of the membranous portion of the urethra a little inferior to the prostate gland. The secretion of these glands precedes ejaculation and adds lubricating and protective mucus to the semen.

3. Prostate gland

Prostate gland is the largest accessory gland of the male reproductive system. It is located immediately inferior to the bladder and internal urethral orifice. It surrounds the first portion of the urethra, known as the *prostatic urethra* (Fig. 11.2-1).

Urinary bladder

Ureter

Seminal vesicle

Ejaculatory duct

Prostate

Bulbo-urethral gland

Vas deferens

Rete testis

Testis

Corpus spongiosum

Urethra

Corpora cavernosa

Glans penis

Fig. 11.2-1. Male reproductive system.

Lobes. The prostate consists of five lobes : two right and left lateral lobes, an anterior lobe, a posterior lobe and a median lobe.

Structure. The prostate is covered by a dense fibrous capsule and consists of glandular units surrounded by fibromuscular tissue that contracts during ejaculation. The glandular tissue consists of tubules which communicate with the urethra by minute orifices.

Functions. It secretes a thin milky fluid which forms 30% the volume of semen and enhances spermatic motility.

III. Ducts of male reproductive system

These include:

Epididymis

It is formed by minute convolutions of the duct of the epididymis, so tightly compacted that they appear solid.
- The efferent duct transports the sperms from the rete testis to the epididymis where they are stored. The sperms can remain viable for a month in the epididymis.
- Secretions of epididymis provide nourishment to the spermatozoa and help them to mature.
- Non-motile spermatozoa become motile after passing through epididymis.

Ductus deferens or vas deferens

It is the continuation of the tail of epididymis. It ends by joining to the duct of seminal vesicle. It serves as a secondary storehouse for spermatozoa which will be released at the time of ejaculation.

Ejaculatory ducts

Each ejaculatory duct is a slender tube that arises by the union of the ductus deferens with the duct of seminal vesicle. The ejaculatory ducts open as minute slit-like opening into the prostatic urethra.

Urethra

The male urethra is a muscular tube (18-20 cm long) that conveys urine from the internal urethral orifice of the urinary bladder to the external urethral orifice at the tip of the glans penis. The urethra also provides an exit for semen (sperms and glandular secretions). The male urethra is divisible into three parts (Fig. 11.2-1) :

Prostatic urethra is embedded within the prostate gland. It is about 3 cm long and extends from the internal urethral orifice to the urogenital diaphragm.

Membranous part is about 1.5 cm long and it passes through the deep perineal space. It is surrounded by the sphincter urethrae externus.

Penile part of urethra runs through the bulb and corpus spongiosum and is about 15 cm long.

IV. Supporting structures of male reproductive system

Spermatic cord

It suspends the testes in the scrotum and contains structures that pass through the inguinal canal to and from the testis viz. ductus deferens, vessels and nerves of the testis.

Scrotum

It is a cutaneous fibromuscular sac (can be considered an outpouching of the lower part of the anterior abdominal wall) which houses testes, epididymis, and the lower ends of the spermatic cords. The smooth muscle layer of the scrotum that is covered by a thin layer of skin disposed in folds or rugae is called the dartos muscle.

The scrotum maintains the temperature lower than the normal body temperature (about 32°C) which is necessary for normal spermatogenesis.

Penis

It is the male copulatory organ and the common outlet for urine and semen.

Parts. Penis can be divided into three parts: root, body and glans penis. The glans penis contains external urethral orifice (meatus) and the sensory end organs that are stimulated during sexual intercourse. The glans penis is covered by prepuce or foreskin formed by the loose skin.

Structure. It is composed of three cylindrical bodies of erectile cavernous tissue—the corpora cavernosa and corpus spongiosum, which are bound together by fibrous strands and covered with skin.

THE TESTES

Gross anatomy

Location. The testes are ovoid bodies suspended by spermatic cords into the scrotum.

Weight. In an adult male, the average weight of each testis is 25 gm (range 10-40 gm). Weight of testis decreases in old age.

Coverings. Each testis, from interior to exterior, is covered by following three layers (Fig. 11.2-2):

i. *Tunica vasculosa.* It is the innermost covering made up of loose connective tissue rich in blood vessels.

ii. *Tunica albuginea.* It is also called capsule of the testis consisting of closely packed collagen fibres intermingling with many elastic fibres.

iii. *Tunica vaginalis* is the outermost covering composed of mesothelial cells.

Blood supply. The arterial blood supply to the testes is by testicular arteries (arise from abdominal aorta).

The venous blood is drained by testicular veins emerging from testes and epididymis and join to form a venous network (pampiniform plexus) consisting of 8-12 veins.

Lymphatic drainage of the testes to lumbar (lateral aortic) and preaortic lymph nodes.

Nerves (innervation) of the testes. The autonomic nerves of the testes arise as testicular plexus of nerves on the testicular artery, which contain vagal *parasympathetic fibres* and *sympathetic fibres* from T_7 segment of the spinal cord.

Structure of testis

Each testis is divided into many lobules by the fibrous septa which project from the mediastinal testis into the tunica albuginea. Each lobule is roughly conical in shape (Fig. 11.2-2A). Each lobule of the testis consists of :

- Seminiferous tubular compartment, and
- Interstitial compartment.

Seminiferous tubular compartment

The seminiferous tubular compartment of each lobule of the testis contains about 2 to 3 seminiferous tubules. The seminiferous tubules constitute about 80 to 90 per cent of the testicular volume.

Each seminiferous tubule is about 80 centimetres long and 150 μm in diameter. It consists of two parts: the convoluted part and the straight part. The convoluted part forms the loops and continues as two straight ends. Near the apex of the lobules the straight ends join one another to form 20-30 larger straight tubules (tubule recti). The straight tubules pass through the fibrous tissue of mediastinal

A

Vas deferens
Head of epididymis
Tunica vasculosa
Tunica albuginea
Tunica vaginalis
Epididymis
Seminiferous tubule
Ductuli efferentes
Tail of epididymis
Septa
Scrotal sac
Duct of epididymis

B

Leydig cell
Seminiferous tubules
Spermatogenic cells
Spermatozoa
Basal lamina
Cell of Sertoli

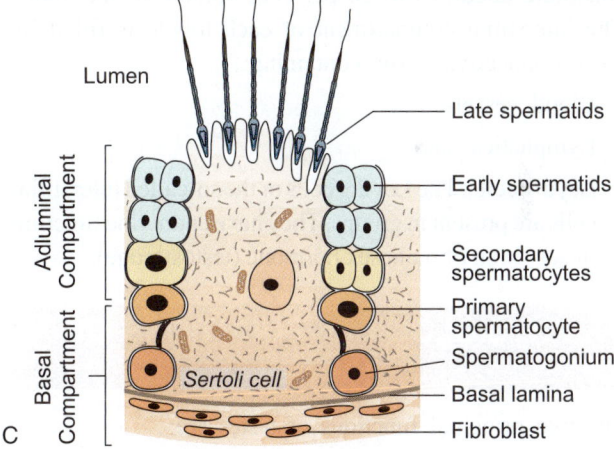

C

Lumen
Late spermatids
Early spermatids
Secondary spermatocytes
Primary spermatocyte
Spermatogonium
Basal lamina
Fibroblast
Sertoli cell
Adluminal Compartment
Basal Compartment

Fig. 11.2-2. *Structure of testis : A, lateral view showing the cut section of testis, epididymis and distal part of spermatic cord; B, histology of testis; C, detailed structure of seminiferous tubule.*

testis and unite to form a network called rete testis. At the upper end of each testis the rete testis gives off 10-20 efferent ductules which continue into the head of epididymis (Fig. 11.2-2A).

Histological structure of seminiferous tubule. Histologically, the wall of seminiferous tubules is comprised of three layers (Fig. 11.2-2B):

1. *Outer capsule or tunica propria*. It consists of fibroelastic connective tissue containing few muscle-like cells (myoid cell). The contraction of myoid cells help in movement of spermatozoa along the wall of the seminiferous tubules.
2. *Basement membrane (basal lamina)*. It is a thin homogenous lamina lying next to the tunica propria.
3. *Epithelial layer* of the seminiferous tubules. This is complex stratified epithelium. The epithelium contains mainly two types of cells:

- Spermatogenic cells lie in between the Sertoli cells. These are arranged in an orderly manner in 4 to 8 layers.
- Sertoli cells are supporting cells. The functions attributed to Sertoli cells are :
  - Physical support and nutrition,
  - Phagocytic function,
  - Maintain blood-testis barrier, and
  - Secrete hormones and substances e.g. inhibin, androgen-binding protein (ABP) and Mullerian duct inhibitory factor (MIF).

Interstitial compartment

The interstitial spaces between the seminiferous tubules constitute about 10 to 20 per cent volume of the testis. The interstitial compartment of each lobule is filled by loose connective tissue containing:

- Blood vessels,
- Lymphatics, and
- Leydig cells. The Leydig cells or the so-called interstitial cells are present in groups. They have endocrine function of secretion of male sex hormone (testosterone).

PHYSIOLOGICAL FUNCTIONS OF TESTES

The two principal functions of testes are:
- Gametogenic function (spermatogenesis), and
- Endocrine function.

SPERMATOGENESIS

Spermatogenesis refers to the process of formation of spermatozoa from the primitive germ cells (spermatogonia).

PHASES OF SPERMATOGENESIS
The phases of spermatogenesis are as follows (Fig. 11.2-3):

1. *Phase of mitotic division of spermatogonia*. Each spermatogonium divides mitotically 5 times to form 32 spermatogonia.

2. *Phase of formation of primary spermatocytes by mitotic division*. The 32 spermatogonia (44 + X + Y) undergo mitosis to form 64 primary spermatocytes (44 + X + Y). Primary spermatocytes are large cells with large nucleus having diploid number of chromosomes (2n).

3. *Phase of formation of secondary spermatocyte by meiotic division*. Each primary spermatocyte undergoes meiotic division:

- After first reduction division (meiosis), the 64 tetraploid primary spermatocytes (4n) are converted into 128 primary spermatocytes with diploid number of chromosomes (2n).
- The 128 primary spermatocytes (meiosis) to form 256 secondary spermatocytes having haploid number of chromosomes (n), i.e. either 22 + X or 22 + Y. Therefore, 50% of sperms will have X chromosome and other 50% will have Y chromosome.

4. *Phase of formation of spermatid*. Each secondary spermatocyte divides mitotically to give rise to two spermatids. Thus, a total of 512 spermatids are formed from a single spermatogonium.

5. *Phase of formation of spermatozoon (spermiogenesis)* The spermatids do not divide further but undergo morphological changes to form sperms or spermatozoa.

Structure of spermatozoon
A fully formed spermatozoon is about 55-65 μm in length. It comprises following parts (Fig. 11.2-4):

1. *Head*. The head is about 4-5 μm long, flattened from anterior to posterior. It is oval when seen from the front. It is surrounded by acrosome.

Acrosome is a thick cap-like structure which covers the anterior two-third part of the head. It contains a number of enzymes (hyaluronidase, proteolytic enzymes and acid phosphatase) which help the sperm in penetrating ovum during fertilization.

2. *Neck*. It is a narrow constricted part. It contains a funnel-shaped basal body and a spherical centriole.

3. *Tail* of the sperm is the motile portion and is also called the flagellum. It can be divided into three parts:

- Middle piece,
- Principal piece, and
- End piece.

Storage of spermatozoa
About 120 million sperms are formed each day. A small quantity of them is stored in the epididymis but most of them are stored in vas deferens and ampulla of vas deferens. They can remain stored maintaining their fertility for about a month.

Fig. 11.2-3. *Phases of spermatogenesis.*

Maturation and capacitation of spermatozoa

Role of epididymis. Epididymis is the site of extra testicular maturation of spermatozoa. When the sperms arrive in the epididymis they are non-motile and acquire some motility only after passing through the epididymis.

Role of seminal vesicles and prostate gland. The secretions of seminal vesicles and the prostate have a stimulating effect on sperm motility, but the spermatozoa become fully motile only after ejaculation.

Role of female genital tract. Spermatozoa acquire ability to fertilize the ovum only after they have been in the female genital tract for some time (1 to 10 hours). This final step in their maturation is called capacitation.

SEMEN

Semen or the seminal fluid refers to the fluid ejaculated during the orgasm at the time of male sexual act.

Characteristic features of seman are :

- *Volume.* The average volume of semen per ejaculation is 2.5-3.5 ml after an abstinence of 2 days. Volume of semen decreases with repeated ejaculations.

Fig. 11.2-4. *Structure of mature human spermatozoon.*

- *Appearance* of semen is milky due to prostatic secretions.
- *Specific gravity* is about 1.028.
- *Reaction* is alkaline with a pH of 7.5. The alkalinity is due to prostatic secretions. The alkaline semen brings the vaginal pH from 3.5-4 to 6-6.5, the pH at which sperms show optimum motility.
- *Nature* of the semen when ejaculated is liquid but soon it coagulates in vitro or in the vagina, and finally undergoes secondary liquefaction after about 15 to 30 minutes.

Components of semen. The semen comprises following components:

- Spermatozoa
- Secretions of seminal vesicles
- Secretion of prostate gland
- Secretion of bulbourethral gland.

ENDOCRINE FUNCTIONS OF TESTES (ANDROGENES)

Testes secrete the following androgens (male sex hormones):

1. *Testosterone.* The most important testicular hormone is testosterone secreted by Leydig cells.

- A normal man secretes 4-9 mg of testosterone daily. Plasma testosterone level in adult males is about 0.65

μg%. More than 98% of secreted testosterone is bound to plasma proteins; and a very small percentage of the plasma testosterone is unbound. The free fraction alone is physiologically active in the target tissues.

2. *Androstenedione* is an important steroid precursor for blood oestrogens in men. It is secreted by the testes at a rate of about 2.5 mg/day.

3. *Dihydrotestosterone (DHT)* is another important androgen present in the blood. Only 20% of the plasma DHT is formed in the testes by the action of 5-α-reductase (from the Sertoli cells) on the testosterone (secreted by Leydig cells). About 80% of the plasma DHT is derived from the peripheral conversion of testosterone.

FUNCTIONS OF ANDROGENS

A. Functions of androgens in fetal period (in utero)

The testosterone is secreted by the fetal testes at about 2nd to 4th month of embryonic life. The functions of androgens in fetal period are:

1. *Effect on sex differentiation in fetus.* Genital differentiation is affected by testosterones.

2. *Effect on descent of testes.* The testes developed in the abdominal cavity are pushed into the scrotum through inguinal canal just before birth. Testosterone is necessary for this descent of testes.

B. Functions of androgens at puberty

1. *Effects on external genitalia.* Testosterone causes pubertal enlargement of penis. Scrotum increases in size and becomes pigmented. Rugal folds appear in scrotal skin.

2. *Effect on accessory sex organs.* Testosterone (with or without DHT) causes enlargement of seminal vesicles. DHT promotes growth of prostate and stimulates prostatic secretions.

3. *Development of male secondary sexual characters* in males is due to this hormone (see Table 11-1-3).

4. *Effects on psyche.* Psychological differentiation. A brief exposure of fetal hypothalamus to androgens (from its own testes) during early embryonic period causes male pattern of sexual behaviour during puberty.

- *Aggresssive behaviour.* Testosterone produces aggressive behaviour and interest in the opposite sex.

5. *Anabolic and general growth promoting effects* are: Testosterone causes nitrogen retention in the body and causes accelerated growth of the body and skeletal muscles in particular.

C. Functions of androgens in adults

1. *Hair growth.* Androgenic patterns of hair growth are

maintained. With increasing age, male baldness may be initiated.

2. *Psyche*. Behavioural attitudes and sexual potency are maintained in postpubertal adults.

3. *Bone*. Bone loss and osteoporosis are prevented by the androgens in adult males.

4. *Spermatogenesis* is maintained in adulthood by testosterone along with FSH.

5. *Haematopoiesis*. Testosterone stimulates erythropoiesis. Therefore, it accounts for the greater haemoglobin concentration and RBC count in males.

6. *Effects on circulating and stored body fats*. Testosterone increases circulating levels of low density lipoprotein (LDL) cholesterol and decreases plasma high density lipoprotein (HDL) cholesterol.

7. *Regulation of gonadotropin secretion*. Androgen suppression of LHRH and LH by negative feedback effect.

CONTROL OF TESTICULAR FUNCTIONS

The two main functions of testes viz. spermatogenesis and secretion of testosterone are controlled by the hypothalamic-hypophyseal-testicular axis.

A. CONTROL OF SPERMATOGENESIS

The hypothalamic-hypophyseal-testicular (seminiferous tubular) axis controlling the spermatogenesis is as follows (Fig. 11.2-5):

Fig. 11.2-5. *Stimulatory and feedback inhibitory control of spermatogenesis.*

I. Stimulatory control

1. *Role of hypothalamus*. At puberty there is a pulsatile release (8 to 14 pulses per day) of gonadotropin releasing hormone (GnRH) from the *hypothalamus*. The GnRH stimulates anterior pituitary to secrete LH and FSH.

2. *Role of anterior pituitary*. The anterior pituitary controls spermatogenesis through the gonadotropic hormones (FSH and LH) and growth hormones.

- *Role of follicular stimulating hormone (FSH)*. FSH stimulates cells of Sertoli which help in conversion of spermatids to sperms. FSH indirectly affects testosterone synthesis by increasing the number of LH receptors on the Leydig cells.

- *Role of LH (also called interstitial cell stimulating hormone, i.e. ICSH)*. The LH stimulates Leydig cells to cause testosterone secretion. The testosterone is required for normal spermatogenesis.

- *Role of growth hormone*. Growth hormone specifically promotes early division of the spermatogonia themselves. In its absence, as in pituitary dwarfs, spermatogenesis is severely deficient or absent.

3. *Role of testicular hormones*. The testosterone acts on both Sertoli cells and germ cells and thus maintains spermatogenesis.

II. Feedback inhibitory control

The rapid speed of spermatogenesis is controlled by following negative feedback mechanisms (Fig. 11.2-5):

- Inhibin secreted by Sertoli cells acts directly on the anterior pituitary and inhibits the secretion of FSH.

- Testosterone and oestradiol inhibit LH secretion by negative feedback mechanism.

B. CONTROL OF TESTOSTERONE SECRETION

In fetus

During fetal life, human chorionic gonadotropin (HCG) secreted by placenta stimulates the development of Leydig cells in the testes of fetus and causes testosterone secretion.

In adults

I. *Stimulatory control*. The hypothalamic-hypophyseal-testicular (Leydig cell) axis controls the secretion of testosterone in adults as (Fig. 11.2-6):

- *Hypothalamus* produces gonadotropin releasing hormone (GnRH) which stimulates anterior pituitary to secrete FSH and LH.

- *Anterior pituitary* controls secretion of testosterone (steroidogenesis) primarily through LH.

- *Leydig cells of testes* have LH receptors located on their plasma membrane. LH binds to these receptors to activate cyclic AMP synthesis which triggers testosterone synthesis and its secretion.

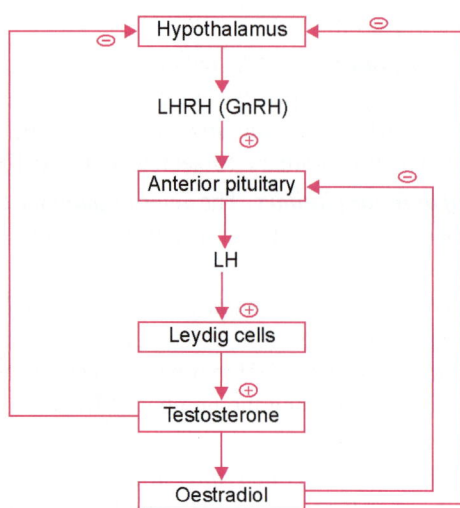

Fig. 11.2-6. *Stimulatory and feedback inhibitory control of secretion of testosterone.*

II. *Feedback inhibitory control.* Plasma testosterone level is maintained at a constant level by a feedback control exerted by testosterone and oestradiol independently to control LH (Fig. 11.2-6).

APPLIED ASPECTS

Some of the important applied aspects, in relation to male reproductive physiology, are:

- Cryptorchidism,
- Hypogonadism in males,
- Hypergonadism in males,

CRYPTORCHIDISM

The testes develop in relation to the lumbar region of the posterior abdominal wall. During fetal life, they gradually descend to the scrotum by the end of the eighth month of gestation. *Cryptorchidism* refers to a condition in which the descent of the testes may fail to occur or may be incomplete.

Characteristic features of cryptorchidism are:

- The undescended testes may lie in the lumbar region, in the iliac fossa, in the inguinal canal, or in the upper part of scrotum.
- Spermatogenesis often fails to occur in cryptorchidism (due to high temperature of the abdominal cavity) resulting in sterility.

HYPOGONADISM IN MALES

Causes. Hypogonadism in males results from absent or deficient testicular functions which may occur in following conditions:

- Congenital non-functioning of testes,
- Underdeveloped testes,
- Cryptorchidism (undescended testes),
- Extirpation of testes, and
- Absence of androgen receptors in testes.

Effects of male hypogonadism depend upon whether the testicular deficiency occurs before or after puberty.

Before puberty hypogonadism leads to permanent sterility, underdevelopment of external genitalia, underdevelopment of secondary sexual characters, and abnormal bone growth.

Hypogonadism *after the onset of puberty leads* to atrophy of accessory sex organs.

HYPERGONADISM IN MALES

Hypergonadism in males results from excessive secretion of male sex hormones (androgens) as occurs in tumours of Leydig cell. It is characterized by:

- Rapid growth of musculature and bones.
- But, the height is less due to early closure of epiphysis.
- There is excessive development of sex organs and secondary sexual characters at an early age.
- The tumours can also secrete oestrogenic hormones which can cause overgrowth of breasts (gynaecomastia).

Female Reproductive System

ANATOMY OF FEMALE REPRODUCTIVE SYSTEM

INTERNAL AND EXTERNAL GENITALIA

The female reproductive system comprises internal and external genitalia which can be organized as (Fig. 11.3-1):

I. Primary sex organs or ovaries

The primary sex organs are a pair of ovaries which correspond with testes in males. The main functions of ovaries are:

- To produce ova, and
- To secrete female sex hormones.

II. Accessory sex organs

The accessory sex organs of females include internal genital organs and external genitalia.

FEMALE INTERNAL GENITALIA

The internal genital organs include uterus, fallopian tubes, and vagina.

I. Uterus

Uterus is a hollow, thick-walled pear-shaped muscular

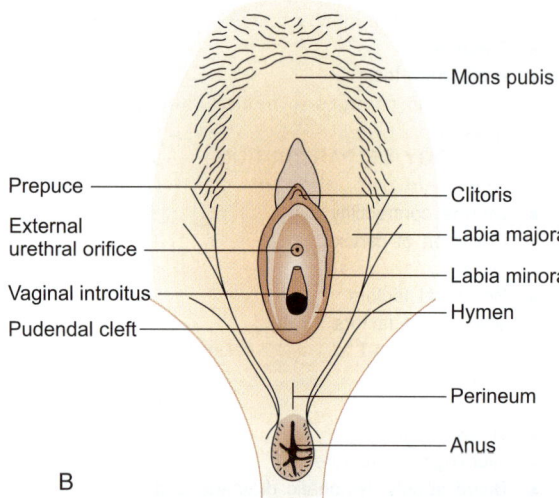

Fig. 11.3-1. *Female reproductive organs : A, lateral view showing position of internal reproductive organs in relation to pelvic viscera; and B, female external genitalia.*

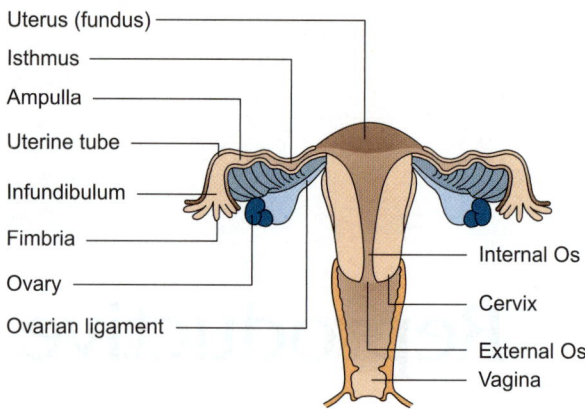

Fig. 11.3-2. *Parts of the uterus and fallopian tube.*

organ, situated in the pelvic cavity between the urinary bladder and rectum. It can be divided into two parts (Fig. 11.3-2):

1. Body of the uterus. It forms upper 2/3rd part of the uterus. Its lower limit is marked by a constriction which corresponds to narrowing of uterine cavity at *internal os*. Body of the uterus can be divided into two parts:

- *Fundus* is the rounded part of the body that lies superior to the openings of the fallopian tubes.
- *Isthmus* is the relatively constricted region of the body (approximately 1 cm long) just above the cervix.

2. Cervix of the uterus. It is the cylindrical lower part which protrudes into the uppermost vagina. It is approximately 2.5 cm long in an adult non-pregnant woman. Its cavity extends from the *internal os* to *external os* which opens into the vagina.

Structure of uterus

The wall of body of uterus consists of three layers (Fig. 11.3-3).

1. Perimetrium is the external serosal layer. It is derived from the peritoneum and covers the superior part of the uterus.

2. Myometrium is the middle muscular layer comprising bundles of smooth muscles amongst which there is connective tissue. Myometrium is about 2 cm thick.

3. Endometrium is inner layer of uterus which consists of epithelial lining and the stroma (Fig. 11.3-4):

- *Epithelial lining* is made up of columnar cells.
- *Stroma* of the endometrium is highly cellular and contains numerous blood vessels and numerous simple tubular uterine glands which are lined by columnar epithelium.

Functional divisions of endometrium. Functionally, the endometrium of body of uterus can be divided into two strata:

1. *Stratum functionale* includes superficial 2/3rd thickness of endometrium which undergoes monthly cyclic changes in preparation for the implantation of fertilized ovum and is shed during menstruation. This portion of endometrium is supplied by long and spiral (coiled) arteries.

2. *Stratum basale* is the deeper 1/3rd layer of endometrium. It does not participate in cyclic changes but functions as regenerative layer. This part of endometrium is supplied by short and straight *basal arteries*.

Structure of cervix of the uterus is somewhat different from that of the body.

1. Perimetrium is the outermost serous layer.

2. Myometrium layer of the cervix is much less muscular as compared to body of uterus, and contains more connective tissue. During childbirth, when the myometrium

Fig. 11.3-3. Histological structure of the body of uterus.

Fig. 11.3-4. Histological structure of the endometrium.

of body of uterus contracts, the myometrium of cervix dilates, consequently the cervical canal becomes large enough for the fetal head to pass through.

3. *Endocervix* refers to the innermost mucosal layer of cervix in contrast to endometrium of the body of uterus. Endocervix is not shed at the time of menstruation. Endocervix consists of:

- *Epithelium.* The mucous membrane of the upper two-thirds of cervical canal is lined by *ciliated columnar epithelium*, but its lower one-third epithelium is non-ciliated columnar. Near the external os the canal is lined by stratified squamous epithelium.
- *Stroma.* The stroma of the cervix is less cellular than that of body of uterus.

Ligaments of uterus

Ligaments are fibrous cords covered with mesothelium and peritoneal folds. These assist in holding the internal reproductive organs in normal position and in anchoring them to the wall and floor of the pelvis. The ligaments of uterus are (Fig. 11.3-5) :

1. *Broad ligaments* are wide peritoneal folds that stretch from the side of the uterus to the side wall and floor of the pelvis on each side.

2. *Round ligaments of uterus* are flattened fibrous cords that extend from the lateral borders of the uterus within the broad ligaments to the connective tissue and skin of the labia majora after passing through the inguinal canals of their respective sides. They help to hold the fundus forward in a slightly anteflexed position.

3. *Uterosacral ligaments* are peritoneal folds that pass from the cervix to the sacrum, and are extending on each side of rectum.

4. *Cardinal ligaments* are enveloping band of fascia that surround the uterine blood vessels as they pass to the vagina and cervix from the lateral pelvis.

5. *Anterior ligament* is the sheath of peritoneum that extends from the urinary bladder to uterus. It does not provide support to the viscera.

6. *Posterior ligament* is the fold of peritoneum reflected from the anterior surface of rectum upon the posterior surface of vagina and uterus. It also does not provide any support to the pelvic floor or viscera.

II. Fallopian tubes

Each fallopian tube (also known as uterine tube) is approximately 10 cm in length and 8 mm in diameter. It has a medial or *uterine end* which is attached to and opens into the uterus and a *lateral end* opens into peritoneal cavity near the ovary.

Parts. Each fallopian tube can be divided into four parts (Fig. 11.3-2):

1. *Uterine or interstitial part* is the most medial part which passes through the thick uterine wall.

2. *Isthmus* is the relatively narrow and thick-walled part which is just next to the uterine part. It is about 2.5 cm in length.

Fig. 11.3-5. *Schematic section to show the relation of female reproductive organs and ligaments of uterus.*

3. *Ampulla* is the next thin-walled and dilated part of the uterine tube. It is the largest part (7 cm) of uterine tube.

4. *Infundibulum* refers to the funnel-shaped lateral end of the tube. It is prolonged into a number of finger-like processes known as fimbria. One fimbria is longer than rest of the fimbriae and is attached to the outer pole of ovary.

Structure. Fallopian tubes consist of same three coats as of the uterus viz. endometrium, myometrium and perimetrium.

Functions. The uterine tubes convey ova, shed by the ovaries, to the uterus. Secretions present in the tubes provide nutrition, oxygen, and other requirements for ova and spermatozoa passing through the tube. Fertilization takes place in the ampulla and the fertilized ovum travels towards the uterus through the tube.

III. Vagina

The vagina is a musculomembranous tube (about 8 to 10 cm long) located anterior to the rectum and posterior to urethra and urinary bladder. Its upper end surrounds the lower part of cervix and forms vaginal recesses around it. These recesses are known as the anterior, posterior and lateral fornices. Its lower end, i.e. vaginal orifice, opens into the vestibule of vagina (the cleft between the labia minora).

Structure. The wall of vagina consists of a mucous membrane, a muscle coat, and an outer fibrous coat or adventitia.

Functions. The vagina serves following functions:
- It serves as the excretory duct for menstrual fluid.
- It forms the inferior part of pelvic (birth) canal.
- It receives the penis and ejaculate during sexual intercourse.

FEMALE EXTERNAL GENITALIA

The external genital organs include mons pubis, labia majora, labia minora, clitoris, vestibule of vagina, bulbs of vestibule and greater vestibular glands (Fig. 11.3-1B).

The synonymous terms vulva and pudendum include all these parts. The vulva serves:
- As sensory and erectile tissue for sexual arousal and intercourse,
- To direct the flow of urine, and
- To prevent entry of foreign material into the urogenital tract.

1. *Mons pubis* is the rounded, fatty prominence anterior to the pubic symphysis, pubic tubercle, and superior pubic rami.

2. *Labia majora* are prominent folds of skin that bound the *pudendal cleft* and thus indirectly provide protection for urethral and vaginal orifices which open into this cleft.

3. *Labia minora* are folds of fat-free, hairless, pinkish skin. They are enclosed in the pudendal cleft and surround the *vestibule of vagina.* They have a core of spongy connective tissue containing erectile tissue and many small blood vessels.

4. *Clitoris* is an erectile organ located where the labia minora meet anteriorly. The clitoris is analogous to male penis, but unlike the penis, the clitoris is not functionally related to the urethra or to urination. It functions solely as an organ of sexual arousal.

5. *Vestibule* is the space between the labia minora that contains the opening of urethra, vagina, and ducts of greater and lesser vestibular glands. The vaginal orifice is surrounded by a thin fold of mucous membrane called *hymen* which is usually ruptured after first intercourse or otherwise. After childbirth, only a few remnants of the *hymen or hymenal caruncles* (tags) are visible.

6. Bulbs of the vestibule are paired masses of erectile tissue which lie along the sides of vaginal orifice under cover of bulbospongiosus muscles. These are homologous with the bulb of the penis and corpus spongiosum.

7. Vestibular glands include a pair each of greater vestibular and lesser vestibular glands. These glands secrete mucus into the vestibule during arousal.

OVARIES

ANATOMY

Gross anatomy

A pair of ovaries are located (one on each side) behind and below the fallopian tubes. The ovaries are ovoid glands with a combined weight of 10-20 gm during reproductive years, which decreases with increasing age. Each ovary is about 3 to 5 cm in length and is attached to the uterus by the broad ligament and round ligament of ovary.

Structure

Histologically, each ovary consists of following parts (Fig. 11.3-6):

1. Germinal epithelium. Germinal epithelium refers to the epithelium lining the outer surface of ovary and consists of a single layer of cuboidal cells. The term germinal epithelium is a misnomer, as it does not produce germ cells.

2. Cortex. The cortex is the outer thick main part of the substance of the ovary. It consists of following tissues:

- Tunica albuginea.
- Stroma.
- Ovarian follicles .

3. Medulla. The medulla is the inner small part of the substance of ovary. It consists of connective tissue in which numerous blood vessels (mostly veins), smooth muscles and elastic fibres are present.

Hilum. The hilum refers to the area where ovary attaches to mesentery. It is the site for entry of blood vessels and lymphatics.

PHYSIOLOGICAL FUNCTIONS OF OVARIES

The two principal functions of ovaries are :
- Gametogenic function, i.e. oogenesis, and
- Endocrine function, i.e. secretion of female hormones called ovarian hormones.

OOGENESIS

Fetal oogenesis

Oogenesis refers to the process of formation of ova from the primitive germ cells.

Primitive germ cells. When the bipotential gonads differentiate into ovaries in genetic female (44 + XX) embryo by 10th week of gestation, the primitive germ cells increase in number by mitosis to form oogonia.

Oogonia are the stem cells from which ova are derived. The oogonia proliferate by mitosis to form primary oocytes.

Primary oocytes, formed from the oogonia, enter a prolonged prophase (*diplotene stage*) of the first meiotic

Fig. 11.3-6. Schematic diagram of the histology of ovary depicting various stages of development of follicles and corpus luteum.

division and remain in this state until ovulation occurs after puberty.

Primordial follicles. The *diploid primary oocytes* become enveloped by single layer of flat granulosa cells and in this form are called *primordial follicles.*

Pubertal oogenesis

- After puberty the oogenesis or formation of ovum occurs in a highly cyclic fashion, once every 28 days till menopause.
- Every month, in each ovary, more than one primordial follicles start undergoing maturation process but only one reaches maturity and the rest undergo atresia at different stages of development. Thus throughout the whole normal reproductive life of about 30 years (from 13 to 42 years) about 450 ova are expelled and the remainder degenerate.
- The different stages of maturation of primordial follicle into graafian follicle (*folliculogenesis*) (Fig. 11.3-7) are:

1. ***Primordial follicles*** are the fundamental reproductive units of ovary. At the time of puberty both ovaries contain about 3,00,000 primordial follicles.

- Each primordial follicle consists of the primary oocyte in prophase of the first meiotic division surrounded by a single layer of spindle-shaped (flat) cells called the granulosa cells.

2. ***Primary follicle.*** The primary follicle is formed when the primordial follicle undergoes following developmental changes (Fig. 11.3-7B):

- *Granulosa cells* become columnar and undergo mitotic division to form a multilayered stratum granulosum.
- *Oocyte enlarges,*
- *Zona pellucida*, a homogeneous membrane, appears.

3. ***Secondary follicle*** is formed from the primary follicle when following changes occur (Fig. 11.3-7C):

- *Granulosa cells* undergo further proliferation.
- *Oocyte* further increases in size upto 100 µ. Its nucleus becomes larger.
- *Theca folliculi* or follicular sheath is formed outside the basal lamina from the spindle-shaped cells from the stroma of cortex in ovary. The theca folliculi consist of an inner rim of secretory cells called *theca interna* and an outer rim of thickly packed fibres and spindle-shaped cells called *theca externa.*

4. ***Tertiary follicle*** is characterized by following features:

- *Formation of antrum.* The granulosa cells start secreting follicular fluid this causes cavity to be formed in the stratum granulosum (cavitation), which is called antrum or follicular cavity. The fluid filled in the antrum is called liquor folliculi which also contains oestrogen (Fig. 11.3-7D).

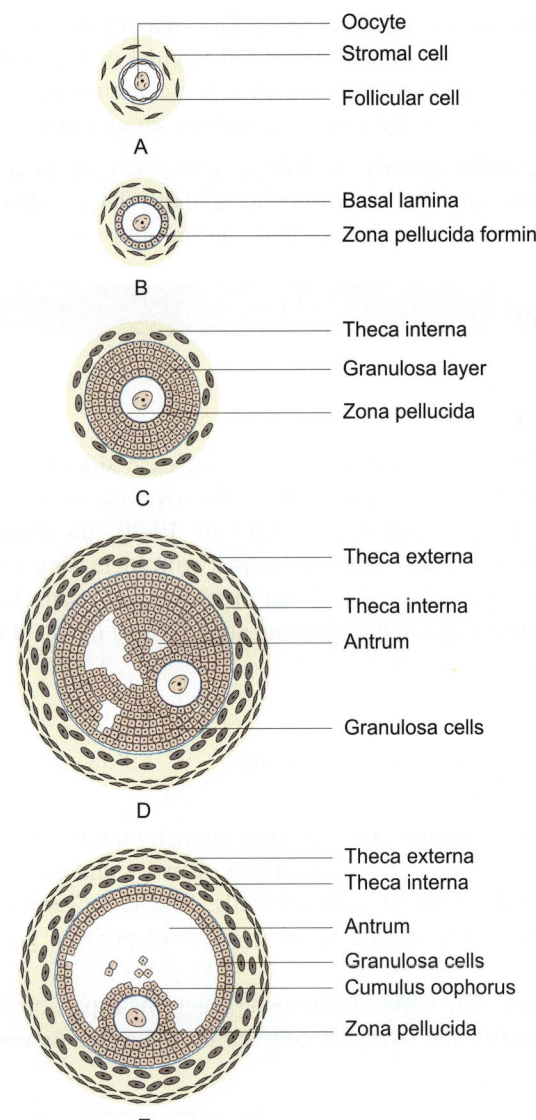

Fig. 11.3-7. *Phases of folliculogenesis.*

ENDOCRINE FUNCTION OF OVARIES

The endocrine function of the ovaries is to produce female sex hormones which include:

- Oestrogens, and
- Progesterone.

OESTROGENS

Oestrogens are C-18 steroids. The naturally occurring oestrogens include:

- *Oestradiol.* It is the principal and physiologically most potent oestrogen. Ovarian oestradiol accounts for more than 90% of the circulating oestrogens.
- *Oestrone.* It is a weak ovarian oestrogen.
- *Oestriol.* It is the degradation product of oestradiol and oestrone. It is the weakest of all naturally occurring oestrogens.

Synthesis, plasma levels, and transport of oestrogens

Sites

In the normal female, oestrogens are mainly secreted by theca interna and granulosa cells of the ovarian follicles. A small quantity is also produced by adrenal cortex, breast, some areas of brain, placenta (during pregnancy), and by Sertoli cells (in males).

Plasma levels

In a normal adult woman the plasma levels of oestrogen vary in different phases of ovarian cycle (Fig. 11.3-8). As shown in Fig. 11.3-8D, there are two peaks of oestrogen secretion. The first occurs just before the ovulation (12-13th day of sexual cycle) and is called *oestrogen surge,* and the second peak occurs in the mid luteal phase. The secretion rate of oestrogen in different phases is:

- In early follicular phase : 36 μg/day,
- Just before ovulation : 380 μg/day, and
- During mid luteal phase : 250 μg/day.

After menopause oestrogen level falls to minimum of 50 μg/day.

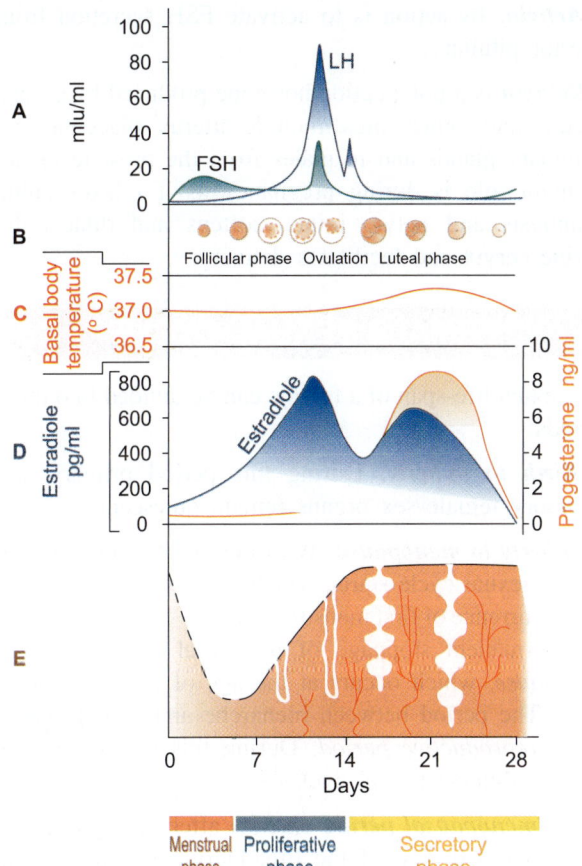

Fig. 11.3-8. *Correlation of plasma concentration of gonadotropins (FSH and LH) (A); ovarian cycle changes (B); basal body temperature (C); ovarian hormones (D); and endometrial changes (E); during female sexual cycle.*

Functions of oestrogens

The functions of oestrogen for descriptive purposes can be grouped as reproductive actions and other actions.

I. Reproductive actions

A. At puberty. At puberty oestradiol is secreted in larger amounts which causes following changes:

1. Growth and development of genital organs

- *Ovaries* increase in size and complete ovarian cycles start.
- *Fallopian tubes* become functional.
- *Uterus.* It enlarges in size, endometrium gets thickened, the rhythmic cyclic changes (proliferative and secretory) occur with onset of menstrual cycle.
- *Cervix* also enlarges and with onset of menstrual cycle, endocervix undergoes cyclic changes.
- *Vagina* increases in size. Its epithelial lining increases in height (from 2-3 layer cuboidal epithelium to 10-12 layers cornified squamous epithelium).
- *External genitalia.* The following changes occur in external genitalia :
  - Increase in size of clitoris,
  - Labia majora and labia minora increase in size and get widened.

2. Appearance of secondary sex characters. Oestrogen is responsible for appearance of secondary sex characters (see page 382):

B. In an adult woman. Oestrogens along with progesterone regulate the ovarian cycle, menstrual cycle and cyclic changes in cervix, vagina and fallopian tubes (see page 403) in non-pregnant state.

- It plays an important role in the maintenance of pregnancy.
- It is important for breast development.

II. Other actions

The other functions of oestrogens include :

1. *Effects on bones.* Oestradiol accelerates the linear growth of bones at puberty.

2. *Effects on metabolism.* Oestrogens cause positive nitrogen balance, and fat deposition in subcutaneous tissues, in the breasts and the thighs.

3. *Water and electrolyte balance.* Oestrogens, like other steroids in general, cause salt and water retention in the body and produce premenstrual tension in some women.

4. *Effects on vasculature.* In general oestrogens have vasodilator and anti-vasoconstrictor effects.

5. *Effects on CNS.* Oestrogens are responsible for oestrous behaviour in animals and also increase the libido in human females.

6. *Effects on skin.* Oestrogens make the skin soft and more vascular. It makes the sebaceous gland secretions thin. Therefore, synthetic oestrogens are used as a part of treatment in acne.

PROGESTERONE

In a normal adult non-pregnant woman progesterone is mainly secreted by corpus luteum and during pregnancy by the placenta. A small amount is also secreted by adrenal cortex.

Plasma levels

In a normal adult woman the plasma levels of progesterone vary with different phases of sexual cycle (Fig. 11.3-8D). *Note.* Throughout the sexual cycle the levels of progesterone are higher than the oestrogens.
During pregnancy the levels of progesterone further rise (see page 406).
After menopause. Progesterone levels fall to its minimum (0.2 ng/ml) or even not detectable.

Functions of progesterone

The physiological actions of progesterone can be grouped as reproductive actions and other actions.

I. Reproductive actions

Reproductive actions are mainly on the reproductive organs primed by oestrogens and these include:

1. *Action on uterus.* The progesterone is responsible for secretory phase of the endometrial cycle and prepares the endometrium to receive the zygote.
   - *Uterine motility.* Progesterone decreases the uterine motility.
2. *Endocervix.* The cervical secretions become thick and viscid, and ferning pattern disappears.
3. *Vagina.* Vaginal epithelium becomes thickened, cornified and infiltrated with leucocytes.
4. *Fallopian tubes.* Progesterone increases the epithelial cell secretions rich in nutritive materials to provide nutrition to shedded ovum, incoming sperm or to zygote if fertilization occurs.
5. *Breast.* Progesterone causes lobular and alveolar growth of breast.
6. *During pregnancy* the main function of progesterone is to maintain the pregnancy (see page 406).

II. Other actions

The other systemic effects of progesterone are:

1. *Thermogenic effect.* Progesterone is known as a thermogenic steroid. It increases the basal body temperature by 0.5°C in postovulatory phase.

2. *Effect on CNS.* Progesterone alters the secretion and release of various neurotransmitters in the hypothalamus and other areas of the brain and thereby decreases the appetite, and produces *somnolence.*

3. *Effect on respiration.* Progesterone increases the sensitivity of the respiratory centre to carbon dioxide stimulation. Due to this fact the partial pressure of Co_2 in arterial blood ($pACO_2$) is slightly less in women during luteal phase of sexual cycle.

4. *Effect on fat metabolism.* Progesterone (particularly C-19 progesterone) decreases the serum HDL. Thus it acts as a proatherogenic agent.

OTHER OVARIAN HORMONES

Besides female sex steroids (oestrogen and progesterone) ovaries also secrete peptide hormones as:

1. ***Inhibin.*** It inhibits the FSH release.

2. ***Activin.*** Its action is to activate FSH secretion from anterior pituitary.

3. ***Relaxin*** is a polypeptide hormone produced by corpus luteum and other sites include uterus placenta and mammary glands and in males from the prostate gland. Its main role is during pregnancy as it relaxes pubic symphysis and pelvic joints, softens and dilates the uterine cervix and facilitates delivery.

FEMALE SEXUAL CYCLE

The sexual life-span of a female can be divided into three periods:

1. ***Birth to puberty.*** During this period primary and accessory female sex organs remain quiescent.

2. ***Puberty to menopause.*** With the onset of puberty the female sexual cycle starts, which repeats every 28 days. The occurrence of first menstrual cycle is called *menarche.* The permanent stoppage of menstrual cycle is called *menopause,* which occurs at the age of about 45 to 50 years. The period between menarche and menopause is called *reproductive period.* During this period females have rhythmical sexual cycles.

3. ***Postmenopausal period*** extends after menopause (45 to 50 years) to rest of the life. During this period the female sexual cycle ceases.

Female sexual cycle refers to monthly rhythmic sexual cycle occurring in females during the normal reproductive period.

Components of human female sexual cycle. During each female sexual cycle, rhythmical changes occur in ovaries and accessory sex organs—uterus, cervix and vagina.

Duration of female sexual cycle is usually 28 days. But under physiological conditions it may vary between 20 and 40 days. Traditionally first day of the menstrual bleeding is taken as the 1st day of female sexual cycle.

OVARIAN CYCLE

Ovarian cycle refers to rhythmic changes occurring in ovaries during each female sexual cycle of about 28 days. During each cycle a single mature ovum is released from the ovary. The ovarian cycle can be divided into three phases:
- Preovulatory phase or follicular phase,
- Ovulation, and
- Postovulatory phase or luteal phase.

1. Preovulatory phase

Preovulatory or follicular phase of the ovarian cycle extends from the 5th day of the cycle till the time of ovulation (which takes place at about 14th day of the cycle). Thus, this phase generally lasts for 8-9 days (but may vary from 10 to 25 days).
- Changes in the ovary during this phase are mostly under the influence of follicular stimulating hormone (FSH) and luteinizing hormone (LH) from the anterior pituitary.
- During this phase of each cycle, some 10-15 primordial follicles start maturing, but only one follicle matures fully and the rest undergo atresia (atrophy) at different stages of development. The process of maturation of follicle is called folliculogenesis (see page 398).

2. Ovulation

Ovulation refers to release of secondary oocyte from the ovary (following rupture of graafian follicle) into the peritoneal cavity. It usually occurs *14 days after the onset* of menstruation.

3. Postovulatory phase

Postovulatory phase is also called luteal phase of ovarian cycle (about 14 days). This phase is characterized by following events (Fig. 11.3-8B):

Formation of corpus luteum. Following ovulation, the outer wall of the graafian follicle collapses and promptly fills with blood forming the so-called corpus haemorrhagicum. Soon, the granulosa cells and theca cells of the follicle lining begin to proliferate, and the clotted blood is rapidly replaced with yellowish lipid-rich *luteal cells.* This process is called *luteinization* and the total mass of the cells is now called *corpus luteum.* LH is responsible for luteinization.

Formation of corpus albicans. If there is no fertilization and pregnancy does not occur, the corpus luteum begins to involute (regress) after 24th day of the sexual cycle and is eventually replaced by a whitish scar tissue, called the corpus albicans.

Corpus luteum of pregnancy. However, if the ovum released is fertilized and pregnancy occurs, then the corpus luteum formed during postovulatory phase persists and serves as the major source of oestrogen and progesterone till the 3rd month of pregnancy when the placenta takes over its endocrine function.

ENDOMETRIAL CYCLE

Endometrial cycle refers to the cyclic changes occurring in the endometrium during active reproductive period (menarche to menopause) in females leading to recurrent monthly bleeding per vaginum (menstruation). These cyclic changes in the endometrium are brought about by the cyclic production of oestrogens and progesterone by the ovaries.

The endometrial cycle of 28 days can be divided into three phases (Fig. 11.3-8E):
- Menstrual phase (1st to 5th day),
- Proliferative phase (6th to 14th day), and
- Secretory phase (15th to 28th day).

For the purpose of better understanding, the menstrual phase is described last of all.

Proliferative phase

Extent of proliferative phase of endometrial cycle is from day 6th to 14th day. It follows the phase of menstruation, after which only a thin basal layer of original endometrium is left.

Hormone responsible for changes in the endometrium during this phase is oestrogen secreted by the developing graafian follicle in the ovary. The proliferative phase of endometrial cycle coincides with the follicular phase of ovarian cycle.

Changes in endometrium, which occur during proliferative phase, are:
1. Thickness of endometrium, which is less than 1 mm at the end of menstrual phase, increases to 3-4 mm at the end of the proliferative phase.
2. Angiogenesis in the stratum functionale leads to proliferation of blood vessels which become the spiral arterioles that profuse the stratum functionale.
3. Endometrial glands are stimulated to grow. The glands contain glycogen but they are nonsecretory.

Secretory phase

Extent of secretory phase (also known as postovulatory phase of endometrial cycle) is from day 15th to 28th day.

CHAPTER 11.3

Hormones responsible for changes in the endometrium during this phase are both oestrogen and progesterone secreted by the *corpus luteum* formed after ovulation. Thus, the secretory phase of endometrial cycle coincides with the luteal phase of ovarian cycle.

Changes in the endometrium, which occur during this phase, are:

- There is elongation and coiling of endometrial mucous glands. These glands become prominent corkscrew-shaped secretory and secrete thick viscous fluid containing glycogen.
- *Blood supply* of endometrium further increases as progesterone promotes spiralling of blood vessels.
- *Thickness* of endometrium increases to 5-6 mm at the end of secretory phase. Thus the thickened endometrium with large amounts of nutrients is ready to provide appropriate conditions for implantation of ovum during this phase.
- *If fertilization does not occur* and there is no pregnancy, the corpus luteum in the ovary involutes to form corpus albicans and on day 26th of the menstrual cycle the levels of oestrogen and progesterone fall suddenly and mark the end of secretory phase of endometrial cycle.

Menstrual phase

The menstrual phase of endometrial cycle is also called bleeding phase. The average duration of this phase is 3-5 days. About 24 hours before the end of menstrual cycle, there is sharp decline in the plasma levels of oestrogen and progesterone, which is responsible for menstrual bleeding. During menstrual phase about 2/3rd of the superficial endometrium is sloughed off and only a thin basal layer (2 mm thick) is left behind.

- *Average amount of blood loss during each* menstrual cycle is 30 ml.
- *Menstrual blood immediately gets clotted inside the uterine cavity but soon gets liquefied* by fibrolysins present in endometrial debris.
- *Endometrial debris* contains necrosed sloughed off tissue, blood, serous fluid and large amount of prostaglandins and fibrolysins.

CYCLIC CHANGES IN CERVIX

The mucosal lining of cervix (endocervix) also shows certain cyclic changes during sexual cycle. These are:

During menstruation phase the mucosa of cervix does not undergo desquamation (shedding off) like that of endometrium.

During proliferative phase (oestrogen phase) the secretions of the mucosal cells of endocervix become thin, watery and alkaline. At the time of ovulation the cervical mucus is thinnest and its elasticity is maximum. It can be

stretched like a long, thin elastic thread upto 8-12 cm (spinnbarkeit effect). The mucus also produces a characteristic fern-like pattern when a drop of mucus is spread on the glass slide and allowed to dry (*Fern test*) (Fig. 11.3-9B).

This characteristic nature of cervical mucus favours the transport of sperms in the female genital tract and makes the conditions favourable for fertilization.

During secretory phase, under the influence of progesterone, cervical secretions decrease in quantity and become thick, tenacious and cellular, and fern pattern is not seen (Fig. 11.3-9C). These changes make a plug and prevent the entry of sperm through cervical canal.

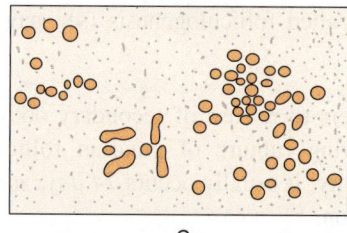

Fig. 11.3-9. *Characteristics of cervical mucus as seen on smear examination during various phases of normal menstrual cycle : A, on 7th day (no fern pattern); B, on 14th day (typical fern pattern); C, on 21st day (fern pattern disappears); and D, 21st day of an unovulatory cycle (fern pattern persists).*

Note. Fern test. The fern pattern of cervical mucus in proliferative phase and its disappearance in secretory phase is indicative of ovulatory cycle, whereas persistence of fern pattern (Fig. 11.3-9D) throughout the cycle indicates anovulatory cycle.

CYCLIC CHANGES IN VAGINA

In proliferative phase, vaginal epithelium becomes thickened (by adding up more and more layers of epithelium) and cornified.

In secretory phase, under the influence of progesterone, vaginal epithelium proliferates and gets infiltrated with leucocytes and the vaginal secretions become thick and viscid.

OTHER CHANGES DURING SEXUAL CYCLE

Hormonal oscillations during sexual cycle though mainly affect ovaries, uterus, cervix and vagina but some changes have also been observed in the fallopian tubes, breast and in the body weight.

HORMONAL CONTROL OF FEMALE SEXUAL CYCLE

The hypothalamo-hypophyseal-gonadal axis regulates the cyclic changes occurring during female sexual cycle. The role of each component of the axis is (Fig. 11.3-10):

Role of hypothalamus and anterior pituitary

Hypothalamus regulates the secretions of gonadotropins (both FSH and LH) through the gonadotropin releasing hormone (GnRH). The gonadotropin releasing hormone (GnRH) is also known as luteinizing hormone releasing hormone (LHRH). It stimulates the anterior pituitary cells to release gonadotropins. Gonadotropins in turn regulate the ovarian cycle, i.e. formation of graafian follicles (folliculosis), ovulation and formation of corpus luteum (see page 401).

Regulation of gonadotropins

The secretion of both FSH and LH is regulated by:

1. Gonadal hormones. The gonadal hormones (oestrogen and progesterone) regulate gonadotropin secretion by their feedback effect (Fig. 11.3-10). Depending on relative plasma level of these hormones the effect may be positive or negative, or both positive and negative.

The feedback effect (positive or negative) of ovarian hormones is brought about by its action either directly on anterior pituitary or through the hypothalamus (Fig. 11.3-10).

Oral contraceptives are the preparations containing high concentration of oestrogen and progesterone. These drugs

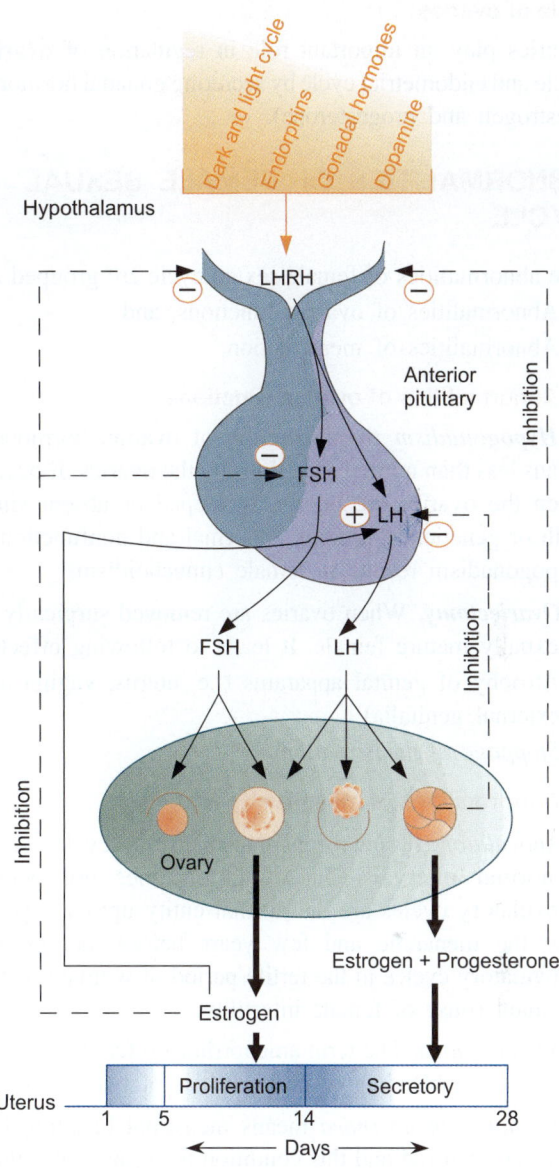

Fig. 11.3-10. *Hypothalamo-hypophyseal-ovarian axis regulating the female sexual cycle through positive and negative feedback mechanisms.*

inhibit gonadotropin release by negative feedback effect and prevent ovulation.

2. Human chorionic gonadotropin (HCG) (see page 405)

3. Prolactin. It is a mammotropic hormone secreted from anterior pituitary during lactation. It inhibits GnRh release and thus lowers the basal secretion of FSH and LH (cause for lactation amenorrhoea).

4. Activin. It is structurally quite similar to inhibin (secreted from ovary). It is synthesized in the cells of anterior pituitary. It stimulates the synthesis and release of FSH by autocrine and paracrine actions.

Role of ovaries

Ovaries play an important role in regulation of ovarian cycle and endometrial cycle by secreting gonadal hormones (oestrogen and progesterone).

ABNORMALITIES OF FEMALE SEXUAL CYCLE

The abnormalities of female sexual cycle are grouped as:
- Abnormalities of ovarian functions, and
- Abnormalities of menstruation.

A. Abnormalities of ovarian functions

1. *Hypogonadism* (hyposecretion of ovarian hormones) means less than normal secretions by the ovaries. It occurs when the ovaries are poorly developed or absent since birth or genetically become abnormal and nonfunctional. Hypogonadism results in female eunuchoidism.

2. *Ovariectomy*. When ovaries are removed surgically in a sexually mature female. It leads to following effects:
- Atrophy of genital apparatus (i.e. uterus, vagina and external genitalia),
- *Stoppage of menstruation.*

B. Abnormalities of menstruation

1. *Anovulatory cycles* means that menstrual cycles occur at normal intervals, but ovulation does not occur. Anovulatory cycles are the normal entity upto 1-2 years after the menarche and few years before menopause. Anovulatory cycles in the fertile period of womanhood is the main cause of female infertility.

2. *Amenorrhoea.* The term amenorrhoea refers to absence of menstrual bleeding or periods. It is of two types :

- *Primary amenorrhoea* means menstrual bleeding has never occurred and this condition is because of failure of sexual maturation.

- *Secondary amenorrhoea* means cessation of menstrual cycles in a woman who previously had normal and regular cycles. Pregnancy is the most common cause of secondary amenorrhoea. Other conditions which result in secondary amenorrhoea are emotional disturbances, environmental changes, hypothalamic and pituitary disorders and certain systemic diseases.

3. *Hypomenorrhoea.* The term refers to scanty menstruation.

4. *Menorrhoea.* It refers to abnormally profuse bleeding during normal regular cycles.

5. *Metrorrhagia.* This condition refers to occurrence of uterine bleeding in between the periods.

6. *Oligomenorrhoea* means infrequent and reduced frequency of menstruation.

7. *Dysmenorrhoea* is the term related to discomfort during menstruation (or painful menstruation).

8. *Premenstrual syndrome* (PMS). About 7-10 days before the end of cycle some women experience symptoms like irritability, lack of concentration, feeling of depression, heaviness, headache and constipation which is called premenstrual syndrome.

PHYSIOLOGY OF PREGNANCY

Physiology of pregnancy is mainly concerned with maternal adaptations to provide ideal atmosphere for fertilization, nutrition to the growing fetus, and safe child-birth. The physiology of pregnancy can be discussed under following headings:
- Fertilization and implantation,
- Formation of placenta and its functions,
- Physiological changes during pregnancy, and
- Applied aspects.

FERTILIZATION AND IMPLANTATION

FERTILIZATION

Fertilization refers to fusion of male and female gametes (i.e. spermatozoon and ovum). It takes place in the middle segment (ampulla) of the fallopian tube. It involves following events:

1. *Transport of gametes*. Before fertilization, the ovum and sperms reach the ampulla for fertilization.

2. *Sperm capacitation*. Sperm capacitation refers to the process that makes a sperm to fertilize an ovum. Sperm capacitation occurs due to removal of certain factors, which normally remain quiescent in male genital tract.

3. *Fusion of gametes*. The fusion of ovum and sperm occurs by penetration of sperm through ovum coverings due to acrosomal reaction which involves release of acrosin (protease enzyme) from anterior membrane of acrosome of the sperm. Only one sperm can enter into the oocyte, and further entry of sperms is prevented by the activation of ovum.

IMPLANTATION

Implantation of a fertilized ovum involves following steps:

1. *Formation of blastocyst*. The fertilized ovum starts dividing immediately and is called morula (16-cell stage) and blastocyst (100-cell stage).

2. *Transportation of blastocyst in uterine cavity*. In next 3-4 days blastocyst is transported into the cavity of the uterus.

3. *Implantation of blastocyst in the endometrium*. The blastocyst then erodes and burrows into the endometrium (implantation) (Fig. 11.3-11). The blastocyst goes deeper and deeper into the uterus mucosa till whole of it lies within the endometrium.

Fig. 11.3-11. *Implantation of blastocyst in the endometrium (A) and decidual reaction (B).*

4. *Decidual reaction.* After implantation the endometrium is called decidua. The stroma cells of endometrium get enlarged, become vacuolated and filled with glycogen and lipids. These cells are called decidual cells. The stored glycogen and lipids are the source of nutrition for the embryo till placenta takes up this function. Therefore this change in stroma cell is called decidual reaction.

PLACENTA AND PREGNANCY TESTS

PLACENTA

Placenta is a temporary organ formed during pregnancy. It is an important link between the mother and the fetus.

- When fully formed, the placenta is a disc-shaped structure, has a diameter of 15-20 cm and weighs about 500 gm.
- After birth of the baby, the placenta is shed off along with the decidua.

The placental membrane

The maternal and fetal blood do not mix with each other. They are separated by a placental membrane, made up of the layers of the wall of the villus. From the fetal side these are (Fig. 11.3-12):

- Endothelium of fetal blood vessels and its basement membrane,
- Surrounding mesenchymal tissue (connective tissue),
- Cytotrophoblast and its basement membrane, and
- Syncytiotrophoblast.

Functions of placenta

The fully functional placenta develops by the end of third month (12 weeks) of pregnancy. Placenta serves mainly three functions:

Fig. 11.3-12. *Structure of placental membrane.*

- Hormone secretion (endocrinal functions of placenta).
- Transport of substances between mother and fetus.
- Protection of the fetus.

A. Hormone secretion

The syncytiotrophoblast of the placenta serves as an endocrine gland. The hormones secreted by the placenta are:

- Human chorionic gonadotropins (HCG),
- Human chorionic somatomammotropins (HCS),
- Human chorionic thyrotropin (HCT),
- Placental progesterone,
- Placental oestrogens, and
- Relaxin.

1. *Human chorionic gonadotropins.* Human chorionic gonadotropin (HCG) is a polypeptide hormone. It is secreted by syncytiotrophoblast soon after fertilization. After fertilization it is detected in the maternal blood as early as 6-8 days after conception, and reaches its peak between 60-90 days of gestation. After this the concentration falls to a very low level and just before labour its level falls to zero. Its approximate peak value in human maternal blood during normal pregnancy is 5 mg/ml.

Physiological effects of HCG. Its actions are similar to LH of anterior pituitary hence also called second *luteotropic hormone.* It maintains the functions of the corpus luteum up to 7 weeks after conception until fetoplacental unit is able to synthesize its own oestrogen and progesterone.

Clinical importance (application) of HCG
The presence of HCG in the urine forms the basis of all the pregnancy tests (see page 406). HCG appears in the urine as early as 10 days after gestation with 99% accuracy.

If fetus dies early then HCG disappears from the blood as well as from the urine.

2. Human chorionic somatomammotropin. The syncytiotrophoblast cells of placenta also secrete large amount of human chorionic somatomammotropin. It functions as maternal growth hormone of pregnancy and causes deposition of protein in the tissues, and bring about nitrogen, calcium and potassium retention.

3. Human chorionic thyrotropin. The physiological role of this substance is not very clear.

4. Placental progesterone.

Plasma concentration. During pregnancy plasma concentration of progesterone rises steadily throughout gestation reaching a maximum plateau at 30-40 weeks of gestation. Just before the onset of labour its level decreases.

Physiological effects of placental progesterone

- It helps to preserve the pregnancy by promoting the growth of endometrium. It converts secretory endometrium of luteal phase of menstrual cycle to decidua during pregnancy.

- Progesterone has a marked inhibitory effect on the contractions of uterus.

- It causes development of alveolar system of mother's breast.

5. Placental oestrogens.

Plasma concentration. Like progesterone, plasma oestrogen (estriol) concentration rises throughout the gestation. Its peak value (14 ng/ml) and secretory curve parallels that of progesterone and maximum *plateau* is reached at 30-40 weeks of gestation.

The plasma concentration of estriol reflects the functional status of fetoplacental maternal unit activity.

Physiological effects.

- It causes growth and development of maternal reproductive organs. Uterus increases in size—weight, length and volume—both by hypertrophy and stretching of myometrium).

- Oestrogen stimulates development of lactiferous ductal system in mammary glands.

- Just before term, oestrogen to progesterone ratio increases and uterus is dominated by oestrogen.

6. Other placental hormones. A number of other substances which are secreted from placenta are:
- Corticotropin releasing hormone (CRH),
- β endorphins, and
- α MSH.

B. Transport of substances between the mother and the fetus

1. Transport of nutrients. The nutritive materials which are transported from mother's blood into the fetus are glucose, fats, amino acids, calcium and inorganic phosphates, potassium, sodium and chloride ions. Substances with molecular weight less than 1000 can cross readily by simple diffusion.

2. Excretion of waste products through placenta. Excretory products, especially urea, uric acid and creatinines, etc., formed in the fetus are transported into the mother's blood and then excreted by mother's kidneys. Thus placenta also acts as fetal kidney.

3. Diffusion of respiratory gases

Oxygen transport. Dissolved oxygen from the maternal sinuses of placenta diffuses into the fetal blood.

Transport of CO_2. CO_2 from fetus is eliminated only through placenta). Thus placenta acts as fetal lungs.

4. Transport of antibodies. Maternal immunoglobulins are transferred into the fetus and are responsible for innate immunity.

Rh agglutinins are easily transported as compared to ABO agglutinins; that is why the effects of Rh incompatibility are more severe.

5. Transport of harmful substances. Certain viruses and many drugs (like nicotine and barbiturates) can easily cross the placental barrier and may produce harmful effect on the fetus. Therefore, as far as possible one should avoid these drugs and smoking during pregnancy.

C. Protection of the fetus

Placenta protects the fetus in many ways:
- It acts as a barrier for certain harmful substances.
- It provides nutrition to the fetus.
- Its hormonal secretion is responsible for proper growth of the fetus.
- Placental progesterone decreases uterine contractions and thus protects the fetus from being expelled.

PREGNANCY TESTS

In an adult healthy woman amenorrhoea is the first sign of pregnancy, but it occurs in many other conditions as well. Therefore, detection of early pregnancy is made possible by certain pregnancy tests. The pregnancy detection tests are based on presence of HCG in the urine of pregnant lady.

Gravindex test

Immunological pregnancy tests are based on antigenic properties of HCG. It gives immediate results.

PHYSIOLOGICAL CHANGES IN MOTHER DURING PREGNANCY

The normal average duration of pregnancy in human beings is 280 days (40 weeks) and is calculated from the first day of the last menstrual period, or 256-270 days from the time of ovulation. As the pregnancy progresses, various types of extra demands are imposed on the mother's body by the growing fetus, which are met with by certain adaptations in almost all the organ systems of the body. These physiological changes include:

I. Changes in genital organs

- To accommodate the growing fetus marked increase in the size of uterus takes place.
- Endocervix gets hypertrophied.
- Mammary glands show hyperplasia of ductal and alveolar tissue. The areola becomes pigmented and many sebaceous glands become prominent in the areola. Nipples also become larger and pigmented.

II. Weight gain

A woman may gain total of 10-12 kg of weight during normal pregnancy, which is contributed by:

- Fetus: 3 kg
- Placenta and amniotic fluid: 1.5 kg
- Uterus and breast enlargement: 1.0 kg
- Increase in blood volume and interstitial fluid: 1.5 kg
- Fat deposition: 3.5 to 4 kg.

PHYSIOLOGY OF PARTURITION

Parturition is the process by which baby is born. It may occur any time between 37th and 40th weeks of gestation. The uterine myometrium and cervix play an important role for this process.

MECHANICS OF PARTURITION

From the functional point of view mechanics of parturition mainly involves:

- uterine contractions, and
- cervical dilatation.

Uterine contractions

The uterus, which remains quiescent during period of pregnancy, becomes progressively more and more excitable towards the end of pregnancy, until finally it begins strong rhythmical contractions with such a force that expel the fetus.

Control or regulation of uterine contractility. The exact cause of increased uterine activity is not known. It is attributed to increased myometrial excitability to oxytocin near term which occurs due to an increase in number of oxytocin receptors on the cells of the uterine smooth muscle during the final weeks of pregnancy and increased synthesis of contractile proteins in the myometrial cells.

Cervical dilatation

Throughout pregnancy cervix remains as a rigid structure, but at the time of parturition certain structural and biochemical changes occur and the cervix becomes soft. This is known as *cervical ripening*. It allows the cervix to stretch when uterine contractions start.

CONTROL OF PARTURITION

The mechanisms responsible for onset of labour in human are still not understood exactly. The control of parturition includes the role of :

- Hormonal factors, and
- Mechanical factors.

A. Hormonal factors

The hormonal changes that initiate the parturition and that cause increased excitability of uterine musculature are:

1. *Activation of fetal hypothalamic-pituitary-adrenal axis.* Resulting in an increase in ACTH secretion few days before parturition. ACTH causes fetal adrenal cortex to secrete large amount of androgens.

The above changes lead to an altered oestrogen-progesterone ratio.

2. *Role of altered oestrogen-progesterone ratio.* The altered oestrogen-progesterone ratio causes:

- An increase in release of oxytocin from maternal posterior pituitary,
- An increase in number of oxytocin receptors in myometrium,
- An increase in prostaglandin synthesis, and
- An increase in synthesis of myometrial contractile proteins.

B. Mechanical factors

Mechanical factors that increase the contractility of uterus include :

1. *Stretch of urterine musculature*. As the pregnancy advances with growing fetus stretch increases leading to uterine contractility.

2. *Positive feedback effect.* Stretching and irritation of cervix is particularly important because of positive feedback effect through initiation of the reflex increase in uterine contractility. The positive feedback mechanism continues until the baby is expelled.

3. *Role of Ferguson reflex.* Once labour is started, the uterine contractions dilate the ripened cervix. The cervical dilatation in turn sets off signals in afferent nerves that increase oxytocin secretion from the posterior pituitary. This is called Ferguson reflex.

Clinical application. The obstetricians frequently induce labour by rupturing the membrane so that the head of the baby stretches the cervix more forcefully than usual and thus initiates it, leading to intitiation of positive feedback effect and Ferguson reflex.

ANATOMY OF BREAST AND PHYSIOLOGY OF LACTATION

ANATOMY OF BREAST

Breastfeeding is the characteristic feature of all the mammals, including human beings. It has evolved as the best method of nourishing the newborn. The mammary glands (the secondary sex organs) play an important role in lactation process.

Mammary glands are present in both the sexes; in males they remain rudimentary. In the female the breasts are small and immature and remain quiescent till puberty. At thelarche i.e., at the time of puberty (9-11 years of age), before the start of menses, the breasts start developing and get enlarged. Thereafter, after the onset of menses (menarche) they grow and develop to their mature size under the influence of oestrogen and progesterone.

Gross appearance

The fully developed breast is a soft, rounded, elevated structure having central dark pigmented area (areola). The central part of areola, projected above the surface, is called nipple. The nipple is perforated at the tip by 15 to 20 minute openings of the lactiferous ducts.

Location and extent. Each breast covers nearly circular space anterior to the pectoralis muscles extending from the second to sixth ribs and from the sternum into the axilla.

Histological structure

Each mammary gland is covered by overlying skin. Deep to skin the entire breast tissue lies in the superficial fascia (i.e. between skin and the deep fascia). The breast tissue consists of discrete masses of glandular tissue present in the connective tissue consisting of stroma and adipose tissue (Fig. 11.3-13).

- *The mammary glands* consist of 15-20 lobes and each lobe has a number of lobules.
- *The glandular tissue* mainly consists of alveoli having secretory cells.
- *The secretions* from these cells are poured by apocrine manner and by exocytosis into the ducts (lactiferous ducts). About 15-20 ducts open at the summit of nipple, and just before opening lactiferous ducts show a dilatation called lactiferous sinus.
- *Around the alveoli,* ductules and lobules are present myoepithelial cells. They squeeze the contents and pour their secretions into the ductules.

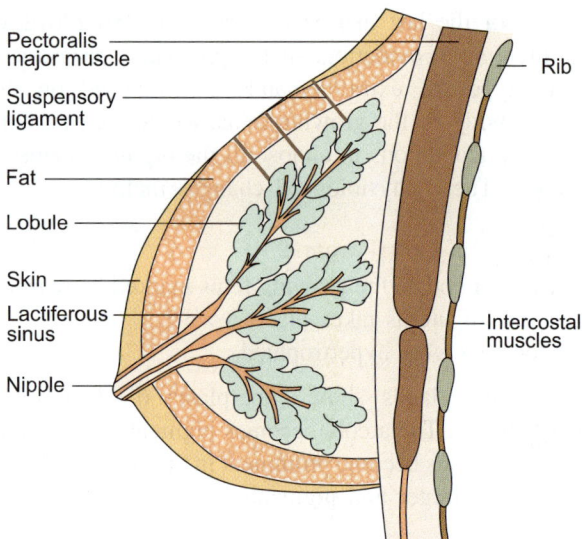

Fig. 11.3-13. Structure of mammary gland (breast).

Blood supply, lymphatic drainage and nerve supply to the breasts

Arterial blood supply is by perforating branches of the internal thoracic artery and thoracic branches of axillary artery and intercostal arteries.

Venous drainage is along the veins corresponding to the arteries supplying the breasts.

Lymphatic drainage. An understanding of the lymphatic drainage of the breast is of the greatest importance in relation to the malignant condition of the breast.

- Most of the lymphatics from the breast drain into *axillary lymph nodes.*
- Some lymphatics also drain into parasternal nodes, intercostal nodes, infraclavicular and supraclavicular nodes.

Nerve supply to the breasts is derived from the 4th, 5th and 6th thoracic spinal nerves which also contain sympathetic fibres. There are numerous somatic sensory nerve endings in the breasts, especially around the nipples. Touch receptors present in the areola region play role in suckling reflex during lactatioin period.

Changes in breast during pregnancy and lactation

Breasts in pregnancy. During pregnancy remarkable growth of both ductal and glandular systems occurs. It is only during first pregnancy that glandular tissue develops fully.

In first half of pregnancy the duct system proliferates and shows extensive sprouting and branching along with growth of stroma and deposition of fat.

In second half of pregnancy there is enormous growth of glandular tissue.

The extensive growth of mammary glands during pregnancy is known as *mammogenesis* or preparation of breast for lactation.

Breasts during lactation. After childbirth the alveolar cells get enlarged and distended and start forming milk (lactogenesis).

Involution of breast. After a normal period of lactation (7 to 9 months), the alveolar epithelium undergoes apoptosis and glands revert back of prepregnant stage.

Control of breast development and growth

Various hormones necessary for full growth and development of mammary glands at various stages are:

1. Oestrogen. It is primarily responsible for ductal growth and fat deposition. It also causes thickening of nipples.

2. Progesterone. The development of glandular tissue mainly depends on progesterone. Both oestrogen and progesterone work best with cooperation of hypo-thalamo-pituitary-adrenal cortex axis.

3. Other hormones including growth hormone, thyroxine, cortisol and insulin enhance overall growth and development of mammary glands at all stages.

4. Corpus luteal and placental hormones, particularly oestrogen, progesterone, human chorionic somato-mammotropic hormone (HCS or HPL), are essential for further growth of breast during pregnancy.

5. Prolactin. It is another very important hormone for development of breasts during pregnancy and lactation. It acts on mammary gland tissue which has already grown under the influence of oestrogen and progesterone.

Human prolactin

Human prolactin is secreted by acidophilic cells of anterior pituitary gland. *During pregnancy* prolactin secretion starts rising from 8th weeks onwards and peak value (200-400 ng/ml) is reached at term. The sources of prolactin during pregnancy are placenta, amniotic fluid and maternal anterior pituitary gland.

Physiological effects of prolactin

1. *Breast growth.* During pregnancy it increases the breast growth particularly of alvealor tissue in the form of alveolar distension, dilatation of mammary vessels, and formation of new capillaries.

2. *Lactogenic effect.* Prolactin acts on the alveolar epithelium and stimulates the secretory activity.

3. *Suppression of ovarian cycle in nursing mothers.* Prolactin inhibits the secretion of gonadotropin releasing hormone (GnRH) from hypothalamus. Therefore, gonadotropin (FSH and LH) secretion from anterior pituitary also decreases. Thus in nursing mothers due to low levels of gonadotropins the ovarian cyclic changes do not occur.

PHYSIOLOGY OF LACTATION

PHASES OF LACTATION

The physiology of lactation can be divided into four phases:

- Preparation of breast for milk secretion (mammo-genesis),
- Synthesis and secretion of milk (lactogenesis),
- Expulsion of milk (galactokinesis), and
- Maintenance of lactation (galactopoiesis).

MAMMOGENESIS

During pregnancy. The breast develops fully and is prepared for milk secretion after delivery (see page 407).

LACTOGENESIS

Stages of lactogenesis

It is the initiation of lactation after childbirth. Immediately after the baby is born, sudden loss of oestrogen and progesterone secretion by the placenta allows the lactogenic effect of prolactin. In this stage:

- The secretion rate increases to 500-750 ml/day, and
- In next 1-7 days the breasts begin to secrete milk instead of colostrum.

Human milk

Types of human milk. The nature and composition varies with postpartum period. Therefore, the human milk is of three types:

1. *Colostrum* is deep yellow-coloured fluid secreted by the mammary glands during first few days of postpartum period.

2. *Transition milk or intermediate milk.* It is secreted from 6th day to 15th day of postpatrum period. The nature and composition of the secretion changes from colostrum to mature milk. Hence it is called transition milk.

3. *Mature milk* is formed from 15th day of postpartum onwards and continues during the whole lactation period (7-9 months).

Composition of human milk. Human milk contains 88.5% water and about 11.5% solids. The solids include both organic and inorganic constituents.

Note. Human milk is balanced diet as it contains first class proteins (caseinogen and lactalbumin), carbohydrates fat, mineral salts and vitamins. Therefore it is an ideal food for the baby.

EXPULSION OF MILK OR GALACTOKINESIS

Though milk is secreted continuously into the alveoli of the breast, but it does not flow continuously from alveoli into the duct system. It depends upon the suckling reflex and some local mechanisms acting within the breast.

Suckling reflex

It is a neuroendocrinal reflex. The characteristic features and mechanism of suckling reflex (Fig. 11.3-14) are:

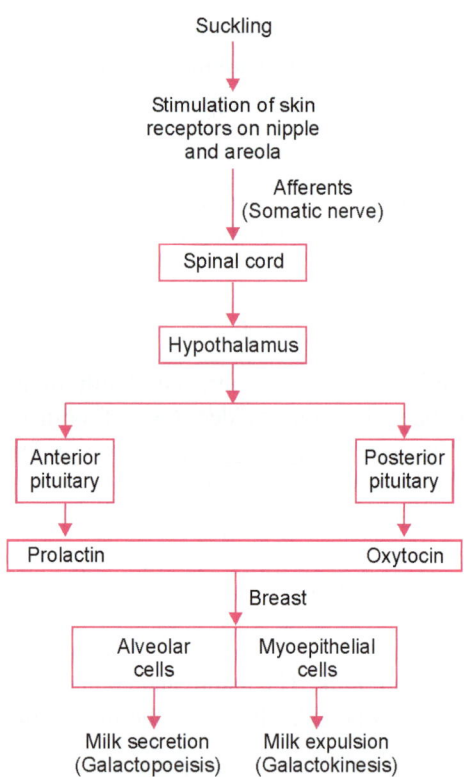

Fig. 11.3-14. *Mechanism of suckling reflex.*

- When baby suckles, the sensory nerve endings or receptors located in skin of areola and nipple get stimulated.
- The sensory impulses are transmitted to the hypothalamus through somatic nerves (from nipple and areola to spinal cord and then to hypothalamus). The activation of hypothalamus causes release of oxytocin and prolactin from pituitary gland.
- The oxytocin is carried to the breasts through blood, where it causes contraction of myoepithelial cells that surround the outer wall of the alveoli, thereby the milk is expressed from alveoli into the ducts. This process is called *milk ejection* or *milk expulsion* or *milk let down*.
- Another important observation is that suckling of one breast causes milk flow in the other breast also.
- Even stimuli such as sight, sound or crying of infant and thought of their infants also cause milk ejection, indicating the psychological component in the neuroendocrine reflex.

MAINTENANCE OF MILK SECRETION OR GALACTOPOIESIS

Maintenance of milk secretion or galactopoiesis depends upon the surge in prolactin secretion. After few weeks of childbirth, prolactin level falls to its basal value, however, in nursing mothers neuroendocrine reflex causes 10-20 fold surge in prolactin secretion, that lasts for one hour. Each time when baby suckles, the impulses from nipple and areolar receptors are transmitted by somatic nerves upto the hypothalamus, which cause 1-20 fold surge in prolactin secretion.

The amount of milk production is related to infant's demand.

IMPORTANCE OF LACTATION

Breastfeeding is being advocated all over the world because of its advantages both for the baby as well as for the mother.

Advantages of breastfeeding to the baby

1. *Balanced diet.* Human milk contains proteins, carbohydrates, fat, mineral salts (calcium and phosphorus) and vitamins. So, it is a natural balanced food for the newborn.

2. *Protection against infections.* Human milk has high count of lymphocytes, neutrophils and macrophages and high content of lysozymes and immunoglobulins. All these substances due to anti-infection property confer non-specific as well as specific immunity.

3. *Easily digestible.* Human milk because of its digestive properties can be easily digested by the newborn babies.

4. *Growth factors.* Growth promoting factors, like epidermal growth factor, insulin and somatomedin-C, are present in the human milk.

5. *Other advantages of breastfeeding* to baby are:

- It is sterile, convenient to give at right temperature. It is inexpensive, and chances of allergy to breast milk are rare.

Advantages of breastfeeding to the mother

1. *Lactational amenorrhoea.* Due to high plasma level of prolactin during lactation, there occurs suppression of FSH and LH. Therefore, after birth of the baby menstruation and ovulation do not start. The period of lactational amenorrhoea is variable (3 months to 3 years). This is the natural way of contraception and birth spacing.

2. *Involution of uterus.* The oxytocin released during each session of breastfeeding also acts on the uterine myometrium, and helps it to involute during postpartum period. The proper involution of uterus protects it against infections.

3. *Protection against breast engorgement.* Breastfeeding does not allow the milk to stagnate, thus preventing the breast engorgement, which is a highly painful condition.

4. *Protection against obesity.* Body fat is used for milk synthesis, therefore, there are less chances of becoming obese after pregnancy.

5. *Emotional bonding* and psychological satisfaction is enhanced by breastfeeding.

6. *Protection against cancer.* Prolonged lactation provides protection against breast cancer.

Physiology of Contraception

11.4

INTRODUCTION

Aims of contraception. Contraception refers to prevention of pregnancy. The aims of contraception are:

- The main aim of contraception is family planning to check the enormous increase in population growth, which is the root cause of socioeconomic problems of poor and developing countries, like India.
- Certain contraceptive measures are important to prevent the sexually transmitted diseases like AIDS.
- Contraceptives are also recommended on medical grounds to control the stress of pregnancy, labour and lactation in women suffering from heart diseases, etc.

Methods of contraception can be broadly grouped as:

- Spacing methods, and
- Terminal methods.

Both types of contraceptive measures are available for use by females as well as males, therefore, these can be described as:

- Contraceptive methods in females, and
- Contraceptive methods in males.

CONTRACEPTIVE METHODS IN FEMALES

SPACING METHODS

The spacing methods increase the gap between two pregnancies. These include:

- Rhythm method,
- Barrier methods,
- Chemical methods, and
- Intrauterine contraceptive devices.

Rhythm method

Rhythm method is also known as *calender method* or *safe period method* or natural method. This method of contraception depends on the time of ovulation. In a woman having regular menstrual cycle, ovulation occurs on 14th day of the cycle. After ovulation, ovum remains viable for 48-72 hours. Similarly, after ejaculation, sperms remain alive for 24-48 hours. Thus pregnancy occurs only if coitus is performed during this period. This is the period of high fertility and is called as *dangerous period.*

Therefore, to avoid pregnancy intercourse should be avoided in the dangerous period. Rest of the cycle, i.e. 5-6 days after bleeding phase of menstrual cycle and 5-6 days before the next cycle is the *safe period* (period of least fertility). This method of contraception is successful only if menstrual cycles are regular and woman knows the exact time of ovulation by keeping a record of basal body temperature.

Disadvantage of this method is that it is the most unreliable method when the menstrual cycles are irregular and time of ovulation is variable.

Barrier methods

Barrier methods of contraception prevent the meeting of ovum and sperms after coitus. These include:

1. *Mechanical barriers.* The mechanical barriers used as contraceptive are diaphargm and cervical caps (Fig. 11.4-1).

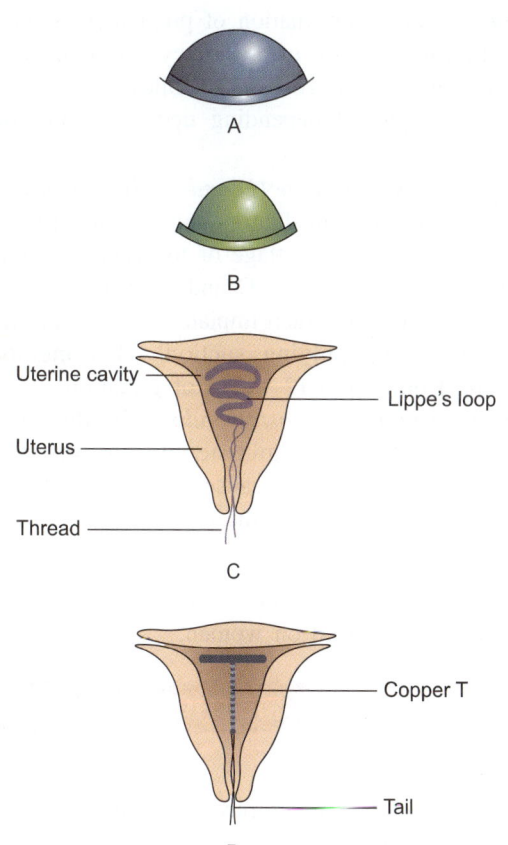

Fig. 11.4-1. Female contraceptive devices: A, vaginal diaphargm; B, cervical cap; C, Lippe's loop; and D, Copper-T.

Labels in figure:
Uterine cavity — Lippe's loop
Uterus
Thread
C
Copper T
Tail
D

Advantages. These devices are inexpensive and usually do not require any medical consultation.

Disadvantages of mechanical barriers include:
• Failures are quite common because chances of displacement of the device are very high.
• Some women get cervicitis (inflammation of cervix) and local irritation.

2. *Chemical barriers.* Chemical barriers refer to spermicidal agents which can destroy the sperms when applied in the female genital tract before coitus. The common spermicidal agents used are Ricinoleic acid (oldest), Nanoxynol-9, and Octoxynol-3.

These spermicidal agents are available in various forms such as foam tablets, pastes, creams, jellies, and vaginal sponges. Vaginal sponge is a polyurethane sponge impregnated with nanoxynol-9. It is available by the trade name 'TODAY'.

3. *Combined methods.* As mentioned above, mechanical barriers (diaphragm and cervical caps) along with spermicidal agents give good protection.

Chemical methods

Chemical methods for contraception are used in various forms like locally applied chemicals (in the form of cream, jellies etc.) and taken as drugs (either orally or in injectable form or as implants).

1. *Oral contraceptives.* Oral contraceptives are steroidal drugs which are most widely used contraceptive measures by the women all over the globe. These are recommeneded in women of younger age group (upto 35 years). In general, oral contraceptives contain synthetic preparation of oestrogen and progesterone and when taken orally they inhibit ovulation. The oral contraceptives are available in differents types of pills:
• Combined pill (classical pill), e.g. MALA-N and MALA-D,
• Sequential pill,
• Minipill, and
• Postcoital (morning after) pill.

2. *Depot preparations* are long-acting drugs and are highly effective. These are available in three forms:
• Injectable preparations,
• Subdermal implants, and
• Vaginal rings.

• *Advantages.* As depot preparations are long-acting drugs, therefore to avoid daily intake of oral pill, these preparations are preferred, and also, the contraceptive effectivity lasts for longer period.
• *Disadvantages* of depot preparation are that sometimes they lead to sterility and alterations in menstrual bleeding pattern.

Intrauterine contraceptive devices

Intrauterine contraceptive devices (IUCDs) are inserted into the uterine cavity for long-term contraception. The devices are usually made up of inert materials like plastic, polythene and metal. These include :

1. *Lippe's loop* (Fig.11.4-1C). It is a serpentine or S-shaped device made up of plastic to which is attached a fine nylon tail. The plastic used is non-toxic and non-tissue reactive. A small amount of *barium sulphate* is also present in the plastic material to allow its radiographic observation. Lippe's loop is available in different sizes.

2. *Copper-T.* Copper-T is the most commonly used IUCD in India. As the name indicates it is made up of copper and its shape resembles the letter T. Like Lippe's loop it is also attached with a nylon thread (tail) (Fig. 11.4-1D).

- *Insertion.* Most ideal time for its insertion is during menstruation or within 10 days of the beginning of menstruation, because the diameter of cervical cavity at this time is greater. It can also be inserted during first week after the delivery.
- *Mechanism of action.* Copper-T prevents implantation and growth of fertilized ovum by evoking aseptic inflammation.

Advantages of IUCDs are:

- This method of contraception is quite safe, effective and reversible. IUCDs can be easily pulled out or removed when contraception is not required.
- Provides long-term contraception without adverse effects.

Disadvantages of IUCDs are:

- In some cases may cause heavy bleeding,
- The IUCD may come out accidently, when not inserted properly, and
- Risks of ectopic pregnancy are there.

TERMINAL METHODS

Terminal method of contraception means permanent sterilization, which can be achieved by following methods.

Surgical methods

1. *Tubectomy* is the permanent method of sterilization in female and is recommended only when the family is completed. In tubectomy operation, fallopian tubes are cut and then cut ends are ligated and buried as shown in Fig. 11.4-2.

2. *Laparoscopic occlusion.* In this procedure the fallopian tubes are occluded using silicon rubber bands, Fallope rings or Hulka-Clemens clips. This method is much quicker and simple and hospitalization is not required.

Fig. 11.4-2. Procedure of tubectomy (female sterilization).

Medical termination of pregnancy

Medical termination of pregnancy (MTP or abortion) is allowed under MTP Act, 1971. Medical pregnancy act has laid down following criteria:

- Conditions in which pregnancy can be terminated,
- The person who can do termination, and
- Place, where it should be performed.

Indications

Indications in which pregnancy can be terminated are:

- *Medical.* When continuation of pregnancy is hazardous to the mother.
- *Eugenic.* When there is substantial risk to the child if born from that pregnancy.
- *Humanitarian grounds.* When pregnancy is the result of rape.
- *Failure of contraceptive measure.*

Methods. Medical termination of pregnancy is possible only in first few months of pregnancy (from 7th week to beginning of second trimester). Following procedures have been employed depending upon the duration of pregnancy:

1. *Dilatation and curettage (D and C).* In this procedure cervix is dilated with dilators and implanted ovum is removed by doing curettage of the endometrium.
2. *Vacuum aspiration.* Like D and C, in this procedure cervix is dilated and then implanted ovum is removed (aspirated) by applying suction. This method is employed only upto 12 weeks of gestation.
3. *Administration of prostaglandins.* In this method prostaglandins are administered into the vagina (intravaginally) which cause uterine contractions resulting in expulsion of the products of conception.

Pregnancy vaccines

Pregnancy vaccines are under experimental trial. These have not yet been tried on women.

CONTRACEPTIVE METHODS IN MALES

SPACING METHODS

The spacing methods of contraception used in males are:
- Natural method,
- Barrier method, and
- Chemical methods.

Natural method or coitus interruptus

It is the oldest method of voluntary fertility control. In this method male withdraws the penis before ejaculation into the vagina and tries to prevent deposition of semen into the vagina. This method needs practice and discipline. The failure rate is high because of following reasons:

- Precoital secretions of the male may contain sperms and even a drop of semen is sufficient to cause pregnancy.
- Slightest mistake in timings of withdrawal may lead to deposition of certain amount of semen.

Barrier methods

Condom is the most widely used barrier by the males all around the world. In India it is known by its trade name *Nirodh* (Fig. 11.4-3). It consists of a fine latex sheath and is electronically tested.

***Fig. 11.4-3.** Condom.*

Mechanism of action. Condom prevents deposition of semen into the vagina thus does not allow the sperms and the ovum to meet.

Advantages

- They are easily available, safe and inexpensive.
- Their use does not require any medical supervision.
- They also provide protection against sexually transmitted diseases.

Disadvantages

- It may slip off or tear off during coitus due to its incorrect use.
- It interferes with sexual sensations.

Chemical methods

Antispermatogenic drugs which inhibit spermatogenesis have been available. These include:

- Male pill (Gossypol)
- *Hormonal preparations.* Various hormonal preparations which can be used as contraceptive measures in males are testosterone, such as testosterone with danazol (17α-ethyl testosterone), and cyproterone acetate.

Tripterygium wilfordii is a special type of wine which reduces the sperm count (mechanism of action is not yet known).

Calcium channel blockers. Calcium channel blockers (e.g. nifedipine) block the Ca^{2+} channels on the cell membrane of the sperms. As a result the sperm membrane

becomes rigid and loaded with cholesterol. The rigid membrane of sperm prevents its binding to the zona pellucida of the ovum.

TERMINAL METHODS

The permanent methods employed for sterilization in males are:

- Vasectomy, and
- Vas occlusion using no scalpel technique.

1. *Vasectomy* is a simple operation in which about one cm piece of vas deferens is removed after clamping. Then both the ends are ligated and sutured so that they face away from each other (Fig. 11.4-4). This procedure reduces the risk of recanalization later on.

Advantages of vasectomy are that it is simpler, faster, less expensive procedure, and no hospitalization is required. It is 100% effective.

2. *No scalpel vas occlusion.* It is a newer technique, which is quite safe, convenient and is acceptable to males. In it an elastomer is injected into the vas deferens, it get hardened in situ within 20 mintues and plug the vas (occlude it). It is an easy procedure, and reversal is possible with 100% efficacy.

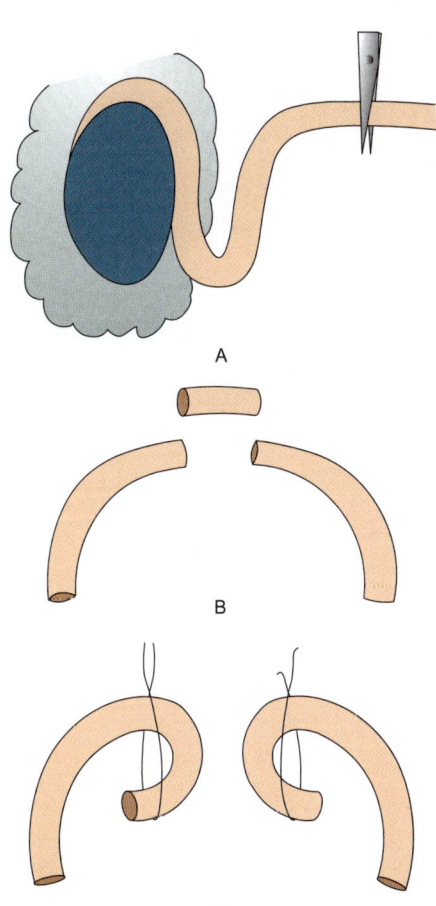

***Fig. 11.4-4.** Procedure of vasectomy (male sterilization).*

Nervous System
and
Special Senses

Organization of Nervous System and Nerve Physiology

12.1

ORGANIZATION OF NERVOUS SYSTEM

Nervous system acts as a control network within the body. The functional units of the nervous system are called *neurons,* which are responsible for the reception and response to changes in the internal and external environment. It is estimated that the human nervous system is composed of more than 100 billion neurons which are linked together in a highly intricate manner. Thus, the various parts of the nervous system are interconnected, but for convenience of description the nervous system can be divided anatomically and functionally into different divisions.

ANATOMICAL DIVISIONS OF THE NERVOUS SYSTEM

The nervous system is broadly classified into two divisions: the central nervous system and the peripheral nervous system (Fig. 12.1-1).

1. *Central nervous system* **(CNS)**, which occupies the central axis of the body, includes brain and spinal cord.

2. *Peripheral nervous system* **(PNS)** is the part of nervous system which lies outside the central nervous system. The PNS consists of peripheral nerves and the ganglia associated with them. Peripheral nerves attached to the brain are called *cranial nerves* (12 pairs), and those attached with spinal cord are called *spinal nerves* (31 pairs).

419

PERIPHERAL NERVOUS SYSTEM

CENTRAL NERVOUS SYSTEM

CRANIAL NERVES

BRAIN

— Cerebrum

— Cerebellum
— Medulla oblongata

SPINAL NERVES

SPINAL CORD

Fig. 12.1-1. *Anatomical divisions of nervous system : the central nervous system; and the peripheral nervous system.*

FUNCTIONAL DIVISIONS OF THE NERVOUS SYSTEM

Functionally, nervous system can be divided into two parts:
- Somatic nervous system, and
- Autonomic nervous system.

Somatic nervous system

Somatic nervous system has two divisions : sensory and motor.

1. *Sensory division* of the somatic nervous system collects the information about the changes that take place in the external environment and interprets the meaning of these changes. The sensory division of the somatic nervous system consists of:

- *Sensory receptors* that receive stimulus from the external environment. The stimulus may be mechanical, chemical, thermal, auditory or visual.
- *Afferent neurons* that carry impulses from the receptors to the brain and spinal cord.
- *Parts of the brain* that primarily deal with the processing of information.

2. *Motor division* of the somatic nervous system executes appropriate actions with the help of skeletal muscles in response to changes in external environment detected by *the sensory* division. It also coordinates the actions of different skeletal muscles of the body.

Motor division of the somatic nervous system consists of neurons that carry signals away from the brain and spinal cord to the skeletal muscles. Somatic nervous system is under voluntary control.

Autonomic nervous system

The word autonomous is taken from the Greek words, the 'autos' meaning self and the 'nomos' meaning control. Thus autonomic nervous system (ANS) is an involuntary system.

Divisions of ANS. The ANS has two main divisions:
- Sympathetic, and
- Parasympathetic, each having a central and a peripheral component.

The ANS collects the information about the changes that take place in the internal environment (i.e. internal viscera), interprets these changes, and guides the action and gets the plan executed with the help of smooth muscles of viscera, cardiac muscles and secretory epithelium of glandular tissues (which are effector organs of ANS). In other words, the ANS is responsible for activities of the organs of digestion, circulation, excretion, respiration and reproduction, as well as of adrenal medulla, sweat, salivary and lacrimal glands. It also controls the activities of smooth muscles of iris, ciliary body and arrectores pilorum.

THE NERVOUS TISSUE

CELLS OF NERVOUS TISSUE

The nervous tissue forming the nervous system is composed of :
- *Neurons,* the functional cells, and
- *Neuroglia,* the supporting cells.

NEURON

Structure

Neurons, or the nerve cells, are the structural and functional units of the nervous system. Neurons vary considerably in size, shape and other features. However, most of them have some major features in common. The basic structure of a neuron is best studied in a spinal motor neuron. A neuron primarily consists of the cell body and processes called *neurites,* which are of two kinds, the dendrites and the axon (Fig. 12.1-2).

Cell body

The cell body of a neuron is also called the *soma* or *perikaryon* and may be round, stellate, pyramidal or fusiform in shape. Like any other cell it consists of a mass of cytoplasm with all its principal constituents surrounded by a cell membrane. The cell body contains a large nucleus with one or two nucleoli but there is no centrosome. The absence of centrosome indicates that the neuron has lost

ability for division. Thus, neurons once destroyed are replaced by neuroglia only. In addition to the general features of a typical cell (page 13), the cytoplasm of a neuron has following distinctive characteristics (Fig. 12.1-2):

Fig. 12.1-2. *Structure of a typical neuron.*

Nissl granules/bodies. These are basophilic granules, seem to be composed of rough surfaced endoplasmic reticulum. The presence of abundant granular endoplasmic reticulum is an indication of the high level of protein synthesis in neurons.

Neurofibrillae. The presence of a network of neurofibrillae in the cytoplasm of the neuron is another distinctive feature. These consist of microfilaments and microtubules. In certain degenerative disease like Alzheimer's disease, the neurofilament protein gets altered, resulting in the formation of *neurofibrillary tangles.*

Pigment granules are seen in some neurons. For example, neuromelanin is present in the neurons of substantia nigra. Aging neurons contain a pigment lipofuscin.

Dendrites

The dendrites are multiple small branched processes. Dendrites contain Nissl bodies and neurofibres. Dendrites are the *receptive processes* of the neuron receiving signals from other neurons via their synapses with axon terminals.

Axon

The axon is the single longer process of the nerve cell. It varies in length from a few microns to one metre. It arises from the conical extension of the cell body called *axon hillock,* which is devoid of Nissl bodies. The part of the axon between the axon hillock and the beginning of myelin sheath is called the *initial segment.* In the axon the cell membrane continues as *axolemma* and the cytoplasm as *axoplasm.* The axon terminates by dividing into a number of branches, each ending in a number of *synaptic knobs* also known as *terminal buttons* or axon telodendria. Synaptic knobs contain microvesicles in which chemical neurotransmitters are stored. *Myelin sheath* is present around the axons in the so-called myelinated nerve fibres (Fig. 12.1-3). Myelin sheath which consists of protein-lipid complex is produced by glial cells called *Schwann cells* which encircle the axon forming around it a thin sleeve. Each Schwann cell provides the myelin sheath for a short segment of the axon. At the junction of any two such segments, there is a short gap, i.e. periodic 1 μm constrictions at about 1 mm distance. These gaps are the *nodes of Ranvier.* There are some axons which are devoid of myelin sheath.

Fig. 12.1-3. *Structure of a myelinated neuron.*

Myelination of axons increases the speed of conduction, but greatly increases their diameter.

Axons perform the specialized function of conducting impulses away from the cell body. They transmit propagated impulses (all or none transmission).

Types of neurons
Neurons have been variously classified as :

I. Depending upon the number of poles
Depending upon the number of poles (from which processes arise), neurons are divided into unipolar, bipolar and multipolar (Fig. 12.1-4).
1. *Unipolar neurons* have a single pole, from which both the processes, axon and dendrite, arise (Fig. 12.1-4A). True unipolar cells are present only in embryonic stage in human being. However, the primary sensory neurons (neurons conveying impulses from a sensory receptor to spinal cord) are *pseudounipolar* (Fig. 12.1-4B).

2. *Bipolar neurons* have two poles, one for axon and other for dendrite (Fig. 12.1-4C). Bipolar neurons are found in the vestibular and cochlear ganglia, and in the nasal olfactory epithelium, and as bipolar cells in the retina.
3. *Multipolar neurons* have many poles. One of the poles gives rise to axon and all others to dendrites (Fig. 12.1-4D). Most vertebrate neurons, especially in the CNS, are multipolar. The dendrites branch profusely to form the dendritic tree.

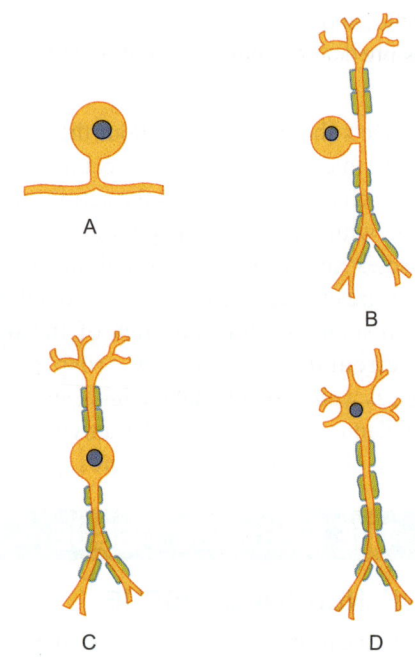

Fig. 12.1-4. *Different types of neurons.*

II. Depending upon the functions
Depending upon the functions the neurons are of two types — motor and sensory.
1. *Motor neurons,* also known as efferent nerve cells, carry the motor impulses from CNS to the peripheral effector organs like muscles, glands and blood vessels. These neurons have very long axon and short dendrites.
2. *Sensory neurons,* also known as afferent nerve cells, carry sensory impulses from periphery to the CNS. These neurons have short axon and long dendrites.

NEUROGLIA

Neuroglia or the glial cells are the supporting cells present within the brain and spinal cord. They are numerous, about 10 times more than the neurons. Glial cells may be divided into two major categories (Fig. 12.1-5):

1. Macroglia

Macroglia or large glial cells are ectodermal in origin. These are of two types:

- *Astrocytes* which may be subdivided into fibrous and protoplasmic astrocytes, and
- *Oligodendrocytes.*

i. Astrocytes. These are small star-shaped cells that give off a number of processes which frequently end in expansions in relation to blood vessels and in relation to the surface of brain. *Fibrous astrocytes* (Fig. 12.1-5A) are seen mainly in the white matter and *protoplasmic astrocytes* (Fig. 12.1-5B) in the gray matter.

ii. Oligodendrocytes. Oligodendrocytes have rounded or pear-shaped bodies with scanty processes (Fig. 12.1-5C). These cells provide myelin sheath to nerve fibres that lie within the brain and spinal cord. Oligodendrocytes give off multiple processes which from myelin sheath on many nieghbouring axons.

2. Microglia

Microglia or the small glial cells are mesodermal in origin. These are the smallest neuroglial cells having flattened cell body and short processes (Fig. 12.1-5D). They are more numerous in gray matter than in white matter. These act as phagocytes and become active after damage to nervous tissue by trauma or disease.

Fig. 12.1-5. Different types of glial cells.

GRAY VERSUS WHITE MATTER

The nervous tissue mass in general is organized into gray and white matter.

GRAY MATTER

Gray matter comprises the cell bodies of neurons and many of their processes (excluding axons). It is found in the outer layer of cortex and other parts of brain and in the core of spinal cord.

The gray matter also composes the ganglion, nucleus, centre and unmyelinated nerve fibres.

WHITE MATTER

White matter, found in the brain, spinal cord, and nerves, is made up of the long axons of the neurons. It contains both myelinated and non-myelinated fibres. However, the preponderance of myelinated fibres gives it a creamy colour, hence the name.

Ganglion

It is an aggregation of neuronal cell bodies located outside the central nervous system. For example :

- *Dorsal root ganglia.* These are composed of cell bodies of the visceral and somatic sensory nerves.
- *Sympathatic and parasympathetic ganglia* of the autonomic nervous system contain the cell bodies of postganglionic visceral efferent nerves.

Nucleus

Nucleus refers to an aggregation of the neuronal cell bodies located inside the central nervous system (brain and spinal cord). The axons (fibres) of the neurons forming nuclei either form a *nerve* (in peripheral nervous system) or a *tract* within the brain or spinal cord. For example :

- *Facial nucleus.* The axons of the cell bodies forming facial nucleus form the facial nerve.
- *Nucleus gracilis.* The axons of the neurons forming nucleus gracilis form the tract inside the central nervous system.

Centre

Centre refers to a group of neurons and synapses regulating certain function. A centre may be located in a nucleus, or ganglion or any other mass of gray matter. Thus, centre refers to a functional entity, while the nucleus and ganglion are anatomical entities. Examples of centres include respiratory control centre, and vasomotor centre located in medulla oblongata.

Peripheral nerve

A compact bundle of axons located outside the CNS is called a nerve. In a nerve the axons are arranged in different bundles called fasciculi (Fig. 12.1-6).

- Each axon or the nerve fibre is covered by *endoneurium* which is bounded internally by basal lamina around the Schwann cells and externally by the relatively impermeable inner basal lamina of the perineurium.
- Each fasciculus is covered by *perineurium.* The cells of perineurium are tightly adherent and act as a barrier to passage of particulate traces, dye molecules or toxins into the endoneurium.
- The whole nerve is covered by *epineurium* which is a tubular sheath formed by areolar membrane. It limits the extent to which the nerve can be stretched by body movements or external pressure, thereby protecting the fragile axons inside the nerve.

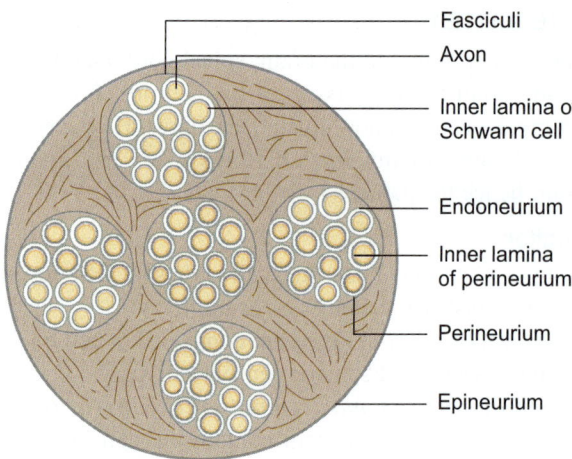

Fig. 12.1-6. *Cross-section of a peripheral nerve.*

Types of nerves

Depending upon the type of nerve impulse transmission, the nerves are of three types :

- Sensory nerves,
- Motor nerves, and
- Mixed nerves.

1. *Sensory nerves* consist of peripheral processes of the neurons which extend upto sensory receptors in the skin. These fibres pass on sensory information to the spinal cord and brain.

2. *Motor nerves* consist of the axons which originate in the brain, spinal cord and autonomic ganglia. They transmit impulses to the effector organs i.e, muscles and glands. Motor nerves are of two types :

- *Somatic motor nerves.* These are involved in voluntary and reflex skeletal muscle contraction.
- *Autonomic nerves* (sympathetic and parasympathetic). These are involved in cardiac and smooth muscle contraction and glandular secretion.

3. *Mixed nerves* consist of sensory as well as motor fibres enclosed within the same sheath of connective tissue.

NERVE PHYSIOLOGY

The main physiological activity of the nerve fibre are :
- Generation of nerve impulse,
- Conduction of nerve impulse, and
- Transmission of impulse at the synapse

GENERATION OF NERVE IMPULSE

EXCITABILITY

Excitability is that property of the nerve fibre by virtue of which it responds by generating a nerve signal (electrical

impulses or the so-called action potentials) when it is stimulated by a suitable stimulus which may be mechanical, thermal, chemical or electrical. In experimental studies, electrical stimulus is more frequently employed since its strength and frequency can be accurately controlled.

RESTING MEMBRANE POTENTIAL

As shown in Fig. 12.1-7A, when two electrodes are placed on the surface of a nerve fibre and connected to a CRO, no potential difference is observed. However, if one of the microelectrodes is inserted inside the nerve fibre (Fig. 12.1-7B), a steady potential difference of –70 mV (inside negative) is observed on the CRO. This is resting membrane potential (RMP) and indicates the resting state of cell also called *state of polarization.*

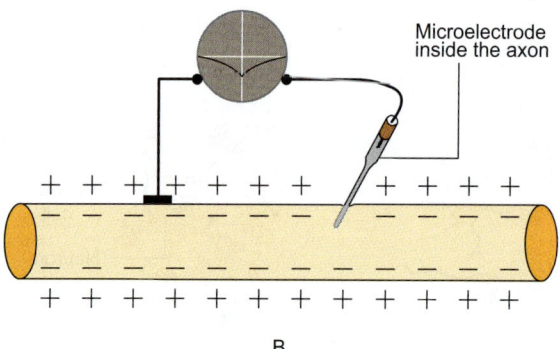

Fig. 12.1-7. *Recording of resting membrane potential.*

ACTION POTENTIAL

The *action potential* may be defined as the brief sequence of changes which occur in the resting membrane potential when stimulated by a threshold stimulus. When the stimulus is subminimal or subthreshold, it does not produce action potential, but does produce some changes in the RMP. There is slight depolarization for about 7 mV which cannot be propagated, since propagation occurs only if the depolarization reaches a firing level of 15 mV (–55 mV). Once the firing level is reached, there occurs action potential, i.e. there occurs abrupt depolarization with propagation (action potential). The adequate strength of stimulus necessary for producing the action potential in a nerve fibre is known as *threshold* or *minimal stimulus.*

Phases of action potential

The action potential basically occurs in two phases: depolarization and repolarization. When the nerve is stimulated, the polarized state (–70 mV) is altered, i.e. RMP is abolished and the interior of the nerve becomes positive (+35 mV) as compared to the exterior. This is called *depolarization phase.* Within no time there occurs reversal to the nearly original potential and this second phase of action potential is called *repolarization phase.*

Ionic basis of action potential

The development of action potential was studied by Hodgkin and Huxley using the *voltage clamp technique.* According to *Hodgkin-Huxley theory,* the sequence of events are (Fig. 12.1-8) :

1. Polarization phase. Resting membrane potential (–70 mV) is due to distribution of more cations outside the cell membrane and more anions inside the cell membrane. At this point though Na⁺ are more in ECF but they cannot enter the cell due to the impermeability of the membrane.

2. Depolarization phase. When threshold stimulus is applied to the cell membrane, at the point of stimulation (Fig. 12.1-8) the permeability of the membrane for Na⁺ ions increases. There occurs a rapid influx of Na⁺ ions into the cell. This rapid entry of Na⁺ leads to depolarization.

3. Repolarization phase. Repolarization occurs due to decrease in further Na⁺ influx and K⁺ efflux through the voltage-gated K⁺ channels which open later than Na⁺ channels but remain activated for prolonged period.

Fig. 12.1-8. *Changes in Na⁺ and K⁺ conductance during action potential.*

Decrease in Na⁺ influx and efflux of K⁺ causes net transfer of positive charge out of the cell that serves to complete the repolarization.

Main characterstics of nerve excitability

1. All or none response. A single nerve fibre always obeys 'all or none law', that is :

- When a stimulus of subthreshold intensity is applied to the axon, then no action potential is produced *(none response);*

- A response in the form of spike of action potential is observed when the stimulus is of threshold intensity; and

- There occurs no increase in the magnitude of action potential when the strength of stimulus is more than the threshold level *(all response).*

This all or none relationship observed between the strength of stimulus and the response achieved is known as 'All or None Law'.

2. Refractory period. Refractory period refers to the period following action potential (produced by a threshold stimulus) during which a nerve fibre either does not respond or responds subnormally to a stimulus of threshold intensity or greater than threshold intensity. It is of two types:

a. *Absolute refractory period (ARP).* It is a short period following action potential during which second stimulus, no matter how strong it may be, cannot evoke any response (another action potential). In other words during absolute refractory period the nerve fibre completely loses its excitability.

b. *Relative refractory period (RRP).* It is a short period during which the nerve fibre shows response if the strength of stimulus is more than normal.

CONDUCTION OF NERVE IMPULSE

Conductivity refers to propagation of nerve impulse (action potential) in the form of a wave of depolarization through the nerve fibre. Normally, in the body, the action potential is transmitted through nerve fibre in one direction. Mechanism of conduction of action potential along an unmyelinated nerve fibre and a myelinated nerve fibre is described below.

Propagation of action potential in an unmyelinated axon

The steps of propagation of action potential along an unmyelinated axon are summarized:

- In the resting phase (polarized state) the axonal membrane is outside positive and inside negative (Fig. 12.1-9A).

- When an unmyelinated axon is stimulated at one site by a threshold stimulus, there occurs action potential at that site, i.e. that site is depolarized. In other words, at that site outside membrane becomes negative and inside positive (reversal of polarity) but the neighbouring areas until now remain in polarized state (Fig. 12.1-9B).

- As ECF and ICF are both conductive to electricity, a current will flow from positive polarized area to negative activated area through ECF and in the reverse direction in ICF (Fig. 12.1-9C). Thus, a *local circuit current* flows between the resting polarized site to the depolarized site of the membrane (current sink).

- This circular current flow depolarizes the neighbouring area of the membrane upto firing level and a new action potential is produced which in turn depolarizes the neighbouring area ahead. Thus, due to successive depolarization of the neighbouring area, the action potential is propagated along the entire length of the axon (Fig. 12.1-9D and E). The portion which depolarizes first also repolarizes first. Thus repolarization also follows the same direction as depolarization (Fig. 12.1.9F).

Propagation of action potential in a myelinated axon

The myelinated nerve fibres have a wrapping of myelin sheath with gaps at regular intervals which are devoid of myelin sheath (nodes of Ranvier). The axonal membrane in the naked area (nodes of Ranvier) bears densely packed ion channels. The myelin sheath acts as an insulator and does not allow the current flow. Therefore, in myelinated nerve fibres the *local circuit of current flow* only occurs from one node of Ranvier to the adjacent node (Fig. 12.1-10). That is, the impulse (action potential) jumps from one node of Ranvier to next. This is known as *saltatory conduction*. Since the impulse jumps from one node to other, the speed of conduction in myelinated fibres is much rapid (50 to 100 times faster) than the unmyelinated fibre.

Orthodromic versus antidromic conduction

Normally, the action potential is propagated in one direction. That is, usually the nerve impulse from the receptors or synaptic junctions travels along the entire length of axon to their termination. This type of conduction is called *orthodromic conduction*. The conduction of nerve impulse in the opposite direction, as seen in the sensory nerve supplying the blood vessels, is called *antidromic conduction*.

Factors affecting conduction velocity

The velocity of conduction in nerve fibres varies from as little as 0.25 m/sec in very small unmyelinated fibres to as high as 100 m/sec in very large myelinated fibres. In general the factors affecting conduction velocity are:

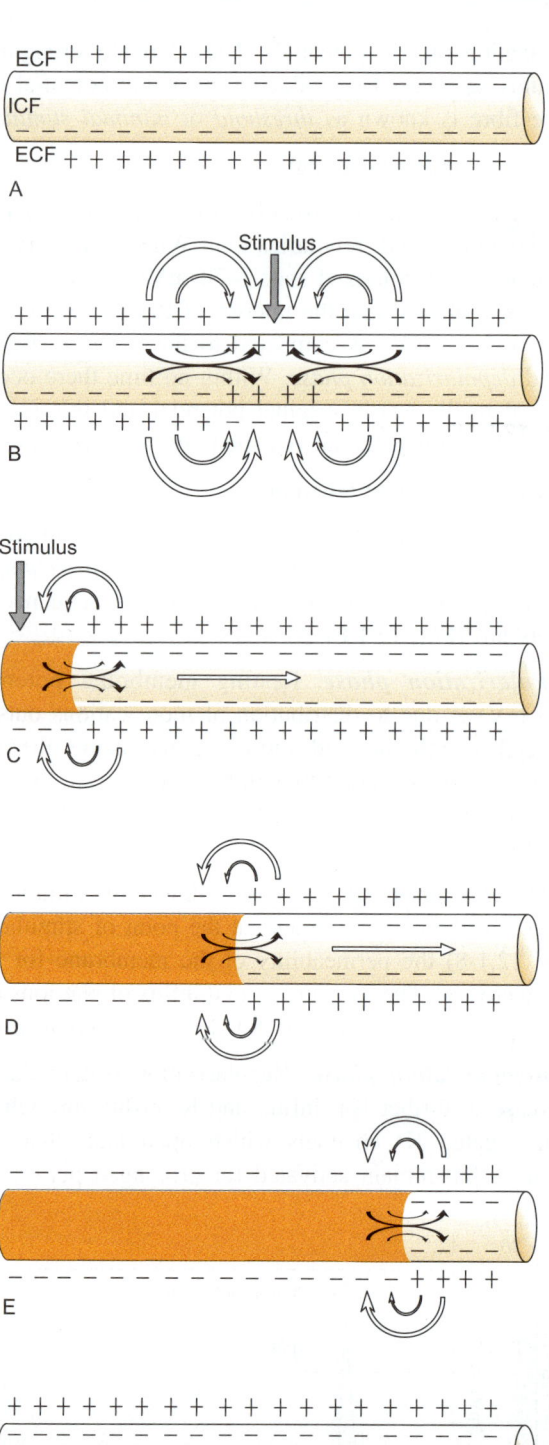

Fig. 12.1-9. *Electrotonic conduction of impulse in an unmyelinated nerve fibre: A, resting phase (polarized state); B, conduction of impulse in both directions when stimulus applied at the middle of nerve fibre; C, when stimulus applied at one end of the nerve fibre; D and E, propagation of impulse in one direction along the nerve fibre; and F, repolarization (occurs in same direction).*

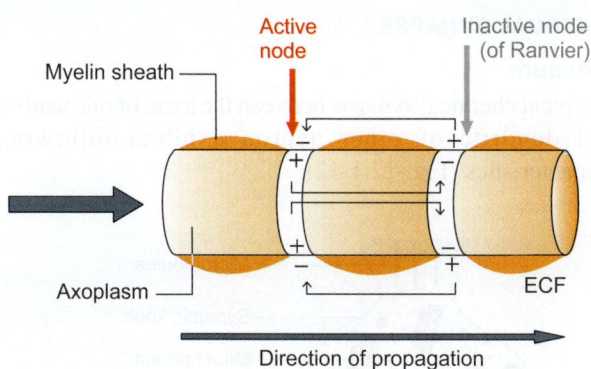

Fig. 12.1-10. *Saltatory conduction along a myelinated nerve fibre.*

1. *Temperature* A decrease in temperature delays conduction, i.e. slows down the conduction velocity.

2. *Axon diameter* affects the conduction velocity through the *resistance offered by the axoplasm* (R_i) to the flow of axoplasmic current. If the diameter of the axon is greater, the axoplasmic resistance (R_i) is lesser and hence the velocity of conduction is higher.

3. *Myelination* increases conduction velocity by its following effects:

- by increasing the axon diameter,
- by the saltatory conduction produced due to its insulating effect (as discussed above).

Conduction velocity and nerve fibre types

Various schemes for classification of nerve fibres on the basis of their diameter and their conduction velocity have been proposed :

1. *Letter classification of Erlanger and Gasser.* This is the best known classification based on the diameter and conduction velocity of nerve fibres. The nerve fibres have been classified into type A, B and C. Their salient features are summarized in Table 12.1-1.

2. *Numerical classification.* Some physiologists have classified sensory nerve fibres by a numerical system into type Ia, Ib, II, III and IV. A comparison of the numerical classification and the letter classification is shown in Table 12.1-2.

TRANSMISSION OF NERVE IMPULSE AT THE SYNAPSE (SYNAPTIC TRANSMISSION)

SYNAPSE: DEFINITION AND TYPES

Definition

The synapse is the anatomic site where the nerve cells communicate among themselves. There is no anatomical connection or continuity between different neurons. They are connected only functionally. So, synapse is the functional junction between two neurons.

Table 12.1-2. Numerical vis-a-vis letter classification of sensory nerve fibres

Numerical classification	Letter classification	Origin
Ia	Aα	Muscle spindle (annulospiral endings)
Ib	Aα	Golgi tendon organ
II	Aβ	Muscle spindle (flower spray endings), touch and pressure
III	Aδ	Pain and cold receptors, some touch receptors
IV	C	Pain, temperature and other receptors.

Table 12.1-1 : Salient features of type A, B and C nerve fibres

Fibre type		Myelinated/ non-myelinated	Fibre diameter (µm)	Conduction velocity (meter/sec)	Spike duration (meter/sec)	Absolute refractory period (meter/sec)	Function Efferent	Afferent
A	α	Myelinated	12–20	70–120	0.4–0.5	0.4–1	Somatic motor	Proprioception
	β	Myelinated	5–12	30–70	0.4–0.5	0.4–1	—	Touch pressure
	γ	Myelinated	3–6	15–30	0.4–0.5	0.4–1	Motor to muscle spindles	—
	δ	Myelinated	2–5	12–30	0.4–0.5	0.4–1		Pain, cold, touch
B	–	Myelinated	< 3	3–15	1.2	1.2	Preganglionic autonomic	
C	–	Non-myelinated	0.4–1.2	0.5–2	2	2	Postganglionic autonomic	Pain, temperature some mechano-receptor reflex responses

Types of synapses

A. Anatomical types

Depending upon the manner an axon terminates on the other neurons, the synapses can be of following types (Fig. 12.1-11):

1. *Axo-dendritic synapse* (Fig. 12.1-11A) is the synapse between axon of a neuron with dendrite of another neuron. It is the most common type of synapse.

2. *Axo-somatic synapse* (Fig. 12.1-11B) refers to the synapse between axon of a neuron with the soma (body) of another neuron.

3. *Axo-axonic synapse* (Fig. 12.1-11C) is the synapse between axon of a neuron with axon of another neuron.

In some parts of the brain (e.g. thalamus) some synapses are seen in which the presynaptic element is dendrite instead of an axon. Such synapses may be *dendro-axonic* or *dendro-dendritic*.

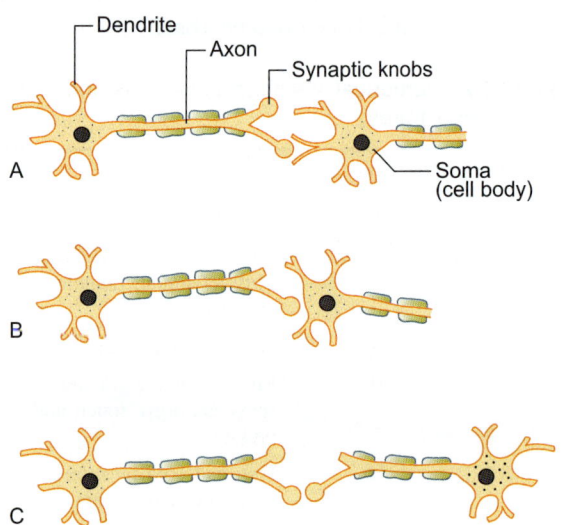

Fig. 12.1-11. *Types of synapses.*

B. Physiological types

Depending upon the process of transmission of impulse, the synapses can be classified as:

1. *Chemical synapses* are those in which transmission is carried out by *neurotransmitter*. Most synapses in human nervous system are of this type.

2. *Electrical synapses* are those in which transmission occurs through gap junctions. Transmission at electrical synapses is essentially an electrotonic conduction between two neurons.

Electrical transmission is seen in a few locations (e.g. within the retina and olfactory bulb) in human nervous system.

3. *Conjoint synapse* refers to a synapse where both the chemical and electrical transmission coexist.

CHEMICAL SYNAPSE

Structure

A typical chemical synapse between the axon of one neuron and dendrite of other neuron exhibits following characteristics (Fig. 12.1-12):

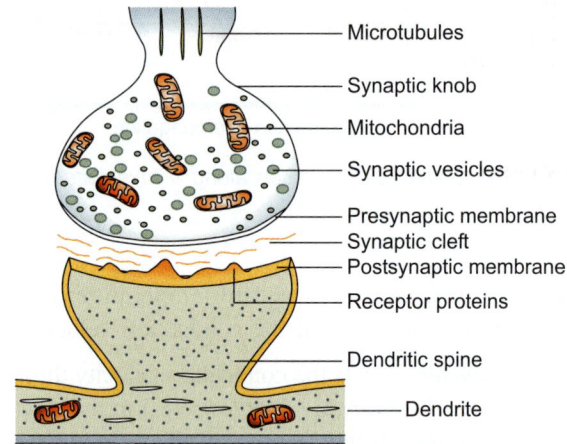

Fig. 12.1-12. *Structure of a chemical synapse.*

Synaptic knob or button. As the axon of neuron approaches the synapse, it loses the myelin sheath and divides into a number of fine branches which end in small swellings called the synaptic knobs or synaptic buttons.

Presynaptic membrane refers to the axonal membrane lining the synaptic knobs.

Synaptic cleft is a small gap (20-40 nm wide) between the pre- and postsynaptic membranes.

Postsynaptic process is the name given to the region of receiving neuron (e.g. dendritic spine) where the synaptic knob synapses.

Postsynaptic membrane is the membrane lining the postsynaptic process.

Process of synaptic transmission

The sequence of events which occur during chemical synaptic transmission are :

- Release of neurotransmitter.
- Development of excitatory post-synaptic potential (EPSP) and inhibitory postsynaptic potential (IPSP).
- Inactivation of neurotransmitter.
- Development of action potential.

NEUROTRANSMITTERS

Definition

Neurotransmitters are the chemical substances which are responsible for transmission of an impulse through a synapse.

Neuromediators or neurohormones. These are chemical substances which are synthesized in neurons and poured into the blood stream through terminals resembling synapses in structure.

Neuromodulators are the chemical substances which are associated with synapses but do not influence synaptic transmission directly.

Physiologically neurotransmitters can be divided into two groups:

- Excitatory neurotransmitters, and
- Inhibitory neurotransmitters.

1. *Excitatory neurotransmitters* can cause an action potential (if the target cell is another neuron), contraction (if the target cell is a muscle), or secretion (if the target cell is a gland).

In the CNS, the excitatory neurotransmitters produce a depolarization of the postsynaptic membrane called the excitatory postsynaptic potential (EPSP). The most common excitatory neurotransmitter within the CNS is glutamate. Other excitatory neurotransmitters are acetylcholine, aspartic acid, etc.

2. *Inhibitory neurotransmitters* reduce or block the activity of the postsynaptic cell. They produce a hyperpolarization of the postsynaptic membrane called the inhibitory postsynaptic potential (IPSP). The most common inhibitory neurotransmitters within the CNS are *glycine* or *gamma-aminobutyric acid* (GABA). Other inhibitory neurotransmitters include dopamine.

Central Nervous System

THE BRAIN

The central nervous system (CNS) consists of the brain and the spinal cord (Fig. 12.2-1). The brain is the largest and most complex mass of nervous tissue in the body. It is contained in cranial cavity and weights about 1380 gm in the adult male and about 1250 gm in the adult female.

Parts of brain

The brain has three parts :

1. *Forebrain* (prosencephalon) comprises :
   - Cerebral hemispheres (telencephalon), and
   - Diencephalon (thalamus plus hypothalamus),
2. *Midbrain* (mesencephalon), and
3. *Hindbrain* (rhombencephalon) comprises :
   - Pons,
   - Medulla oblongata, and
   - Cerebellum

Spinal cord traced upwards becomes medulla oblongata. Above the medulla, a broad bridge, the pons, connects the two hemispheres of the cerebellum which lie behind the pons and medulla. The midbrain connects the forebrain with hindbrain.

Medulla oblongata, pons and midbrain together constitute the *brain stem*.

THE CEREBRUM

EXTERNAL FEATURES

Cerebrum consists of two cerebral hemispheres which are separated from each other in the upper part by a median longitudinal fissure in which the *falx cerebri* (a fold of dura mater) invaginates. In the lower part the two cerebral hemispheres are connected by the largest white commissure called *corpus callosum*.

Sulci and gyri

The surface of cerebral hemisphere is covered by a thin layer (2-4 mm thick) of gray matter called the cerebral cortex. The entire surface of cerebral hemisphere is folded with intervening grooves of fissures. The folds or

Fig. 12.2-1. *Diagrammatic depiction of parts of central nervous system.*

convolutions are called gyri, and the intervening fissures are called sulci. The cerebral cortex follows the contour of the sulci and gyri of the hemisphere. As a result of the folding of the cerebral surface, the cerebral cortex acquires a much larger surface area (about 2200 cm^2).

LOBES AND FUNCTIONAL AREAS

Each cerebral hemisphere is divided into four lobes (Fig. 12.2-2) :
- Frontal lobe,
- Parietal lobe,
- Temporal lobe, and
- Occipital lobe.

FRONTAL LOBE

The frontal lobe lies in front of the central sulcus and above the posterior ramus of the lateral sulcus (Fig. 12.2-2). It forms about one-third of cortical surface. On the basis of functions, the frontal lobe is subdivided into two main areas:
- Precentral cortex, and
- Prefrontal cortex.

I. Precentral cortex

Precentral cortex refers to posterior part of the frontal lobe that includes lip of central sulcus, precentral gyrus, and posterior part of superior, middle and inferior frontal gyri. The precentral cortex is also called excitomotor area of cortex.

Nowadays the motor cortex and sensory cortex are together known as *sensorimotor cortex.*

Areas in precentral cortex

The precentral cortex includes following important areas:
- Primary motor area (Brodmann's area 4),
- Premotor area (Brodmann's areas 6, 8, 44 and 45), and
- Supplementary motor area.

1. *Primary motor area (area 4).* It lies in the precentral gyrus extending into the paracentral lobule on the medial surface (Fig. 12.2-2). Different parts of the contralateral half of the body are represented separately in more or less inverted order. Those parts of the body which carry out the most skilled movements, e.g. the fingers and thumb have the largest areas of cortical representation. The body is represented upside down (however face is not represented in inverted manner) (Fig. 12.2-3A).

Functions. It is concerned with initiation of voluntary movements of the contralateral half of the body and initiation of speech.

2. Premotor area. Premotor area lies anterior to the primary motor area and includes Brodmann's areas 6, 8, 44 and 45.
- *Area 6.* It abuts on the primary motor cortex both above and behind. Cells from this area contribute fibres to pyramidal tracts. Topographical organization of this area is roughly the same as that of primary motor cortex.
- *Area 8.* It is also called frontal eyefield. It lies anterior to area 6. It is concerned with control of eye movements.
- *Area 44 and 45 or Broca's motor speech area.* It is special region of premotor cortex situated in inferior frontal gyrus.

Functions. This area, specially in dominated hemisphere (left hemisphere in right-handed person), is concerned with movements of those structures which are responsible for the production of voice and articulation of speech.

II. Prefrontal cortex

Location. Prefrontal cortex also called prefrontal lobe or orbitofrontal cortex is the anterior part of frontal lobe lying anterior to area 8 and 44 (Fig. 12.2-2).

Major areas. Prefrontal cortex has different Brodmann's areas such as 9 to 14, 23, 24, 29, 32 and 44 to 47.

PARIETAL LOBE

Parietal lobe (Fig. 12.2-2) lies between the central sulcus and parieto-occipital sulcus and upper part of first imaginary line.

Areas of parietal lobe

Functionally parietal lobe can be divided into three parts:
- Primary sensory area (which corresponds to Brodmann's areas 3, 1 and 2),
- Secondary sensory area, and

Fig. 12.2-2. *Left cerebral hemisphere showing lobes, sulci, gyri and functional areas : A, superolateral surface; B, medial surface; and C, inferior surface.*

- Sensory association areas (Brodmann's areas 5 and 7).

Primary sensory area (first somatic sensory area)

Location. The first somatic sensory area (SI) occupies the posterior wall of the central sulcus, the postcentral gyrus and the postcentral part of the paracentral lobule (Fig. 12.2-2).

Major areas. It includes Brodmann's area 3, 1 and 2.

Topographical organization. The primary sensory cortex receives sensory inputs from the opposite half of the body. The representation of the body within this area is similar to that already noted in primary motor cortex (page 433, Fig. 12.2-3B).

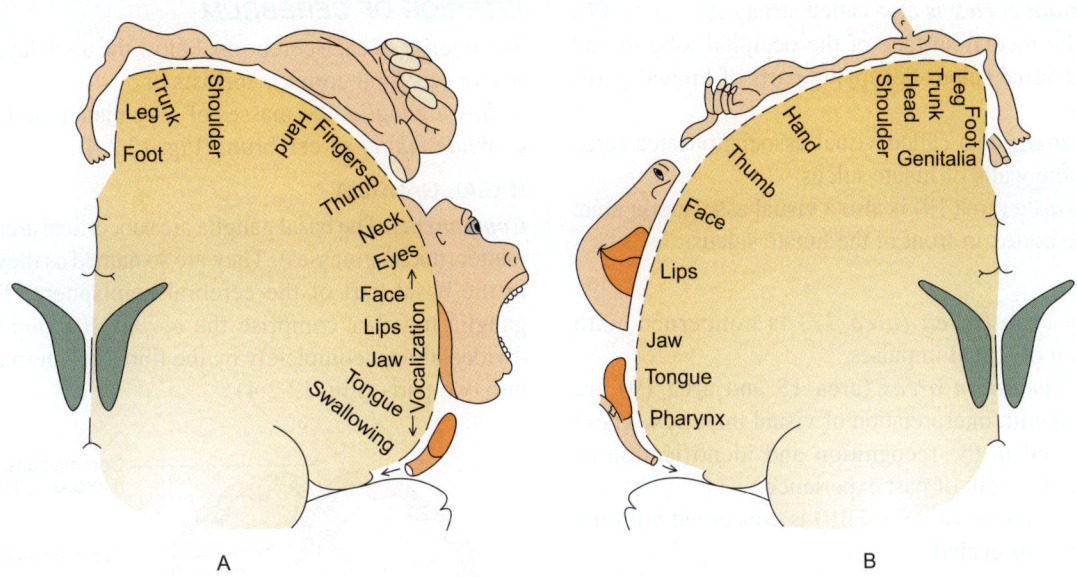

Fig. 12.2-3. *Topographic representation (homonuculus) of motor (A) and sensory (B) areas in cerebral cortex.*

Secondary sensory area

Location. Secondary sensory area, also called second somatic sensory area (SII), is situated in postcentral gyrus below the area of face of first somatic sensory area. Most of it is buried in the superior wall of the sylvian fissure (lateral cerebral sulcus).

Topographical representation. The secondary sensory (SII) area receives sensory impulses from primary sensory area (SI) as well as from thalamus directly. Like SI, the SII area also manifests a dermatomal (point-to-point) sequence of representation (although there is more overlap). Thus the body is represented twice in the somatic sensory cortex, i.e. in area SI as well as in area SII

Sensory association areas

The sensory association areas include area 5 and 7. The area 40 is higher association area.

TEMPORAL LOBE

Temporal lobe (Fig. 12.2-2) lies below the posterior ramus of lateral sulcus and its continuation the second imaginary line.

Areas of temporal lobe

The major areas in the temporal lobe are (Fig. 12.2-2):

Primary auditory area

Primary auditory area, also called audiosensory area, includes Brodmann's area 41 and 42 and forms the centre for hearing.

Functions. This area perceives the nerve impulses as sound, i.e. auditory information such as loudness, pitch, source and direction of sound.

Auditory association area

Auditory association area corresponds to Brodmann's areas 22, 21 and 20.

Area 22, also called Wernicke's area, is a sensory speech centre situated in the posterior part of superior temporal gyrus behind the area 41 and 42, in the categorical hemisphere, i.e. dominant hemisphere.

Functions. It is concerned with:

- Interpretation of the meaning of what is heard, and
- Comprehension of spoken language and the formation of ideas that are to be articulated in speech.

Areas 21 and 20

Location. Areas 21 and 20 are located in the middle and inferior temporal gyrus, respectively.

Functions. These areas receive impulses from primary area and are concerned with interpretation and integration of auditory impulses.

Lesions of these areas impair auditory, short-term memory without impairing visual memory.

OCCIPITAL LOBE

Occipital lobe lies behind the parieto-occipital sulcus and its continuation down an imaginary line (Fig. 12.2-2).

Areas of occipital lobe

Occipital lobe is mostly formed of sensory and association areas. It contains visual cortex having three areas (Fig. 12.2-2):

- Primary visual cortex (area 17),
- Visual association area (area 18), and
- Visual association area or occipital eyefield (area 19).

Primary visual cortex is also called striate area (area 17). It lies on the medial surface of the occipital lobe in and near the calcarine sulcus occupying parts of lingual gyrus and cuneus.

Peristriate area, also called visual association area (area 18), lies in the walls of lunate sulcus.

Parastriate area (area 19) is also a visual association area. It lies in the cortex in front of the lunate sulcus.

Functions

- *Primary visual area (area 17)* is concerned with perception of visual impulses.
- *Visual association areas* (area 18 and area 19) are concerned with interpretation of visual impulses. These are involved in the recognition and identification of objects in the light of past experience.
- *Occipital eyefield area* (area 19) is concerned with the movements of eyeball.

SUMMARY OF CORTICAL FUNCTIONAL AREAS

Classically, cortical functional areas are subdivided into following areas (Fig. 12.2-2):

Motor areas include:

- Primary motor area (Brodmann's area 4),
- Premotor area (area 6),
- Frontal eye field (area 8),
- Supplementary motor area.

Sensory areas include:

- Primary somaesthetic areas (area 3, 1 and 2).
- Secondary (supplementary) somaesthetic area,
- Somaesthetic association areas (area 5, 7 and higher association area 40).

Auditory areas include:

- Primary auditory area (area 41) or auditory area I,
- Auditory association area (area 42) or auditory area II,
- Higher auditory association area (area 22).

Visual areas include:

- Primary visual area (area 17) or visuostriate area of visual area I,
- Visual association area 18 (peristriate area), and
- Visual association area 19 (parastriate area).

Speech areas include:

Motor speech area comprises:

- Anterior area (Broca's area) or areas 44, 45, and
- Superior area.

Sensory speech areas comprise:

- Area 39 (or reading centre),
- Area 40, and
- Area 22 (Wernicke's area)

Smell area is:

- Area 28.

Gustatory area is:

- Area 43.

INTERIOR OF CEREBRUM

The interior of each cerebrum, below the thick layer of gray matter (cerebral cortex), consists of :

- *Basal ganglia*, the masses of gray matter, and
- *White matter* of cerebrum (Fig. 12.2-4).

BASAL GANGLIA

Components. The basal ganglia are subcortical areas of gray matter (nuclear masses). They are so named as they develop in the basal part of the cerebral hemisphere. The basal ganglia together comprise the *corpus striatum* which is divided almost completely by the fibres of internal capsule into two parts (Fig. 12.2-4) :

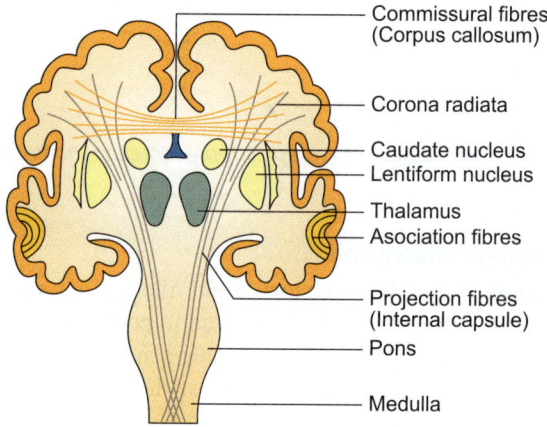

Commissural fibres (Corpus callosum)

Corona radiata

Caudate nucleus
Lentiform nucleus

Thalamus
Asociation fibres

Projection fibres (Internal capsule)

Pons

Medulla

Fig. 12.2-4. *Frontal view of coronal section of cerebrum showing basal ganglia and white matter in the interior.*

1. *Caudate nucleus* (medial part), and
2. *Lenticular nucleus* (lateral part), which is further subdivided into two parts :
   - Putamen (an outer part), and
   - Globus pallidus (the inner part).

Connections. There are connections between the individual members of the basal ganglia and between them and cerebral cortex, the thalamus and the reticular formation of brain stem.

Functions. The basal ganglia form part of a complex known as the *extrapyramidal system,* and control the voluntary movements which are initiated by the motor cortex (upper motor neurons which form the pyramidal system). The extrapyramidal system makes the movements precise and harmonious.

Disorders of basal ganglia (extrapyramidal system) cause diseases with involuntary movements such as:

- *Parkinsonism,* characterized by a triad of akinesia, rigidity and tremors.
- *Chorea,* characterized by irregular, semi-purposive often jerky movements.
- *Athetosis,* characterized by slow, writhing movements.

WHITE MATTER OF CEREBRUM

Passing through, between and around the subcortical masses of gray matter of cerebrum, are tracts of white fibres. The white fibres of cerebrum are of three types (Fig. 12.2-4):

- Association fibres,
- Commissural fibres, and
- Projection fibres.

1. *Association fibres.* Association fibres connect the different gyri of the same hemisphere (Fig. 12.2-4):

2. *Commissural fibres.* Commissural fibres connect the corresponding parts of two cerebral hemispheres with each other. There are five bundles of commissural fibres (Fig. 12.2-4).

- Corpus callosum,
- Anterior commissure,
- Posterior commissure,
- Habenular commissure, and
- Hippocampal commissure.

3. *Projection fibres.* Projection fibres connect the cerebral hemispheres with other parts of CNS, e.g. thalamus, brain stem and spinal cord. Projection fibres include the afferent and efferent tracts contained in corona radiata and internal capsule.

Corona radiata. Corona radiata (fountain of fibres) refers to that part of projection fibres that radiates from the upper end of internal capsule to cerebral cortex (Fig. 12.2-4). It contains both the ascending and descending fibres.

Internal capsule. Internal capsule is a thick curved band of projection fibres (ascending and descending) that occupy the space between the thalamus and caudate nucleus medially, and the lentiform nucleus laterally. Superiorly, it fans out as corona radiata and inferiorly, the fibres descend into the crus cerebri. The inernal capsule can be divided into following parts :

- Anterior limb,
- Genu,
- Posterior limb,
- Retrolenticular of caudal part, and
- Sublentiform part.

Applied aspect. Internal capsule fibres are densely crowded in a narrow area. Pyramidal fibres being compressed in this little space, are particularly vulnerable to effects of even a pinpoint vascular lesion.

- Damage to internal capsule from infarction and haemorrhage is a common form of stroke, resulting in loss or decrease in sensations and movements of the opposite half of the body (*hemianaesthesia and hemiplegia*).

- Most common cause of hemiplegia is the thrombosis or rupture of one of the striate branches of middle cerebral artery which passes through the anterior perforated substance to supply the internal capsule.

DIENCEPHALON

The diencephalon consists of :

- Thalamus, and
- Hypothalamus.

THALAMUS

The thalamus is a large ovoid structure placed immediately lateral to the third ventricle (Figs. 12.2-5 and 12.2-6).

- *Posterior end* (or pole) is expanded and is called pulvinar.
- *Dorsal or superior surface* of the thalamus is convex and forms the part of floor of the central part of lateral ventricle (Fig. 12.2-6).

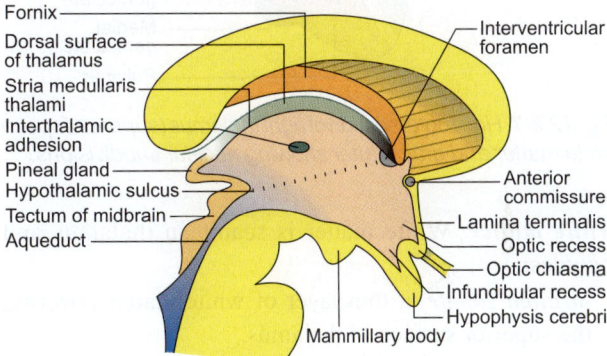

Fig. 12.2-5. *Median section through the brain showing medial surface of thalamus and hypothalamus.*

Fig. 12.2-6. *Coronal section through the brain passing through the basilar part of pons showing the relations of ventral surface of thalamus and subthalamic structures.*

- *Medial surface* forms the greater part of the lateral wall of third ventricle and is lined by ependyma. The medial surfaces of the two thalami are connected by a short bar of gray matter called the *interthalamic adhesion.* Inferiorly, the medial surface is separated from the hypothalmus by *hypothalamic sulcus* (Fig. 12.2-5).
- *Lateral surface* of thalamus is related to the posterior limbs of internal capsule.

Internal structure

Like other parts of brain, thalamus consists of gray matter (mainly) and white matter (Fig. 12.2-7).

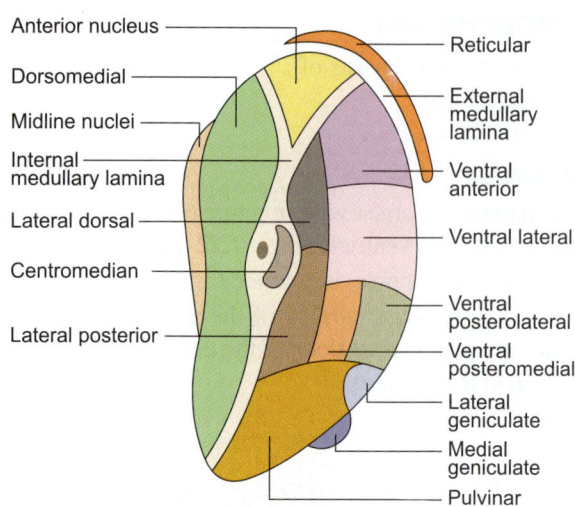

Fig. 12.2-7. *Horizontal section of right thalamus (superior aspect) white matter and gray matter showing nuclear subdivisions.*

White matter. White matter is scanty in thalamus and includes:

- *Stratum zonale*, a thin layer of white matter covering the superior surface of thalamus.
- *External medullary lamina* is a thin layer of white matter covering the lateral surface of thalamus. It consists of thalamocortical and corticothalamic fibres.
- *Internal medullary lamina* is a Y-shaped sheet of white matter placed vertically in the gray matter of thalamus. It consists mainly of internuclear thalamic connections.

Gray matter. Gray matter of thalamus is divided into three masses of nuclei by the Y-shaped internal medullary lamina.

- Anterior group of nuclei,
- Lateral group of nuclei, and
- Medial group of nuclei.

Functionally, the thalamic nuclei can be grouped under two divisions:

- Non-specific projection nuclei, and
- Specific projection nuclei.

Functions and connections

Various functions of thalamus along with the connections through which these functions are mediated are summarized below :

1. *Sensory relay centre*. Almost all the sensory impulses (except olfactory) reach the thalamic nuclei, which relay them to the cerebral cortex by thalamic radiations (ascending thalamocortical system). Because of this, thalamus is usually considered the *head ganglion* of all the sensory system.

2. *Centre for integration of sensory impulses*. The thalamus also forms a major centre for integration and modification of peripheral sensory impulses before the impulses are projected to specific areas of cerebral cortex.

Because of this, thalamus is usually considered as a *functional gateway* of cerebral cortex.

3. *Crude centre for perception of sensations*. Thalamus also acts as a crude centre for sense perception. Pain sensation is perceived in the thalamus itself. Whether a sensation is pleasant or unpleasant and agreeable or disagreeable, is the function of thalamus.

4. *Centre for integration of motor function*. Thalamus receives the output from the basal ganglia and the cerebellum before projecting it to the motor cortex, thereby helping in integration of motor functions by unconscious regulation of muscle tone.

5. *Role in arousal and alertness reaction*. Majority of non-specific ascending impulses from RAS are relayed to thalamus before proceeding to cortex. Through these fibres the thalamus is involved in controlling the level of consciousness and maintaining state of alertness and wakefulness.

6. *Role in emotional aspect of behaviour*. Because of intimate connections between thalamus and frontal cortex and hypothalamus, the thalamus is involved in subjective feeling of various emotions.

7. *Role in language*. Thalamus is also concerned with language (speech) function. Integration between different cortical parts by subcortical connections in the thalamus helps to achieve speech.

8. *Role in synchronization of electroencephalogram*. Thalamus also plays an important role in the genesis of synchronization of electroencephalogram (EEG).

9. *Centre for integration of visceral and somatic function*. Thalamus receives somatic as well as autonomic sensations, and is also connected with hypothalamus. Because of this it also acts as a centre for integration of visceral and somatic functions.

10. *Centre for sexual sensations*. Thalamus also acts as a centre for perception of sexual sensations.

11. *Centre for reflex activity*. All the sensory fibres relay in thalamus, so it forms the centre for many reflex activities.

Applied aspects

Thalamic syndrome. The thalamic syndrome is a disturbance of emotional responses to sensory experience characterized by symptoms and signs which occur on the opposite side of the body. These include:

1. *Astereognosis* occurs due to loss fo tactile localization, tactile discrimination and stereognosis.
2. *Thalamic over-reaction,* i.e. the threshold for pain, touch and temperature is decreased and the sensations become exaggerated and disagreeable.

- Ataxia, decreased muscle tone and profound muscular weakness.
- Involuntary movements

HYPOTHALAMUS

The hypothalamus is a bilateral diencephalic diffuse nuclear mass situated below the thalamus. It is the most important organ of integration in the homeostatic control of internal environment.

Subdivisions and nuclei of hypothalmus

For convenience of description the hypothalamus can be divided as:

From medial to lateral into two zones:

- Medial zone, and
- Lateral zone.

From anterior to posterior, the hypothalmic nuclear mass is arranged in four regions (Fig. 12.2-5):

- Preoptic region,
- Supraoptic region,
- Tuberal region, and
- Mammillary region.

Connections of hypothalamus

The hypothalamus serves as the main integrator of the autonomic nervous system and is concerned with visceral functions, and is, therefore, connected to other areas having a similar function. These include the various parts of the limbic system, the reticular formation, and autonomic centres in the brain stem and spinal cord.

Apart from its neural connections, the hypothalamus also acts by releasing secretions into the blood stream, and into the CSF.

Functions of hypothalamus

1. *Autonomic functions* subserved by the hypothalamus are:

i. *Cardiovascular regulation,* through cardiovascular control centres in the reticular regions of medulla and pons (see page 196).

ii. *Regulation of peristaltic and secretomotor functions of alimentary tract.*

2. *Endocrinal functions* include :

i. *Control of anterior pituitary.* Hypothalamus does the following functions through the releasing hormones:

- Controls the metabolism by controlling thyroid gland.
- Through its influence over adrenal cortex, controls the metabolism of different foodstuffs and maintains electrolyte balance.
- Keeps the gonads inhibited till the physical growth is complete. After physical growth is complete this inhibition is removed so that gonads start functioning and gametes are produced (propagation of species).
- Controls the formation of milk by the breasts by controlling prolactin secretion.

ii. *Regulation of posteior pituitary functions.* Neural control of posterior pituitary with the secretion of antidiuretic hormone (ADH) in regulation of water balance by controlling water excretion by kidneys.

iii. *Regulation of uterine contractility and regulation of milk ejection from the breast.* Oxytocin secretion increases the contractility of uterus especially at end of the pregnancy and thus helps during parturition. It also contracts the myoepithelial cells that surround the alveoli of breast and cause milk ejection. When the baby suckles the breast, signals from nipple to hypothalamus cause reflex oxytocin release which causes expulsion of milk through nipples (see page 410).

3. *Control of circadian rhythm* (biological clock). Circadian rhythm refers to rhythmic fluctuations in certain physiological parameters of the body. These are called circadian rhythms because they often show 24-hour cycles (circadian—around a day).

Common rhythmic variations in homeostatic regulatory mechanism are:

- Rhythmic secretion of ACTH,
- Rhythmic secretion of growth hormone,
- Rhythmic secretion of melatonin,
- Sleep-wake cycles,
- Body temperature rhythm,
- Rhythmic gonadotropin secretion.

4. *Regulation of food intake* by two centres namely, the *feeding centre* and *the satiety centre.*

Normally, the feeding centre is always active and its activity is inhibited by satiety centre after food intake.

5. *Regulation of sexual behaviour and reproduction.* In animals, hypothalamus plays an important role in maintaining the sexual functions, especially in females. A decorticate female animal will have regular oestrous cycle provided the hypothalamus is intact.

6. *Emotional and instinctual behaviour.* The emotional and instinctual behaviour is mainly regulated by limbic cortex. The two centres in hypothalamus involved in such a behaviour and emotional changes are called *reward centre* and *punishment centre.*

7. *Regulation of body temperature.* The hypothalamus acts as principal integrating centre for heat regulation. By adjusting a balance between heat production and heat loss, it helps to maintain body temperature at 37°C. Hypothalamus accomplishes this function by two centres: *heat loss centre,* and *heat gain centre.*

8. *Role in regulation of water balance.* Regulates water balance of the body by two mechanisms:

- *Through thirst centre* by controlling water intake, and
- *Through osmoreceptors* in supraoptic nucleus by controlling water loss.

Applied aspects

Disturbances in hypothalamic lesions include :

- Autonomic disturbances.

- Disturbances of body temperature regulation.
- Sleep disturbances due to lesions in mammillary body and anterior hypothalamus.
- Endocrine abnormalities, e.g. hypogonadism, and hypothyroidism.
- Disturbance in sexual functions due to involvement of mid-hypothalamus.
- Disturbance of body water balance due to damage to supraoptic nuclei or infundibular stalk, characterized by excessive thirst and polyuria.
- Emotional disturbances leading to sham rage due to lesions in ventromedial and posterolateral parts.

BRAIN STEM

The brain stem consists (from below upwards) of the medulla oblongata, pons and midbrain (Fig. 12.2-8).

MEDULLA OBLONGATA

The medulla oblongata is conical in shape and connects the pons above and to the spinal cord below.

External features

Surface of medulla exhibits (Fig. 12.2-8):

- *Median fissure*, present in the centre of anterior surface of medulla, is continuous below with the anterior median fissure of spinal cord.
- *Pyramids* are two swellings, one each present on either side of median fissure. These are composed of bundles of nerve fibres that originate in large nerve cells in the precentral gyrus of the cerebral cortex.
- *Olives* are oval-shaped elevations, present one on each side just posterior to the pyramids. These are produced by the underlying olivary nuclei.
- *Inferior cerebellar peduncles*, which connect the medulla to cerebellum, are present behind the olives.
- *Gracilis and cuneatus tubercles* (produced by the medially placed underlying nucleus gracilis and nucleus cuneatus, respectively) are present on the posterior surface of the inferior part of the medulla oblongata.
- *Cranial nerves* 9th, 10th, 11th and 12th emerge from the surface of medulla.

Internal structure

The main features of the internal structure of the medulla oblongata are most easily reviewed by examining cross-sections at following levels:

- The level of pyramidal decussation (Fig. 12.2-9A), and
- Transverse section at the level of sensory decussation (Fig. 12.2-9B).

Functions

1. *Pathway for ascending and descending tracts.* The medulla oblongata forms the main pathway for the ascending and descending tracts of spinal cord (see page 472 and 475).

2. *House of vital centres.* The medulla oblongata houses many important centres which control the vital functions of the body:

- *Respiratory centres* (inspiratory and expiratory) control the normal rhythmic respiration (page 240)
- *Vasomotor and cardiac centres* control the blood pressure and functions of heart and vascular system (page 196)
- *Deglutition centre* controls the pharyngeal and oesophageal phase of deglutition (page 267)
- *Vomiting centre* is responsible for inducing vomiting in disorders of gastrointestinal tract.
- *Superior and inferior salivary nuclei*, located in the medulla, control the salivary secretion (page 453).

3. *Cranial nerve nuclei* located in the medulla control following functions:

- *Twelfth cranial (hypoglossal) nerve* controls the movements of tongue,
- *Eleventh cranial (accessory) nerve* controls the movements of shoulder.
- *Tenth cranial (vagus) nerve* controls the functions of important viscera viz heart, lungs and GIT.
- *Eighth cranial nerve* controls the auditory function (cochlear division of the nerve has the relay in medulla oblongata) and vestibular function (medial and inferior vestibular nuclei extend through much of the medulla).

PONS

The pons is situated on the anterior surface of the cerebellum below the midbrain and above the medulla oblongata (Fig. 12.2-8).

Internal structure

Internally pons is divisible into two parts (Fig. 12.2-10):

1. *Ventral (basilar) part of the pons* contains:

- *Transverse fibres*, laterally form the middle cerebellar peduncle.
- *Vertical fibres*, present in the pons, are of two types:
  - Corticopontine fibres, and
  - Corticospinal fibres
- *Pontine nuclei* are the groups of neurons which are scattered amongst the nerve fibres.

2. *Dorsal (tegmental) part of pons* contains:

- Decussations of trapezoid body,
- Nuclei of 5th, 6th, 7th and 8th cranial nerves,
- Pontine reticular formation, and
- A number of descending and ascending tracts.

The most prominent ascending tracts are the four lemnisci: medial, trigeminal, spinal and lateral.

Functions

Pons subserves following functions:

1. Connecting pathway between cerebral cortex and cerebellum.

Fig. 12.2-8. *Gross anatomy of brain stem: A, ventral aspect; and B, dorsal aspect.*

2. Pathway for ascending and descending tracts of spinal cord and medulla oblongata.

3. Joining station for medial lemniscus with fibres of 5th, 7th, 9th and 10th cranial nerves.

4. Contains pneumotaxic and apneustic centres for regulation of respiration (page 240).

MIDBRAIN

The midbrain is a narrow part of the brain that connects forebrain to hindbrain (Fig. 12.2-8).

Posterior surface of midbrain exhibits (Fig. 12.2-8B):

- *Superior colliculi,* two rounded swellings, one on each side of midline.

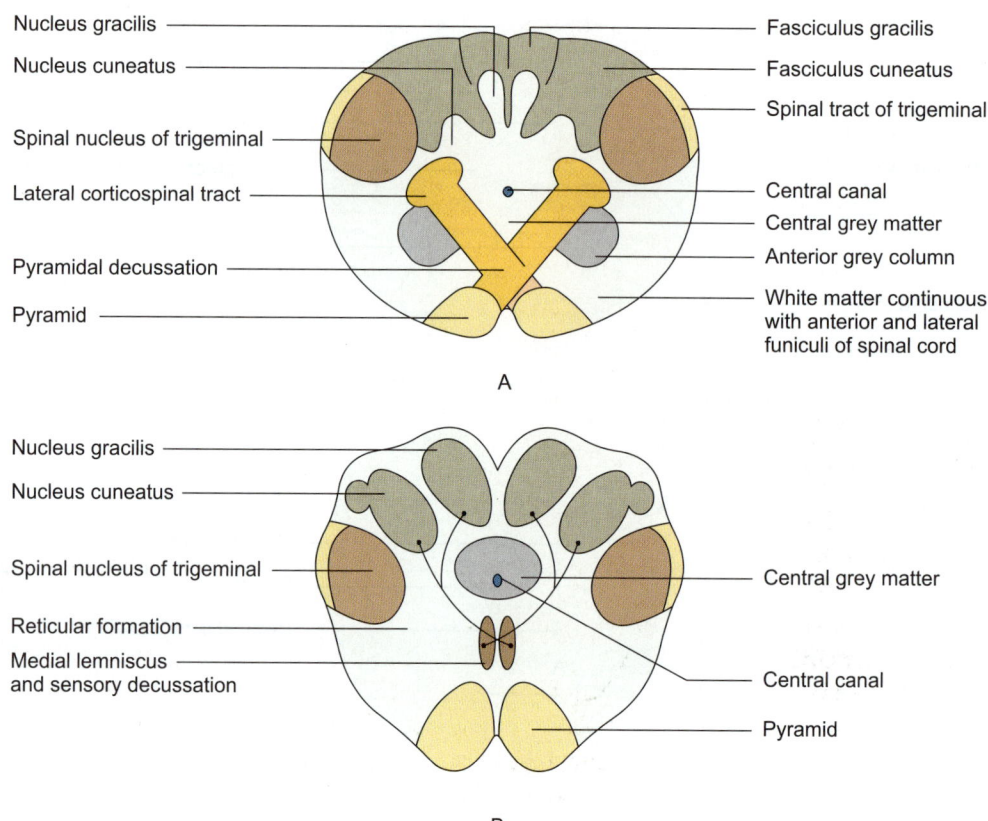

Fig. 12.2-9. *Main features of internal structure of medulla oblongata exhibited by transverse section at the level of :*
A, pyramidal decussation; and B, sensory decussation.

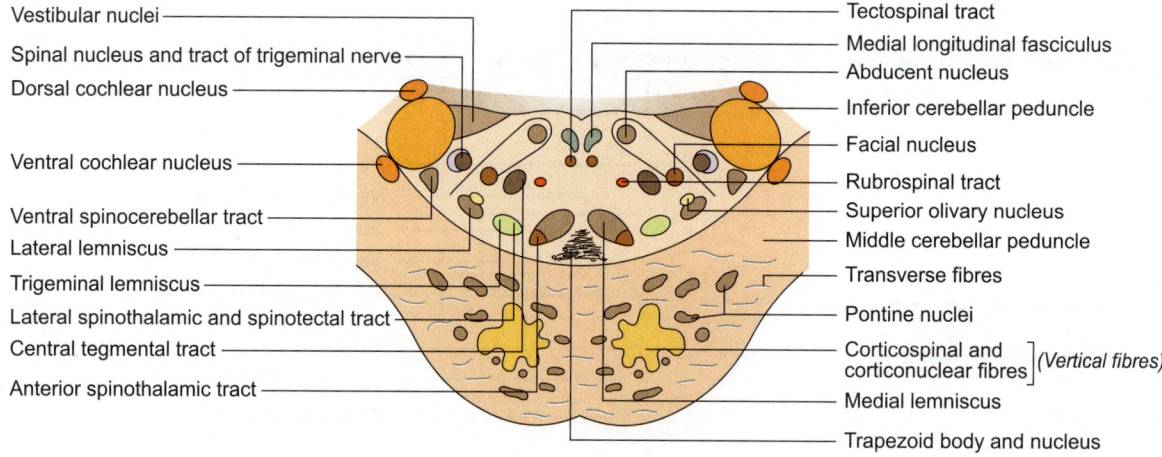

Fig. 12.2-10. *Internal structure of pons.*

- *Inferior colliculi,* two rounded swellings, one on each side of the midline located below the superior colliculi.

Internal structure

Internally for convenience of description the midbrain can be divided into two parts (Fig. 12.2-11):

1. Tectum. It consists of superior and inferior colliculi.

2. Cerebral peduncles. Each cerebral peduncle, in turn, consists of three parts, which from anterior to posterior side are:

i. *Crus cerebri* (or basis pedunculi). It consists of large mass of vertically running descending fibres from cerebral cortex which include frontopontine fibres, corti-

Fig. 12.2-11. *Internal structure of mid brain exhibited by transverse section at the level of superior colliculi.*

cospinal and corticonuclear fibres and temporopontine, parietopontine and occipitopontine fibres (occupying the lateral one-sixth of crus).

ii. *Substantia nigra* is a mass of pigmented gray matter (therefore appears dark in colour).

iii. *Tegmentum* of the two sides is continuous across the midline. It contains following important masses of gray matter and nerve fibres:

- Red nucleus,
- Nuclei of 3rd, 4th and 5th cranial nerves,
- Reticular formation of midbrain,
- Fibre bundles of the tegmentum, and
- Three decussations.

HINDBRAIN

The hindbrain consists of

- Pons (described above),
- Medulla oblongata (described above), and
- Cerebellum.

CEREBELLUM

Gross anatomy

Cerebellum, the largest part of hindbrain, consists of two lateral parts called the *cerebellar hemispheres* connected in the midline by a narrow central region called the *vermis*. The cerebellum is thrown into numerous transverse folds called folia. The surface of the cerebellum presents three main fissures (Fig. 12.2-12):

- *Primary fissure*. It is V-shaped, with open being forwards. It forms the posterior limit of the anterior lobe.
- *Horizontal fissure* separates the superior surface of the cerebellum from its inferior surface.

- *Posterolateral fissure* is situated anteriorly on the inferior surface of the cerebellar hemisphere and separates the posterior lobe from the flocculonodular lobe.

Vermis

Vermis is so named because it resembles a worm which is bent on itself to form a complete circle. It consists of following parts: lingula, central lobule, culmen, declive, folium, tuber, pyramis, uvula and nodule (Fig. 12.2-13).

Anatomical divisions

Anatomically the cerebellum has been divided into three lobes:

1. Anterior lobe is that part of cerebellum which lies in front of the primary fissure on the superior surface (Figs. 12.2-12 and 12.2-13).

2. Posterior lobe is that part of cerebellum which lies between the primary fissure and posterolateral fissure.

3. Flocculonodular lobe is that part of the cerebellum which lies anterior to the posterolateral fissure on the inferior surface. It consists of (Figs. 12.2-12 and 12.2-13):

- *Nodule*, which is rostral part of the vermis, and
- *Floculli*, which are irregular shaped masses attached to nodule on each side. They are almost completely separated from the rest of cerebellum.

Histological structure

Histologically, cerebellum consists of (Fig. 12.2-14):

- Cerebellar cortex (outer gray matter layer),
- White matter (formed by afferent and efferent nerve fibres of cerebellum) forming medullary core, and
- Deep cerebellar nuclei (masses of gray matter embedded in the medullary core).

I. Cerebellar cortex

Microscopically the gray matter of cerebellar cortex

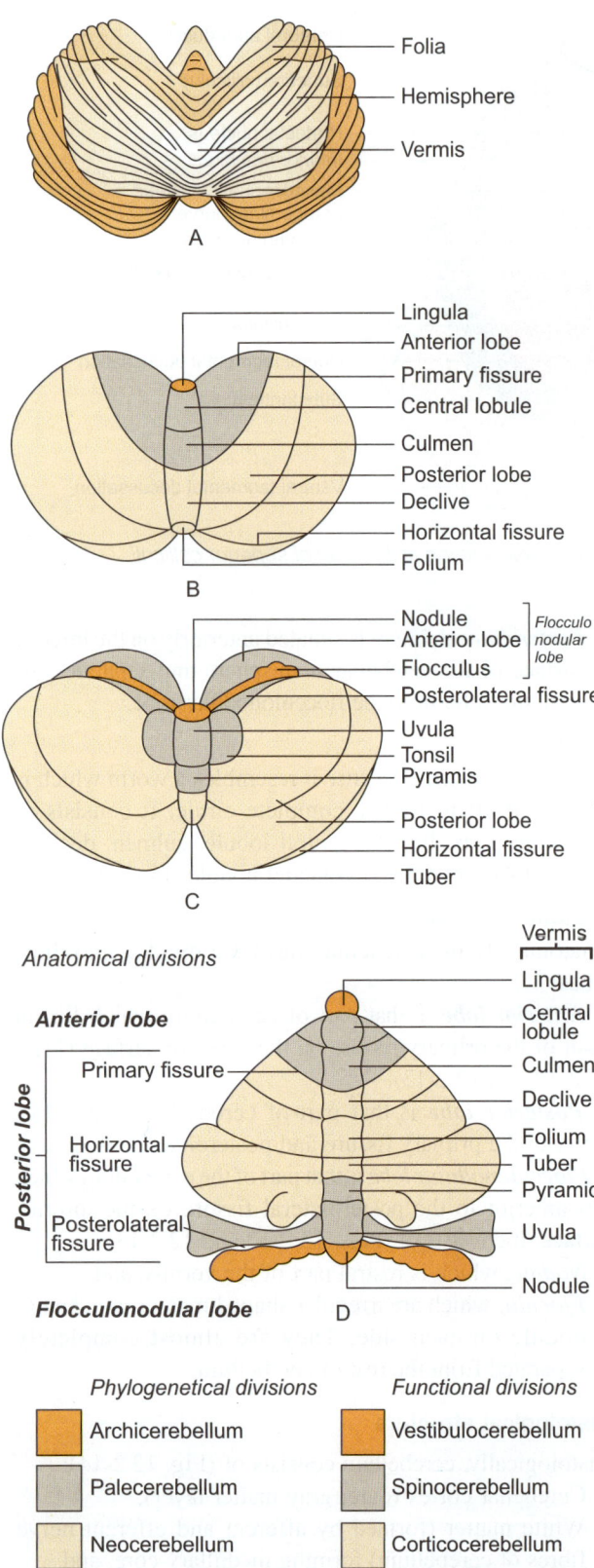

Lobes of cerebellum	Part of vermis	Part of hemisphere
Anterior lobe	Lingula	No lateral projection
	Central lobule	Alae
	Culmen	Anterior quadrangular lobule
	Primary fissure	
Posterior lobe	Declive	Posterior quadrangular lobule
	Folium	Superior similunar lobule
	Horizontal fissure	
	Tuber	Inferior semilunar lobule
	Pyramis	Biventral lobule
	Uvula	Tonsil
	Posterolateral fissure	
Flocculo-nodular lobe	Nodule	Flocculus

Fig. 12.2-13. *Lobes of cerebellum and parts of vermis and hemisphere forming them.*

consists of five main types of neurons (stellate cells, basket cells, Purkinje cells, granule cells and Golgi cells) which are arranged in three layers:

- **Molecular layer** (most superficial) is composed of two types of neurons (stellate and basket cells) and unmyelinated nerve fibres.
- **Purkinje cell layer.** It is composed of a single layer of large flask-shaped Purkinje cells and dendrites of Purkinje cells.
- **Granule cell layer** consists of granule and Golgi cells, with their processes, and sensory mossy fibres with their synaptic glomeruli.

II. White matter of cerebellum

The cerebellar cortex, i.e. outer gray matter surrounds inner medullary core of white matter (an arrangement opposite to what is seen in spinal cord). White matter is formed by both afferent and efferent fibres. These fibres can be classified in three groups:

1. *Projection fibres* of the cerebellum leave or enter the cerebellum. These are arranged in three bundles:

- *Inferior cerebellar peduncle* consists of fibres connecting cerebellum with medulla,
- *Middle cerebellar peduncle* contains the fibres which connect cerebellum with pons, and
- *Superior cerebellar peduncle* which connects the cerebellum with midbrain.

2. *Association fibres* connect different regions of the same cerebellar hemisphere.

3. *Commissural fibres* connect the areas of two halves of cerebellar cortex with each other.

III. Deep cerebellar nuclei

Within the white matter of medullary core of cerebellum

Fig. 12.2-12. *Gross anatomy of cerebellum: A, Superior surface showing folia; B and C, Superior and Inferior surface showing lobes, fissures and parts of vermis; and D, Schematic diagram show parts of vermis and hemispheres.*

Fig. 12.2-14. *Histology of cerebellar cortex.*

are embedded four pairs of masses of gray matter called deep cerebellar nuclei.

1. *Dentate nucleus*
2. *Emboliform nucleus*
3. *Globossus nucleus*
4. *Fastigial nucleus*

Functions of cerebellum

1. Control of body posture and equilibrium. Vestibulocerebellum which includes flocculonodular lobe as its principal component and nucleus fastigii (as its effector nucleus) and vermal region of the cerebellum are concerned with control of body posture and equilibrium.

2. Control of muscle tone and stretch reflexes. Spinocerebellum regulates the postural reflexes by modifying muscle tone. It facilitates the gamma motor neurons in the spinal cord. The γ motor neurons reflexly modify the activity of α motor neurons and thus regulate the muscle tone. Thus cerebellum forms an important site of linkage of α-γ systems responsible for muscle tone.

3. Control of voluntary movements. Cerebellum is not able to initiate any motor activity, but coordinates movements initiated by the motor cortex.

Control of movements by cerebellum includes regulation of time, rate, range (extent), force and direction of muscular activity.

4. Other functions of cerebellum. Recent studies have shown the importance of the cerebellum as:

i. *Influence on autonomic system.* It has been postulated that the cerebellum may influence autonomic functions and thus respiratory, cardiovascular, pupillary and urinary bladder responses.

ii. *Influence on conduction in ascending sensory pathway* may be exerted by the cerebellum through the reticular formation and thalamus.

iii. *Control of eyeball movements.* The oculomotor, trochlear and abducent nuclei which supply extraocular muscles of eye movements are brought under the cerebellar control through vestibular nuclei. Medial longitudinal fasciculus is involved in these connections.

Cerebellar lesions

Common signs observed in patients with cerebellar dysfunction due to lesions of cerebellum are:

1. Disturbances in tone and posture include :

i. *Atonia or hypotonia.* Hypotonia refers to reduction and atonia to loss of tone in muscles. It occurs due to reduction of the facilitatory neocerebellar output to the descending inhibitory reticular formation.

ii. *Attitude changes.* Trunk is bent with concavity towards the affected side; this is because the weight of the body is thrown on the unaffected leg.

iii. *Deviation movement.* The arm held straight out in front of the body deviates laterally when the eyes are closed. In bilateral lesions both arms deviate.

iv. *Effect on deep reflexes.* The deep or tendon reflexes become weak and pendular.

2. *Disturbances in equilibrium.* The patient suffering from disturbance of equilibrium walks on a wide base, sways from side to side (drunken-like gait), and is unable to maintain the upright posture due to involvement of vestibular system.

3. *Disturbances in movements* include :

i. *Ataxia*, i.e. lack of coordination of movements, is the hallmark of cerebellar disorder.

ii. *Intention tremors* become evident during purposeful movements, and diminish or disappear with rest. These tremors become more marked as the hand approaches the object, i.e. are observed at the end of movement and are coarse, oscillating, to and fro and rhythmic.

iii. *Nystagmus* refers to regular and rhythmic to and fro involuntary oscillatory movements of the eyes, occurring due to incoordination of extraocular muscles.

iv. *Dysarthria* or scanning speech occurs due to inco-ordination of various muscles and structures involved in speech.

SPINAL CORD

ANATOMY OF SPINAL CORD

Gross anatomy

- The spinal cord (Fig. 12.2-15) extends from the upper border of the first cervical vertebra to the lower border of the first lumbar vertebra.
- Its upper end becomes continuous with medulla oblongata and its lower end called *conus medullaris* becomes continuous with a fibrous cord called *filum terminale*.
- The spinal cord, like the brain, is surrounded by three meninges: the dura mater, the arachnoid mater, and the pia mater.

Internal structure

As seen on cross-section (Fig. 12.2-16) the spinal cord presents inner gray matter and outer white matter. Gray matter is constituted by the nerve cell bodies, dendrites and parts of axons, while white matter is formed by the myelinated and unmyelinated nerve fibres.

1. Spinal gray matter

In transverse section the gray matter of spinal cord forms an H-shaped mass in the centre of which is present a canal called the spinal canal. The *spinal gray* matter exhibits following parts:

Dorsal horn or posterior gray column refers to the posterior horn-like projection of the H-shaped gray matter in each lateral half of the cord.

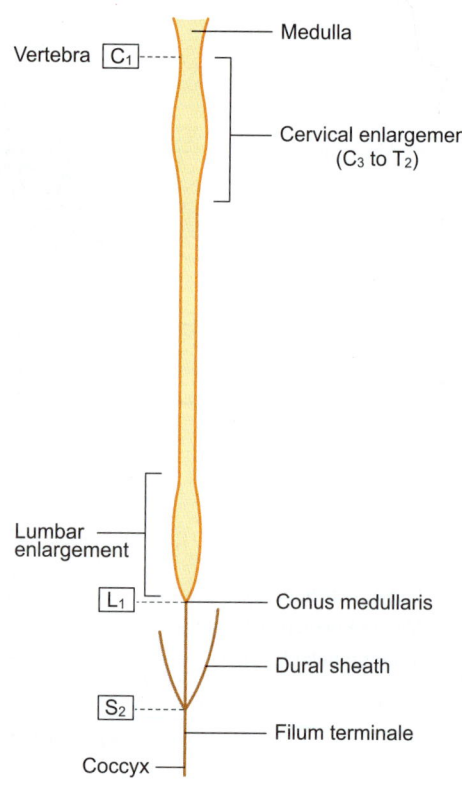

Fig. 12.2-15. *Gross appearance of spinal cord and its relations with vertebrae.*

Ventral horn or anterior gray column refers to the anterior projection of the gray matter in each lateral half of the cord.

Lateral horn or intermediate horn or lateral column refers to small lateral projection between the ventral and dorsal gray columns, present in the thoracic segments and first two lumbar segments only.

Gray commissure is the part of the gray matter which connects the two (right and left) symmetrical halves of spinal gray matter across the midline. It is traversed by the central canal.

Neurons in spinal gray matter

Neurons in ventral horn. The ventral horn neurons of spinal gray matter are involved in motor functions and send motor nerve fibres to the muscles and other effector organs.

Neurons in dorsal horn. The dorsal horn neurons of spinal gray matter are involved in sensory functions.

Neurons in the lateral horn. The lateral horn cells of spinal gray matter extend from T_1 to L_2 segments and from S_2 to S_4 segments of the spinal cord.

2. White matter of spinal cord

White matter is formed by the nerve fibres which are arranged as ascending and descending tracts (described later). In general, the white matter of spinal cord is divided into right and left halves, in front by a deep *anterior median*

Fig. 12.2-16. *Cross section of thoracic segment of spinal cord.*

fissure, and behind by the *posterior median septum* (Fig. 12.2-16). In each half the spinal white matter exhibits following parts:

- Posterior funiculus or posterior white column
- Anterior funiculus or anterior white column
- Lateral funiculus
- Anterolateral funiculus
- Ventral (anterior) white commissure
- Dorsal (posterior) white commissure.

Note. Tracts of spinal cord are described along with the tracts of the brain stem (see page 438).

Spinal segments and spinal nerves

Spinal segments

Spinal cord, though a continuous structure, can be considered to consist of 31 spinal segments, each giving attachment to rootlets of the ventral and dorsal root, of each spinal nerve (Fig. 12.2-17). The 31 segments of spinal cord correspond symmetrically to 31 spinal nerves and are named as:

- *8 Cervical segments* give attachment to 8 cervical nerves,
- *12 Thoracic segments* give attachment to 12 thoracic nerves,
- *5 Lumbar segments* give attachment to 5 lumbar nerves,
- *5 Sacral segments* give attachment to 5 sacral nerves, and
- *1 Coccygeal segment* gives attachment to 1 coccygeal nerve.

Spinal nerves

Each spinal nerve is a mixed nerve formed by union of two roots: a dorsal (sensory) root and a ventral (motor) root (Fig. 12.2-17).

1. *Dorsal nerve root.* The dorsal nerve root is formed by several rootlets. All sensory fibres reach the spinal cord

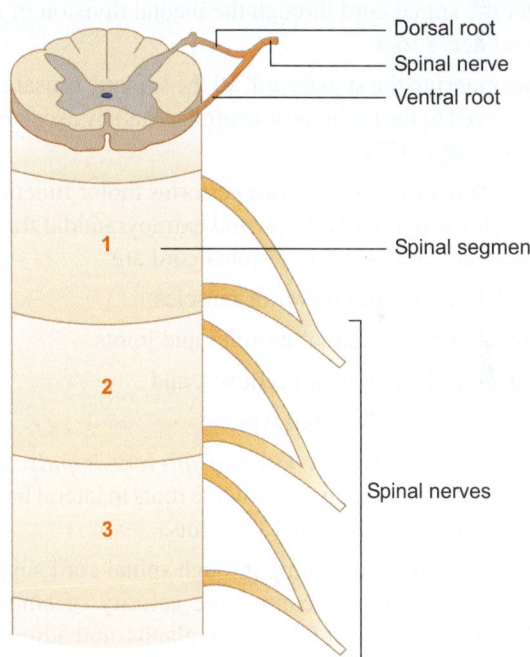

Fig. 12.2-17. *Scheme to illustrate the concept of spinal segment and roots of spinal nerve.*

through dorsal nerve roots. Each dorsal nerve root is marked by a swelling called dorsal nerve root ganglion or spinal ganglion. Dorsal root ganglion is composed of T-shaped unipolar neurons with peripheral and central processes.

Peripheral processes of dorsal root ganglion cells extend upto sensory receptors in the skin. The area of the skin supplied by a spinal nerve is called *dermatome*.

Central processes of dorsal root ganglion cells constitute the dorsal nerve root which is attached to spinal cord through various rootlets. Each rootlet just before entering the spinal cord divides into medial and lateral divisions.

2. *Ventral nerve root.* The ventral nerve root is composed of axons of motor neurons present in the ventral gray horn. The ventral root also contains the autonomic fibres originating from the lateral (intermediate) horn of the spinal gray matter (lamina VII).

FUNCTIONS OF SPINAL CORD

1. *Sensory functions.* All the somatic afferent impulses enter the spinal cord through the dorsal nerve root as:

- The fibres mediating *thermal and pain sensations* enter the spinal cord through the lateral division of dorsal nerve root, and

- The fibres conveying all *other sensory impulses* and proprioceptive impulses (touch, deep pressure, joint sense, vibration sense) from muscles, tendons and joints enter the spinal cord through the medial division of the dorsal nerve root.

After entering the spinal cord, all the somatic sensations are conveyed to the brain (post-central gyrus) by ascending tracts (see page 472).

2. *Motor functions.* Spinal cord performs motor functions through the pyramidal tracts and extrapyramidal tracts. Motor functions served by spinal cord are:

- Control of tone and power of muscles,
- Control of movement of muscles and joints,
- Control of deep (tendon) reflexes, and
- Control of superficial reflexes.

3. *Autonomic functions.* *Visceral afferent impulses* in spinal cord travel through dorsal nerve roots to lateral horns of T_1 to L_2 and S_2 to S_4 spinal segments.

Autonomic efferents travelling through spinal cord supply the visceral organs and control the activity of smooth muscles, heart, glands of GIT, sweat glands, and adrenals. The spinal cord also regulates the body temperature. In other words, spinal cord helps in maintaining the optimal internal environment of the body through its autonomic function.

LESIONS OF SPINAL CORD

Complete transection of spinal cord

The effects (symptoms and signs) produced by complete transection of the spinal cord occur in following three stages:

A. *Stage of spinal shock.* Spinal shock refers to cessation of all the functions and activity below the level of the section immediately after injury. *Characteristic effects during shock* are summarized:

1. *Motor effects* include:
- Paralysis of the muscles below the level of section.
- Loss of tone in the paralysed muscles. So the muscles become atonic or flaccid. This is called state of flaccid paralysis.
- Areflexia, i.e. all the superficial and deep reflexes are markedly decreased or lost.
2. *Sensory effects.* All the sensations are lost below the level of transections.
3. *Vasomotor effects.* The sympathetic vasoconstrictor fibres leave the spinal cord between T_1 and L_2. Therefore, depending upon the site of lesion, the vasomotor effects produced are:
- Extremities are cold and blue (cyanotic).
- Skin becomes dry and scaly and bedsores may develop.
4. *Visceral effects* produced are:
- Retention of urine.
- Constipation
- Penis becomes flaccid and erection becomes impossible.

B. *Stage of reflex activity.* After about 3 weeks period, depending largely upon the general health of the patient, the reflex activity begins to return to the isolated segments of spinal cord below the level of lesion. Various developments which take place are :
- Smooth muscles regain functional activity first of all.
- Sympathetic tone of the blood vessels is regained.
- Skeletal muscle tone then recovers slowly after 3 to 4 weeks.
- Reflex activity begins to return after few weeks of recovery of muscle tone.

C. *Stage of reflex failure.* The failure of reflex activity may occur when general condition of the patient starts deteriorating.

Peripheral Nervous System

The peripheral nervous system is that part of nervous system which lies outside the central nervous system (CNS). It consists of peripheral nerves and the ganglia associated with them. A peripheral nerve may consist of one, two or all the following three divisions :
- *Somatic sensory division,*
- *Somatic motor division, and*
- *Autonomic division.*

Somatic system connects the CNS to the skin and skeletal muscles, while the autonomic fibres connects the CNS to visceral organs such as the heart, stomach, intestine, various glands and smooth muscles in the body. The peripheral nervous system includes :
- *Cranial nerves, and*
- *Spinal nerves.*

CRANIAL NERVES

There are twelve pairs of cranial nerves which arise from the brain (Fig. 12.3-1). Some of them are sensory bringing impulses to the brain, others are motor, carrying impulses from the brain to periphery, while a few are mixed containing both motor and sensory fibres.

Fig. 12.3-1. *Undersurface of brain showing attachment of the various cranial nerves.*

Cranial nerves are designated either by a number or a name. The numbers indicate the order in which the cranial nerves arise from the front to the back of brain, and the names which describe their nature, function, or distribution. The twelve cranial nerves include :

Number	Name	Nature
I	Olfactory nerve	Sensory
II	Optic nerve	Sensory
III	Oculomotor nerve	Motor
IV	Trochlear nerve	Motor
V	Trigeminal nerve	Mixed
VI	Abducens nerve	Motor
VII	Facial nerve	Mixed
VIII	Vestibulocochlear nerve	Sensory
IX	Glossopharyngeal nerve	Mixed
X	Vagus nerve	Mixed
XI	Accessory nerve	Motor
XII	Hypoglossal nerve	Motor

I. OLFACTORY NERVE

Each olfactory nerve consists of about 15-20 nerve filaments. It is a sensory nerve associated with sense of smell. For details (see page 501)

II. OPTIC NERVE

The optic nerve is a sensory nerve associated with sense of vision. For details (see page 485)

III. OCULOMOTOR NERVE

Functional components

The oculomotor nerve is entirely motor in function having three functional components :

- *Somatic efferent component* is concerned with the movements of eyeball and supplies all the extraocular muscles except the lateral rectus and superior oblique.

- *General visceral efferent* (parasympathetic) component of nerve is meant for accommodation and constriction of pupil. It supplies the ciliary muscle and sphincter pupillae muscle.
- *General somatic afferent* component is associated with propioceptive impulses from the extraocular muscles supplied. Thus, although the III nerve is a motor nerve, some sensory fibres are present.

Nucleus

The nuclear complex of the oculomotor nerve is situated in the midbrain (Fig. 12.3-2). It has two motor nuclei:
- *Main motor nucleus* is composed of five subnuclei each supplying a muscle.
- *Accessory motor nucleus* (Edinger-Westphal nucleus) sends preganglionic parasympathetic fibres along the other oculomotor fibres.

Course and distribution

Each third nerve (Fig. 12.3-3) emerges from the midbrain, runs forward through the cavernous sinus. In the anterior part of cavernous sinus it divides into superior and inferior divisions which enter the orbit through the middle part of superior oblique fissure (Fig. 12.3-4).
Superior division supplies the superior rectus and levator palpebral superioris muscle.
Inferior division divides into three branches :

- Nerve to medial rectus,
- Nerve to inferior rectus, and
- Nerve to inferior oblique, which gives off the *motor root* containing preganglionic parasympathetic fibres to *ciliary ganglion.*

Fig. 12.3-2. *Scheme to show the cranial nerve nuclei as projected on to the posterior surface of brain stem.*

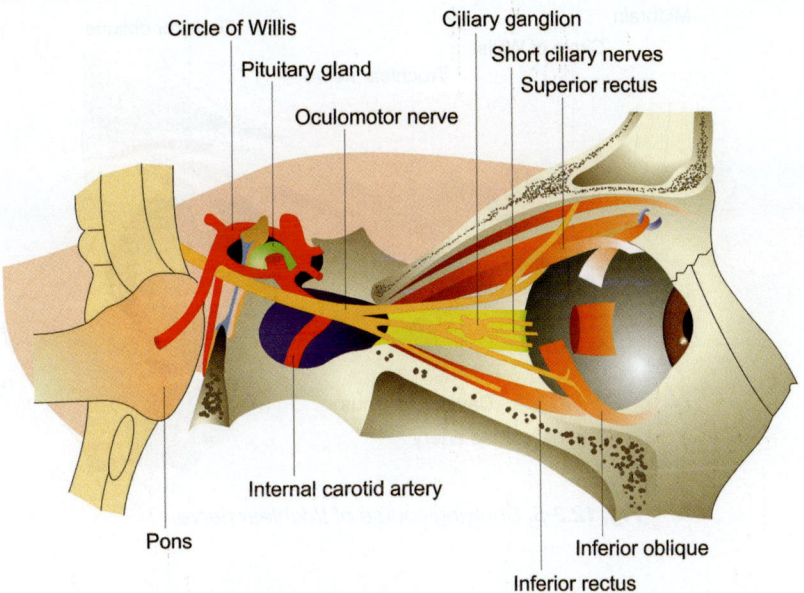

Circle of Willis
Pituitary gland
Oculomotor nerve
Ciliary ganglion
Short ciliary nerves
Superior rectus
Internal carotid artery
Pons
Inferior oblique
Inferior rectus

Fig. 12.3-3. *Showing the course of oculomotor nerve.*

Lacrimal nerve
Frontal nerve
Superior ophthalmic vein
Trochlear nerve
Lateral rectus
Oculomotor nerve
Nasociliary nerve
Abducent nerve
Oculomotor nerve

Superior rectus
Levator palpebrae superioris
Superior oblique
Medial rectus
Optic nerve
Ophthalmic artery
Annulus of Zinn
Inferior rectus
Superior orbital fissure
Inferior ophthalmic vein

Fig. 12.3-4. *Apical part of orbit showing origin of extraocular muscles and structures passing through superior oblique fissure and optic canal.*

IV. TROCHLEAR NERVE

Functional components

The trochlear nerve is entirely motor in function having two functional components :

- *Somatic efferent* component is concerned with the movement of eyeball through the superior oblique muscle.
- *General somatic afferent* component carries propioceptive impulses from the superior oblique muscle. These impulses are relayed to the mesencephalic nucleus of the trigeminal nerve.

Nucleus

Nucleus of trochlear nerve is located in midbrain caudal to and continuous with third nerve nuclear complex (Fig. 12.3-2).

Course and distribution

The trochlear nerve (Fig. 12.3-5), after emerging from the dorsal aspect of midbrain, winds around it and runs forward through the cavernous sinus. In the anterior part of cavernous sinus it rises up, enters the orbit through the lateral part of superior oblique fissure (Fig. 12.3-4) and ends by supplying the superior oblique muscle.

VI. ABDUCENS NERVE

Sixth cranial nerve is described before fifth cranial nerve, as like third and fourth nerve it also supplies extraocular muscle.

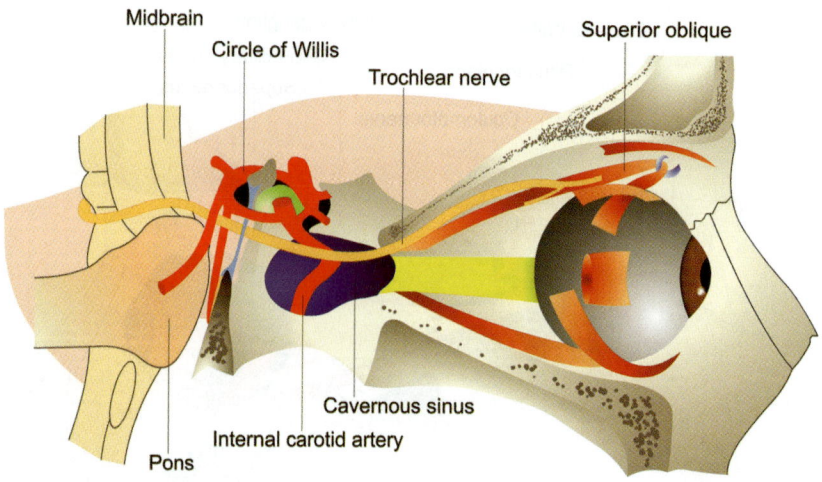

Fig. 12.3-5. *Showing course of trochlear nerve.*

Functional components

The abducens nerve is small entirely motor nerve having two functional components :
- *Somatic efferent* component, for lateral movement of the eyeball.
- *General somatic afferent,* component for propioceptive impulses from the lateral rectus muscle. These impulses ultimately reach the mesencephalic nucleus of trigeminal nerve.

Nucleus

The abducens nucleus is situated in the lower part of pons, close to midline, beneath the floor of fourth ventricle. It lies in line with nuclei of fourth and third nerves above and with nucleus of hypoglossal nerve below (Fig. 12.3-2).

Course and distribution

The abducens nerve emerges from the junction of pons (Fig. 12.3-1) and runs forwards, upwards and slightly laterally. At the sharp upper border of petrous temporal bone, the nerve bends forward at right angle and enters the cavernous sinus through its posterior wall (Fig. 12.3-6). In the cavernous sinus the nerve runs forward and leaves the sinus to enter the orbit through the middle part of superior oblique fissure within the annulus of Zinn (Fig. 12.3-4). In the orbit, the nerve runs forward and enters the ocular surface of the lateral rectus muscle (Fig. 12.3-6).

V. TRIGEMINAL NERVE

The trigeminal (fifth cranial) nerve is the largest cranial nerve and contains both sensory and motor fibres.

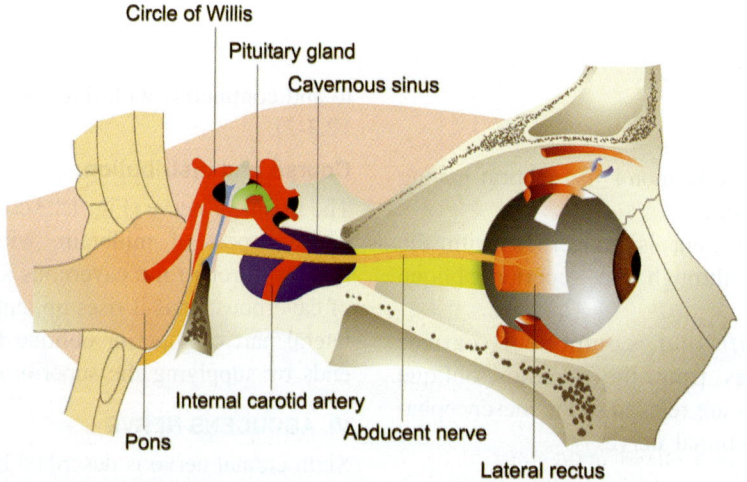

Fig. 12.3-6. *Showing course of sixth cranial nerve.*

Nuclei

The trigeminal nerve has four nuclei (Fig. 12.3-2):

1. **Main sensory nucleus** lies in the upper part of pons.
2. **Spinal nucleus** extends from below the main sensory nucleus in the pons, through the whole length of the medulla oblongata into the upper two segments of the spinal cord.
3. **Mesencephalic nucleus** extends from the midbrain down in the pons upto the main sensory nucleus.
4. **Motor nucleus** is situated in the upper part of pons medial to the main sensory nucleus.

Functional components

Trigeminal nerve is a mixed nerve, having two functional components :

1. **General somatic afferent** component is constituted by sensory nuclei which receive the sensory fibres from trigeminal nerve as below :

- *Main sensory nucleus* receives fibres carrying sensations of touch and pressure.
- *Spinal nucleus* receives fibres carrying sensations of pain and temperature.
- *Mesencephalic nucleus* receives fibres carrying proprioceptive impulses from the facial and extraocular muscles and muscles of mastication.

2. **Branchial efferent (motor) component** for muscles of mastication and certain muscles in the floor of mouth.

Course and distribution

The trigeminal nerve emerges from the anterior aspect of pons as a small motor root and large sensory root (Fig. 12.3-1). It passes forwards and joins the trigeminal (gasserian) ganglion.

Trigeminal ganglion is the sensory ganglion of the fifth cranial nerve. It is homologous with the dorsal root ganglion of a spinal nerve.

Division of trigeminal nerve. It has three divisions (Fig. 12.3-7) :

1. *Ophthalmic division or nerve.* It consists of sensory fibres that bring impulses to the brain from the surface of eye, the lacrimal gland, skin of upper eyelid, forehead, and anterior part of scalp (Fig. 12.3-8). Main branches are lacrimal nerve, frontal nerve and nasociliary nerve.

2. *Maxillary division or nerve.* It is also a sensory nerve and consists of the fibres which bring impulses to the brain from the area of cheek, upper lip, upper gums, upper teeth and mucous lining of palate (Fig. 12.3-8). It ends by dividing into two terminal branches : infraorbital and zygomatic nerve.

3. *Mandibular nerve.* It is a mixed nerve formed by the union of two trunks—the large sensory and small motor.

Fig. 12.3-7. *Showing course of trigeminal nerve.*

Fig. 12.3-8. *Area of face and scalp supplied by three divisions of trigeminal nerve : A, ophthalmic nerve; B, maxillary nerve; and C, mandibular nerve.*

- *Sensory trunk* consists of the fibres which bring impulses from the lower lip, lower jaw, lower gums, lower teeth and skin of scalp behind the ear (Fig. 12.3-8).
- *Motor root* supplies the muscles of mastication, tensor tympani muscles and certain muscles of the floor of mouth.

VII. FACIAL NERVE

Functional components

The facial (seventh cranial) nerve is both a motor and sensory nerve. It consists of three functional components:

- *Special visceral efferent* component for facial expression and elevation of hyoid bone.
- *General visceral efferent* component is concerned with parasympathetic supply of the lacrimal gland, submandibular and sublingual salivary glands.
- *Special visceral afferent* for taste sensation from the tongue.

- *General somatic afferent* from the skin of external ear. These fibres end in spinal nucleus of trigeminal nerve.

Nuclei

The facial nerve has three nuclei (Fig. 12.3-2).

1. *Main motor nucleus* is located deep in the pons. Special visceral efferent fibres arise from this nucleus. The part of nucleus that supplies the muscles of upper part of face receives corticonuclear fibres from both cerebral hemispheres and that supplies to the lower part of face receive corticonuclear fibres from the opposite cerebral hemisphere only (Fig. 12.3-9).

Cerebral cortex

UMN lesions (supranuclear)

Paralysis of lower face on the oppposite side

Nuclear ⎤
          ⎬ LMN lesions
Infranuclear ⎦

Paralysis of upper as well as lower face on the same side

UMN lesion   LMN lesion

Fig. 12.3-9. Facial nerve nucleus, connections vis-a-vis supply to upper and lower part of face and facial expression defects associated with lesion of 1, upper motor neuron; and 2, lower motor neuron.

2. *Parasympathetic nuclei* are :
- *Superior salivatory nucleus* which sends preganglionic (general visceral) fibres for submaxillary and sublingual salivary glands.
- *Lacrimatory nucleus.* It sends preganglionic (general visceral) fibres for innervation of the lacrimal gland.

3. *Sensory nucleus* is formed by the upper part of the *nucleus tractus solitarius* which belong to the special visceral efferent group. It receives afferents fibres carrying sensation of taste.

Course and distribution

The two roots (motor and sensory) of facial nerve emerge from the junction of pons and medulla (Fig. 12.3-10). These roots then run laterally and forward and enter the internal *acoustic meatus,* where it joins to form single trunk. The *geniculate ganglion* associated with the nerve is formed by cell bodies of the *sensory neurons* carrying impulses from the skin of external ear.

Branches and course of the nerve within petrous part of temporal bone is shown in Fig. 12.3-10 and its extracranial course and branches after emerging from the stylomastoid foramen are shown in Fig. 12.3-11.

VIII. VESTIBULOCOCHLEAR NERVE

Functional component and nuclei

The vestibulocochlear nerve consists of two divisions, both made of *special somatic afferent fibres.* The sensory nuclei include :

1. *Vestibular nuclei* are four in number, which are situated partly in the medulla and partly in the pons, immediately beneath the lateral part of the floor of fourth ventricle (Fig. 12.3-2).

2. *Cochlear nuclei* are two in number, dorsal and ventral. They are located on the dorsal and ventral aspects of the inferior cerebellar peduncle, respectively in the upper part of the medulla (Fig. 12.3-2).

Course and distribution

The vestibulocochlear nerve arises from the medulla (Fig. 12.3-1). It consists of two divisions :

1. *Vestibular nerve* consists of the central processes of bipolar neurons while cell bodies are located in the *vestibular ganglion* near the vestibule and semicircular canals of the ear. The peripheral processes of these neurons innervate the vestibular receptors in the semicircular ducts and saccule and utricle of the inner ear. These receptors are sensitive to changes in the position of head. The impulses they initiate pass into the cerebellum, where they are used in reflexes associated with the maintenance of equilibrium.

2. *Cochlear nerve* consists of the central processes of bipolar neurons of spiral ganglia. The peripheral processes of these neurons innervate the *organ of Corti* (hearing receptors). Impulses from the cochlear nerve pass through the pons and medulla oblongata on their way to temporal lobe (auditory cortex) for interpertation. For details see page 500.

IX. GLOSSOPHARYNGEAL NERVE

Functional components and nuclei

Glossopharyngeal nerve is a mixed nerve having following nuclei and functional components (Fig. 12.3-12).

1. *Special visceral (branchial) efferent.* Fibres arise from the *nucleus ambiguus,* which is an elongated not clearly defined (hence the name ambiguos, nucleus that extends

Fig. 12.3-10. *The course and distribution of branches of facial nerve within the facial canal in the petrous part of temporal bone.*

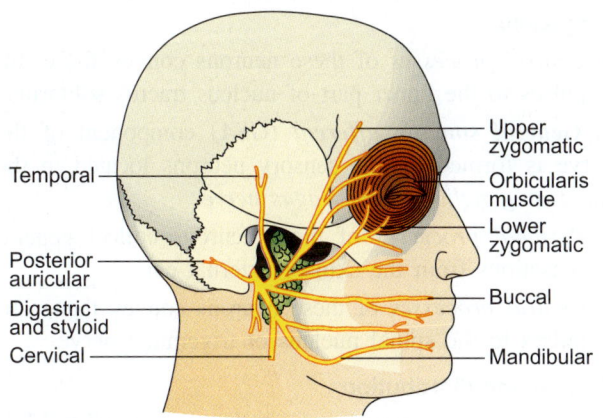

Fig. 12.3-11. *Branches of facial nerve after emerging from the stylomastoid foramen.*

throughout the length of medulla (Fig. 12.3-2). The special visceral efferent fibres arising from it supply only one muscle—the *stylopharyngeous.*

2. General visceral efferent fibres, which arise from the *inferior salivatory nucleus,* is located in the pons, immediately caudal to superior salivatory nucleus and just above the upper end of the dorsal nucleus of vagus (Fig. 12.3-2). The preganglionic parasympathetic fibres arising from this nucleus relay in the *otic ganglion;* and the postganglionic fibres supply the parotid gland (Fig. 12.3-13).

3. **General visceral afferent (GVA)** component of the glossopharyngeal nerve is formed by sensory neurons located in the *superior ganglion* of glossopharyngeal nerve.

- *Peripheral processes* of these neurons collect general sensations (touch, pain and temperature) from the posterior 1/3rd of the tongue, pharynx and carotid body.
- *Central processes* of these neurons relay these sensations to the spinal nucleus of trigeminal nerve.

4. **Special visceral afferent** (SVA) component of ninth cranial nerve is formed by the sensory neurons located in the *inferior ganglion* of the nerve.

Fig. 12.3-12. *Functional components and nuclei of IX (glossopharyngeal) nerve.*

- *Peripheral processes* of these neurons collect taste sensation from the posterior 1/3rd of tongue.
- *Central process* of these neurons relay the taste sensation to the nucleus of tractus solitarius, located in the medulla (Fig. 12.3-2).

Course and distribution

Glossopharyngeal nerve arises from the medulla (Fig. 12.3-1). Course and distribution of its fibres described above in the functional components is depicted in Fig. 12.3-13.

Fig. 12.3-14. Functional components and nuclei of vagus.

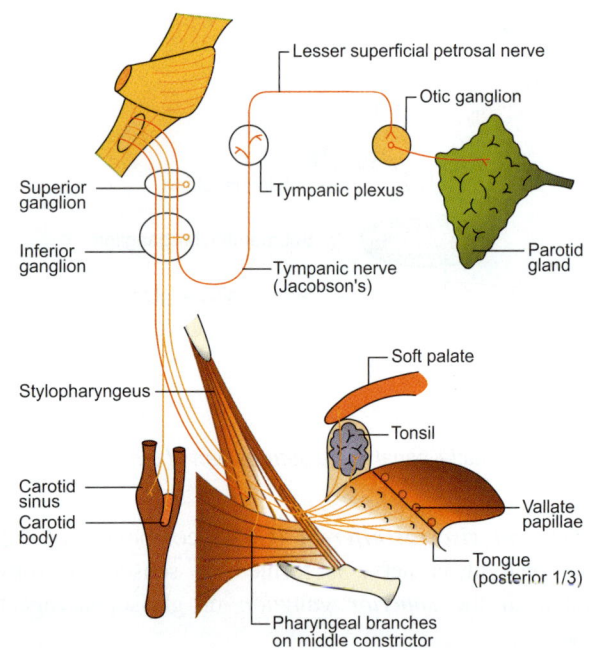

Fig. 12.3-13. Course and distribution of glossopharyngeal nerve.

X. VAGUS NERVE

Functional components and nuclei

Vagus nerve is a *mixed nerve* having following functional components and associated nuclei (Fig. 12.3-14):

1. Special visceral efferent (SVE) fibres arise from the *nucleus ambiguos* and supply muscles of pharynx and larynx.

2. General visceral efferent (GVE) fibres arise from the *dorsal nucleus of vagus* also called *motor nucleus of vagus,* which is elongated and extends in most of the length of medulla (Fig. 12.3-2).

- *Preganglionic parasympathetic fibres* arising from the dorsal vagus nucleus relay in the small ganglia situated close to or within the walls of viscera supplied.
- *Postganglionic parasympathetic fibres* arising from the small ganglia supply the heart, lungs, GIT upto the junction of right 2/3rd and left 1/3rd of transverse colon (Fig. 12.3-15).

3. General visceral afferent (GVA) component of vagus nerve is formed by the sensory neurons located in *inferior ganglion of* the nerve.

- *Peripheral processes* of these neurons collect sensations from the pharynx, trachea, oesophagus and thoracic and abdominal viscera.
- *Central processes* of these neurons convey the impulses to *nucleus tractus solitarius* and dorsal nucleus of vagus.

4. Special visceral afferent (SVA) component of the vagus nerve is formed by the sensory neurons located in the *inferior ganglion of the vagus nerve.*

- *Peripheral processes* of these neurons bring taste sensations from the posterior-most part of the tongue and epiglottis.
- *Central processes* of these neurons convey these impulses to the upper part of nucleus tractus solitarius.

5. General somatic afferent (GSA) component of the nerve is formed by the sensory neurons located in the *superior ganglion of the vagus nerve.*

- *Periphal processes* of these neurons collect general sensations from the skin of external ear.
- *Central processes* of these neurons convey these impulses to the spinal nucleus of trigeminal nerve.

Course and distribution

The vagus nerve originates from the medulla (Fig. 12.3-1), and extends downward through the neck into the abdomen. Course and distribution of its various branches carrying different fibres described above in the functional components are shown in Fig. 12.3-15.

XI. ACCESSORY NERVE

Functional components and nuclei

1. Special visceral efferent (SVE) fibres arise from the *nucleus ambiguos* and from the *cranial root* of the nerve. These fibres are distributed through the vagus nerve to supply :

- *Muscles of palate* except tensor palati which is supplied by mandibular division of trigeminal nerve.

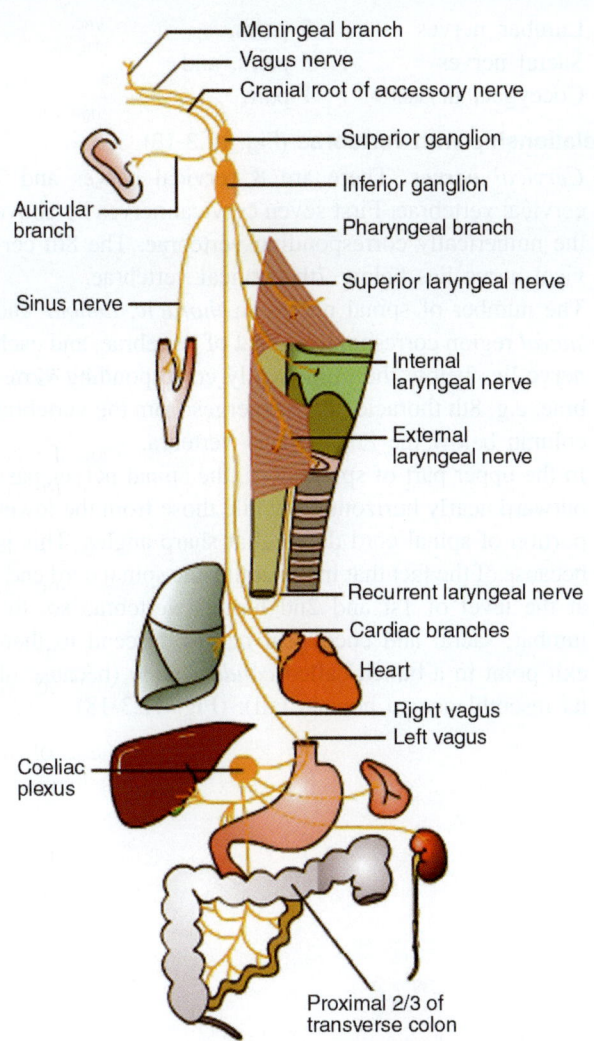

Fig. 12.3-15. Distribution of vagus nerve.

Fig. 12.3-16. Course and distribution of accessory nerve.

XII. HYPOGLOSSAL NERVE

Functional components and nuclei

Hypoglossal nerve is a motor nerve having following functional components and associated nuclei :

1. **General somatic efferent (GSE)** component is formed by the nerve fibres arising from the *hypoglossal nucleus,* which is an elongated column extending throughout the length of medulla oblongata in the para- median plane (Fig. 12.3-2). These fibres supply all the intrinsic and extrinsic muscles of the tongue except the platoglossus which is supplied by the cranial root of accessory nerve through the vagus nerve.

2. **General somatic afferent (GSA)** component is formed by the sensory fibres which carry proprioceptive impulses from muscles of the tongue. The location of the neurons of origin of these fibres is uncertain.

- *Muscles of pharynx* except stylopharyngeus which is supplied by the glossopharyngeal nerve.
- *Muscles of larynx.*

2. **General somatic efferent (GSE)** component of the nerve is formed by the motor fibres arising from the *spinal nucleus of accessory nerve,* which is located in the lateral part of the anterior gray column of the upper five cervical spinal segments. These fibres form the *spinal root* of the nerve.

Course and distribution

The accessory nerve originates as two roots (Fig. 12.3-1):

1. **Cranial root** of the accessory nerve arises from the medulla and joins the vagus nerve. As mentioned above it carries motor impulses to muscles of palate, larynx and pharynx (Fig. 12.3-16).

2. **Spinal root** of the nerve arises from the spinal cord and descends into the neck and supplies motor fibres to trapezius and sternocleidomastoid muscles (Fig. 12.3-16).

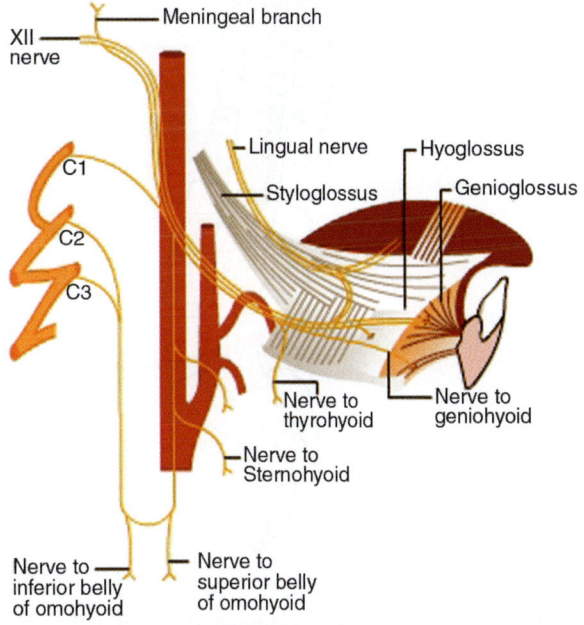

Fig. 12.3-17. Course and distribution of hypoglossal nerve.

Course and distribution

Hypoglossal nerve arises from the medulla by ten to fifteen rootlets (Fig. 12.3-1). It leaves the cranial cavity through the hypoglossal canal and extends downward in the neck upto the level of angle of mandible. Then it passes forward into the tongue and supplies the muscles that move the tongue in speaking, chewing, and swallowing. Course and distribution of nerve are depicted in Fig. 12.3-17.

SPINAL NERVES

GENERAL CONSIDERATIONS

There are 31 pairs of spinal nerves which originate from the spinal cord. They are grouped together in five groups. Nerves belonging to different groups are named according to the regions of vertebral column with which they are associated. Various groups of spinal nerves are as below:

- Cervical nerves : 8 pairs,
- Thoracic nerves : 12 pairs,
- Lumbar nerves : 5 pairs,
- Sacral nerves : 5 pairs, and
- Coccygeal nerves : 1 pair.

Relationship with vertebrae (Fig. 12.3-18)

- *Cervical nerves.* There are 8 cervical nerves and 7 cervical vertebrae. First seven cervical nerves lie above the numerically corresponding vertebrae. The 8th cervical nerve lies below 7th cervical vertebrae.
- The number of spinal nerves in *thoracic, lumbar* and *sacral* region corresponds to that of vertebrae, and each nerve lies below the numerically corresponding vertebrae, e.g. 8th thoracic nerve emerges from the vertebral column below the 8th thoracic vertebra.
- In the upper part of spinal cord, the spinal nerves pass outward nearly horizontally while those from the lower portion of spinal cord descend at sharp angles. This is because of the fact that in the adults the spinal cord ends at the level of 1st and 2nd lumbar vertebrae so, the lumbar, sacral and coccygeal nerves descend to their exit point in a bunch called *cauda equina* (because of its resemblance to horse's tail). (Fig. 12.3-18).

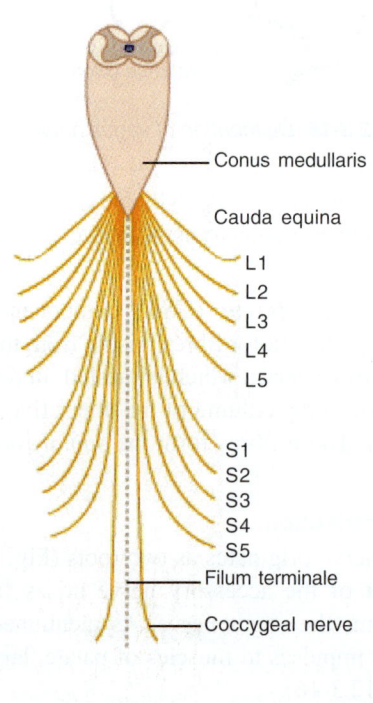

Fig. 12.3-18. A: Lateral view showing relationship of the spinal cord to the vertebral column. Note the site of origin of each spinal nerve in the cord and its point of exit from the vertebral column; B : Formation of cauda equina.

DESCRIPTION OF A TYPICAL SPINAL NERVE

A typical spinal nerve is a mixed nerve, i.e., consists of sensory and motor nerve fibres.

Origin of spinal nerve

Each spinal nerve arises by two roots, a ventral root and a dorsal root from the spinal cord (Fig. 12.3-19).

Ventral root (motor root) consists of efferent fibres which are axons of the motor neurons present in the gray matter of anterior or ventral horn of the spinal cord. These convey motor impulses from the spinal cord to the periphery.

Dorsal root (sensory root) consists of the afferent fibres which carry impulses from the periphery to the spinal cord. The cell bodies of these fibres are located outside the spinal cord in a swelling on the dorsal root called the *dorsal root ganglion.* The dendrites of these sensory neurons conduct impulses inward from peripheral parts of the body, while their axons extend through the dorsal root into the spinal cord, where they form synapses with dendrites of other neurons.

The ventral and dorsal roots join to form the a spinal nerve just before leaving the canal through the intervertebral foramen.

Course and distribution of a spinal nerve

Immediately after emerging from the intervertebral foramen, each spinal nerve gives a recurrent meningeal branch and divides into posterior ramus and an anterior ramus each containing both sensory and motor fibres (Fig. 12.3-19) :

- *Recurrent meningeal branch* re-enters the vertebral canal to innervate the meninges.
- *Posterior ramus* passes posteriorly around the vertebral column and supplies the muscles and skin of the back.
- *Anterior ramus* is larger than the posterior ramus. It runs anteriorly to supply the skin and muscles over the anterolateral part of the body. In its initial course the anterior ramus of 1st thoracic to 3rd lumbar spinal nerve is connected to a sympathetic ganglion by gray and white rami communicants (Fig. 12.3-19).

PLEXUSES OF SPINAL NERVES

The anterior rami of spinal nerves (except for theoracic nerves from T_3 to T_{11}) join together and/or branch to form a network of nerves known as nerve plexuses. In this way the body structures get supply from more than one spinal nerve and, therefore, damage to one spinal nerve does not cause loss of function of a region.

There are five plexuses of mixed nerves formed on each side of the vertebral column. These include :
- Cervical plexus,
- Brachial plexus,
- Lumbar plexus,

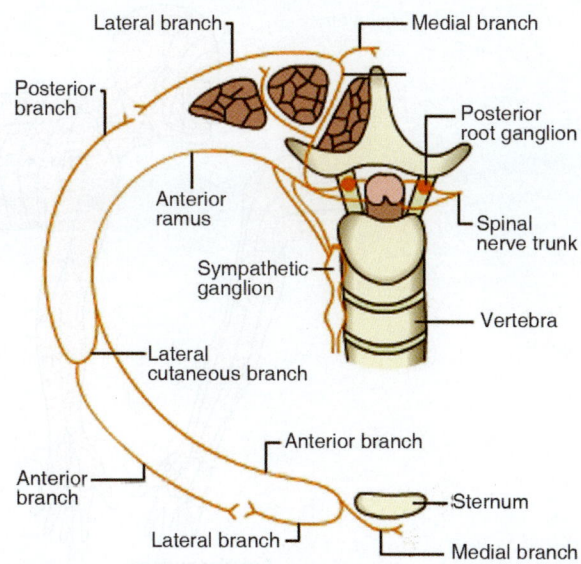

Fig. 12.3-19. *Diagram of typical spinal nerve showing scheme of branching and relationship to spinal cord, sympathetic ganglion and vertebral column.*

- Sacral plexus, and
- Coccygeal plexus.

Dermatome

Dermatome refers to area of the skin supplied by a single segment of spinal cord. Thus, each spinal cord segment is related to the body in a segmental way by its spinal nerves (Fig. 12.3-20).

Cervical plexus

The cervical plexuses lie deep in the neck on either side, opposite the 1st, 2nd, 3rd and 4th cervical vertebrae under cover of sternocleidomastoid muscle. The ventral rami of first four cervical (C1, C2, C3 and C4) nerves unite with each other to form the cervical plexus (Fig. 12.3-21).

Branches. Many branches arise from the cervical plexus.
- *Cutaneous branches* are superficial, supply the skin of neck upto the level of sternum and back and side of head.
- *Muscular branches* are deep and supply the muscles of neck.
- *Phrenic nerve* (C3, C4, C5) is the only motor supply to diaphragm.

Brachial plexus

The brachial plexus is situated in the neck and shoulder above and behind the subclavian vessels and in the axilla. Its construction is as below (Fig. 12.3-22).

Roots are constituted by the anterior rami of lower four cervical nerves and a large part of first thoracic nerve (C5 to C8 and T1).

Trunks are formed by union of roots :

Fig. 12.3-20. Dermatome distribution of body.

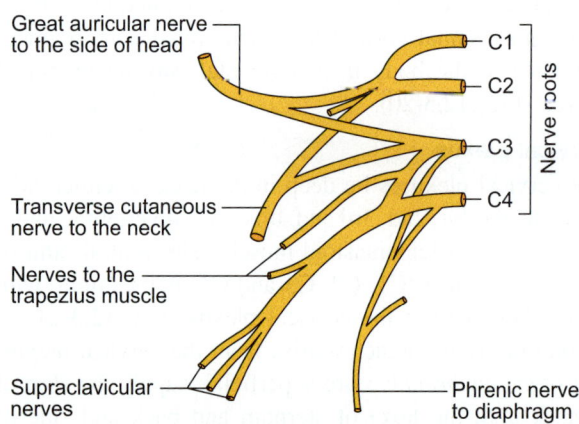

Fig. 12.3-21. The cervical plexus.

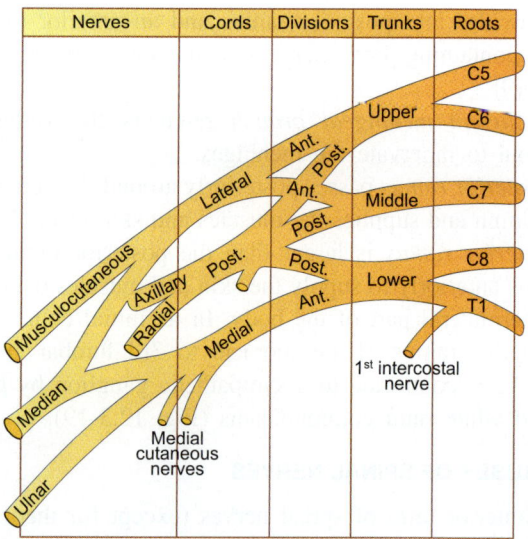

Fig. 12.3-22. The brachial plexus.

- *Upper trunk* is formed by union of roots of C5 and C6.
- *Middle trunk* is formed by roots of C7.
- *Lower trunk* is formed by roots of C8 and T1.

Divisions. Each trunk divides into ventral and dorsal division (which ultimately supply the anterior and posterior aspects of limbs).

Cords are formed by union of divisions :

- *Lateral cord* is formed by union of ventral divisions of upper and middle trunks.
- *Medial cord* is formed by the ventral division of the lower trunk.

- *Posterior cord* is formed by union of dorsal divisions of all the three trunks.

Branches of brachial plexus are many and supply the skin and muscles of upper limbs and some of the chest muscles. The major branches of brachial plexus are (Fig. 12.3-23) :

Fig. 12.3-23. *Main nerves of arm : A, anterior view; and B, posterior view.*

- *Axillary nerve (C5, C6).* It supplies the deltoid muscle, shoulder joint and overlying skin.
- *Musculo cutaneous nerve (C5, C6, C7)* which supplies muscles of the arms on the anterior side and skin of forearm.
- *Ulnar nerve (C7, C8, T1).* It supplies muscles of the forearm and hands, and the skin of hands.
- *Median nerve (C5, C6, C7, C8, T1).* It supplies muscle of the forearm and hands, and skin of the hand.
- *Radial nerve (C5, C6, C7, C8, T1).* It supplies muscles of the arm on the posterior aspect, and the skin of forearm and hands.

Lumbar plexus

The lumbar plexus is formed by the ventral rami of upper four lumbar (L1, L2, L3 and L4) nerves (Fig. 12.3-24). It is located in front of the transverse processes of lumbar vertebrae and behind the psoas major muscle.

Branches from the lumbar plexus supply mostly the muscles of thigh. The largest branches are :

- *Obturator nerve* which supplies the adductor muscles of thigh,
- *Femoral nerve* is a motor and sensory nerve to the structures of thigh.

Sacral plexus

The sacral plexus is formed by union of ventral rami of first four sacral nerves (S1, S2, S3 and S4), along with the lumbosacral trunk (derived from the few fibres of L4 and all fibres of L5) (Fig. 12.3-24).

Branches. Apart from the sciatic and pudendal nerves (main branches), sacral plexus gives off several branches that supply skin and muscles in the lower extremity (Fig. 12.3-25).

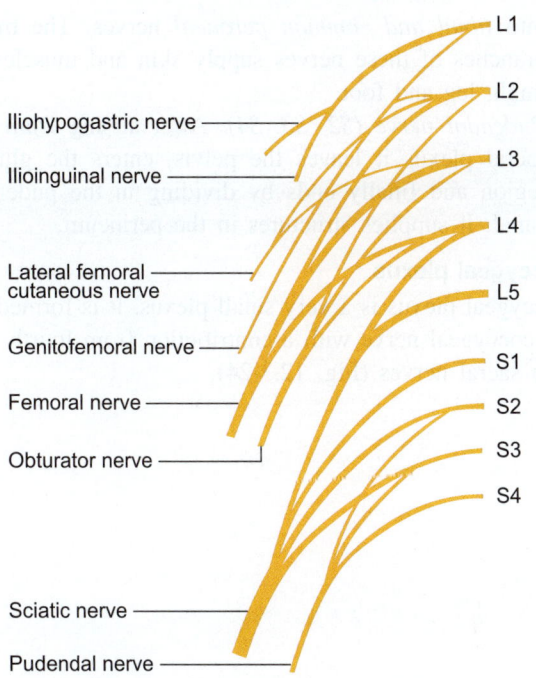

Fig. 12.3-24. *Lumbar, sacral and coccygeal plexuses.*

Anterior view   Posterior view

Fig. 12.3-25. *Main nerves of the lower limb.*

- *Sciatic nerve (L4, L5, S1, S2, S3).* It is the largest and longest nerve in the body. It passes downward into the buttock and descends into the thigh, where it divides into *tibial and common peroneal* nerves. The many branches of these nerves supply skin and muscles of thigh, leg and foot.

- *Pudendal nerve (S2, S3, S4).* After arising from the sacral plexus it leaves the pelvis, enters the gluteal region and finally ends by dividing in the pudendal canal. It supplies structures in the perineum.

Coccygeal plexus

Coccygeal plexus is a very small plexus. It is formed by the coccygeal nerve with a contribution from fourth and fifth sacral nerves (Fig. 12.3-24).

Branches from coccygeal plexus supply the skin in the region of coccyx, and some muscles of floor of pelvis.

THORACIC NERVES

Ventral rami (anterior branches) of thoracic spinal nerves do not make any plexus. These branches pass as *intercostal nerves* out into the intercostal spaces to supply the intercostal muscles and upper abdominal muscles. They also receive sensory impulses from the skin of thorax and abdomen.

Autonomic Nervous System

ANATOMICAL CONSIDERATIONS
- Autonomic nervous system: divisions
- General organization of ANS
- Neurons of ANS
- Anatomy of sympathetic nervous system
- Anatomy of parasympathetic nervous system

PHYSIOLOGICAL CONSIDERATIONS
- Autonomic neurotransmitters and receptors
- Functions of ANS
- Differences between sympathetic and parasympathetic systems

APPLIED ASPECTS
- Autonomic failure
- Horner's syndrome

ANATOMICAL CONSIDERATIONS

DIVISIONS OF AUTONOMIC NERVOUS SYSTEM

The word autonomous is taken from Greek words the *autos* meaning 'self' and the *nomos* meaning 'control'. Thus, ANS is an involuntary system. Since it controls the vegetative functions it is also called vegetative system.

Autonomic nervous system has two main divisions:

1. *Sympathetic division*, also called thoracolumbar division, consists of thoracic and lumbar chains of sympathetic ganglia.

2. *Parasympathetic division*, also called craniosacral division, consists of the ganglia associated with 3rd, 7th, 9th, and 10th cranial nerves.

GENERAL ORGANIZATION OF THE AUTONOMIC NERVOUS SYSTEM

The autonomic nervous system (ANS) is organized as:

I. Autonomic areas in the cerebral hemispheres

The autonomic areas controlling visceral functions located in the cerebral hemisphere are:

Higher brain centres, such as the limbic cortex, parts of the cerebral cortex, can influence the activity of autonomic nervous system by sending signals to the hypothalamus and lower brain area.

Hypothalamus is the site of integration of somatic, autonomic and endocrine functions. Such an integration is essential for maintenance of homeostasis during stresses like extreme hot, extreme cold, stress of surgical operation, stress of injuries and haemorrhage and so on.

Since hypothalamus plays an important role in the regulation of autonomic acitivity, it has been called the main ganglion of the ANS. However, it is now known that the limbic cortex is equally important in the regulation of the ANS.

II. Autonomic centres in the brain stem

These are located in the reticular formation and in the general visceral nuclei of cranial nerves.

General visceral nuclei of cranial nerves

These include both general visceral afferent and efferent nuclei.

General visceral afferent nucleus is represented by the *nucleus of solitary tract* present in the medulla. It receives fibres carrying general visceral sensations through the vagus and glossopharyngeal nerves. This nucleus plays an important role in reflex control of respiratory and cardiovascular functions.

Fibres of taste (special visceral afferents) carried by the facial, glossopharyngeal and vagus nerves end in the upper part of the nucleus of the solitary tract which is sometimes called *gustatory nucleus.*

According to some authorities some general visceral afferents end in the dorsal vagal nucleus.

General visceral efferent nuclei. These nuclei give origin to preganglionic fibres that constitute the cranial parasympathetic outflow. The general visceral efferent nuclei include:

- Edinger-Westphal nucleus (of oculomotor nerve) situated in the midbrain,
- Salivary nucleus (superior and inferior) located in the pons, and
- Dorsal nucleus of vagus present in the medulla.

III. Autonomic centres in the spinal cord

These are located in the intermediolateral grey column of spinal cord at two levels:

1. *Thoracolumbar outflow.* Neurons present in the thoracic and upper two or three lumbar segments of spinal cord (T_1 to L_3) constitute the preganglionic neurons of sympathetic nervous system (thoracolumbar outflow).

2. *Craniosacral outflow.* Neurons present in the second, third and fourth sacral segments of spinal cord (S_2 to S_4) are the preganglionic neurons of the sacral part of parasympathetic system, which along with the cranial part constitute the craniosacral outflow.

IV. Peripheral part of ANS

This is made up of all autonomic nerves and ganglia throughout the body. In fact, autonomic fibres are intimately related to different cranial and spinal nerves.

NEURONS OF ANS

Unlike in motor nerves, where a single motor neuron travels all the way from spinal cord or cranial nuclei to the muscle, the autonomic efferent pathway from the spinal cord or cranial nuclei is made of two neurons: the preganglionic and postganglionic.

Preganglionic neurons. The cell body of the preganglionic neuron is located either in the brain stem or spinal cord. The axon of this visceral motor neuron projects as a thinly myelinated preganglionic fibre to an autonomic ganglion.

Postganglionic neuron. The body of the postganglionic neuron is located in the autonomic ganglion and sends an unmyelinated axon, the postganglionic fibre, to visceral effector cells.

In general, sympathetic ganglia are located close to the central nervous system, whereas parasympathetic ganglia are located close to the effector tissues. Therefore, sympathetic pathway has short preganglionic fibres and long postganglionic fibres, whereas para-sympathetic pathway has long preganglionic fibres and short postganglionic fibres.

ANATOMY OF SYMPATHETIC NERVOUS SYSTEM

Sympathetic preganglionic neurons

The cell bodies of sympathetic preganglionic neurons are located in the intermediolateral horn of the spinal cord from level T_1 to L_2. The myelinated axons of these visceral motor neurons leave the spinal cord via the ventral root and then pass via the white rami communicantes to the paravertebral ganglia of the sympathetic trunk (Fig. 12.4-1). After reaching the sympathetic trunk preganglionic fibres may pass to one of the following three destinations:

- They may terminate in the ganglion at the level of entrance by synapsing with an excitor cell in the ganglion (Fig. 12.4-2).
- They may travel up or down in the sympathetic trunk to terminate in the ganglia located at a higher or lower level (Fig. 12.4-2).
- They may travel through the sympathetic trunk and exit without synapsing via splanchnic nerve and terminate in a prevertebral ganglion (Fig. 12.4-2).

Preganglionic fibres that innervate the adrenal medulla travel through the sympathetic trunk, exit without synapsing via greater splanchnic nerve and end directly on the cells of suprarenal medulla. These medullary cells may be regarded as modified sympathetic excitor cells that secrete epinephrine and norepinephrine into the blood stream. These secretory cells of the adrenal medulla are derived embryologically from nervous tissue and are analogous to postganglionic neurons.

Sympathetic ganglia

Sympathetic ganglia are of three types:

- Paravertebral ganglia,
- Prevertebral or collateral ganglia, and
- Peripheral or terminal ganglia.

Paravertebral ganglia. Paravertebral ganglia are arranged along the entire length of two sympathetic trunks (right and left placed on either side of vertebral column throughout its length). Paravertebral ganglia of sympathetic trunk are divided into:

- *Cervical ganglia.* These are three in number: superior, middle and inferior.
- *Thoracic ganglia.* These are 11-12 in number.
- *Lumbar ganglia* are 4 in number.

Note. In all there are 22 or 23 ganglia on each trunk.

The inferior cervical ganglion and the first thoracic

Fig. 12.4-1. *General arrangement of somatic part of nervous system (on left) compared with autonomic part of nervous system (on right).*

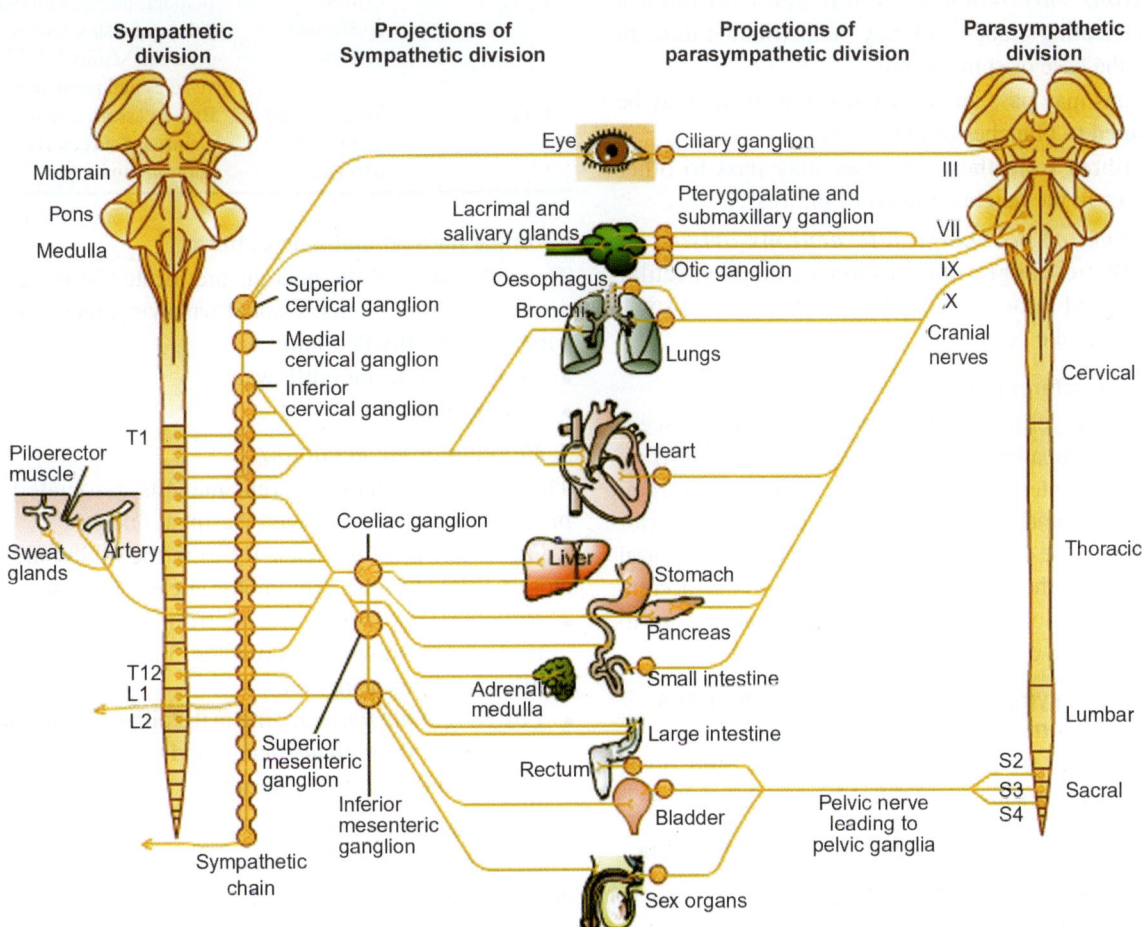

Fig. 12.4-2. *Efferent part of autonomic nervous system: Parasympathetic (on right) and sympathetic (on left),*

ganglion are often fused to form a large stellate ganglion. The two sympathetic trunks end below by joining together to form a single ganglion, the *ganglion impar*.

Prevertebral or collateral ganglia are three in number (coeliac ganglion, inferior mesenteric ganglion and superior mesenteric ganglion).

Peripheral or terminal ganglia are located within or close to structures innervated by them. Heart, bronchi, pancreas, and urinary bladder are innervated by the terminal ganglia.

Postganglionic sympathetic neurons

Sympathetic postganglionic neurons are located primarily in ganglia on the sympathetic trunks. Some are located in the prevertebral ganglia and the peripheral autonomic plexus (Figs. 12.4-1 and 12.4-2). Axons arising from these neurons behave in one of the following ways:

- *The axons may pass through a grey ramus communicantes* and re-enter ventral root to reach a spinal nerve (Fig. 10.5-1). In the spinal nerve the postganglionic fibres travel through its branches to innervate sweat glands and arrectores pilorum muscles of the skin in the region to which spinal nerve is distributed.
- *The axons may reach a cranial nerve* through a communicating branch and may be distributed through it as in the case of spinal nerve.
- The axons may pass into a vascular branch and may be distributed to branches of the vessel.
- Some fibres from these plexuses may pass to other structures in the neighbourhood of the vessel.
- *The axons of postganglionic neurons arising* in sympathetic ganglia may travel through vascular branches and through autonomic plexus to reach some viscera (e.g. the heart).

Sympathetic afferent fibres

The afferent myelinated fibres travel from the viscera through the sympathetic ganglia without synapsing (Fig. 12.4-1). They enter the spinal nerve via the white rami communicantes and reach their cell bodies in the posterior root ganglia of the corresponding spinal nerve. The central axons then enter the spinal cord and may form the afferent component of a local reflex arc. Others may pass up to higher autonomic centres in the brain.

Distribution of sympathetic preganglionic neurons and postganglionic fibres

The distribution of preganglionic neurons and post-ganglionic fibres is shown in Table 12.4-1 and Fig. 12.4-2.

ANATOMY OF PARASYMPATHETIC NERVOUS SYSTEM

Parasympathetic preganglionic neurons

The parasympathetic fibres form the *craniosacral outflow*, consisting of cranial parasympathetic outflow and sacral parasympathetic outflow.

Table 12.4-1. Distribution of sympathetic preganglionic neurons and postganglionic fibres

Segmental level of preganglionic neurons	Area of distribution	Final distribution of postganglionic fibres
T_1, T_2	Head and neck	Dilator pupillae muscle, superior and inferior, Muller's muscles of eyelids, blood vessels, and sweat glands.
T_3, T_4	Thoracic viscera	Heart, oesophagus, trachea, bronchi, and lungs.
T_5 to T_9	Upper limb	Blood vessels, sweat glands, and arrectores pilorum muscles.
T_{10} to L_2	Lower limb	Blood vessels, sweat glands and arrectores pilorum muscles.
T_6 to T_{12}	Upper abdominal viscera	GIT, liver, spleen adrenal capsule, medulla, and urinary tract.
L_1, L_2	Lower abdominal viscera	Bladder, uterus, fallopian tubes (or testes, vas deferens, seminal vesicles and prostate).
T_1 to T_{12}	Thoracic and abdominal parieties	Blood vessels, sweat glands and arrectores pilorum muscles

I. Cranial parasympathetic outflow

The cell bodies of the neurons are located in the general visceral efferent nuclei. Cranial parasympathetic outflow can be further divided into:

- Midbrain or tectal outflow, and
- Bulbar outflow.

1. Midbrain or tectal outflow

The general visceral efferent nucleus associated with midbrain outflow is Edinger-Westphal nucleus.

Edinger-Westphal nucleus. It lies in the midbrain and is closely related to the oculomotor nucleus complex.

- *Preganglionic fibres* arising from Edinger-Westphal nucleus pass through oculomotor (3rd cranial) nerve and relay in ciliary ganglion.
- *Postganglionic fibres* arising in the ciliary ganglion pass through the short ciliary nerves and supply the sphincter pupillae and the ciliary muscle.

2. Bulbar outflow

The general visceral efferent nuclei associated with bulbar outflow are:

i. Superior salivary nucleus. *Preganglionic fibres* arising from superior salivary nucleus enter the facial (7th cranial) nerve and ultimately relay in *submandibular ganglion*.

Postganglionic fibres pass to submandibular and sublingual salivary glands to which they are secretomotor.

ii. Lacrimal nucleus of 7th cranial nerve sends preganglionic fibres to the *pterygopalatine* (spheno-palatine) ganglion. The postganglionic fibres reach the lacrimal gland to which they are secretomotor.

iii. Inferior salivary nucleus sends preganglionic fibres into the glossopharyngeal (9th cranial) nerve. These fibres relay in the otic ganglion, from where the postganglionic fibres go to parotid gland to which they are secretomotor.

iv. Dorsal (motor) nucleus of the vagus. About 75 per cent of all parasympathetic fibres arise from dorsal nucleus. *Preganglionic fibres* travelling in the vagus nerve end in ganglia (or nerve plexuses) closely related to the visceral organs such as heart, lungs, bronchi, oesophagus, stomach, small intestine and large intestine up to two-thirds of transverse colon.

Postganglionic fibres arise in these ganglia, and run a short course to supply smooth muscles and glands in these organs.

II. Sacral parasympathetic outflow

Preganglionic fibres. Cell bodies of the preganglionic neu-rons, of sacral parasympathetic outflow, are located in the intermediolateral grey horn of second, third and fourth sac-ral segments (S_2, S_3 and S_4) of spinal cord (Fig. 12.4-2). Their axons form the preganglionic fibres which pass out through the ventral spinal root of corresponding nerves. These axons leave the spinal nerves to form the pelvic splanchnic nerves which end in the pelvic autonomic plex-uses.

Postganglionic fibres. The postganglionic neurons are located in the pelvic autonomic plexuses close to or within the viscera. Their axons (postganglionic fibres) run a very short course to supply the concerned pelvic viscera. These fibres also supply the rectum, the sigmoid colon, the descending colon and the left one-third of transverse colon.

Parasympathetic afferent fibres

The afferent myelinated fibres travel from viscera to their cell bodies located either in the sensory ganglia of the cranial nerves or in the posterior root ganglia of the sacrospinal nerves. The central axons then enter the central nervous system and take part in the formation of local reflex arc, or pass to higher centres of the ANS.

PHYSIOLOGICAL CONSIDERATIONS

AUTONOMIC NEUROTRANSMITTERS AND RECEPTORS

Neurotransmitters of ANS

Parasympathetic fibres
1. Preganglionic fibres: acetylcholine
2. Postganglionic fibres: acetylcholine

Sympathetic fibres
1. Preganglionic fibres: acetylcholine
2. Postganglionic fibres:
- Adrenergic fibres : Norepinephrine (mainly), or epinephrine
- Cholinergic fibres : Acetylcholine (the postganglionic sympathetic cholinergic nerve fibres supplying sweat glands, blood vessels in heart and skeletal muscles).

Autonomic receptors

The autonomic neurotransmitters (acetylcholine or nor-epinephrine) produce their effects on the organs by combining with specific protein molecules known as receptors, which are of following types:

1. Cholinergic receptors

On the basis of their pharmacologic properties, these are of two types:

i. Nicotinic receptors. These receptors are located in/at autonomic ganglia of sympathetic and parasympathetic nervous system, neuromuscular junction, and adrenal medulla.

The receptors at these locations are similar but not identical.

Activation. Nicotinic receptors are activated by acetyl-choline (ACh) and nicotine.

Effect. These receptors produce excitation.

Blockage. Ganglion blockers (e.g. hexamethonium, trimethaphan) block the nicotinic receptors for ACh in the autonomic ganglia, but not at the neuromuscular junction.

ii. Muscarinic receptors. These receptors are located in the heart, smooth muscles (except vascular smooth muscle) and glands.

Activation. These receptors are activated by acetylcholine (ACh) and muscarine.

Effects produced by their stimulation is :
- *Inhibitory in the heart,* e.g. decreased heart rate, and decreased conduction velocity in AV node.
- *Excitatory* in smooth muscle and glands (e.g. increased gastrointestinal motility and increased secretion).

Blockage. Muscarinic receptors for acetylcholine are blocked by atropine.

2. Adrenergic receptors

On the basis of their pharmacologic properties, adrenergic receptors are of two types:
- *Alpha (α) adrenergic receptors* (which are of further two types: α_1 and α_2), and
- *Beta (β) adrenergic receptors* (which are of further three types: β_1, β_2 and β_3).

i. α_1 receptors are located on vascular smooth muscles of skin and splanchnic regions, gastrointestinal and bladder sphincters, and radial muscles of the iris.

Effect. These receptors produce excitation, e.g. contraction or constriction.

SECTION 12

ii. α_2 receptors are located in presynaptic nerve terminals, platelets, fat cells, and walls of the gastrointestinal tract.

Effect. Often produce inhibition (e.g. relaxation or dilatation).

iii. β_1 receptors are located in the sinoatrial (SA) node, atrioventricular (AV) node, and ventricular muscles of the heart.

Effect. These receptors produce excitation (e.g. increased heart rate, increased conduction velocity and increased contractility).

iv. β_2 receptors are located on vascular smooth muscle of skeletal muscle, bronchial smooth muscle, walls of the gastrointestinal tract, and bladder.

Effect. These receptors produce relaxation (e.g. dilation of vascular smooth muscle, dilation of bronchioles, and relaxation of bladder wall).

v. β_3 receptors. These receptors are located on the adipose tissue and cause lipolysis.

Note. The type of adrenergic receptors present in various organs and the effects produced by their stimulation are depicted in Table 12.4-2.

Table 12.4-2 : Responses of effector organs to sympathetic and parasympathetic stimulation

S. No.	Effector organ	Parasympathetic effect	Sympathetic effect — Receptor type	Sympathetic effect — Response
1.	**Eyes**			
	• Dilator pupillae muscle	—	α	Contraction (mydriasis)
	• Sphincter pupillae muscle	Contraction (meiosis)	—	—
	• Ciliary muscle	Contraction (produces accommodation for near vision)	β_2	Relaxes (flattens lens for far vision)
2.	**Heart**			
	• SA node	↓ Heart rate, vagal arrest	β_1 & β_2	↑ Heart rate
	• Atria	↓ Contractility, ↓ Conductivity	β_1 & β_2	↑ Contractility ↑ Conductivity
	• A-V node and conduction system	↓ Conduction velocity	β_1 & β_2	↑ Conduction velocity
	• Ventricles	↓ Contractility	β_1 & β_2	↑ Contractility
3.	**Arterioles**			
	• Coronary		α_1 & α_2 β_2	Constriction Dilatation
	• Cutaneous and mucosal	No supply	α_1 & α_2	Constriction
	• Skeletal muscle	No supply	α_1 β_2	Constriction Dilatation
	• Cerebral	Dilatation	α_1	Constriction
	• Pulmonary	Dilatation	α_1 β_2	Constriction Dilatation
	• Abdominal viscera	No supply	α_1	Constriction
	• Renal	No supply	α_1 & α_2 β_1 & β_2	Constriction Dilatation
	• Salivary glands	Dilatation	α_1 & α_2	Constriction
4.	**Systemic veins**	No supply	α_1 & α_2 β_2	Constriction Dilatation
5.	**Lungs**			
	• Bronchial muscles	Contraction	β_2 α_1	Relaxation Inhibition
	• Bronchial glands	Stimulation	β_2	Stimulation
6.	**Salivary glands**	Stimulation (profuse watery secretion)	α_1	Stimulation (thick viscous secretion)
7.	**Stomach**			
	• Motility and tone	Increases	α_1, α_2, β_2	Decreases
	• Sphincters	Relaxation	α_1	Contraction
	• Secretion	Stimulation	α_2	Inhibition
8.	**Gall bladder**	Contraction	β_2	Relaxation

Table 12.4-2. Contd...

S. No.	Effector organ	Parasympathetic effect	Sympathetic effect	
			Receptor type	Response
9.	*Liver*	—	α_1, β_2	Glycogenolysis
10.	*Pancreas*			
	• Exocrine glands	Stimulates secretion	α_1	Inhibits secretion
	• Endocrine glands	—	α_2	Inhibits insulin secretion
			β_2	Stimulates glucagon
11.	*Spleen capsule*		α_1	Contraction
			β_2	Relaxation
12.	*Adrenal medulla*	Secretion of epinephrine and norepinephrine		
13.	*Urinary bladder*			
	• Detrusor muscle	Contraction	β_2	Relaxation (usually)
	• Sphincter	Relaxation	α_1	Contraction
14.	*Uterus*	Variable	α_1	Contraction (pregnant)
			β_2	Relaxation (non-pregnant)
15.	*Male sex organ*	Erection	α_1	Ejaculation
16.	*Lacrimal glands*	Secretion		
17.	*Skin*			
	• Pilomotor muscle	—	α_1	Contraction (erection of hair)
	• Sweat glands	Generalized (cholinergic sweating)	α_1	Localized (adrenergic) sweating
18.	*Nasopharyngeal glands*	Secretion	—	—
19.	*Adipose tissue*	—	α_1, β_1, β_3	Lipolysis, release of FFA
20.	*Juxtaglomerular cells*	—	β_1	Increased renin secretion
21.	*Pineal gland*	—	β_1	Increased melatonin synthesis and secretion
22.	*Skeletal muscles*	—	β_2	Increased glycogenolysis
23.	*Basal metabolic rate*	—	β_2	Increased
24.	*Mental activity*	—		Increased

FUNCTIONS OF AUTONOMIC NERVOUS SYSTEM : EFFECTS OF AUTONOMIC NERVE IMPULSES ON EFFECTOR ORGANS

General principles

- ANS controls the various vegetative functions which are beyond voluntary control and thus plays an important role in maintaining the constant internal environment (homeostasis).
- Most of the visceral organs have dual innervation, i.e. are supplied by both sympathetic and parasympathetic divisions of ANS. The two divisions produce anta-gonistic effects on each organ and provide a very fine degree of control over the effector organ.
- Some of the visceral organs are innervated by one division of ANS only; e.g.
  - Uterus, adrenal medulla and most of the arterioles are innervated by sympathetic division only.
  - Glands of stomach and pancreas are innervated by parasympathetic division only.
- In the case of sphincter's muscles, both adrenergic and cholinergic innervations are excitatory, but one supplies the constrictor component of the sphincter and other the dilator.
- *Effects of acetylcholine,* i.e. of localized cholinergic discharge are generally discrete and shortlasting, because ACh is rapidly removed from the nerve endings due to high concentration of acetylcholine esterase at cholinergic nerve endings.
- *Effects of norepinephrine* are more prolonged than ACh, as it spreads further. In the blood, epinephrine and dopamine come from the adrenal medulla, while norepinephrine diffuses from the adrenergic nerve endings.

CHAPTER 12.4

Effects of stimulation of sympathetic and parasympathetic divisions of ANS

Responses of effector organs to autonomic nerve impulses are summarized in Table 12.4-2.

DIFFERENCES BETWEEN SYMPATHETIC AND PARASYMPATHETIC SYSTEMS

As summarized in Table 12.4-2, sympathetic and parasympathetic systems produce antagonistic effects on each organ of the body. The main differences between sympathetic and parasympathetic systems are depicted in Table 12.4-3.

Autonomic failure

Types. Autonomic failure is of two types:

- *Primary autonomic failure* from unexplained (primary) autonomic neuronal degeneration.
- *Secondary autonomic failure* occurs secondary to some general medical disorders. Diabetes mellitus is the most common cause of secondary autonomic dysfunction.

Features of autonomic failure (primary or secondary) are:

Table 12.4-3. Main differences between sympathetic and parasympathetic system

Feature	Sympathetic system	Parasympathetic system
Location	Cell bodies of preganglionic neurons are located in intermediolateral horn of T_1 to L_2 or L_3 spinal segments, so also called thoracolumbar outflow.	Cell bodies of preganglionic neurons are located in: • *Cranial nuclei* associated with 3rd, 7th, 9th and 10th cranial nerves (cranial outflow), and • Intermediolateral horn of S_2 to S_4 spinal segments (sacral outflow). So, it is also called craniosacral outflow.
Components and ganglia	• Components are consolidated. • Ganglia are linked up to form a chain.	• Components are isolated. • Ganglia remain isolated.
Preganglionic fibres	Are short, myelinated and end in paravertebral or prevertebral ganglia	Are long, myelinated and end on short postganglionic neurons located on or near the viscera.
Postganglionic fibres	• Long • Non-myelinated	• Short • Myelinated
Neurotransmitter • Preganglionic fibres • Postganglionic fibres	• Cholinergic • Mostly adrenergic	• Cholinergic • Cholinergic
Area of effect	Preganglionic fibres branch, enter several ganglia and transmit nerve impulse to many postganglionic fibres. So, sympathetic activity is spread over many segments.	Preganglionic fibres do not branch, each enters a single ganglion and transmits nerve impulses to a single postganglionic fibre. Therefore, parasympathetic activity is localized, i.e. target is usually a single organ or system.
Functions	Mass sympathetic discharge usually occurs in threatening situation, i.e. it prepares the individual to cope with the emergency. It causes flight or fight reactions characterized by: • Dilatation of pupil • Increased heart rate • Increased blood pressure (providing better perfusion of the vital organs and muscles). • Constriction of cutaneous arterioles (which limits blood loss from wounds, if any) • Increased alertness and arousal due to decreased threshold in the reticular formation. • Increased blood glucose and FFA levels (supplying more energy). Because of these actions sympathetic system is also sometimes called *catabolic nervous system*.	Unlike sympathetic nervous system, the functions of parasympathetic system are discrete and each function is separately regulated. This system is concerned with vegetative aspect of day-to-day living. For example, its action favours: • Digestion and absorption of food, increased activity of intestinal musculature and increased gastric secretion and pyloric relaxation, • Micturition, • Pupillary constriction, and • Bradycardia. Since, parasympathetic system decreases the rate of metabolism, it is also called *anabolic nervous system*.

- *Cardiovascular features* include tachycardia and orthostatic hypotension.

- *Sudomotor features* are anhidrosis and heat intolerance.

- *Gastrointestinal features* include constipation, occasional diarrhoea and dysphagia.

- *Urinary features* are nocturia, frequency, urgency, incontinence and retention of urine.

- *Reproductive* organ problems include erectile and ejaculation failure.

- *Ocular* features include miosis and enophthalmos.

Horner's syndrome

Horner's syndrome refers to ipsilateral *oculosympathetic paresis* due to any cause. Its common causes are Pancoast's tumour of the lung, malignancy of cervical lymph nodes pressing on the cervical sympathetic chain.

Clinical features of Horner's syndrome are :

- *Ptosis* (drooping down of upper eyelid) due to paralysis of Muller's muscle of upper eyelid.

- *Miosis* (small pupil) due to paralysis of dilator pupillae muscle.

- *Facial anhidrosis,* i.e. reduced sweating on the ipsilateral face and neck.

Somatosensory System, Somatomotor System and Reflexes

12.5

SOMATOSENSORY SYSTEM
Sensation, receptors and sensory transductions
- Sensations
- Receptors
- Sensory transduction

Neural pathway (transmission of sensations)
- Dorsal column sensory pathway
- Anterolateral sensory pathway
- Dorsolateral column sensory pathway
- Pathway of sensations from face and oral cavity

Role of thalamus and sensory cortex
- Encoding : recognition of types of sensation

SOMATOMOTOR SYSTEM
Introduction
Components of somatic motor control system
- Highest level of motor control
- Middle level of motor control
- Lowest level of motor control

Skeletal muscles : the effector organ of somatic motor system
- Motor unit
- Muscle sensors
- Muscle tone

REFLEX ACTIVITY
Anatomical aspects
- Reflex arc

Spinal cord reflexes
- Stretch reflex
- Golgi tendon reflex
- Withdrawal reflex

SOMATOSENSORY SYSTEM

SENSATIONS, RECEPTORS AND SENSORY TRANSDUCTION

SENSATION

Sensory division of the human nervous system is concerned with collection of the information about outside world and changes occurring within the body itself. Sensation refers to conscious perception of sensory information reaching the brain. Sensations may be broadly classified into two groups:

1. Special senses. These include visual sensations, auditory sensations, gustatory (taste sensation), and olfactory (smell) sensations. These have been discussed in detail in chapter 12.7.

2. Somaesthetic senses. These, depending upon their point of origin, can be classified into three types:

A. *Exteroceptive sensations* also known as cutaneous sensations arise from the surface of the body and these include :

- Tactile sensation,

- Pressure sensation,

- Pain sensation, and

- Temperature sensation.

B. *Visceral sensations* arise from the viscera, i.e. internal organs and are called visceral sensations.

C. *Proprioceptive and kinaesthetic sensations* arise from the muscles, tendons and joints. These include:

i. *Proprioceptive sensations*: These are concerned with the physical state of the body, i.e. the sense of position, tendon

470

and muscle sensations, deep pressure and sense of equilibrium.

ii. *Kinaesthetic sensations* or kinaesthesia: It is the conscious recognition of rate of movement of different parts of the body. Kinaesthetic sensations include both:

- Conscious kinaesthetic sensations, and
- Unconscious kinaesthetic sensations.

RECEPTORS

Sensory receptors are specialized cells that receive stimuli from the external or internal environment and transduce these signals into neural signals. A *stimulus* is a change of environment of sufficient intensity to evoke a response in an organism.

Receptors for somatic sensations

A. Receptors for cutaneous sensations include :

1. *Mechanoreceptors* or receptors of touch, pressure and vibration sensation provide information about these stimuli to skin. In general, these receptors consist of an unmyelinated axon surrounded by lamellated connective tissue corpuscles. These include (Fig. 12.5-1):

Fig. 12.5-1. *Sensory receptors.*

- Pacinian corpuscles
- Meissner's corpuscles
- Merkel's discs
- Ruffini's end organs
- Hair end organs
- Krause's end bulbs
- Free nerve endings

2. *Thermoreceptors*. Thermoreceptors are responsible for detecting temperature sensation. Separate receptors exist for encoding warm and cold sensations and are called warm receptors and cold receptors respectively. Free nerve endings of unmyelinated C fibres form the *warm receptors* and that of *small myelinated* Aδ fibres form the *cold receptors*.

Location. Thermoreceptors are located in the skin of all parts of the body. However, density of thermoreceptors is greatest in the lips, moderate in the fingertips, and least in the skin of trunk.

3. *Nociceptors*. Nociceptors or pain receptors refer to special type of free nerve endings of :

- Aδ myelinated nerve fibres, and
- C unmyelinated nerve fibres.

Location. High density of pain receptors is present in the superficial layers of skin and in many deeper tissues like periosteum, joints, arterial wall and falx and tentorium in the cranium.

B. Receptors for propioceptive and kinaesthetic sensations

The receptors concerned are called *proprioceptors* and include:

- Muscle spindle or stretch receptors (see page 478),
- Joint receptors located in the joint capsules and ligaments around the joints. Ruffini's end organs are the most important receptors for this function. A few pacinian corpuscles are also involved,
- Golgi tendon organ (see page 478), and
- Vestibular receptors (see page 494).

SENSORY TRANSDUCTION

Sensory transduction refers to the phenomenon of transduction of environmental signals into neural signals by the receptors. Steps of sensory transduction are:

- Arrival of stimulus to receptor,
- Production of generator or receptor potential, and
- Production of action potential in sensory nerve.

1. *Arrival of stimulus to receptor.* The stimulus arriving at the given sensory receptor may be in the form of:

- *Mechanical force* causing depression of the skin which stimulates mechanoreceptors,
- *Cold or warm temperature* stimulating thermoreceptors.

2. *Production of receptor potential.* When a stimulus excites the receptor, it changes the potential across the membrane of the receptors. This change in the potential is called receptor or generator potential.

Mechanism of development of receptor potential

The change in membrane potential in a receptor is caused by a change in permeability of membrane of the unmyelinated terminals to Na⁺. The resultant influx of Na⁺ causes development of generator or receptor potential.

3. *Production of action potential in a sensory nerve.* The receptor potential developed in unmyelinated nerve ending (transducer region) depolarizes the sensory nerve at the first node of Ranvier (spike generator region) by electrotonic depolarization current sink action. When the receptor potential rises above the threshold level (i.e. above 10 mV), it brings the membrane potential of the first node of Ranvier to the firing level causing production of action potential, which is propagated in the nerve fibre (Fig. 12.5-2). Thus, the first node of Ranvier (spike generator region) converts the graded response of the receptor into action potential. Greater the magnitude of receptor potential, greater is the rate of discharge of action potentials in the nerve fibre.

C
H
A
P
T
E
R

12.5

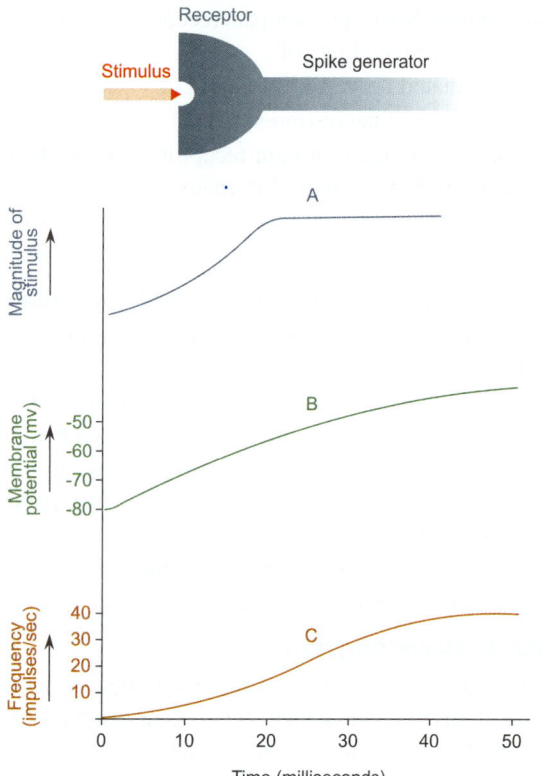

Fig. 12.5-2. Mechanism of development of generator potential and its relationship with intensity of stimulus: A, stimulus to mechanoreceptors causes its deformation which opens up channels which are permeable to Na⁺ causing membrane depolarization; B, the generator potential (receptor potential) follows the time course; and C, the frequency of action potential. Note the magnitude of generator potential and frequency of action potential are proportionate to the magnitude of stimulus.

NEURAL PATHWAY (TRANSMISSION OF SENSATIONS)

The transduced signals from the sensory receptor ultimatey reach the thalamus and sensory cortex through the neural pathway. Pathways in somatosensory system are formed by a chain of three neurons which constitute the spinal nerves, ascending sensory tracts and relay stations.

ASCENDING SENSORY TRACTS

The major ascending sensory tracts in the spinal cord have been grouped as:

- Dorsal (posterior) column sensory pathway,
- Anterolateral sensory pathway, and
- Dorsolateral column sensory pathway.

Dorsal column sensory pathway

Dorsal column sensory pathway (Fig. 12.5-3) in man is well developed and wholly myelinated.

First order neurons are formed by Aα (Ia), and Aβ (II) fibres which enter the spinal cord at medial division of dorsal nerve roots. These carry sensations of fine touch, tactile localization, two-point discrimination, vibration, pressure with intensity discrimination and sense of position and proprioception. These fibres run in the spinal cord through *dorsal column* as fasciculus gracilis and fasciculus cuneatus (Fig. 12.5-3) to end in the *nucleus gracilis* and *nucleus cuneatus*, respectively. Many fibres of the dorsal columns, on their way up, terminate or relay in the dorsal grey horn.

Second order neurons arise from the nucleus gracilis and nucleus cuneatus located in medulla oblongata. These decussate in the medulla as *internal arcuate fibres* and ascend up in the brain stem as medial lemniscus. The fibres of *medial lemnisci terminate* in the *ventroposterior lateral* (VPL) nucleus of thalamus.

Third order neurons are from the *ventroposterior lateral nucleus* of thalamus. These ascend to the sensory cortex through the thalamic radiations.

Anterolateral pathway

First order neurons of anterolateral pathway are formed by Aδ (III) and (IV) fibres which enter the spinal cord as lateral division of the dorsal nerve root. These carry sensations of pain, temperature and crude touch. After entering the spinal cord these fibres separate into short ascending and descending branches. They finally terminate on the *nucleus proprius* of the spinal cord. Some sensory afferents end on the short interneurons in the *substantia gelatinosa* which connect them to nucleus proprius.

Second order neurons arise from the nucleus proprius and cross in the anterior commissure of the spinal cord to the opposite side in anterior and lateral white column in which they run upward to the brain as anterior and lateral spinothalamic tracts, respectively.

Anterior spinothalamic tract mainly carries sensation of crude touch, tickle and itch etc. Higher up in the brain stem, the anterior spinothalamic tract joins the medial lemniscus of thalamus.

Lateral spinothalamic tract consists of the fibres carrying pain and temperature sensation, and higher up in the brain stem is called the spinal lemniscus (Fig. 12.5-4).

Anterolateral pathways terminate in two areas:

- Throughout *reticular nuclei* of brain stem.
- Spinal and medial lemnisci terminate in the *ventrobasal complex* and *intralaminar* nuclei of thalamus.

Third order neurons arise from the ventrobasal complex of thalamus and carry tactile signals to the somatic sensory area of the cortex along with the fibres of dorsal column.

Dorsolateral column pathway

Dorsolateral column pathways carry proprioceptive impulses arising from the muscles and joint receptors of the lower part of the body to the cerebellum. Recent investigations have shown that touch may also reach the cerebellum through these pathways.

Fig. 12.5-3. Dorsal column sensory pathways. Fibres carrying touch, pressure and proprioceptive sensations are arranged as fasciculus gracilis and fasciculus cuneatus in dorsal column of spinal cord.

C H A P T E R   1 2 . 5

First order neurons are located in the posterior root ganglia. Their peripheral processes receive impulses from muscle spindles, Golgi tendon organs and other proprioceptive receptors. Some fibres are related to end organs concerned with exteroceptive sensations (touch and pressure).

Second order neurons are located in the junctional area between the ventral and dorsal grey column (laminae V, VI and VII) in the lumbar and sacral segments of spinal cord. Their axons form the:

• Ventral spinocerebellar tract, and

• Dorsal spinocerebellar tract.

Pathway of sensations from face and oral cavity

The sensations of touch, pain and temperature from the face and oral cavity including teeth, and proprioceptive information from the jaw muscles are carried by trigeminal nerve.

First order neurons are located in the *trigeminal ganglion*, which is equivalent to dorsal nerve root ganglia in the spinal cord. The peripheral processes of these neurons form three divisions of the trigeminal nerve: ophthalmic, maxillary and mandibular which innervate different areas of the facial skin (Fig. 12.3-8). The central processes of these neurons of trigeminal ganglia terminate in different components of trigeminal sensory nucleus as (Fig. 12.5-5):

Principal sensory trigeminal nucleus, located in the pons, receives fibres carrying *tactile* sensations.

Spinal nucleus is elongated and extends down to the upper spinal cord. It receives fibres carrying *pain* and *tempe-rature* sensations.

Mesencephalic nucleus, which extends from the pons into midbrain, receives fibres carrying *proprioceptive* information.

Second order neurons are located in the above described three components of the sensory trigeminal nucleus. Axons

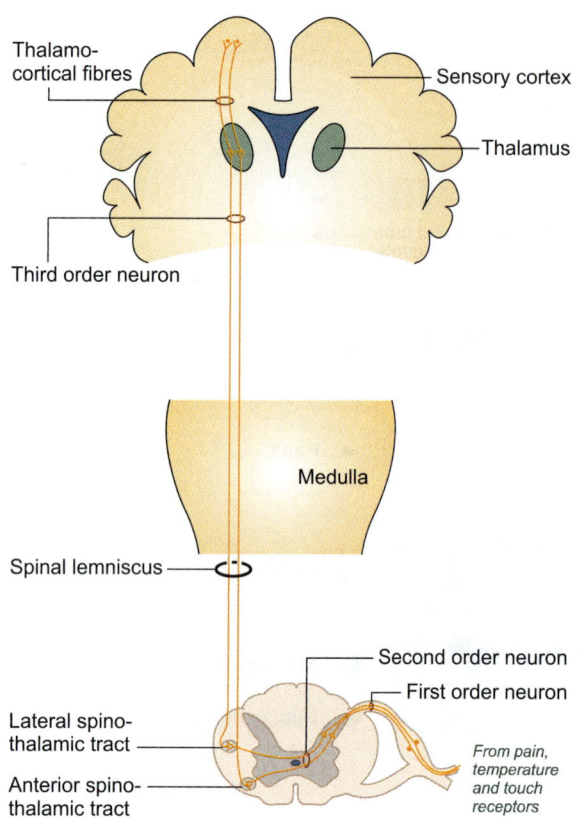

Fig. 12.5-4. *Course of anterior and lateral spinothalamic tracts.*

Fig. 12.5-5. *Termination of central processes of trigeminal ganglion in three components of sensory nucleus of trigeminal nerve.*

of these neurons cross to the opposite side and ascend as *trigeminal lemniscus* to the ventroposterior medial (VPM) nucleus of thalamus.

Third order neurons are located in the VPM nucleus of thalamus. All the sensations reaching this nucleus are carried primarily to sensory area of cerebral cortex by fibres passing

through the posterior limb of internal capsule *(superior thalamic radiations)*.

ROLE OF THALAMUS AND SENSORY CORTEX

Thalamus

Third order neurons of sensory pathway are located in the *ventral posterior nucleus* of thalamus. Role of thalamus in sensory system is as below :

- Serves as *relay cortex* for all sensations,
- *Integrates* sensory impulses, and also
- Acts as *crude centre* for sense perception.

Sensory cortex

The sensory cortex includes primary sensory area, secondary sensory area and sensory association area located in parietal lobe (for details see page 433 and Fig. 12.2-2).

Encoding: Recognition of type of sensation

As discussed above, the sensory receptors transduce all forms of sensory stimuli into a common type of neural signal, i.e. action potentials which are carried by the peripheral nerves and sensory tracts in the spinal cord and brain stem to the sensory cortex. The question arises how does brain differentiate between the action potentials generated from a touch receptor and a pain receptor and interpret the sensation accordingly. It is believed that the sensory receptors themselves act as peripheral analysers.

SOMATOMOTOR SYSTEM

The execution, planning, coordination and adjustments of the movements of the body are under the influence of different parts of the nervous system which together constitute the somatic motor system, which is organized as three-tier system consisting of highest level of motor control, middle level of motor control, and lowest level of motor control (Fig. 12.5-6).

1. *Highest level of motor control* involves activities of various areas of cerebral cortex. It is mainly concerned with generation of the idea of voluntary movements (motor plan) and issuing the motor commands for their execution.

2. *Middle level of motor control* involves activities of various subcortical centres such as basal ganglia, some brain stem nuclei and cerebellum. The middle level of motor control is concerned with developing and perfecting each motor programme and subprogramme for bringing out a motor act. It also supervises the implementation of motor programme.

3. *Lowest level of motor control* is exerted by cranial nerve nuclei in brain stem and the spinal cord. The spinal cord contains the final common pathway through which a movement is executed.

Fig. 12.5-6. *Integration of highest, middle and lowest level of motor control system.*

Feedback signals to CNS from the proprioceptors in muscles, joints, skin and other sensory receptors are used to adjust the motor commands during somatic motor activity.

In view of the above background, the somatic motor control system is discussed in detail under following headings:

- Components of somatic motor control system,
- Skeletal muscles: the effector organ of somatic motor system,
- Reflexes, and
- Regulation of posture and equilibrium.

COMPONENTS OF SOMATIC MOTOR CONTROL SYSTEM

I. HIGHEST LEVEL OF MOTOR CONTROL

The highest level of motor control is exerted through motor cortex and two major descending pathways emerging from the motor areas.

Motor cortex

Areas of motor cortex include (Fig. 12.2-2):

- *Primary motor cortex* (Brodmann's area 4).
- *Premotor cortex,* (it includes Brodmann's area 6, 8, 44 and 45), and
- *Supplementary motor cortex.*

(also see page 431)

Functional role of motor cortex in control of voluntary movements

- *Supplementary motor cortex* is responsible for generating the idea for a movement.

- *Primary motor cortex* is responsible for execution of movement.

Premotor cortex coordinates the voluntary activity.

Plasticity property of motor cortex. The motor system 'learns by doing', and performance improves with repetition. This involves synaptic plasticity. The motor cortex shows plasticity. This has been confirmed by PET and functional MRI (fMRI) in intact experimental animals and humans.

Descending motor pathways from motor cortex

A. Pyramidal tracts include the tracts which are constituted by the axons that transmit motor signals directly from the cortex to spinal cord (*corticospinal tracts*) and cranial nerve nucleus (*corticobulbar tracts*). Corticospinal fibres are divided into two tracts (Fig. 12.5-7).

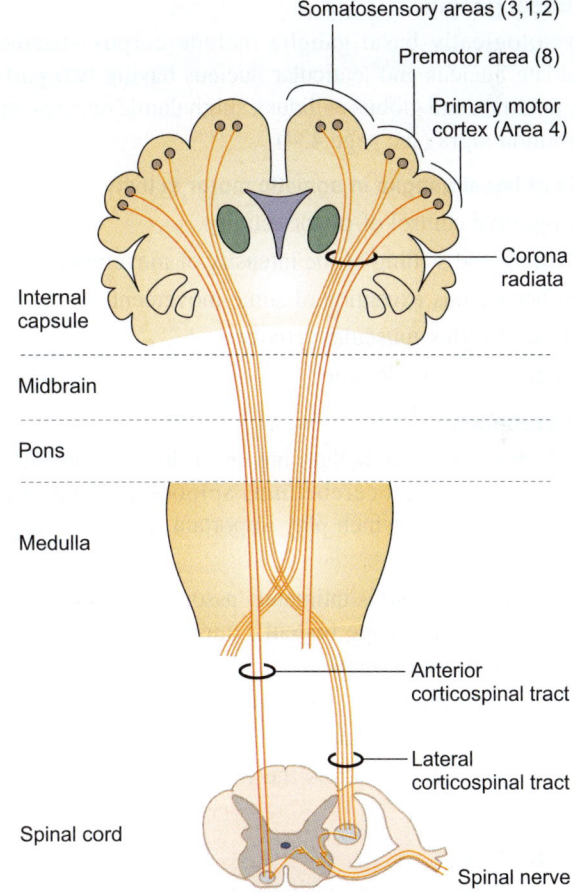

Fig. 12.5-7. *Pathway of corticospinal (pyramidal) tracts.*

- *Lateral corticospinal tract* is constituted by the 80% of fibres which cross the midline in the medullary pyramids. These fibres are responsible for making skilled precision movements (e.g. the muscles that move the fingers and hands and the muscles that produce speech) (*lateral motor system*).

- *Anterior corticospinal tract* is formed by 20% uncrossed fibres which descend ipsilaterally in the ventral white column of the spinal cord. These fibres ultimately cross the midline but only at the level where they synapse. This pathway controls the axial (trunk muscles) and proximal limb muscles that are concerned with posture and equilibrium (*medial motor system*).

B. *Extrapyramidal tracts*. Extrapyramidal pathways are chiefly concerned with regulation of muscle tone, posture and equilibrium.

II. MIDDLE LEVEL OF MOTOR CONTROL

The middle level of motor control specifies the postures and movements necessary to carry out the desired acts. It involves activities of basal ganglia, cerebellum and brain stem.

A. Basal ganglia

Physiologically basal ganglia include corpus striatum (caudate nucleus and lenticular nucleus having two parts, e.g. putamen and globus pallidus), subthalamic nucleus and substantia nigra (see page 434).

Role of basal ganglia in somatic motor activity

- Cognitive control of motor activity
- Timing and scaling of the intensity of movements
- Subconscious execution of some movements
- Control reflex muscular activity
- Control the muscle tone

B. Cerebellum

Functionally, the cerebellum has been divided into three divisions: vestibulocerebellum, spinocerebellum and corticocerebellum, which play important role in different motor activities.

- *Corticocerebellum* is intimately associated with control of timing, rate, range (extent), duration, direction and strength of a movement.
- *Vestibulocerebellum* is responsible for control of body posture and equilibrium.
- *Spinocerebellum* controls the muscle tone and stretch reflex.

C. Brain stem

Reticular formation and vestibular nuclei are important components of the motor control system present in the brain stem.

Reticular formation. The *motor control centres* within the reticular formation are a relay station for all descending motor commands, except those requiring the greatest precision, which are transferred directly from the cortex to spinal cord.

Vestibular nuclei. The vestibular system reflexes :

- Maintain tone in antigravity muscles,

- Coordinate the adjustments made by the limbs and trunk to maintain balance, and
- Adjust the position of the eyes to maintain visual fixation when the position of head changes.

III. LOWEST LEVEL OF MOTOR CONTROL

The lowest level of motor control is exerted by motor nuclei of cranial nerves and spinal cord. The spinal cord contains the *final common pathway* through which a movement is executed.

Spinal cord

Motor neurons of spinal cord present in ventral horn are:

1. *Alpha motor neurons*. These are responsible for contraction of muscles in upper limbs, trunk and lower part of the body.

2. *Gamma motor neurons*. These neurons innervate the intrafusal fibres of the muscle spindles and are responsible for maintenance of muscle tone.

3. *Interneurons*. The interneurons actually receive the bulk of synaptic input that reaches the spinal cord, either as incoming sensory information or signals descending from higher centres in the brain.

4. *Renshaw cells*. These are inhibitory neurons which play an important role in synaptic inhibition at the spinal cord.

Motor functions served by spinal cord are:

- Control of movement of muscles and joints,
- Control of tone and power of muscles,
- Control of deep (tendon) reflexes, and
- Control of superficial reflexes.

SKELETAL MUSCLES: THE EFFECTOR ORGAN OF SOMATIC MOTOR SYSTEM

The motor activity, be it in the form of walking, physical labour, skilled work like typing, performing surgical operations or even expression of thoughts and feelings through gesture or speech, is a result of highly co-ordinated movements produced by the skeletal muscles. The skeletal muscles, thus, form the effector organ of the somatic motor system. The physiology of skeletal muscle has been discussed in Chapter 5.2. However, certain aspects which need elaboration of skeletal muscle as effector organ and are relevant to complete the study of somatic motor system are:

- Motor unit,
- Muscle sensors (proprioceptors), and
- Muscle tone.

Motor unit

The motor unit is the functional module used by the motor control system to carry out a movement. The movement produced by a skeletal muscle basically depends upon the pattern and ratio of discharge of motor neurons supplying the muscle. A *motor unit consists* of single motor neuron and the muscle fibres that it innervates.

Muscle sensors

Muscle sensors refer to the proprioceptors present in the muscles, tendons of muscles, joints, ligaments and fasciae. Proprioceptors are the receptors which give information about change in position of different parts of the body in space, especially joints or tension of muscles at any given moment. The muscle sensors are:

- Muscle spindle,
- Golgi tendon organ,
- Pacinian corpuscle, and
- Free nerve endings.

In addition to the above proprioceptors, the labyrinth also contains proprioceptors (see page 494).

1. *Muscle spindle.* Muscle spindles are *stretch receptors* present in the skeletal muscles. Each skeletal muscle contains muscle spindles of variable number depending upon the task performed.

2. *Golgi tendon organs* are high threshold stretch receptors present in the tendons. They are supplied by group Ib afferent fibres and detect muscle tension.

3. *Pacinian corpuscles* are pressure receptors situated in fasciae throughout the muscles, tendons, joints and periosteum. They are supplied by *group II afferent fibres* and detect *vibration.*

4. *Free nerve endings* are basically pain receptors situated in the muscles, tendons, fasciae and joints. They are supplied by *group III and IV afferent fibres* and detect noxious stimuli.

Muscle tone

Definition. Muscle tone is defined as resistance offered to active or passive stretch. In other words, muscle tone refers to sustained partial state of contraction of the muscle under resting condition, i.e. a state of partial tetanus. The muscle tone is present in all the muscles, but is well pronounced in the extensor muscles, i.e. antigravity muscles.

Basis of muscle tone. The muscle tone is purely a function of myotactic (stretch reflex), occurring due to low frequency and asynchronous discharge of γ motor neurons. The discharge is out of phase with each other which ultimately merges to produce smooth muscle contraction.

Anomalies of muscle tone are hypotonia and hypertonia.

1. *Hypotonia* refers to decrease in muscle tone. The hypotonic or also called flaccid muscle offers little or no resistance to stretching. The muscles are generally hypotonic when the rate of γ efferent discharge is low, i.e. when stretch reflex becomes hypoactive.

2. *Hypertonia* refers to increase in muscle tone. The hypertonic or spastic muscle offers high resistance to stretch. The muscles are generally hypertonic when the rate of γ- efferent discharge is high, i.e. when stretch reflex becomes hyperactive. Hypertonia is of two types:

- *Spasticity* refers to hypertonia which is confined to only one group of muscles. For example, lesions of internal capsule and upper motor neuron lesions produce spasticity.
- *Rigidity* refers to hypertonia which involves both groups of muscles, i.e. extensor as well as flexors equally. For example, lesions of basal ganglia produce rigidity.

REFLEX ACTIVITY

ANATOMICAL ASPECTS

A reflex is an involuntary response to a peripheral nervous stimulation. In other words, it is a mechanism by which sensory impulse is automatically converted into a motor effect through the involvement of CNS. It is a type of protective mechanism which tries to protect the body from irreparable damage.

Reflex arc

The pathway for a reflex activity is called reflex arc. It consists of (Fig. 12.5-8):

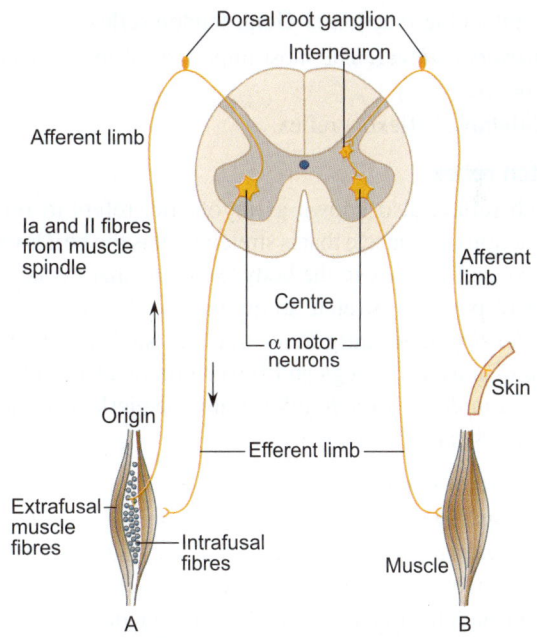

Fig. 12.5-8. Components of reflex arc in monosynaptic (A) and disynaptic (B) reflexes.

- Afferent limb,
- Centre, and
- Efferent limb.

1. *Afferent limb* of each reflex arc consists of a receptor and an afferent or sensory nerve. *Afferent neuron* carries sensory input from the receptor to the centre. The afferent neurons enter the CNS via the dorsal roots or cranial nerves and have their cell bodies in the dorsal root ganglia or in the homologous ganglia on the cranial nerves.

2. Centre. This is the part of CNS (spinal cord or brain) where afferent limb ends and either synapses directly with efferent motor neuron or establishes connection with the efferent neuron via interneurons (internuncial or intercalated neurons).

3. Efferent limb of a reflex arc consists of an efferent or motor nerve and an effector organ.

- *Efferent nerve* transmits motor impulses from the centre to the effector organ.
- *Effector organ* may be in the form of a muscle or a gland which shows the response to the stimulus.

SPINAL CORD REFLEXES

Spinal cord reflexes enhance the ability of the motor control system to produce a coordinated movement. According to the receptors from which they originate the spinal cord reflexes can be categorized into muscle reflexes and cutaneous reflexes.

Muscle reflexes. Two important reflexes which originate in muscles are:

- Stretch reflex, and
- Lengthening reaction or Golgi tendon reflex.

Cutaneous reflexes. The most important of the cutaneous reflexes is:

- Withdrawal (flexor) reflex.

Stretch reflex

Stretch reflex, also known as myotactic, refers to reflex contraction of a muscle that is stretched. It is the best known monosynaptic reflex in the body. *Stimulus* that evokes the reflex response is 'stretch' to the muscle. *Stretch reflex is well developed* in antigravity muscles such as extensor group of muscles of legs and flexor groups of muscles of arm. *Examples of stretch reflexes* are knee jerk, ankle jerk, biceps jerk, and triceps jerk.

Reflex arc of stretch reflex *(Fig. 12.5-8)*

1. Afferent limb consists of receptor *muscle spindle* and *afferent nerve* fibres emerging from the muscle spindle. Which travel along the spinal nerve and enter the spinal cord through the dorsal root and send branches to α-motor neuron that goes to the muscle from which the Ia originated.

2. Centre. Centre for stretch reflex is the ventral grey horn area where the afferent nerve ends and synapses directly with the α-motor neuron. Thus, α-motor neuron is the final common pathway, serving as both integrating centre and efferent pathway.

3. Efferent limb consists of :

- *Efferent nerve.* The axons of α-motor neurons form the efferent nerve fibres which leave the spinal cord through the ventral root and supply the skeletal muscle fibres.

- *Effector organs.* Both extensor and flexor muscles exhibit stretch reflexes.

Reciprocal innervation in stretch reflex

The stretch reflex is characterized by reciprocal innervation, i.e. excitation of one group of muscles is associated with inhibition of the antagonistic group of muscles on the same side, allowing the agonistic muscles to contract without interference. Reciprocal innervation is one of the important features of both flexor and extensor reflexes.

Functions of stretch reflex

1. Role in maintaining muscle tone.
2. Role in maintaining posture.
3. Role in control of voluntary movement.

Golgi tendon reflex (disynaptic reflex)

The Golgi tendon reflex, also called 'inverse stretch reflex', is a disynaptic reflex. The receptors involved are the Golgi tendon organs.

Physiological role or the functions of Golgi tendon reflex are:

- *Protective function.* Historically, this reflex has been described as a protective reflex in which a strong and potentially damaging muscle force reflexively inhibits the muscle, causing the muscle to lengthen instead of trying to maintain the force and risking damage.
- *Regulation of tension during normal muscle activity*

Clasp-knife reflex refers to an exaggerated form of the Golgi tendon reflex, which can occur with disease of the corticospinal tracts (hypertonicity or spasticity). For example, when the arm is hypertonic, the increased sensitivity of the muscle spindles in the extensor muscles (triceps) causes resistance to flexion of the arm. Eventually, tension in the triceps increases to the point at which it activates Golgi tendon reflex, causing triceps to relax and the arm to flex closed like a jack knife, hence the name clasp-knife reflex. The physiological name for it is *lengthening reaction,* because it is the response of a spastic muscle to lengthening.

Withdrawal reflex (polysynaptic reflex)

Definition. Withdrawal reflex, also known as flexor reflex, is a cutaneous reflex which occurs in response to nociceptive (pain) stimuli and is characterized by removal of a body part from painful stimulus.

Receptors for withdrawal reflex are *nociceptors* located in free nerve endings of Aδ and C fibres.

Pathway (reflex arc) of withdrawal reflex (Fig. 12.5-9):

- The pain fibres carrying impulses, upon entering the spinal cord, synapse on many interneurons. Some of these also convey information to CNS. Others form several reflex pathways.

   – Some of the interneurons project onto α-motor neurons

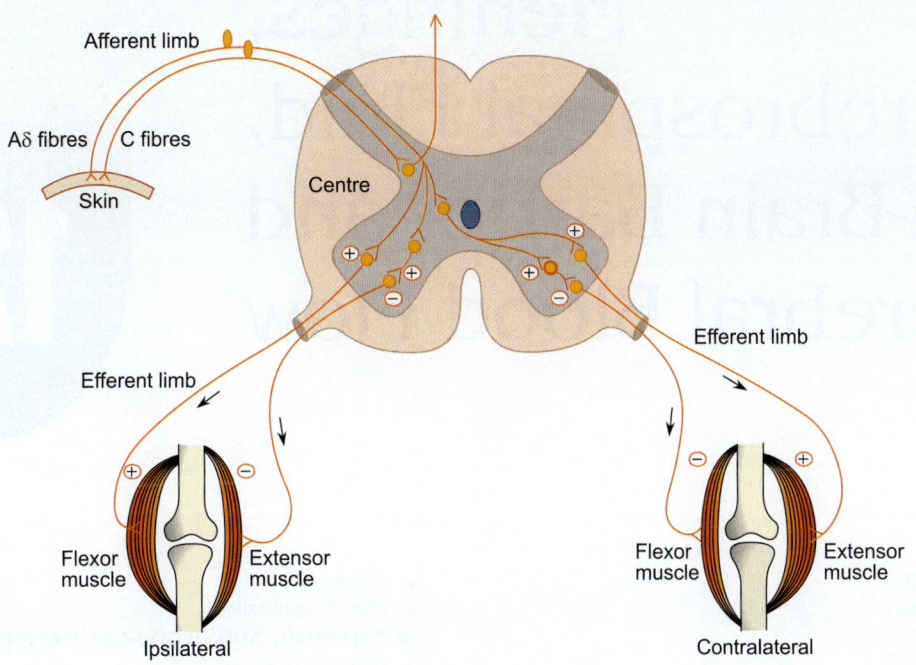

Fig. 12.5-9. *Reflex arc of polysynaptic reflex (withdrawl reflex or crossed extensor reflex).*

on the ipsilateral side and stimulate the flexors which withdraw the limbs.

– Some of the interneurons form inhibitory pathway and terminate on α-motor neurons supplying the extensor muscles on the ipsilateral side producing their relaxation. This is called reciprocal innervation which ensures that the flexion movement is not impeded by contraction of the extensors.

– Some of the interneurons cross to the opposite side of spinal cord and end on the α-motor neurons supplying the extensors on contralateral side. In case of need, this pathway produces extension of the opposite limbs (crossed extensor reflex).

Effector organs. The effector organs of the withdrawal reflex are the skeletal muscles that cause withdrawal of the limb i.e. flexor responses.

Meninges, Cerebrospinal Fluid, Blood-Brain Barrier and Cerebral Blood Flow

12.6

MENINGES
- Pia mater
- Arachnoid mater
- Dura mater

CEREBROSPINAL FLUID
- Composition, volume and pressure
- Formation, circulation and absorption

- Functions
- Clinical applications

BLOOD-BRAIN AND BLOOD-CSF BARRIERS
- Blood-brain barrier
- Blood-CSF barrier

CEREBRAL BLOOD FLOW
- Normal cerebral blood flow

MENINGES OF THE BRAIN

The brain is enclosed within the cranial cavity by three concentric connective tissue layers: pia mater, arachnoid mater and dura mater, which constitute the meninges of the brain (Fig. 12.6-1).

Pia mater

Pia mater, covering closely and continuously the external surface of the brain, is a thin and highly vascular membrane.

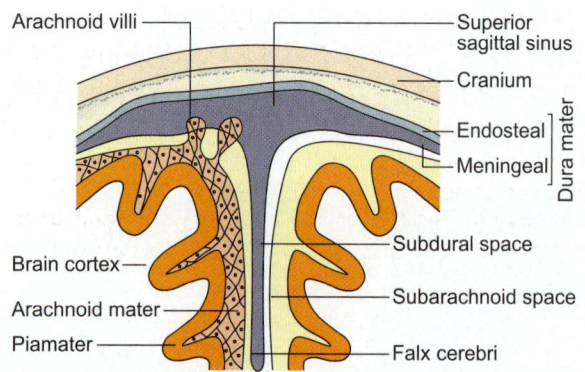

Fig. 12.6-1. Meninges of brain.

Folds of pia mater enclose tufts of capillaries called choroid plexuses to form tela choroidea in relation to ventricles of brain.

Arachnoid mater

Arachnoid mater is connected to the pia mater by many filamentous fibres. Subarachnoid space between these two layers is filled with cerebrospinal fluid (CSF).

Dura mater

Dura mater is composed of two layers: outer endosteal and inner meningeal. These are fused except where folds form (e.g. falx cerebri) or venous sinuses (e.g. superior sagittal sinus) are enclosed between them. *Subdural space* separates the dura mater from arachnoid mater. The arachnoid mater has minute protrusions (*arachnoid villi*) which pass through fenestrae in the dura mater and project into the venous sinuses to allow escape of CSF into venous sinuses.

CEREBROSPINAL FLUID

Cerebrospinal fluid (CSF) cushions the brain and along with blood-brain barrier, the buffering function of neuroglia, and regulation of CNS circulation controls the extracellular environment of neurons. Within the substance of brain in the *ventricular system,* there are series of spaces filled with CSF.

Composition, volume and pressure of CSF

Composition of CSF. The extracellular fluid within the CNS communicates directly with the CSF. Thus, the composition of CSF indicates the composition of the extracellular environment of the neurons in the brain and spinal cord. The composition of CSF vis-a-vis blood is depicted in Table 12.6-1. The CSF differs from blood in having a lower concentration of K^+, glucose, and protein and a higher concentration of Na^+ and Cl^-. CSF normally lacks blood cells. The increased concentration of Na^+ and Cl^- enables the CSF to be isotonic to blood, despite the much lower concentration of proteins in the CSF.

Table 12.6-1. Composition of CSF vis-a-vis blood

Constituent	Lumbar CSF	Blood
Na^+ (mEq/L)	148	136-145
K^+ (mEq/L)	2.9	3.5-5
Cl^- (mEq/L)	120-130	100-106
Glucose (mg/dl)	50-75	70-100
Protein (mg/dl)	15-45	6.8×10^3
pH	7.3	7.4

CSF volume and pressure. The cranial cavity contains about 140 ml CSF.

The volume of CSF within the cerebral ventricles is approximately 40 ml, and that in the subarachnoid space is about 100 ml. The pressure in the CSF column is about 120 to 180 mm H_2O when a person is recumbent. Rate of CSF formation (about 0.35 ml/minute) is independent of CSF pressure as well as systemic blood pressure.

Formation, circulation, and absorption of CSF

Formation of CSF. The CSF is mainly formed by the choroidal plexuses, which are covered by specialized ependymal cells. The *choroidal plexuses* are located in the cerebral ventricles (lateral, third and fourth). About 500 ml of CSF is secreted per day.

Circulation of CSF (Fig. 12.6-2). CSF formed in the lateral ventricles passes through the interventricular foramina (of Monro) into the third ventricle. Thence the fluid flows through the cerebral aqueduct (of Sylvius) into the fourth ventricle. From fourth ventricle, some CSF passes into the central canal of spinal cord, but most escapes into the subarachnoid space (surrounding the brain and spinal cord) through the median aperture (foramen of Magendie) of fourth ventricle and the two lateral apertures of fourth ventricle (foramina of Luschka).

Subarachnoid cistern refers to the regions where subarachnoid space is distended to form pools of CSF. An example is the *lumbar cistern* which surrounds the lumbar and sacral spinal roots below the level of termination of spinal cord. The lumbar cistern is the target for lumbar puncture, a procedure used clinically to sample the CSF.

Absorption of CSF. A large part of CSF is removed by bulk flow through the valvular *arachnoid villi* into the dural venous sinuses in the cranium. Unlike rate of formation, the absorption rate of CSF is a direct function of the CSF pressure.

Functions of CSF

- *Protection to CNS* by acting as a 'water-jacket', as it absorbs shock in the event of blow.
- *Removal of waste products* of brain metabolism.
- *Regulates extracellular environment* for the neurons of central nervous system.
- *Transports* hormones and hormone-releasing factors.

Clinical applications

Hydrocephalus

Hydrocephalus refers to an abnormal accumulation of CSF in the cranium.

Causes of hydrocephalus include:
- Obstruction to CSF circulation,
- Excessive production of CSF, and
- Interference with absorption of CSF.

Lumbar and cisternal puncture

Lumbar puncture refers to tapping of CSF from lumbar cistern. CSF examination is required in many disorders of CNS. It is performed by inserting a needle in between the L_2 and L_3 or L_3 and L_4 vertebrae.

Cisternal puncture refers to tapping of CSF from cisterna magna. To do this, a needle is passed through the posterior atlanto-occipital membrane forwards and upwards to a depth of 4.5 cm from the surface.

BLOOD-BRAIN BARRIER AND BLOOD-CSF BARRIER

Blood-brain barrier

Blood-brain barrier restricts the movement of large molecules and highly charged ions from the blood into the brain and spinal cord. It is formed by CNS capillary endothelial cells, their intercellular junctions, and a relative lack of vesicular transport. Most substances that must cross the blood-brain barrier are not lipid soluble and therefore cross by specific carrier-mediated transport system.

Some areas of the brain do not have a blood-brain barrier, e.g. posterior pituitary and circumventricular organs. The absence of blood-brain barrier in these regions is consistent

Dura mater
Superior sagittal sinus
Arachnoid villus
Choroid plexus
Lateral ventricle
Foramen of Monro
Third ventricle
Aqueduct of Sylvius
Fourth ventricle
Foramen of Magendie
Central canal
Pia mater
Arachnoid membrane
Subarachnoid space
Dura mater

Fig. 12.6-2. *Circulation of cerebrospinal fluid. Arrows indicate the direction of flow.*

with their physiological functions. These leaky regions are isolated from the rest of the brain by specialized ependymal cells called *tanycytes.*

Disruption of blood-brain barrier occurs in a variety of pathological situations such as brain tumours and bacterial meningitis etc. This fact can be exploited radiologically by introducing into the circulation a substance that normally cannot penetrate the blood-brain barrier. If the substance can be imaged, its leakage into the region occupied by the brain tumour can be used to demonstrate the distribution of tumour.

Blood-CSF barrier

The capillaries that traverse the choroidal plexuses are freely permeable to plasma solutes. However, a barrier (blood-CSF barrier) exists at the level of epithelial cells that make up the choroid plexuses. This barrier is responsible for carrier-mediated active transport.

CEREBRAL BLOOD FLOW

Functioning of the brain is closely related to the level of cerebral blood flow. Total cessation of blood flow to the brain causes unconsciousness within 5 to 10 seconds because of the decrease in oxygen delivery and the resultant cessation of metabolic activity.

Normal cerebral blood flow in an adult averages 50 to 65 ml/100 gm, or about 750 to 900 ml/min. Thus, the brain receives approximately 15 per cent of the total resting cardiac output.

Special Senses

SENSE OF VISION

ANATOMY OF EYEBALL AND ITS ACCESSORY ORGANS

Sense of vision is a complex function of the visual apparatus consisting of two eyeballs, visual pathway and their central connections. In addition to these essential organs, there are accessory organs which are necessary for the protection and functioning of the eyeball.

ACCESSORY ORGANS OF THE EYE AND ORBIT

Accessory organs of the eye include eyebrows, eyelids, conjunctiva, lacrimal apparatus and extraocular muscles.

Eyebrows

The two eyebrows are arched structures placed horizontally over the superciliary ridge of the frontal bone, separated from each other by a smooth hairless prominent area known as glabella. The surface of the eyebrows is covered by hair which project obliquely from the skin and form an important part of the eyebrows. They protect the eyeball from sweat, dust and other foreign bodies.

Eyelids

The eyelids are mobile tissue curtains placed in front of the eyeballs. These act as shutters protecting the eyes from injuries and excessive light. These also perform an important function of spreading the tear film over the cornea and conjunctiva.

   Eyelashes are short curved hair present on the lid margins (free edges of the eyelids).

Structure. From anterior to posterior the eyelid consists of following layers (Fig. 12.7-1)

1. *Skin.* It is elastic and very thin.
2. *Subcutaneous loose areolar tissue.*
3. *Layer of striated muscles.* It consists of orbicularis oculi muscle which closes the lids. In addition, the upper eyelid also contains levator palpebrae superioris muscle which raises the upper eyelids.
4. *Submuscular areolar tissue.* The nerves and vessels of the eyelids lie in this layer.
5. *Fibrous layer.* It is the framework of the lids and consists of two parts : the central *tarsal plate* and the peripheral *septum orbitale*.

6. *Layer of nonstriated muscle* fibres is formed by palpebral muscle of Muller.
7. *Conjunctiva.* The lids on their inner surface are lined by a thin mucous membrane called the palpebral conjunctiva.

Conjunctiva

The conjunctiva is a translucent mucous membrane which lines the posterior surface of the eyelids and anterior aspect of the eyeball upto limbus.

Parts. Conjunctiva consists of following parts (Fig. 12.7-2) :

1. *Palpebral conjunctiva* lines the posterior surface of the eyelids.
2. *Bulbar conjunctiva* covers the anterior part of eyeball upto the limbus.
3. *Fornices.* Superior and inferior conjunctival fornices are the cul-de-sacs formed at the junction of bulbar conjunctiva with the palpebral conjunctiva.
4. *Plica semilunaris* is a pinkish crescentric fold of conjunctiva present in the medial canthus.

Lacrimal apparatus

The lacrimal apparatus (Fig. 12.7-3) comprises the structures concerned with the formation (main lacrimal gland and accessory lacrimal glands) and drainage (lacrimal passages: puncta, canaliculi, lacrimal sac and nasolacrimal duct) of tears.

Fig. 12.7-1. Structure of upper eyelid.

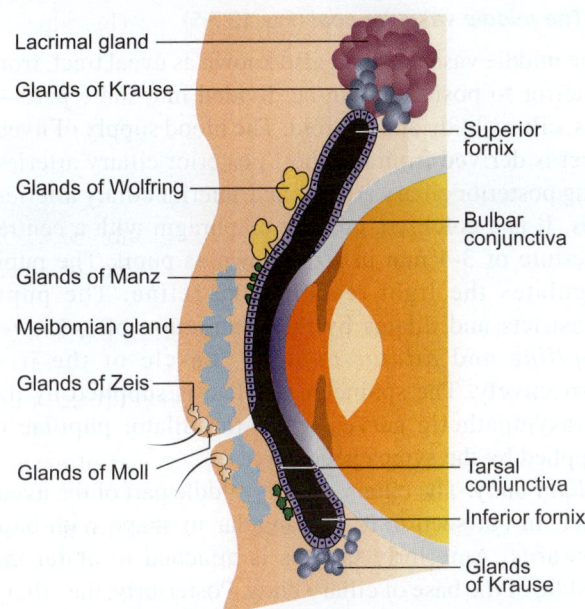

Fig. 12.7-2. Parts of conjunctiva.

Fig. 12.7-3. The lacrimal apparatus.

Main lacrimal gland

The main lacrimal gland is situated at the upper and outer angle of the orbit, in a depression known as the fossa for the lacrimal gland. It consists of an upper orbital and a lower palpebral part. Each gland is about the size and shape of an almond. It is composed of secretory epithelial cells. The ducts of lacrimal gland which are about 12 in number open in the superior fornix. The gland secretes tears composed of water, salt and lysozyme (a bactericidal enzyme).

Accessory lacrimal glands

These are microscopic glands situated beneath the palpebral conjunctiva between fornix and edge of the tarsal plate.

Lacrimal passages

1. *Lacrimal puncta.* These are two small rounded or oval openings situated on a small elevation called *lacrimal papilla,* about 6 mm from the inner canthus on each eyelid margin.

2. *Lacrimal canaliculi.* These are narrow tubular passages which join the puncta to lacrimal sac.

3. *Lacrimal sac.* It lies in the lacrimal fossa located in the anterior part of medial orbital wall. The sac continues with the nasolacrimal duct inferiorly.

4. *Nasolacrimal duct (NLD).* It is a membranous canal about 15-18 mm long. It extends from the lower part of lacrimal sac to inferior meatus of the nose. Direction of NLD is downwards, backwards and laterally. Hasner's valve, which prevents reflux from the nose is present at the lower end of NLD.

Extraocular muscles (Fig. 12.7-4)

A set of six extraocular muscles (4 recti and 2 obliques) control the movements of each eye. These muscles are attached to the outer coat of the eyeball at one end and to the walls of the orbital cavity at the other end. The extraocular muscles include :

- Medial rectus
- Lateral rectus
- Superior rectus
- Inferior rectus
- Superior oblique
- Inferior oblique

Fig. 12.7-4. Extraocular muscles.

Orbit

The bony orbits are quadrangular truncated pyramids situated between the anterior cranial fossa above and the maxillary sinuses below. Seven bones take part in its formation. It has four walls (medial, lateral, superior and inferior), a base and an apex.

THE EYEBALL

Each eyeball is a cystic structure kept distended by the pressure inside it.

Dimensions of an adult eyeball

Anteroposterior diameter	: 24 mm
Horizontal (transverse) diameter	: 23.5 mm

Vertical diameter	: 23 mm
Circumference	: 75 mm
Volume	: 6.5 ml
Weight	: 7 gm

Coats of the eyeball

The eyeball comprises three coats: outer (fibrous coat), middle (vascular coat) and inner (nervous coat) (Fig. 12.7-5).

1. The outer fibrous coat

It is a dense strong wall which protects the intraocular contents. Anterior one sixth of the fibrous coat is transparent and is called cornea. The posterior 5/6th opaque part is called sclera. Junction of the cornea and sclera is called limbus.

Cornea. The cornea is a transparent, avascular, watchglass-like structure with a smooth shining surface. The average diameter of the cornea is 11-12 mm. Its thickness in the central part is 0.52 mm and in the peripheral part 0.67 mm.

Nerve supply of cornea is purely sensory, derived from the ophthalmic division of the 5th cranial nerve.

Sclera. The sclera is a strong, opaque, white fibrous layer. It is a relatively avascular structure about 1 mm in thickness. It is pierced by nerves and vessels entering the eyeball. Histologically, sclera consists of three layers : episcleral tissue, sclera proper and lamina fusca.

2. The middle vascular coat (Fig. 12.7-5)

The middle vascular coat, also known as uveal tract, from anterior to posterior, can be divided into three parts—iris, ciliary body and choroid. The blood supply of uveal tract is derived from the short posterior ciliary arteries, long posterior ciliary arteries and anterior ciliary arteries.

Iris. It is a coloured, circular diaphragm with a central aperture of 3-4 mm in size known as pupil. The pupil regulates the light reaching the retina. The pupil constricts and dilates by the contraction of *sphincter pupillae* and *dilator pupillae* muscle of the iris, respectively. The sphincter pupillae is supplied by the parasympathetic nerves while the dilator pupillae is supplied by the sympathetic nerves.

Ciliary body. The ciliary body is middle part of the uveal tract. In cut section it is triangular in shape with base forwards. Anteriorly the iris is attached to about the middle of the base of ciliary body. Posteriorly, the ciliary body becomes continuous with the choroid.

The ciliary body contains a non-striated muscle called the *ciliary muscle* which is supplied by parasympathetic fibres and takes part in the process of accommodation of the eye.

There are about 70-80 finger-like projections from the ciliary body. These are called *ciliary processes* and are the site of aqueous humour production—a watery fluid which maintains the intraocular pressure of the eyeball.

Fig. 12.7-5. *Gross anatomy of eyeball.*

Choroid. It is a dark brown highly vascular layer situated in between sclera and retina. It supplies nutrition to the outer layers of retina.

3. The inner nervous coat (retina) (Fig. 12.7-6)

Retina, the innermost tunic of the eyeball, is a thin, delicate, transparent membrane. It is the most highly developed tissue of the eye. It is concerned with the visual functions.

Gross anatomy. Grossly, retina can be divided into optic disc, macula lutea and the peripheral retina.

Ora serrata is the anterior serrated termination of the retina.

Macula lutea (yellow spot) is a comparatively dark area situated at the posterior pole temporal to the optic disc. Its central depressed area of 1.5 mm in diameter is called *fovea centralis,* which is the most sensitive part of the retina. Visual acuity is maximum in this part of retina.

Optic disc. It is a well-defined circular, pink coloured disc of 1.5 mm diameter. It has only nerve fibre layer, so it does not excite any visual response. It produces *blind spot* in the field of vision.

Interior of the eyeball

Interior of the eyeball contains, from anterior to posterior— the aqueous humour, lens and vitreous.

Aqueous humour

It is a watery fluid present in the anterior and posterior chambers of the eyeball. *Anterior chamber* is the space bounded anteriorly by the back of cornea and posteriorly by the anterior surface of iris. *Posterior chamber* is the space between the front of crystalline lens and back of iris. Through pupil, anterior and posterior chambers communicate with each other.

Crystalline lens

The lens is a transparent, biconvex, crystalline structure placed between the iris and the vitreous. It is suspended from the ciliary body by the suspensory ligament or zonules of Zinn. Refractive power of the lens is about 15-16 D.

Lens is elastic in nature and its power changes with accommodation. Elasticity of the lens gradually decreases with the age. It is a vascular structure and derives its nutrition from the aqueous humour.

Vitreous humour

Vitreous humour is an inert, transparent, jelly-like structure that fills the posterior four-fifths of the cavity of eyeball. It serves the optical function. It consists of 90% water, some salts and mucoproteins.

RETINA AND VISUAL PATHWAY

Structure of retina

Retina consists of ten layers, which from without inwards, are as follows (Fig. 12.7-7) :

1. *Layer of pigment epithelium.* It is a single layer of hexagonal cells containing melanin pigments.

2. *Layer of rods and cones.* Rods and cones are end organs of vision and are also known as photoreceptors.

3. *External limiting membrane.* It is a thin fenestrated membrane.

4. *Outer nuclear layer.* It consists of nuclei of the rods and cones.

5. *Outer plexiform layer.* It consists of connections of axons of rods and cones with the dendrites of the bipolar cells.

6. *Inner nuclear layer.* It consists of nuclei of bipolar cells, which constitute first order neurons of vision.

7. *Inner plexiform layer.* It consists of synapses of the axons of the bipolar cells with the dendrites of the ganglion cells.

8. *Ganglion cell layer.* It consists of ganglion cells.

9. *Nerve fibre layer.* It consists of axons of the ganglion cells which pass through lamina cribrosa to form the optic nerve.

10. *Internal limiting membrane.* It separates the retina from the vitreous.

A

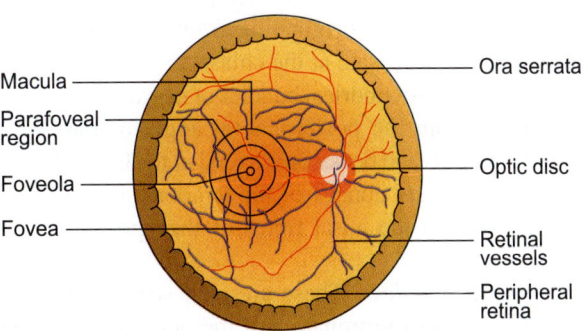

B

Fig. 12.7-6. *Gross anatomy of retina*

1. **Pigmented epithelium** — Optic nerve fibres
2. **Layer of rods and cones** — Rod — Cone
3. **External limiting membrane**
4. **Outer nuclear layer** — Cone nucleus — Rod nucleus
5. **Outer plexiform layer**
6. **Inner nuclear layer** — Horizontal cell — Bipolar cell
   Amacrine cell
7. **Inner plexiform layer** — Parasol ganglion cell
8. **Ganglion cell layer** — Ganglion cell
9. **Nerve fibre layer**
10. **Internal limiting membrane**

Fig. 12.7-7. *Microscopic structure of retina.*

Visual pathway

Each eyeball acts as a camera; it perceives the images and relays the sensations to the brain (occipital cortex) via visual pathway which comprises optic nerve, optic chiasma, optic tract, geniculate body and optic radiations (Fig. 12.7-8).

1. *Optic nerve.* Each optic nerve (second cranial nerve) starts from the optic disc and extends upto the optic chiasma. It is the continuation backward of the nerve fibre layer of retina, which consists of the axons of the ganglion cells. The optic nerve is about 47-50 mm in length.
2. *Optic chiasma.* It is a flattened structure lying above the pituitary fossa. Fibres originating from the nasal halves of the retina decussate at the chiasma.
3. *Optic tracts.* These are cylindrical bundles of nerve fibres which originate from the posterolateral angle of the chiasma and outwards and backwards to end in the lateral geniculate bodies. They consist of the temporal fibres of the same side and the nasal fibres of the opposite side.
4. *Lateral geniculate bodies.* These are oval structures situated at the posterior termination of the optic tracts. The fibres of the optic tracts end in the lateral geniculate bodies and nerve fibres of the optic radiations originate from them.

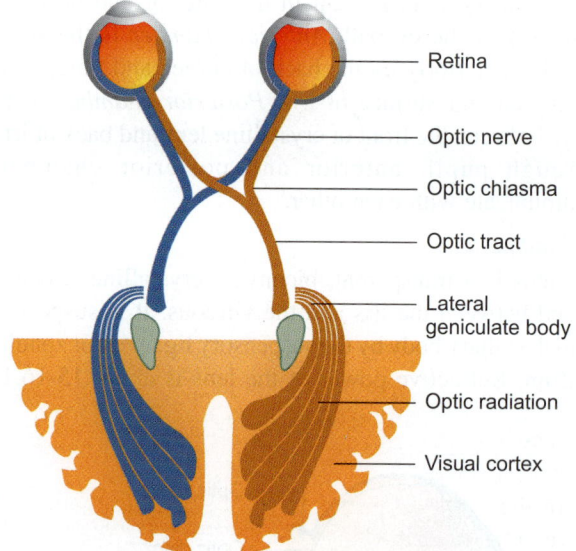

— Retina
— Optic nerve
— Optic chiasma
— Optic tract
— Lateral geniculate body
— Optic radiation
— Visual cortex

Fig.12.7-8. *Components of visual pathway.*

5. *Optic radiations.* These extend from the lateral geniculate bodies to the visual cortex.
6. *Visual cortex.* It is located on the medial aspect of the occipital lobe, above and below the calcarine fissure. It is subdivided into the visuosensory area (striate area 17) that receives the fibres of the radiations, and the

surrounding visuopsychic area (peristriate area 18 and parastriate area 19).

PHYSIOLOGY OF EYE AND VISION

Function of the eyes is to provide sense of sight (vision), which is the choicest gift from the Almighty to humans and other animals. The eyeballs are able to perform their function with the help of following physiological activities.

1. Maintenance of clear media of the eye.
2. Maintenance of normal intraocular pressure.
3. Neurophysiology of vision.
4. Mechanism of sight.
5. Physiology of binocular vision.

MAINTENANCE OF CLEAR MEDIA OF THE EYE

The main factor responsible for transparency of the refractive media of the eye is their avascularity. The structures forming refractive media of the eye from anterior to posterior are as below :

1. *Tear film.* It keep the cornea moist and provides oxygen and nutrients.
2. *Cornea.* It forms the main refracting medium of the eye.
3. *Aqueous humour.* It is a clear watery fluid filling the anterior chamber and posterior chamber of the eye.
4. *Crystalline lens.* It is a biconvex lens which has been provided with a unique mechanism of changing its power (*accommodation*). Due to this characteristic it helps in sharp focussing of the images of the objects present at varying distances from the eye.
5. *Vitreous humour.* It is clear jelly-like material which in addition to being a refractive medium also helps in maintaining the shape of the eyeball.

MAINTENANCE OF NORMAL INTRAOCULAR PRESSURE

Aqueous humour and intraocular pressure

Aqueous humour

The aqueous humour is a clear watery fluid filling the anterior chamber (0.25 ml) and posterior chamber (0.06 ml) of the eyeball. In addition to its role in maintaining a proper intraocular pressure it also plays an important metabolic role by providing substrates and removing metabolites from the avascular cornea and the lens.

Aqueous humour is derived from plasma within the capillary network of ciliary processes. It flows from the posterior chamber into the anterior chamber through the pupil. From the anterior chamber the aqueous is drained out by two routes:

- Trabecular (conventional outflow), and
- Uveoscleral (unconventional) outflow.

Maintenance of intraocular pressure

The intraocular pressure (IOP) refers to the pressure exerted by intraocular fluids on the coats of the eyeball. The normal IOP varies between 10 and 21 mm of Hg (mean 16 ± 2.5 mm of Hg). The normal level of IOP is essentially maintained by a dynamic equilibrium between the formation and outflow of the aqueous humour. In glaucoma interaocular pressure rises.

NEUROPHYSIOLOGY OF VISION

Neurophysiology of vision is a complex phenomenon which is still poorly understood. The main mechanisms concerned with vision are as follows:

1. Initiation and transmission of visual sensation

Light falling upon the retina initiates photochemical changes in the visual pigments of rod and cone cells. The photochemical reaction initiates the visual sensation in the form of changes in electrical potential which are transmitted through the bipolar cells to the ganglion cells and along the fibres of the optic nerve to the brain.

Photoreceptors

- Rods and cones (*photoreceptors*) are the end organs of vision which transform light energy into visual (nerve) impluse.
- Rods contain a photosensitive substance, visual purple (*rhodopsin*), and subserve the peripheral vision and vision of low illumination (scotopic vision).
- Cones also contain a photosensitive substance and are primarily responsible for highly discriminatory central vision (photopic vision) and colour vision.
- There are about 120 million rods and 6.5 million cones.

Structure of photoreceptor. Each photoreceptor consists of a cell body and nucleus (which lie in the outer nuclear layer).

Visual pigments

Rhodopsin (visual purple). Rhodopsin is the photosensitive visual pigment present in the discs of the rods' outer segments. It consists of a protein opsin (called scotopsin) and a carotenoid called retinal (the aldehyde of vitamin A).

The absorption spectrum of rhodopsin lies within the narrow limits of 493-505 nm. It absorbs primarily yellow wavelength of light, transmitting violet and red to appear purple by transmitted light; it is therefore also called visual purple.

Cone pigments. Cone pigments are somewhat different from the rhodopsin, in that they respond to specific wavelength of light, giving rise to colour vision. These differences are present in the opsin portion of the molecule, whereas the chromophore 11-cis-retinal remains the same.

Light-induced changes

Light falling upon the retina is absorbed by the visual

pigments and initiates *photochemical changes* which in turn trigger a sequence of events that cause phototransduction.

2. Visual perception

It is a complex integration of light sense, form sense, sense of contrast, and colour sense.

The light sense

It is awareness of the light. The minimum brightness required to evoke a sensation of light is called the *light minimum*. It should be measured when the eye is dark adapted for at least 20-30 minutes.

The human eye in its ordinary use throughout the day is capable of functioning normally over an exceedingly wide range of illumination by a highly complex phenomenon termed as the *visual adaptation*. The process of visual adaptation primarily involves :

- *Dark adaptation* (adjustment in dim illumination), and
- *Light adaptation* (adjustment to bright illumination).

Dark adaptation. It is the ability of the eye to adapt itself to decreasing illumination. When one goes from bright sunshine into a dimly-lit room, one cannot perceive the objects in the room until some time has elapsed. During this period eye is adapting to low illumination. The time taken to see in dim illumination is called *dark adaptation time*. The rods are much more sensitive to low illumination than cones. Therefore, rods are used more in dim light (*scotopic vision*) and cones in bright light (*photopic vision*).

Dark adaptation curve plotted with illumination of test object in vertical axis and duration of dark adaptation along the horizontal axis shows that visual threshold falls progressively in the darkened room for about half an hour until a relative constant value is reached (Fig. 12.7-9).

The form sense

It is the ability to discriminate between the shapes of the objects. Cones play a major role in this faculty. Therefore, form sense is most acute at the fovea, where there are maximum number of cones and decreases very rapidly towards the periphery (Fig. 12.7-10). Visual acuity recorded by Snellen's test chart is a measure of the form sense.

The colour sense

Colour sense is the ability of the eye to discriminate between colours excited by light of different wave-lengths. Some broad facts about colour vision are:

- Colour vision is a function of cones and thus better appreciated in photopic vision.
- There are three different types of cones viz. red sensitive, green sensitive and blue sensitive, which combinedly perform the function of colour vision.
- All colours are a result of admixture in different proportion of three primary colours: the red (723-647

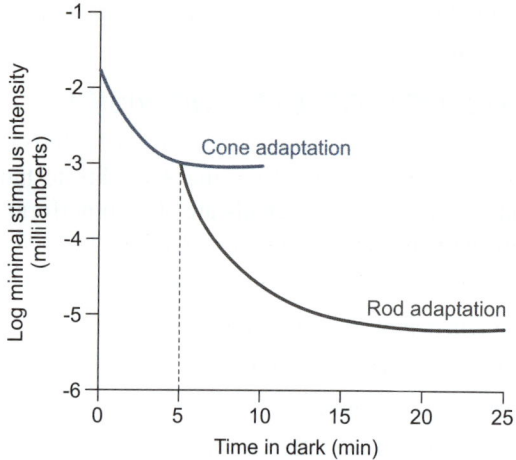

Fig. 12.7-9. *Dark adaption curve.*

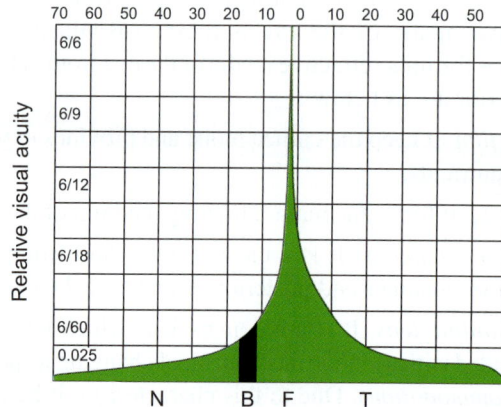

Fig. 12.7-10. *Visual acuity (form sense) in relation to regions of retina: N (Nasal retina); B, Blind spot; F, Fovea region and T, Temporal retina*

nm), green (575-492 nm), and blue (492-450 nm) (Young-Helmholtz theory).

Contrast sensitivity

Contrast sensitivity is the ability to perceive slight changes in luminance between regions which are not separated by definite borders and is just as important as the ability to perceive sharp outlines of relatively small objects.

MECHANISM OF SIGHT

As described on page 483, the functioning of the eye as an optical instrument can be compared with a camera (Fig. 12.7-11) as below :

- *Eyelids* act as shutter of the camera.
- *Cornea and crystalline lens* act as focussing system of the camera.
- *Iris* acts as diaphragm which regulates the size of the aperture (*pupil*) and therefore the amount of light entering the eye.
- *Choroid* helps in forming the darkened interior of the camera.

Fig. 12.7-11. *Sense of sight in many ways similar to close circuit colour TV system.*

- *Retina* acts as light-sensitive plate or film on which image is formed.

The optic nerve and its connections convey the details of the image to the occipital region of the cerebral cortex where they are processed before reaching consciousness.

Optics of eye : image formation

The optics of eye is very complex. However for understanding it has been simplified. The focussing structures of eye (cornea and crystalline lens) form a convex lens of +60 D which focus the light rays on the sensitive layer of retina (Fig. 12.7-12). Optically normal eye is called *emmetropic accommodation.*

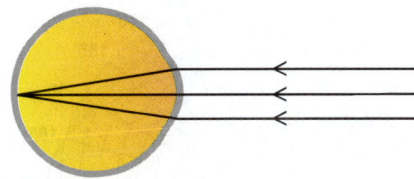

Fig. 12.7-12. *Refraction in an emmetropic eye.*

Accommodation

Our eyes have been provided with a unique mechanism by which we can even focus the diverging rays coming from a near object on the retina in a bid to see clearly (Fig. 12.7-13). This mechanism is called accommodation. In it there occurs :

- Increase in the power of the crystalline lens,
- Constriction of pupil, and
- Convergence of eyeballs.

Changes in the curvature of lens surface. The principal change in the lens during accommodation is seen in the

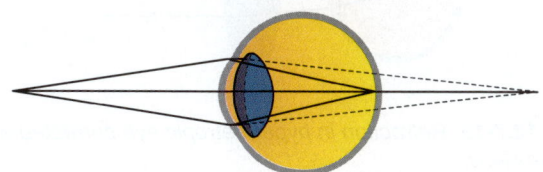

Fig. 12.7-13. *Effect of accommodation on divergent rays entering the eye.*

anterior surface of the lens as compared to posterior surface. As the refractive index of lens (1.39) is more than the refractive index of aqueous and vitreous, increase in convexity of the lens increases its dioptric power and thus allows the near objects to be focussed clearly on the retina. ***Pupillary constriction and convergence of eyes.*** In addition to the changes in the lens and zonular system the pupil constricts and the eyes converge, almost simultaneously. These changes occur in a bid to achieve clear vision for near objects.

Common defects of the image-forming mechanism

Emmetropia

Emmetropia (optically normal eye) can be defined as a state of refraction, when the parallel rays of light coming from infinity are focused at the sensitive layer of retina with the accommodation being at rest (Fig. 12.7-12).
Ametropia. Ametropia (a condition of refractive error) is defined as a state of refraction, when the parallel rays of light coming from infinity (with accommodation at rest) are focussed either in front or behind the sensitive layer of retina, in one or both the meridia. The ametropia includes myopia, hypermetropia and astigmatism.
Hypermetropia. Hypermetropia (hyperopia) or long-

sightedness is the refractive state of the eye wherein parallel rays of light coming from infinity are focussed behind the retina with accommodation being at rest (Fig. 12.7-14).

Optical correction. Basic principle of treatment of hypermetropia is optical correction with convex (plus) lenses, so that the light rays are brought to focus on the retina (Fig. 12.7-15).

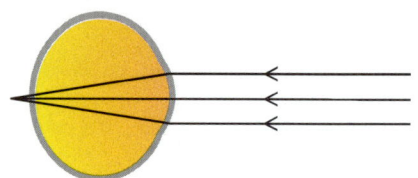

Fig. 12.7-14. Refraction in hypermetropic eye.

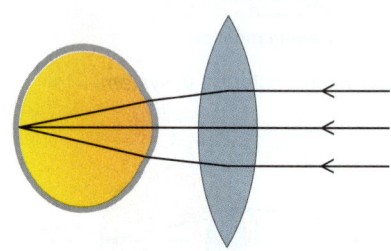

Fig. 12.7-15. Refraction in hypermetropic eye corrected with convex lens.

Myopia. Myopia or short-sightedness is a type of refractive error in which parallel rays of light coming from infinity are focussed in front of the retina when accommodation is at rest (Fig. 12.7-16).

Optical correction. Basic principles of treatment of myopia is optical correction with concave (minus) lenses, so that clear image is formed on the retina (Fig. 12.7-17).

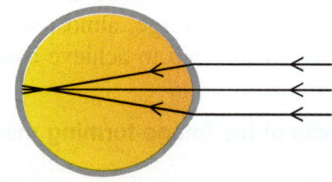

Fig. 12.7-16. Refraction in myopic eye.

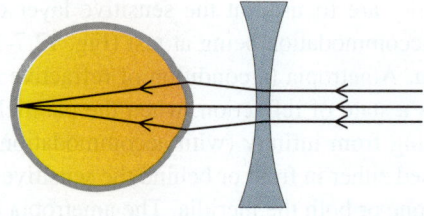

Fig. 12.7-17. Refraction in myopic eye corrected with concave lens.

Astigmatism. Astigmatism is a type of refractive error wherein the refraction varies in the different meridia. Consequently, the rays of light entering the eye cannot converge to a point focus but form focal lines.

Presbyopia. Presbyopia (eyesight of old age) is not an error of refraction but condition of physiological insufficiency of accommodation, leading to failing vision for near.

Since, we usually keep the book at about 25 cm, so we can read comfortably up to the age of 40 years. After the age of 40 years, the near point of accom-modation recedes beyond the normal reading or working range. This condition of failing near vision is due to age-related decrease in the amplitude of accommodation.

Treatment of presbyopia is the prescription of appropriate convex glasses for near work.

BINOCULAR SINGLE VISION AND FIELD OF VISION

Binocular single vision

When a normal individual fixes his visual attention on an object of regard, the image is formed on the fovea of both the eyes separately, but the individual perceives a single image. This state is called binocular single vision. It is a conditioned reflex which is not present since birth but is acquired during first 6 months and is completed during first few years. The process of its development is complex and partially understood.

Field of vision

The visual field is a three-dimensional area that can be seen around an object of fixation. The extent of normal visual field with a 5 mm white colour object is superiorly 60°, inferiorly 70°, nasally 60° and temporally 90° (Fig. 12.7-18).

Fig. 12.7-18. Extent of normal visual field.

PHYSIOLOGY OF PUPIL

Light reflex

When light is shone in one eye, both the pupils constrict. Constriction of the pupil to which light is shone is called *direct light reflex* and that of the other pupil is called *consensual (indirect) light reflex.* Light reflex is initiated by rods and cones.

Pathway of light reflex (Fig. 12.7-19). The *afferent fibres* extend from retina to the pretectal nucleus in the midbrain. These travel along the optic nerve to the optic chiasma where fibres from the nasal retina decussate and travel along the opposite optic tract to terminate in the contralateral pretectal nucleus, while the fibres from the temporal retina remain uncrossed and travel along the optic tract of the same side to terminate in the ipsilateral pretectal nucleus.

Internuncial fibres connect each pretectal nucleus with Edinger-Westphal nuclei of both sides. This connection forms the basis of consensual light reflex.

Efferent pathway consists of the parasympathetic fibres which arise from the Edinger-Westphal nucleus in the midbrain and travel along the third (oculomotor) cranial nerve. The preganglionic fibres enter the inferior division of the third nerve and via the nerve to the inferior oblique reach the ciliary ganglion to relay. Postganglionic fibres travel along the short ciliary nerves to innervate the sphincter pupillae.

SENSE OF HEARING

FUNCTIONAL ANATOMY

THE EAR

The mechanism of hearing is closely associated with the mechanism of equilibrium, therefore, the inner ear acts as an organ of hearing and equilibrium. For hearing, the sound waves have to pass through the three subdivisions of the ear, which are (Fig. 12.7-20):

- External ear,
- Middle ear, and
- Internal ear.

External ear

The external ear consists of the pinna (auricle) and the external auditory meatus.

Pinna or auricle consists of a single convoluted plate of elastic cartilage covered by skin. In humans, the pinna is not moveable.

Functions. The pinna collects and reflects the sound waves into the external auditory canal.

External auditory meatus extends from the pinna to the tympanic membrane. It is lined with skin, which secretes wax (from the ceruminous glands) and oil (from the sebacious glands).

Fig. 12.7-19. *Pathway of light reflex.*

Labels: Ciliary ganglion; Third nerve; Optic tract; Central grey matter; Aqueduct; Lateral geniculate body; Edinger-Westphal nucleus; Pretectal nucleus; Posterior commissure

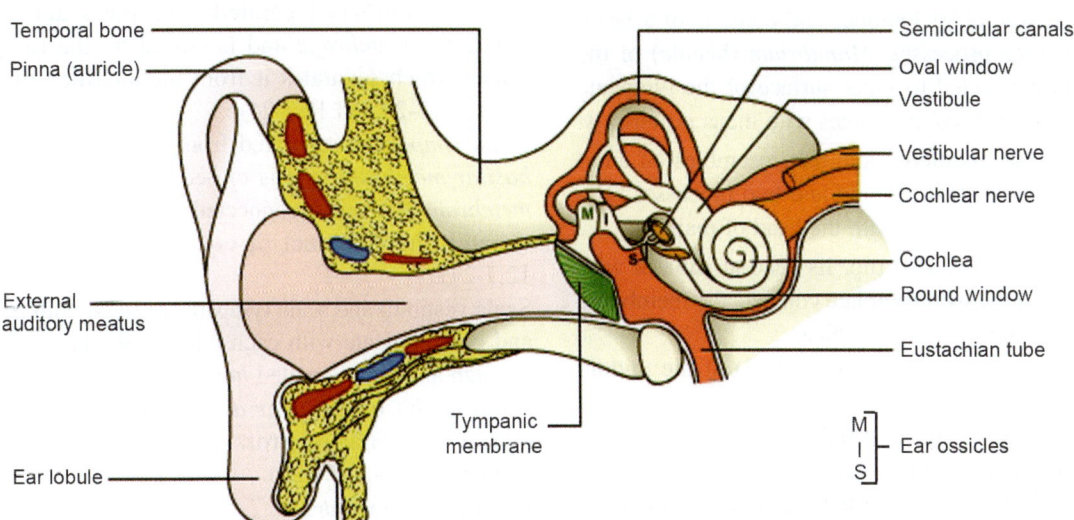

Labels: Temporal bone; Pinna (auricle); External auditory meatus; Ear lobule; Tympanic membrane; Semicircular canals; Oval window; Vestibule; Vestibular nerve; Cochlear nerve; Cochlea; Round window; Eustachian tube; M I S Ear ossicles

Fig. 12.7-20. *Structure of three subdivisions of the ear.*

Middle ear

The middle ear or the tympanic cavity is an air-filled rectangular space in the petrous part of temporal bone. It consists of following structures :

Tympanic membrane is a cave-shaped structure with concavity directed towards the external auditory meatus. Point of maximum convexity is called umbo. It consists of connective tissue covered with skin on the outside and mucous membrane on the inside.

Eustachian tube or the pharyngotympanic tube connects the middle ear cavity with pharynx. Air can pass through this tube into the middle ear. Therefore, it serves the function of equalization of pressure on two sides of tympanic membrane.

Ear ossicles. The three ear ossicles (auditory ossicles) include malleus, incus and stapes. They are attached to each other by ligaments and form a chain (Fig. 12.7-21).

***Fig. 12.7-21.** Ear ossicles and their parts.*

- *Malleus.* It resembles hammer and consists of a head, neck and three processes. *Manubrium* (handle) of the malleus is connected to inner surface of the tympanic membrane, and *head* articulates with incus posteriorly.
- *Incus.* It is the middle ossicle that resembles an anvil in shape. It consists of a body and two processes. The body of incus articulates with the head of malleus.
- *Stapes.* It resembles a stirrup. Its head articulates with the incus, and the oval footplate contacts the membrane of the oval window of the cochlea.

Windows. Medial wall (labyrinthine wall) of the middle ear contains two windows :

- *Oval window* (fenestra vestibuli) is present above, in which footplate (face plate or stapes) is attached. It leads to the vestibule of the internal ear and transmits the sound vibrations of the ossicles to the perilymph of scala vestibuli.

- *Round window* (fenestra cochlea) is present in the lower part, and is closed by a thin membrane called *secondary tympanic membrane*. It accommodates the pressure waves transmitted to the perilymph of the scala tympani.

Muscles. The middle ear contains two muscles: the tensor tympani and stapedius. Both muscles of the middle ear act simultaneously and reflexly in response to loud sound and attenuate the sound.

Internal ear

The internal ear or labyrinth is situated in the petrous part of the temporal bone. It consists of bony labyrinth and membranous labyrinth (Fig. 12.7-22). *Bony labyrinth* consists of three parts: vestibule, semicircular canals and the cochlea. *Membranous labyrinth* is lodged within the bony labyrinth. The inner ear can be divided into two main parts—vestibular apparatus, and auditory receptor apparatus. The vestibular apparatus is concerned with equilibrium.

Auditory apparatus

The auditory apparatus is formed by the *duct of cochlea* which lies within the bony cochlea.

Bony cochlea is a spiral tube which in humans has a two and three-fourths turns around a central bone called the *modiolus*. Around the modiolus and winding spirally like the thread of a screw, is a thin plate of bone called *osseous spiral lamina*. It divides the bony cochlea incompletely, and gives attachment to the basilar membrane. Two membranes (basilar membrane and Reissner's membrane) divide the bony cochlea into three compartments (Fig. 12.7-23):

- Scala vestibuli,
- Scala media (membranous chochlear duct), and
- Scala tympani.

Scala vestibuli is separated from the scala media by *Reissner's membrane* and is closed by the footplate of stapes which separates it from the air-filled middle ear (Figs. 12.7-23 and 12.7-24).

Scala tympani is separated from the scala media by the *basilar membrane* and is closed by *secondary tympanic membrane*. It is also connected with subarachnoid space through the aqueduct of cochlea (Figs. 12.7-23 and 12.7-24).

Scala vestibuli and scala tympani are filled with perilymph and communicate with each other at the apex of cochlea through an opening called *helicotrema*.

Scala media or *cochlear duct* or *membranous cochlea* appear triangular on cross-section. Its three walls are formed by (Fig. 12.7-23):

- Basilar membrane,
- Reissner's membrane, and
- Stria vascularis.

Fig. 12.7-22. *Structure of inner ear: A, left bony labyrinth; B, left membranous labyrinth; and C, cut section of bony labyrinth.*

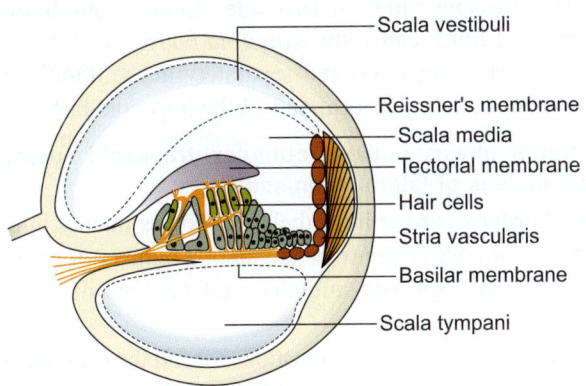

Fig. 12.7-23. *Vertical section through cochlea showing scala vestibuli, scala media (cochlear duct) and scala tympani. Note the location of organ of Corti over the basilar membrane in the cavity of cochlear duct.*

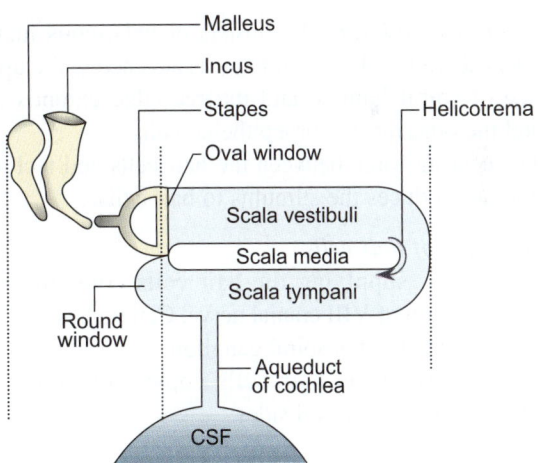

Fig. 12.7-24. *Diagrammatic depiction of arrangement of perilymphatic system, three compartments of cochlea (scala vestibuli, scala media, and scala tympani), and ear ossicles of the middle ear. Note the CSF passes into scala tympani through aqueduct of cochlea.*

Perilymph and endolymph

Perilymph is the fluid present in the scala tympani and scala vestibuli compartments of the cochlea. Its composition is similar to extracellular fluid (ECF) in that it is high in Na⁺ and low in K⁺.

Endolymph is the fluid present within the scala media or the membranous cochlea. Its composition is similar to intracellular fluid (ICF) in that it is high in K⁺ and low in Na⁺. It is secreted by the stria vascularis which forms the lateral wall of scala media.

Organ of Corti

The organ of Corti, the sense organ of hearing, is situated on the top of the basilar membrane in the scala media (Fig. 12.7-25). It contains the auditory receptors or the peripheral receptors of sense of hearing. Important components of the organ of Corti are :

1. Rods of Corti. These are two projections (inner and outer rods) from the basilar membrane into the scala

C H A P T E R 12.7

media. In between the two rods is the *tunnel of Corti* which contains a fluid called *cortilymph*. The exact function of the rods and cortilymph is not known.

2. *Hair cells*. Hair cells are receptor cells that transduce sound energy into electrical energy. Two groups of hair cells lie on the basilar membrane—inner hair cells and outer hair cells these are responsible for *detecting the presence of sound*.

3. *Supporting cells* (Fig. 12.7-25) : These support the hair cells.

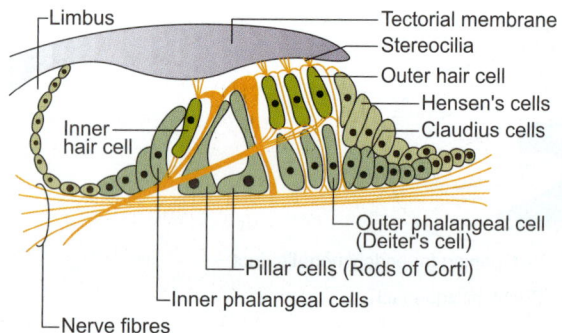

Fig. 12.7-25. *Structure of organ of Corti. Note the connections between tectorial membrane and cilia of hair cells.*

4. *Tectorial membrane*. It consists of gelatinous matrix with delicate fibres. This membrane is attached to the upper surface of spiral lamina, and its free edge extends just beyond the outermost neuroepithelial cells.

The shearing force between the hair cells and tectorial membrane produces the stimulus to hair cells.

Nerve supply of hair cells

Afferent fibres supplying the hair cells constitute the cochlear division of VIII cranial nerve. Cell bodies of these fibres are located in the spiral ganglion.

Efferent fibres to the hair cells come from both the ipsilateral and contralateral sides.

AUDITORY PATHWAYS

Auditory pathways comprise following relay stations (Fig. 12.7-26):

Spiral ganglion

First order neurons are the bipolar cells of the *spiral ganglion*.

- *Dendrites* of these bipolar cells constitute the afferent fibres innervating the hair cells.
- *Axons* of these bipolar cells form the cochlear division of VIII cranial nerve. The cochlear nerve ends in the cochlear nuclei in medulla.

Cochlear nuclei

Second order neurons have their cell bodies in the

Fig. 12.7-26. *Central auditory pathways.*

cochlear nuclei which are situated in the medulla. There are two cochlear nuclei: dorsal and ventral. The axons of second order neurons from cochlear nuclei pass medially in the dorsal part of pons.

- The crossing fibres of two sides form a conspicuous mass of fibres called the *trapezoid body*.
- Some crossing fibres run separately in the dorsal part of pons and do not form part of the trapezoid body.

Superior olivary nucleus complex, trapezoid nucleus and nucleus of lateral lemniscus

Third order neurons have their cell bodies mainly in the *superior olivary complex* (made up of a number of nuclei) and also in trapezoid nucleus, and nucleus of lateral lemniscus.

The fibres from these collections ascend through *lateral lemniscus* and ascend to the midbrain and terminate in the inferior colliculus.

Inferior colliculus

Fourth order neurons have their cell bodies in *inferior colliculus* where the fibres of lateral lemniscus terminate. Fibres arising in the inferior colliculus enter the inferior brachium to reach the medial geniculate body.

Medial geniculate body

Fifth order neurons have their cell bodies in the medial geniculate body where most of the fibres arising in inferior colliculus terminate. Fibres arising in the medial geniculate body form the *acoustic radiation* which ends in the acoustic area of the cerebral cortex.

Auditory cortex

Major areas constituting auditory cortex present in the temporal lobe are:

- Primary auditory cortex (areas 41 and 42), and
- Auditory association areas (areas 22, 21 and 20).

PHYSIOLOGY OF HEARING

Hearing, i.e. detection of sound waves, may serve to warn of impending danger or localize friends. But most importantly, audition allows social communication. Physiology of audition can be discussed under following headings:

- Stimuli or sound waves,
- Conduction of sound waves,
- Transduction of sound waves,
- Neural transmission of signals, and
- Encoding of signals.

STIMULI OR SOUND WAVES

Stimuli for the receptors of hearing are sound waves. Sound is a form of energy produced by a vibrating object. A sound wave consists of alternating phases of compression and rarefaction of molecules of the medium (air, liquid, or solid) in which it travels.

Physical properties of sound

Physical properties of sound and certain terms which are frequently used in audiology and acoustics are (Fig. 12.7-27).

Fig. 12.7-27. *Characteristics of sound wave: A, pure tones; B, increase in amplitude (intensity) of sound wave thus the sound is louder; C, increase in frequency (pitch); D, complex waveform due to mixture of pure tones and overtones; determines the quality of sound (timbre); and E, aperiodic irregular waveform (noise).*

1. *Speed of sound.* Speed or velocity of the sound waves is different in different media. *In the air*, at 0° C, at sea level, sound travels at a rate of approximately 330 m/sec (1100 ft/sec).
2. *Frequency of sound* refers to number of waves per second.
- The *unit* of frequency is hertz (Hz).
- Range of human hearing is approximately 20-20,000 Hz.
- Range of average speaking voice is approximately 2000-5000 Hz.
3. *Amplitude (intensity) of sound* is the strength which determines its loudness. The intensity of sound is measured in terms of maximum pressure change at the tympanic membrane which is more commonly expressed as *sound pressure level* (SPL). The unit of SPL is decibel (dB).
4. *Pure tone.* A single frequency sound is called a pure tone, e.g. a sound of 25-50 or 100 Hz
5. *Complex sound* refers to that with more than one frequency. For example, human voice is a complex sound.
6. *Pitch.* It is the subjective sensation produced by frequency of sound. Higher the frequency greater is the pitch.
7. *Overtones.* A complex sound is a mixture of pure tones. The lowest frequency at which a source vibrates is called *fundamental (or primary) frequency.* All other frequencies which are multiples of the fundamental frequency are called *overtones* or *harmonics.*

CONDUCTION OF SOUND WAVES

Role of external ear

External ear captures the sound waves.

Pinna collects and reflects the sound waves into the external auditory meatus.

External auditory meatus conducts the sound waves to tympanic membrane. Its S-shaped course helps in amplifying the sound waves.

Role of middle ear

Conduction of sound stimulus by tympanic membrane to ear ossicles. The sound waves that pass through the pinna and external auditory meatus strike the tympanic membrane and enable it to vibrate. Eustachian tube does the function of equalization of pressure on two sides of tympanic membrane. The vibrating tympanic membrane causes the ear ossicles to vibrate.

Conduction of sound waves mechanically from middle ear to inner ear. Tympanic membrane vibrations are transmitted and amplified through the middle ear by movement of ossicles associated with an *impedance matching mechanism.* The to and fro movements of the footplate of stapes at the oval window transmits the sound waves to inner ear by setting up fluid waves in the perilymph of the scala vestibuli (Fig. 12.7-28).

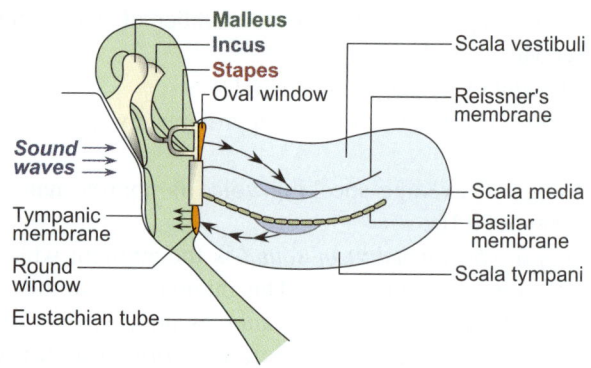

Fig. 12.7-28. *Diagrammatic depiction of the mechanism of vibrations of basilar membrane produced by in and out motion of stapes (for details see text).*

TRANSDUCTION OF SOUND WAVES

Transduction of mechanical sound wave into electrical signal occurs in the organ of Corti of inner ear. Steps involved in the process of transduction are:

Vibration of basilar membrane. Sound waves entering the inner ear from the oval window spread along the scala vestibuli as a travelling wave. As the sound energy passes from scala vestibuli to scala tympani, it causes the basilar membrane to vibrate.

Stimulation of the hair cells. The up-and-down movements of the basilar membrane in turn cause the organ of Corti to vibrate up and down. The bending of stereocilia stimulates (excites) the hair cells.

Membrane potential changes in the hair cells

The movements of hair cells of organs of Corti cause their depolarization and development of receptor potential leading to generation of action potential in the neuron. In this way sound wave is transduced into electrical signal.

NEURAL TRANSMISSION OF SIGNALS

The electrical signals from hair cells are transmitted through a complex auditory pathway (Fig. 12.7-26) to the auditory cortex.

NEURAL PROCESSING OF AUDITORY INFORMATION

In the auditory cortex the sound wave in the form of nerve impulse is processed and perceived. Neural processing of auditory information involves:

- Encoding of frequency (pitch determination),
- Encoding of intensity (determination of loudness),
- Feature detection, and
- Localization of sound in space.

APPLIED ASPECTS

Noise and masking

Noise. Noise is defined as an aperiodic complex sound. There are three types of noise :

- *White noise.* In this all frequencies are in audible spectrum. It is used for masking.
- *Narrow-band noise.*
- *Speech noise.* It is a noise having all frequencies in the speech range (300-3000 Hz).

Masking refers to a phenomenon in which the presence of one type of sound decreases the ability of the ear to hear another type of sound.

Hearing loss, deafness and tinnitus

Hearing loss refers to impairment of hearing and its severity may vary from mild to profound.

Deafness is labelled when there is little or no hearing at all.

Types of hearing loss. Hearing loss can be of two types:

- Conductive hearing loss,
- Sensorineural hearing loss.

Tinnitus

Tinnitus refers to ringing sensation in the ear. It is caused by irritative stimulation of either the inner ear or the vestibulocochlear nerve.

THE SENSE OF SMELL

The sense of smell or olfaction is well developed in animals like dog and rabbit to give warning of the environmental dangers. Such animals are called *macrosomatics.* In humans, apes and monkeys (primates) the sense of smell is comparatively less developed, but still it is important for pleasure and for enjoying the taste of food. Therefore, the humans and primates are called *microsomatics.*

SITE OF OLFACTION

The olfactory stimuli are detected by specialized receptors located on the free nerve endings of the olfactory nerves which are located in the olfactory mucosa of nose in human beings.

Olfactory mucosa

In humans, the olfactory mucosa is confined to upper one-third of nasal cavity (Fig. 12.7-29).

Histologically, the olfactory mucosa consists of three types of cells—receptor cells, supporting cells and basal cells. Receptor cells are bipolar neurons which lie between the supporting (sustentacular) cells.

Nerve supply of olfactory mucosa

- *Special sensory nerves* innervating the olfactory mucosa are 15-20 bundles of olfactory nerve fibres (1st cranial nerve) which convey sense of smell.

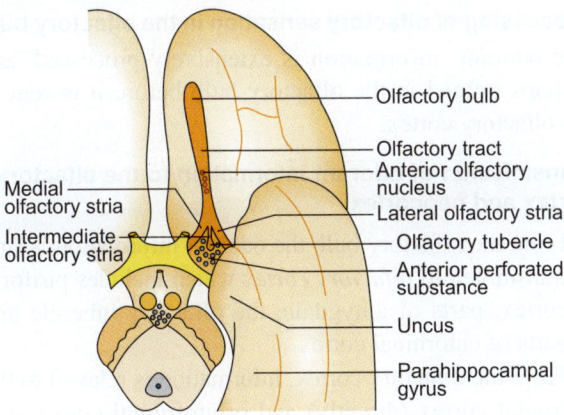

Fig. 12.7-30. *Olfactory bulb and olfactory tract.*

Fig. 12.7-29 Location of olfactory mucosa (A) and histological features of olfactory mucosa (B).

- *General sensory nerves* supplying the olfactory mucosa are branches of trigeminal nerve (V cranial nerve). The irritative character of some odorants results from stimulation of free nerve endings of the trigeminal nerve.

OLFACTORY PATHWAYS

Olfactory pathways comprise:

1. *Olfactory nerves*. About 15-20 olfactory nerve filaments which consist of the axons of the bipolar olfactory neurons which pierce the cribriform plate on either side to reach olfactory bulb.

2. *Olfactory bulb* (Fig. 12.7-30). It is an oval flattened strip of gray matter lying on the cribriform plate which receives the olfactory nerve filaments. The olfactory bulb contains three types of cells: mitral cells, tufted cells, and interneurons (granule cells and periglomerular cells). The mitral and tufted cells constitute 2nd order neurons. *Axons of the mitral and tufted cells* leave the olfactory bulb and run in the olfactory tract.

3. *Olfactory tract*. It lies in the olfactory sulcus on the orbital surface of the frontal lobe and proceeds backwards from each olfactory bulb to the region of anterior

perforated substance on the base of brain where it divides into lateral, intermediate and medial olfactory striae (Fig. 11.3-32).

4. *Olfactory cortex*. It includes the anterior olfactory nucleus, prepiriform cortex, olfactory tubercle and amygdala. All these are parts of limbic system.

PHYSIOLOGY OF OLFACTION

Odoriferous stimuli

The odoriferous (smell-producing molecules) stimuli enter the nasal cavity while breathing. The odorant molecules must dissolve in the mucous layer (lining the olfactory mucosa) before they can come in contact with olfactory receptors.

***Types of odorant stimuli*.** There seems to be over 50 *primary smell sensations*. Although the olfactory capability of humans is somewhat limited compared with that of macrosomatic animals, nevertheless humans are able to perceive more than 10,000 different odorous molecules.

Olfactory receptors

The cilia of the olfactory neurons are specialized for odour detection. They have specific receptors for odorants.

Steps in transduction in the olfactory receptor neurons

1. *Binding of odorant molecule to receptors*. It has been suggested that the mucous layer covering the olfactory mucosa contains one or more odorant-binding proteins (OBP) that concentrate and transfer the odorant molecules to the receptors present on the cilia of olfactory neurons.

2. *Depolarization receptor potential*. The interaction of an odorant with its receptor produces a depolarizing receptor potential.

3. *Action potentials*. The receptor potential depolarizes the initial segment of the axon to threshold leading to the generation of action potentials in the sensory axon and the *transmission of signal to olfactory bulb*.

Processing of olfactory sensation in the olfactory bulb

The odorant information is extensively processed, and perhaps refined in the olfactory bulb before it is sent to the olfactory cortex.

Transmission of odorant information to the olfactory cortex and neocortex

- From the olfactory bulb the odorant information is first transmitted to *olfactory cortex* which includes piriform cortex, parts of amygdala, the olfactory tubercle and parts of entorhinal cortex.
- From the olfactory cortex, information is relayed to the frontal cortex (directly) and orbitofrontal cortex (via thalamus).

Factors influencing olfactory function

1. *Threshold of olfactory receptors*. The threshold of olfactory receptors varies from substance to substance. For example, methyl mercaptan, a substance which gives garlic its characteristic odour, has extremely low threshold.

2. *Intensity/concentration of the odour*. The concentration of an odoriferous substance must be changed by about 30% before a difference can be detected.

3. *Adaptation*. Olfactory sensation adapts very rapidly with continued exposure to an odour.

APPLIED ASPECTS

1. *Anosmia and hyposmia*. Anosmia is total loss of sense of smell while hyposmia refers to diminished olfactory sensitivity.

2. *Paraosmia or dysosmia*. It refers to distortion or perversion of smell. In it, person interprets the odours incorrectly. Often these persons complain of disgusting odours.

SENSE OF TASTE

Sense of taste (gustation) is a chemical sense that is stimulated by food and drink. Taste must be distinguished from flavour, which includes the olfactory, tactile, and thermal attributes of food in addition to taste.

SITE OF TASTE

The taste (gustatory) stimuli are detected by specialized chemoreceptors called taste receptors or taste cells. The taste receptors are clustered in the taste buds located on the tongue, palate, pharynx, epiglottis, and upper third of oesophagus.

Tongue, the main site of taste detection, contains numerous taste buds on its dorsal surface. The mucous membrane of the dorsal surface of tongue exhibits numerous papillae, which increase the surface area of the mucosa available for taste receptors. The taste buds are located in the walls of these papillae.

Taste bud

It consists of cluster of cells with a small opening (taste pore) in the surface. It consists of following cells (Fig. 12.7-31):

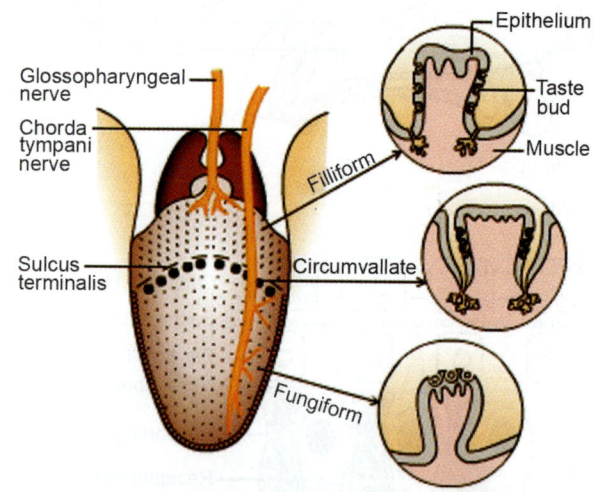

Fig. 12.7-31. *Structure and distribution of papillae on the tongue and arrangement of tastebuds in the three types of papillae. Innervation by the cranial nerves is also indicated.*

1. *Receptor cells*. These are modified epithelial cells elongate, bipolar-shaped and extend from the epithelial opening of the taste bud to its base. The taste cells are innervated by sensory neurons (primary gustatory afferent fibres) at its basal pole.

2. *Basal replacement cells*. These are small round cells present at the bottom of taste bud (Fig. 12.7-32).

3. *Supporting cells*. In addition to taste cells and basal cells, the taste buds contain supporting or sustentacular cells.

Fig. 12.7-32. *Structure of a taste bud.*

Innervation. The special sensory nerve fibres innervating the taste cells come from the branches of the facial, glossopharyngeal and vagus nerve (7th, 9th and 10th

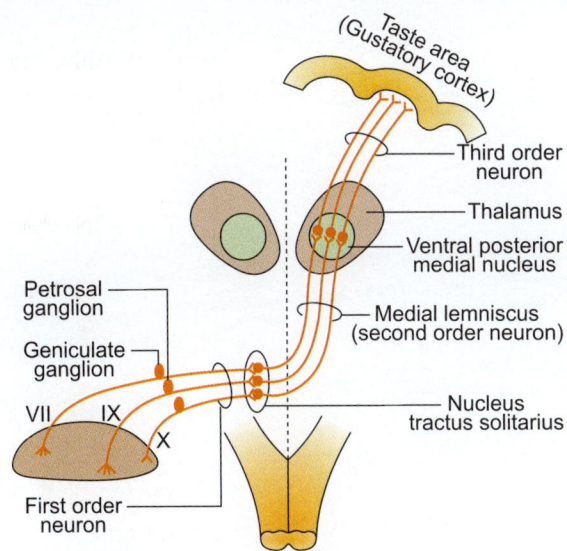

Fig. 12.7-33. *The taste pathways.*

cranial nerve, respectively). The tactile and temperature receptors of the mouth, tongue, and pharynx are innervated by the trigeminal nerve (5th cranial nerve).

TASTE PATHWAYS

The taste pathways consist of three orders of neurons (Fig. 12.7-33):

First order neurons. The cell bodies of the first order neurons innervating the taste cells in taste buds are located in different ganglia of the 7th, 9th and 10th cranial nerves as:

Termination of first order neurons. Ultimately all the taste fibres, travelling in different cranial nerves join the tractus solitarius to terminate in the nucleus of tractus solitarius (Fig. 12.7-33).

Second order neurons. The cell bodies of second order neurons are located in the *nucleus of tractus solitarius (NTS)* in the medulla. Axons of second order neurons cross the midline to join the medial lemniscus and terminate with 5th cranial nerve fibres (carrying pain, touch, and temperature fibres) in the ventral posterior medial nucleus of thalamus.

Third order neurons. Their cell bodies are located in the *thalamus*. Axons of third order neurons proceed to terminate in the inferior part of the postcentral gyrus, i.e. the part of sensory cortex.

PHYSIOLOGY OF TASTE

Gustatory stimuli

Types of stimuli and most sensitive areas of tongue

Conventionally four basic types of taste sensations have been described: *sweet, salt, sour* and *bitter*. All other taste

sensations (hundreds in humans) are assumed to result from various combinations of these primary (basic) taste sensations.

Substances producing primary (basic) taste sensations

1. *Sweet sensation* is produced by a number of organic molecules including sugars, glycols, alcohols, aldehydes, esters, etc. Tip of the tongue was considered the area most sensitive to sweet stimuli.

2. *Salty sensation* is produced by the anions of ionizable salts especially the sodium chloride. The front half of each side of the tongue was thought to be the area most sensitive to salty stimuli.

3. *Sour sensation*. It is produced by acids. The posterior half of each side of the tongue was the area considered most sensitive to sour stimuli.

4. *Bitter sensation* is produced by alkaloids such as quinine, caffeine, nicotine and strychnine.

Transduction of gustatory stimuli

Transduction of gustatory stimuli into electrical signals is initiated at the level of receptors. The taste receptors are chemoreceptors which are stimulated by substances dissolved in the mouth by saliva. The dissolved substances act on the microvilli of taste receptors exposed in the taste pore of taste buds. This interaction typically depolarizes the cell. This causes the development of *receptor potential* in the receptor cell which in turn generates action potential in the sensory nerves.

Transmission of information about taste to the cortex

Each sensory fibre contacts a number of taste cells and each taste cell synapses with numerous sensory fibres. Thus the electrical activity recorded from a single sensory fibre represents the input of many taste cells. As described in the taste pathway (Fig. 12.7-33), the signals carried by sensory fibres travel through several different nerves to the gustatory cortex.

Encoding of taste information

The identity of a taste stimulus appears to be encoded in the gustatory cortex by a unique pattern of inputs from many separate fibres that provide components of the patterns for different stimuli.

Sensation of flavours

The multitude of different sensation of flavours that one experiences results from a combination of gustatory, olfactory and somatosensory inputs.

Abnormalities of taste sensations

1. *Ageusia* refers to absence of taste sensation.

2. *Hypogeusia* refers to diminished taste sensitivity.

3. *Dysgeusia* refers to disturbed sense of taste.

Index

◆ **T** ◆